Health Professional as Educator

Principles of Teaching and Learning

Susan B. Bastable, EdD, RN
Professor and Chair
Department of Nursing
Le Moyne College

Pamela Gramet, PT, PhD
Associate Professor
Department of Physical Therapy Education
Upstate Medical University

Karen Jacobs, EdD, OTR/L, CPE, FAOTA
Clinical Professor
Department of Occupational Therapy
Boston University

Deborah L. Sopczyk, PhD, RN
Dean
School of Health Sciences
Excelsior College

JONES & BARTLETT
L E A R N I N G

P9-DGD-542

World Headquarters

Jones & Bartlett Learning
40 Tall Pine Drive
Sudbury, MA 01776
978-443-5000
info@jblearning.com
www.jblearning.com

Jones & Bartlett Learning Canada
6339 Ormindale Way
Mississauga, Ontario L5V 1J2
Canada

Jones & Bartlett Learning International
Barb House, Barb Mews
London W6 7PA
United Kingdom

Jones & Bartlett Learning books and products are available through most bookstores and online booksellers. To contact Jones & Bartlett Learning directly, call 800-832-0034, fax 978-443-8000, or visit our website, www.jblearning.com.

Substantial discounts on bulk quantities of Jones & Bartlett Learning publications are available to corporations, professional associations, and other qualified organizations. For details and specific discount information, contact the special sales department at Jones & Bartlett Learning via the above contact information or send an email to specialsales@jblearning.com.

This publication is designed to provide accurate and authoritative information in regard to the Subject Matter covered. It is sold with the understanding that the publisher is not engaged in rendering legal, accounting, or other professional service. If legal advice or other expert assistance is required, the service of a competent professional person should be sought.

Production Credits
Publisher: David Cella
Associate Editor: Maro Gartside
Editorial Assistant: Teresa Reilly
Production Manager: Julie Champagne Bolduc
Production Assistant: Sean Coombs
Marketing Manager: Grace Richards
Manufacturing and Inventory Control Supervisor: Amy Bacus
Composition: Publishers' Design and Production Services, Inc.
Cover Design: Kristin E. Parker
Cover Image: © Denis Tevekov/Dreamstime.com
Printing and Binding: Malloy, Inc.
Cover Printing: Malloy, Inc.

Library of Congress Cataloging-in-Publication Data

Health professional as educator : principles of teaching and learning / Susan B. Bastable . . . [et al.].
    p. ; cm.
  Includes bibliographical references and index.
  ISBN 978-0-7637-9278-7 (alk. paper)
  1. Patient education. 2. Health education. I. Bastable, Susan Bacorn.
  [DNLM: 1. Health Personnel. 2. Teaching. 3. Education, Professional. 4. Learning. 5. Patient Education.
6. Professional Role. W 18]
  R727.4.H425 2011
  613—dc22

2010038295

6048
Printed in the United States of America
14   10 9 8 7 6

To the past, present, and future students and professional colleagues from the various healthcare disciplines who have shared, and will continue to share, their experiences, insights, and perspectives on teaching and learning.

and

In loving memory of
Doris (Dorrie) Williams Bacorn, RN (1918–2007)
cherished mother of Susan B. Bastable

Contents

Part One: Perspectives on Teaching and Learning

1 Overview of Education in Health Care 1
Susan B. Bastable
Pamela R. Gramet

2 Ethical, Legal, and Economic Foundations of the Educational Process 25
M. Janice Nelson
Catherine V. Caldicott

Part Two: *Characteristics of the Learner*

Part Three: Techniques and Strategies for Teaching and Learning

Foreword

During the next decade, health care in the United States will be experiencing the most significant change since the founding of Medicare and Medicaid in the 1960s. Health reform will drive much greater integration of healthcare providers and settings of care, improved efficiency of care processes, and a higher level of accountability for clinical and administrative outcomes. All of this will take place within the context of highly technical, complex care provided by a team of healthcare professionals using sophisticated clinical and information tools to an increasingly diverse population of patients.

Health Professional as Educator recognizes these sea changes and builds on Susan Bastable's three successful editions of *Nurse as Educator*, which have given nurses invaluable methods for partnering with patients and serving the community.

Health Professional as Educator is a comprehensive guide that addresses all of the practical issues health professionals confront as they strive to provide effective patient/family education. The book could not be more timely, as health professionals work to enhance their patients' ability to self-manage their care, educate family members to support the daunting complexity of treatment protocols, and understand the needs of the learners who have highly variable levels of healthcare literacy and cultural requirements.

The authors have anticipated and explored all the dimensions of teaching and learning in this important text. While including the fundamentals of learning theories and teaching methods, *Health Professional as Educator* also focuses on critical issues such as readiness to learn, learning styles, health literacy, and teaching people with disabilities, all based on the latest research and theoretical underpinnings.

All health professionals will benefit from the content and format of this book and will be fully prepared to embrace the opportunities of health reform to improve patient safety, engage patients and families, and reduce costs. Well-informed patients and family members who partner with a team of highly effective health educators will be at the center of positive change in health care.

Nancy M. Schlichting
President and CEO
Henry Ford Health System
Detroit, Michigan

Preface

This text is written for health professionals—physical therapists, occupational therapists, pharmacists, social workers, nutritionists, respiratory therapists, physician assistants, nurses, physicians, and many other members of the healthcare workforce—who are involved on a daily basis in educating clients, fellow colleagues, and/or prospective members of their respective disciplines. No matter who their audience may be, health professionals are expected to educate individuals to assist them in achieving independence. This role expectation involves helping clients and their significant others to manage self-care activities as well as promoting the growth and development of staff and students to deliver high-quality, safe, and cost-effective care to the consumers they serve.

The recent healthcare reform movement, the technological advances in health care, the changing demographics of the population, the increased interest of consumers in health and wellness, the rise in chronic illnesses, and many other factors have resulted in a growing demand for health professionals to meet the public's increasing need and desire for health care. These trends, to name just a few, have given rise to the recognition of consumer health literacy as a significant concern, the increasing importance of client education for the improvement of health outcomes, and the growing need for continuing education to sustain a well-prepared professional workforce of healthcare providers. This text is a timely resource to address these pressing issues.

Educating others has been an essential component of health professional practice for many years, yet the majority of health providers acknowledge that they have not had the formal preparation to successfully and securely assume the teaching role. In today's healthcare arena, practice requirements mandate that health professionals possess the knowledge and skills necessary to educate various audiences in a variety of settings with efficiency and effectiveness as well as with competency and confidence.

This text was written to assist health professionals to understand the many principles of teaching and learning. It is comprehensive in scope and depth of information, taking into consideration the basic foundations of the teaching–learning process, the needs and characteristics of learners, the appropriate techniques and strategies for instruction, and the methods to evaluate the achievement of changes in learner behavior. In essence, this text addresses the components that pertain to the education process and answers the questions who, what, where, when, how, and why.

The chapters in this text reflect a balance between current theoretical perspectives on teaching and learning and the application of these theories and models to practice. Many current as well as classic references are included to bolster any claims made. Also, the changing role of the health professional and consumer is acknowledged with respect to the accountability and responsibility for teaching and learning. No longer should the health professional function as the "giver of information" when teaching but as the "guide by the side" and the "facilitator" in partnership with the consumer, who must assume a much greater role in learning. This new educational paradigm of interdependence between the teacher and the learner is emphasized throughout the chapters.

The text is divided into three parts. Part I focuses on the perspectives on teaching and learning; Part II focuses on the many characteristics of the learner; and Part III emphasizes the techniques and strategies for teaching and learning. Although all topics covered in this text are essential to the complete understanding of the teaching and learning process, some unique aspects include: the ethics of the student/teacher and client/teacher relationship highlighted in Chapter 2; a review of motor learning integrated into the content of learning theories in Chapter 3; the approaches to educating learners with disabilities in Chapter 9; and the importance of new technology as a tool for pedagogy but not a substitute for the role of the educator as described in Chapter 13. In addition, case studies in every chapter address interprofessional education and interdisciplinary collaboration efforts to enhance teaching and learning.

Accompanying this text is a companion Web site that offers various resources for instructors and students. Faculty will find tools to assist them with the delivery of content as well as with the assessment and evaluation of students who are learning the educator role. Students will find materials to help them achieve learning objectives. In addition, this book can be used not only in a specific course on teaching and learning, but as a reference throughout a curriculum that integrates client education in multiple courses. Also, it is an invaluable reference in all practice settings where the health professional is involved in client and staff education.

This text for health professionals is intended for use by faculty teaching in academic programs, by direct care providers practicing in any setting as caregivers, by staff development and in-service educators, and by upper-level undergraduate and graduate students who are to become the future professionals of tomorrow. No matter what their role or status, it is an ethical, moral, and in many cases a legal responsibility of health providers to teach others with proficiency and expertise.

Acknowledgments

A special appreciation is extended to the original authors of chapters in the *Nurse as Educator* text whose valuable work provided the foundation for revision of information and addition of new material by the editor and co-editors of this textbook, which is more broadly designed for use by professionals in various healthcare disciplines. We value and recognize the contributions of everyone involved in this significant undertaking.

Also, many thanks are offered to the entire publishing staff in the Health Professions division of Jones & Bartlett Learning, in particular David Cella, Publisher, Maro Gartside, Associate Editor, and Julie Bolduc, Production Manager, for their technical expertise, organizational skills, expert advice, and administrative support throughout the process of launching this publication. They are truly a wonderful, talented team!

Also instrumental in the preparation of this manuscript are the librarians who worked behind the scenes in locating the references used for each chapter. Specifically, Cathleen Scott, science librarian at Le Moyne College, and Jim Capodagli, librarian at Upstate Medical University, are recognized for their significant efforts devoted to data collection.

Nancy Schlichting, President and CEO of the Henry Ford Health System, is gratefully acknowledged for her insightful remarks expressed in the Foreword, which highlight the need for a well-educated workforce of health professionals to meet the public's need for high-quality, safe, and cost-effective care.

And last, but certainly not least, sincere gratitude goes to our families and colleagues for their unwavering support, endless patience, and consistent encouragement over the many months of research, writing, and editing. They sacrificed a great deal on our behalf to make this text a reality.

Contributors

Margaret M. Braungart, PhD
Professor Emeritus, Center for Bioethics and
  Humanities
Upstate Medical University Health System
Syracuse, New York

Richard G. Braungart, PhD
Professor Emeritus, Maxwell School of
  Citizenship and Public Affairs
Syracuse University
Syracuse, New York

Catherine V. Caldicott, MD, FACP
Associate Professor, Center for Bioethics and
  Humanities
Upstate Medical University Health System
Syracuse, New York

Michelle A. Dart, MSN, PNP, CD
Pediatric Associates
Syracuse, New York

**Kirsty Digger, MS, RN, CEN, Doctoral
Candidate**
Lecturer, Department of Nursing
State University of New York at New Paltz
New Paltz, New York

Julie A. Doody, MS, RN
Nurse Administrator, Wellness Center for
  Health and Counseling
Le Moyne College
Syracuse, New York

Nancy Wolcott Doyle, MS, OTR/L
OT Doctoral Student
Boston University
Boston, Massachusetts

Kathleen Fitzgerald, MS, RN CDE
Patient Educator
St. Joseph's Hospital Health Center
Syracuse, New York

Diane S. Hainsworth, MS, RN-C, ANP
Clinical Case Manager – Oncology (retired)
Upstate University Hospital
Upstate Medical University Health System
Syracuse, New York

Sharon Kitchie, PhD, RN, ACNS-BC
Patient Education and Interpreter Services
  Director
Upstate University Hospital
Upstate Medical University Health System
Syracuse, New York
Adjunct Faculty, Nursing Division
Keuka College
Keuka Park, New York

M. Janice Nelson, EdD, RN
Professor and Dean Emeritus, College of
  Nursing
State University of New York
Upstate Medical University Health System
Syracuse, New York

Eleanor Richards, PhD, RN
Professor Emeritus, Department of Nursing
State University of New York at New Paltz
New Paltz, New York

Kay Viggiani, MS, RN, CNS
Associate Professor (retired) and Adjunct,
    Nursing Division
Keuka College
Keuka Park, New York

Priscilla Sandford Worral, PhD, RN
Coordinator of Nursing Research
Upstate University Hospital
Upstate Medical University Health System
Syracuse, New York

About the Editors

Susan Bacorn Bastable, EdD, RN, earned her MEd in community health nursing and her EdD in curriculum and instruction in nursing at Teachers College, Columbia University, in 1976 and 1979 respectively. She received her diploma from Hahnemann Hospital School of Nursing (now known as Drexel University of the Health Sciences) in Philadelphia in 1969 and her bachelor's degree in nursing from Syracuse University in 1972.

Dr. Bastable is currently Professor and founding Chair of the Department of Nursing at Le Moyne College in Syracuse, New York. She began her academic career in 1979 as Assistant Professor at Hunter College, Bellevue School of Nursing, in New York City where she remained on the faculty for two years. From 1987 to 1989, she was Assistant Professor in the College of Nursing at the University of Rhode Island. In 1990, she joined the faculty of the College of Nursing at Upstate Medical University of the State University of New York (SUNY) in Syracuse, where she was Associate Professor and Chair of the Undergraduate Program for 14 years. In 2004, she assumed her present leadership position at Le Moyne and has successfully established an RN-BS completion program, created an innovative 4-year undergraduate Dual Degree Partnership in Nursing with the associate's degree program at St. Joseph's College of Nursing in Syracuse, and instituted an MS program and two post-MS certificate programs with tracks in nursing education and nursing administration.

Dr. Bastable has taught undergraduate courses in nursing research, community health, and the role of the nurse as educator, and courses at the master's and post-master's level in the academic faculty role, curriculum and program development, and educational assessment and evaluation. For the past 29 years, she has been a consultant and external faculty member for Excelsior College (formerly known as Regents College of the University of the State of New York). Her clinical practice includes experience in community health, oncology, rehabilitation and neurology, occupational health, and medical/surgical nursing.

Dr. Bastable is the recipient of the 1996 President's Award for Excellence in Teaching at Upstate Medical University; the SUNY 1999 Chancellor's Award for Excellence in Teaching; the 2002 Award for Nursing Excellence as well as the 2008 Lifetime Achievement Award from District #4 of the New York State Nurses Association; and the 2001 Distinguished Achievement Award in Nursing Education from the Nursing Education Alumni Association of Teachers College, Columbia University. Also in 2001, she was inducted into the Nursing Education Alumni Association's Hall of Fame at Teacher's College, Columbia University.

She is a member of numerous nursing education advisory boards, serves as a consultant on curriculum and program development, and is the author of two other textbooks on the principles of teaching and learning.

Pamela Gramet, PT, PhD, is currently associate professor in the Department of Physical Therapy Education at Upstate Medical University in Syracuse, New York. During her tenure at Upstate, she has also served in a variety of administrative positions including department vice chair, department chair, and academic coordinator of clinical education.

Dr. Gramet earned her doctoral degree in child and family studies from Syracuse University, her master of science degree in education from Stony Brook University, and her bachelor of science in physical therapy, magna cum laude, from Ithaca College. She holds advanced certifications in neurodevelopmental treatment, teaching improvement, clinical instruction, and board leadership.

Dr. Gramet has more than 30 years of teaching experience, and her areas of expertise include education theory and practice, clinical education, neurologic physical therapy, professionalism, and complementary and alternative medicine. Dr. Gramet was a member of the American Physical Therapy Association task force that developed the first national Clinical Performance Instruments (CPIs) for assessment of physical therapist and physical therapist assistant student clinical performance. She was also a founding member of the New York Physical Therapy Clinical Education Consortium. Over the years, Dr. Gramet has developed and taught numerous workshops on clinical teaching skills for clinical instructors. She was instrumental in developing the curriculums for both the master's degree program and the professional and post professional doctoral physical therapy programs at Upstate Medical University. She has served as a curriculum consultant for several graduate physical therapy programs.

Dr. Gramet is a recipient of the President's Award for Excellence in Teaching and received Certificates of Appreciation from the New York Physical Therapy Association and the American Physical Therapy Association. She is also a recipient of the Outstanding Academic Coordinator of Clinical Education Award and a Certificate of Excellence from the Clinical Education Consortium. Dr. Gramet's research interests include education, clinical teaching, and the professional and psychosocial aspects of physical therapy.

Karen Jacobs, EdD, OTR/L, CPE, FAOTA, is a past president and vice president of the American Occupational Therapy Association (AOTA). She is a 2005 recipient of a Fulbright Scholarship to the University of Akuryeri in Akuryeri, Iceland; is the 2009 recipient of the Award of Merit from the Canadian Association of Occupational Therapists (CAOT); and received the Award of Merit from the American Occupational Therapy Association in 2003.

Dr. Jacobs is a clinical professor of occupational therapy and the program director of the distance education post professional occupational therapy programs at Boston University. She has expertise in the development and instruction of online and on-campus graduate courses. In addition, she has faculty appointments at Stony Brook University in Stony Brook, New York, and the University of Indianapolis in Indianapolis, Indiana.

Dr. Jacobs earned a doctoral degree at the University of Massachusetts, a master of science at Boston University, and a bachelor of arts at Washington University in St. Louis, Missouri.

Dr. Jacobs's research examines the interface between the environment and human capabilities. In particular, she examines the individual factors and environmental demands associated with increased risk of functional limitations among populations of university and middle-school-aged students, particularly in notebook computing, backpack use, and the use of games such as WiiFit (http://blogs.bu.edu/kjacobs/). Most recently, she is co-developing with Dr. Nancy Baker at the University of Pittsburgh the Telerehabilitation Computer Ergonomics System (*tele-CES*) for computer users with arthritis. The *tele-CES* is a remote systematic ergonomics program aimed at substantially reducing work disability among workers with any type of arthritis.

In addition to being an occupational therapist, Dr. Jacobs is also a certified professional ergonomist (CPE) and the founding editor-in-chief of the international, interdisciplinary journal *WORK: A Journal of Prevention, Assessment and Rehabilitation* (IOS Press, The Netherlands), which celebrates its 20th anniversary this year. Dr. Jacobs is the chairperson of the Ergonomics for Children in Educational Environments Technical Committee (ECEE) for the International Ergonomics Association (IEA) and the program chair for the Environment Design Technical Group for the Human Factors and Ergonomics Society (HFES). Dr. Jacobs has a small business that provides consulting services in ergonomics and entrepreneurship.

Deborah Sopczyk, **PhD, RN**, earned a baccalaureate in nursing from the State University of New York at Plattsburgh, a master of science in nursing from the State University of New York at Buffalo, and a doctoral degree in social welfare from the State University of New York at Albany. Dr. Sopczyk has more than 30 years of experience in higher education and is currently the dean of the School of Health Sciences at Excelsior College in Albany, New York. She has also taught at D'Youville and Trocaire Colleges, both in Buffalo, New York. Dr. Sopczyk is an expert in adult and distance education. Her clinical practice areas include child health, pediatric oncology, and family violence.

Part One

Perspectives on Teaching and Learning

Chapter 1

Overview of Education in Health Care

Susan B. Bastable

Pamela R. Gramet

CHAPTER HIGHLIGHTS

Historical Foundations for the Teaching Role of Health Professionals

Social, Economic, and Political Trends Affecting Health Care

Purposes, Goals, and Benefits of Client and Staff Education

The Education Process Defined

Role of the Health Professional as Educator

Barriers to Teaching and Obstacles to Learning
  Factors Affecting the Ability to Teach
  Factors Affecting the Ability to Learn

Questions to Be Asked About Teaching and Learning

State of the Evidence

KEY TERMS

❑ education process
❑ teaching/instruction
❑ learning
❑ patient education

❑ staff education
❑ barriers to teaching
❑ obstacles to learning

OBJECTIVES

After completing this chapter, the reader will be able to

1. Discuss the evolution of the teaching role of health professionals.
2. Recognize trends affecting the healthcare system.
3. Identify the purposes, goals, and benefits of client and staff/student education.
4. Compare the education process to healthcare practice.

5. Define the terms *education process*, *teaching*, and *learning*.
6. Identify reasons why client and staff/student education is an important duty for health professionals.
7. Discuss the barriers to teaching and the obstacles to learning.
8. Formulate questions that health professionals in the role of educator should ask about the teaching–learning process.

Education in health care today—both patient education and staff/student education—is a topic of utmost interest to health professionals in every setting in which they practice. Teaching is an important aspect of the professional role for the majority of health professionals. The current trends in health care are making it essential that clients be prepared to assume responsibility for self-care management. Also, these trends make it imperative that health professionals in the workplace be accountable for the delivery of high-quality care. The focus is on outcomes that demonstrate the extent to which clients and their significant others have learned essential knowledge and skills for independent care, or that staff and students have acquired the up-to-date knowledge and skills needed to competently and confidently render care to the consumer in a variety of settings.

According to Carpenter and Bell (2002), the need for nurses to teach others and to help others learn will continue to increase in the healthcare environment. This is certainly true for all health professionals. Because there are so many changes occurring in the healthcare system, health professionals are increasingly finding themselves in challenging, constantly changing, and highly complex positions. Health professionals in the role of educators must understand the forces, both historical and present day, that have influenced and continue to influence their responsibilities in practice.

One purpose of this chapter is to shed light on the historical evolution of teaching as part of the health professional's role. Another purpose is to offer a perspective on the current trends in health care that make the teaching of clients a highly visible and required function of healthcare delivery. This chapter also addresses the continuing education efforts required to ensure ongoing practice competencies of health personnel.

In addition, this chapter clarifies the broad purposes, goals, and benefits of the teaching–learning process; focuses on the philosophy of the health professional–client partnership in teaching and learning; identifies barriers to teaching and obstacles to learning; and highlights the status of research in the field of patient education as well as staff and student education. The focus is on the overall role of the health professional in teaching and learning, no matter who the audience of learners may be. Health professionals must have a basic prerequisite understanding of the principles and processes of teaching and learning to carry out their professional practice responsibilities with efficiency and effectiveness.

Historical Foundations for the Teaching Role of Health Professionals

"Patient education has been a part of health care since the first healer gave the first patient advice about treating his (or her) ailments" (May, 1999 p. 3). Although the term patient education was not specifically used, considerable efforts by the earliest healers to inform, encourage, and caution patients to follow appropriate hygienic and therapeutic measures occurred even in prehistoric times

(Bartlett, 1986). Since the early healers—physicians, herbalists, midwives, and shamans—did not have a lot of effective diagnostic and treatment interventions, it is likely that education was, in fact, one of the most common interventions (Bartlett, 1986).

From the mid-1800s through the turn of the 20th century, described as the formative period by Bartlett (1986), several key factors influenced the growth of patient education. The emergence of the nursing profession, the surplus of physicians, technological developments, the patient–caregiver relationship, the spread of tuberculosis, and the growing interest in the welfare of mothers and children all had an impact on patient education (Bartlett, 1986). In nursing, Florence Nightingale was a resolute advocate of the educational responsibilities of district nurses and authored Health Teaching in Towns and Villages, which advocated for school teaching of health rules as well as health teaching in the home (Monterio, 1985).

The number of physicians swelled during this time, and the surplus was made worse by the urbanization of the population and technological changes such as the development of the automobile and telephone. The population shift and technological advances contributed to decreasing the amount of time physicians spent making house calls to rural patients (Starr, 1982). Because care was then less time consuming, fewer physicians were needed. The invention of the stethoscope, ophthalmoscope, and laryngoscope contributed to increasing the social distance between patients and physicians and thus changed the dynamics of the physician–patient relationship (Reiser, 1978). For example, instead of putting their head on patients' chests to hear the heart beating, physicians began using an instrument (a cold stethoscope) to hear the heartbeat. This lessened the amount of touching that occurred during a visit and encouraged a more detached relationship. Evidence suggests that during this time some physicians were uncomfortable with patients questioning them,

and they also discouraged self-care activities by patients to keep patients coming to them for care (Bartlett, 1986).

The chronic illness of tuberculosis required patients to take medication over long periods of time. This was not consistent with the traditional medical approach of making a diagnosis and prescribing therapy, so education took on an important role (Bartlett, 1986). The first Society for the Prevention of Tuberculosis strongly emphasized education measures (Bartlett, 1986). In support of maternal and child health, the Division of Child Hygiene was established in New York City in 1908 (Bartlett, 1986). Here, public health nurses provided instruction to mothers of newborns in the lower East Side on how to keep their infants healthy.

The period from 1930 through 1960 is described as a time of relative quiet for patient education. Education continued to occur as a part of clinical encounters, but it was overshadowed by the rising technological orientation of medicine (Bartlett, 1986). The first references in the literature to patient education began to appear in the early 1950s (Falvo, 2004). In 1953, the Veterans Administration (VA) hospitals issued a technical bulletin titled *Patient Education and the Hospital Program*. This bulletin identified the nature and scope of patient education and provided guidance to all hospital services involved in patient education (Veterans Administration, 1953). At the same time, members of the National Tuberculosis Association started teaching patients and their families about the disease and its treatment (Breckon, 1982).

In the 1960s and 1970s, patient education began to be seen as a specific entity where emphasis was placed on educating individual patients rather than providing general public health education. Developments during this time, such as the civil rights movement, the women's movement, and the consumer and self-help movement, all affected patient education (Bartlett, 1986; Nyswander, 1980;

Rosen, 1977). In the early sixties, voluntary agencies and the Public Health Service funded several patient and family education projects dealing with congestive heart failure, stroke, cancer, and renal dialysis, and hospitals in a variety of states also became involved in various education programs and projects (Public Health Service, 1971). In 1964, the American Medical Association held the First National Conference on Health Education Goals where a noteworthy outcome was the development of an objective focusing on educating individuals to have better accountability for maintaining their own health (Falvo, 2004).

Concerned that patient education was being provided only occasionally and that patients were not routinely being given information that would allow them to participate in their own health care, the American Public Health Association formed a multidisciplinary Committee on Educational Tasks in Chronic Illness in 1968 that recommended a more formal approach to patient education (Public Health Service, 1971). One of the committee's seven basic premises was the suggested use of an educational prescription that would base teaching on individual patient needs and be included as part of the patient's record. This was one of the first times that the documentation of patient education was mentioned (Falvo, 2004). The committee developed a model that defined the educational processes necessary for patient and family education that could be used with any illness by any member of the healthcare team (Health Services and Mental Health Administration, 1972).

In 1971, two significant events occurred: A publication from the Department of Health, Education and Welfare titled *The Need for Patient Education* emphasized a concept of patient education that provided information about disease and treatment as well as teaching patients how to stay healthy, and President Nixon in a message to Congress used the term *health education* (Falvo, 2004). Nixon later appointed the President's Committee on Health Education that recommended hospi-

tals offer health education to families of patients (Bartlett, 1986; Weingarten, 1974). Although the terms *health education* and *patient education* were used interchangeably, this recommendation had a great impact on the future of patient education because a health education focal point was established in what was then the Department of Education and Welfare (Falvo, 2004). As a result of this committee's recommendations, the American Hospital Association (AHA) appointed a special committee on Health Education (Falvo, 2004). The AHA committee believed that it was a responsibility of hospitals as well as other healthcare institutions to provide educational programs for patients and that all health professionals were to be included in patient education. Through these health education programs, hospitals could contribute to important healthcare goals such as improved quality of patient care, reduced healthcare costs, shorter lengths of stay, fewer admissions and readmissions to inpatient facilities, and better utilization of outpatient services (AHA, 1976). In 1978, the AHA established the Center for Health Promotion (Bartlett, 1986). The concept of patient education expanded during this era, affecting the healthcare delivery system as well as the patient (Falvo, 2004). Also, the healthcare system began to pay more attention to patient rights and protections involving informed consent (Roter, Stashefsky-Margalit, & Rudd, 2001).

Patient education was a significant part of the AHA's *A Patient's Bill of Rights*, affirmed in 1972 and first published in 1973 (AHA, 1973). This document outlines patients' rights to receive current information about diagnosis, treatment, and prognosis in understandable terms as well as information that enables them to make informed decisions about their health care. The *Patient's Bill of Rights* also guarantees a patient's right to respectful and considerate care. The adoption of this bill of rights promoted additional growth in the concept of patient education because it came to be seen as a "patient right" as well as an obligation and legal responsibility of health professionals. In addition, patient education was recognized as a condition of quality care and as a factor that could affect the efficiency of the healthcare system (Falvo, 2004).

In the 1970s, insurance companies also dealt with issues surrounding patient education (Bartlett, 1986). They began to see the possible positive impact patient education could have on the costs of health care. Several papers, publications, and brochures, such as *White Paper. Patient Health Education*, approved by the Board of Governors of the Blue Cross Association in 1974, *Report from the Committee on Health Education to the Health Insurance Benefits Advisory Council of the Department of Health, Education, and Welfare*, and *Financing In-Hospital Patient Education: Proposed Criteria* by the Health Insurance Association of America, dealt with how patient education could be included as a part of medical care (Bartlett, 1986).

Further support and validation of patient education as a right and expectation of quality health care came as a result of the 1976 edition of the *Accreditation Manual for Hospitals* published by the Joint Commission on Accreditation of Healthcare Organizations, now known as Joint Commission (Falvo, 2004). This edition of the manual broadened the scope of patient education to include outpatient as well as inpatient services and specified that criteria for patient education should be established. Patients had to receive information about their medical problem, prognosis, and treatment. The manual further stated that evidence be provided that patients understood the information they were given and that final progress notes included the specific instructions the patient and family received (Joint Commission on Accreditation of Healthcare Organizations, 1976).

In the 1980s, national health education programs once again came into vogue as healthcare trends focused on disease prevention and health promotion. This was a logical response to the cost-containment efforts occurring in health care at that time. The U.S. Department of Health and Human Services' *Healthy People 2000: National Health Promotion and Disease Prevention Objectives*, issued in 1990 and building on the U.S. Surgeon General's *Healthy People* report of 1979, established important goals for national health promotion and disease prevention in 22 areas (U.S. Department of Health and Human Services [USDHHS] Office of Disease Prevention and Health Promotion, 2000). Establishing educational and community-based programs was one of the priority areas in this document. Following *Healthy People 2000, Healthy People 2010* built on the previous two initiatives and provided a framework for health prevention for the nation. Specific objectives in 28 focus areas support the two overarching goals of increasing the quality and years of healthy life and eliminating health disparities (USDHHS, 2010). These goals and objectives include the development of effective health education programs to assist individuals to recognize and change risk behaviors, to adopt or maintain healthy practices, and to make appropriate use of available services for health care. Patient education is a fundamental component of these far-reaching national initiatives.

In recognition of the importance of patient education by nurses, the Joint Commission (JC), formerly the Joint Commission on Accreditation of Healthcare Organizations (JCAHO), established nursing standards for patient education as early as 1993. These standards, known as mandates, describe the type and level of care, treatment, and services that agencies or organizations must provide to receive accreditation. Required accreditation standards have provided the impetus for nursing service managers to emphasize unit-based clinical staff education activities for the improvement of nursing care interventions to achieve expected client outcomes (JCAHO, 2001). Nurses are to achieve positive outcomes of patient care through teaching activities that must be patient centered and family oriented. More recently, the JC expanded its expectations to include an interdisciplinary team approach in the provision of patient education as well as evidence that patients and their significant others participate in care and decision making and understand what they have been taught. This requirement means that providers must consider the literacy level, educational background, language skills, and culture of every client during the education process (Cipriano, 2007; Davidhizar & Brownson, 1999; JCAHO, 2001).

In the mid-1990s, the Pew Health Professions Commission (1995), influenced by the dramatic changes surrounding health care, published a broad set of competencies it believes would mark the success of the health professions in the 21st century. Shortly thereafter, the commission released a fourth report as a follow-up on health professional practice in the new millennium (Pew Health Professions Commission, 1998). The fourth report offers recommendations that affect the scope and training of all health professional groups, as well as a new set of competencies for the 21st century. Many of the competencies pertain to the teaching role of health professionals. These competencies for the practice of health care include the need for health professionals to do the following:

- Embrace a personal ethic of social responsibility and service
- Provide evidence-based, clinically competent care
- Incorporate the multiple determinants of health in clinical care
- Rigorously practice preventative health care
- Improve access to health care for those with unmet health needs
- Practice relationship-centered care with individuals and families
- Provide culturally sensitive care to a diverse society
- Use communication and information technology effectively and appropriately
- Continue to learn and help others learn

In 2006, the Institute for Healthcare Improvement announced the 5 Million Lives campaign. The campaign's objective is to reduce the 15 million incidents of medical harm that occur in U.S. hospitals each year. Such an ambitious campaign has major implications for teaching patients and their families as well as staff and students the ways they can improve care to reduce injuries, save lives, and decrease costs of health care (Berwick, 2006).

Another recent initiative is the formation of the Sullivan Alliance to recruit and educate health professionals to deliver culturally competent care to the public they serve. Effective health care and health education of patients and their families depend on a sound scientific base and cultural awareness in an increasingly diverse society. This organization's goal is to increase the racial and cultural mix of health professional faculty, students, and staff, who are sensitive to the needs of clients of diverse backgrounds (Sullivan & Bristow, 2007).

Accomplishing the goals and meeting the expectations of these various organizations call for a redirection of education efforts. Since the 1980s, the role of the health professional as educator has undergone a paradigm shift, evolving from what once was a disease-oriented approach to a more prevention-oriented approach. In other words, the focus is on teaching for the promotion and maintenance of health (Roter et al., 2001). Education, once done as part of discharge plans at the end of hospitalization, has expanded to become part of a comprehensive plan of care that occurs across the continuum of the healthcare delivery process (Davidhizar & Brownson, 1999).

As described by Grueninger (1995), this transition toward wellness entails a progression "from disease-oriented patient education (DOPE) to prevention-oriented patient education (POPE) to ultimately become health-oriented patient education (HOPE)" (p. 53). Instead of the traditional aim of simply imparting information, the emphasis is now on empowering patients to use their potentials, abilities, and resources to the fullest (Glanville, 2000). Along with supporting patient empowerment, health professionals must be mindful to continue to ensure the protection of "patient voice" and the therapeutic relationship in patient education against the backdrop of ever-increasing productivity expectations and time constraints (Roter et al., 2001).

Today, the vast majority of health professionals consider the education of clients, families, colleagues, students, and others to be part of their professional responsibility. It was not until recently, however, that many of the professions formally identified the responsibility of teaching in their professional documents. According to Breslow (1985), every student of medicine learns that *doctor* means teacher, yet it was only in 1975 that the House of Delegates of the American Medical Association (AMA) adopted a formal statement that addressed patient education as an integral part of high-quality health care (AMA, 1976). This statement by the AMA emphasizes the responsibility of physicians in conducting patient education, but it also recognizes the responsibility of nurses, dietitians, and other health professionals in this area. It stresses the "team effort" aspect of patient education as well as the patient's responsibility for patient education outcomes (Falvo, 2004).

In the 1970s, the fields of pharmacy, dietetics, and physical therapy also published formal statements on their role in patient education. The *Statement on Pharmacist-Conducted Patient Counseling*, published in 1976 by the American Society of Hospital Pharmacists, delineates the role of pharmacists in educating patients about their medications (American Society of Hospital Pharmacists, 1976). A position paper by the American Dietetic Association in 1976 recommends that dietitians counsel individuals and families in nutritional principles, dietary plans, and food selections, adapting plans to the individual's lifestyle. It also recommends that dieticians record dietary history in medical records and compile or develop educational materials to use as aids in nutrition counseling (American Dietetic Association, 1976). In 1958, an early article recognizing the importance of teaching as a fundamental part of treatment appeared in the physical therapy literature, but the first accreditation criteria related to the teaching role of physical therapists were developed by the American Physical Therapy Association in 1978 (May, 1999). This document states that the physical therapy graduate should be able to "apply basic educational concepts of learning theories in designing, implementing and evaluating learning experiences in order to teach patients and families and to design and implement community education in-service programs" (American Physical Therapy Association, 1978, p. B-7).

Nursing is unique among the health professions in that patient education has long been considered a major component of standard care given by nurses. Since the mid-1800s, when nursing was first acknowledged as a unique discipline, the responsibility for teaching has been recognized as an important role of nurses as caregivers. The focus of nurses' teaching efforts is on the care of the sick and promotion of the health of the well public, as well as educating other nurses for professional practice.

As early as 1918, the National League of Nursing Education (NLNE) in the United States (now the National League for Nursing [NLN]) observed the importance of health teaching as a function within the scope of nursing practice. Two decades later, this organization recognized nurses as agents for the promotion of health and the prevention of illness in all settings in which they practiced (NLNE, 1937). By 1950, the NLNE had identified course content in nursing school curricula to prepare nurses to assume the role of teachers of others. So, too, the American Nurses Association (ANA) has for years put forth statements on the functions, standards, and qualifications for nursing practice, of which patient teaching is a key element. In addition, the International Council of Nurses (ICN) has long endorsed the nurse's role as educator to be an essential component of nursing care delivery. Today, all state nurse practice acts (NPAs) include teaching within the scope of nursing practice responsibilities. Nurses, by legal mandate of the NPAs, are expected to provide instruction to consumers to assist them to maintain optimal levels of wellness and manage illness.

A variety of other health professions also identify their commitment to patient education in their professional documents (Falvo, 2004). Standards of practice, practice frameworks, accreditation standards, guides to practice, and practice acts of many health professions delineate the educational responsibilities of their members. In addition, professional workshops and continuing education programs routinely address the skills needed for quality patient and staff education. Although specific roles vary according to profession, contemporary patient education clearly echoes Bartlett's (1986) assertion that it "must be viewed as a fundamentally multidisciplinary enterprise" (p. 146).

In addition to providing patient education, health professionals are also responsible for educating their colleagues. Another role of today's health professional educator is one of training the trainer—that is, preparing staff through continuing education, in-service programs, and staff development to maintain and improve their clinical skills and teaching abilities. Health professionals must be prepared to effectively perform teaching services that meet the needs of many individuals and groups in different circumstances across a variety of practice settings.

Health professional educators also serve as clinical instructors for students in the practice setting. Many health professionals function as clinical instructors, preceptors, and mentors to ensure that students meet their expected learning outcomes. However, evidence indicates that some health professionals in the clinical and academic settings feel inadequate as mentors and preceptors as a result of poor preparation for their role as teachers. This challenge of relating theory learned in the classroom setting to the practice environment requires health professionals not only to be up-to-date with clinical skills and innovations in practice, but also to possess the knowledge and skills of the principles of teaching and learning. Knowing the practice field is not the same thing as knowing how to teach the field. The role of the clinical educator is a dynamic one that requires the teacher to actively engage students to become competent and caring professionals (Gillespie & McFetridge, 2006).

Social, Economic, and Political Trends Affecting Health Care

In addition to the professional and legal standards various organizations and agencies have put forth, many social, economic, and political trends nationwide that affect the public's health have focused attention on the role of the health professional as teacher and the importance of client and staff education. The following are some of the significant forces influencing nursing practice in particular and healthcare practice in general (Birchenall, 2000; Bodenheimer, Lorig, Holman, & Grumbach, 2002; Cipriano, 2007; De-Silets, 1995; Glanville, 2000; USDHHS, 2000; Zikmund-Fisher, Sarr, Fagerlin, & Ubel, 2006):

- As discussed earlier, the federal government published *Healthy People 2010: Understanding and Improving Health* and will soon publish *Healthy People 2020*, setting forth national health goals and objectives for the next decade. Achieving these national priorities would dramatically cut the costs of health care, prevent the premature onset of disease and disability, and help all Americans lead healthier and more productive lives. Health professionals play an important role in making a real difference by teaching clients to attain and maintain healthy lifestyles.

- The growth of managed care has resulted in shifts in reimbursement for healthcare services. Greater emphasis is placed on outcome measures, many of which can be achieved primarily through the health education of clients.

- Health providers are recognizing the economic and social values of reaching out to communities, schools, and workplaces to provide education for disease prevention and health promotion.

- Politicians and healthcare administrators alike recognize the importance of health education to accomplish the economic goal of reducing the high costs of health services. Political emphasis is on productivity, competitiveness in the marketplace, and cost-containment measures to restrain health service expenses.

- Health professionals are increasingly concerned about malpractice claims and disciplinary action for incompetence. Continuing education, either by legislative mandate or as a requirement of the employing institution, has come to the forefront in response to the challenge of ensuring the competency of practitioners. It is a means to transmit new knowledge and skills as well as to reinforce or refresh previously acquired knowledge and abilities for the continuing growth of staff.

- Consumers are demanding increased knowledge and skills about how to care for themselves and how to prevent disease. As people are becoming more aware of their needs and desire a greater understanding of treatments and goals, the demand for health information is expected to intensify. The quest for consumer rights and responsibilities, which began in the 1990s, continues into the 21st century.

- Demographic trends, particularly the aging of the population, require the health professions to emphasize self-reliance and maintenance of a healthy status over an extended life span. As the percentage of the U.S. population older than age 65 years climbs dramatically in the next 20 to 30 years, the healthcare needs of the baby-boom generation of the post–World War II era will increase as people deal with degenerative illnesses and other effects of the aging process.

- Among the major causes of morbidity and mortality are those diseases now recognized as being lifestyle related and preventable through educational intervention. In addition, millions of incidents of medical harm occur every year in U.S. hospitals so that it is imperative that clients, staff, and students be educated about preventive measures to reduce these incidents (Berwick, 2006).

- The increase in chronic and incurable conditions requires that individuals and families become informed participants to manage their own illnesses. Client teaching can facilitate an individual's adaptive responses to illness and disability.

- Advanced technology increases the complexity of care and treatment in home and community-based settings. More rapid hospital discharge and more procedures done on an outpatient basis force clients to be more self-reliant in managing their own health. Patient education assists them to follow through with self-management activities independently.

- To improve health outcomes nationwide, healthcare providers increasingly recognize client health literacy as an essential skill. Health professionals must attend to the education needs of their clients to be sure that clients adequately understand the information required for independence in self-care activities that promote, maintain, and restore their health.

- Many healthcare providers believe, and this belief is supported by research, that client education improves compliance and, hence, health and well-being. Better understanding by clients and their families of the recommended treatment plans can lead to increased cooperation, decision making, satisfaction, and independence with therapeutic regimens. Health education enables patients to solve problems they encounter outside the protected care environments of hospitals, thereby increasing their independence.

- An increasing number of self-help groups exist to support clients in meeting their physical and psychosocial needs. The success of these support groups and behavioral change programs depends on the health professional's role as teacher and advocate.

Health professionals recognize the need to develop their expertise in teaching to keep pace with the demands of patient and staff education. As they continue to define their role, body of knowledge, scope of practice, and professional expertise, they realize, more than ever before, the significance of their role as educators. Health professionals have many opportunities to carry out health education. Interestingly, the health professions included in the Gallup honesty and ethics poll (nurses, pharmacists, and physicians) comprised three of the four top-rated professions in the poll. Close to two thirds of Americans rated these professions very high or high in this area (Saad, 2008). The trusting relationship generated between the health professional and client facilitates the exchange of health education information.

Purposes, Goals, and Benefits of Client and Staff Education

The purpose of patient education is to increase the competence and confidence of clients for self-management. The goal is to increase the responsibility and independence of clients for self-care. This can be achieved by supporting clients through the transition from being dependent on others to being self-sustaining in managing their own care and from being passive listeners to active learners. An interactive, partnership education approach provides clients the opportunity to explore and expand their self-care abilities (Cipriano, 2007).

The single most important action of health professionals as educators is to prepare clients for self-care. If clients cannot independently maintain or improve their health status when on their own, health professionals have failed to help them reach their potential (Glanville, 2000). The benefits of client education are many. For example, effective teaching by a health professional can do the following:

- Increase consumer satisfaction
- Improve quality of life
- Ensure continuity of care
- Decrease client anxiety
- Effectively reduce the complications of illness and the incidence of disease
- Promote adherence to treatment plans
- Maximize independence in the performance of activities of daily living
- Energize and empower consumers to become actively involved in the planning of their care

Because clients must handle many health needs and problems at home, a need to educate people on how to care for themselves—both to get well and to stay well—truly exists. Illness is a natural life process, but so is humankind's ability to learn. Along with the ability to learn comes a natural curiosity that allows people to view new and difficult situations as challenges rather than as defeats. As Orr (1990) observes, "Illness can become an educational opportunity ... a 'teachable moment' when ill health suddenly encourages [patients] to take a more active role in their care" (p. 47). This observation remains relevant today.

Numerous studies document the fact that informed clients are more likely to comply with medical treatment plans, find innovative ways to cope with illness, and be less likely to experience complications. Overall, clients are more satisfied with care when they receive adequate information about how to manage for themselves. One of the most frequently cited complaints by patients in litigation cases is that they were not adequately informed (Reising, 2007).

Just as the need exists to teach clients to become participants and informed consumers to achieve independence in self-care, the need also exists for staff to be exposed to up-to-date information with the ultimate goal of enhancing their practice. The purpose of staff and student education is to increase the competence and confidence of health professionals to function independently in providing care to the consumer. The goal of education efforts is to improve the quality of care delivered by health professionals. In turn, the benefits to health professionals in their role as educators include increased job satisfaction when they recognize that their teaching actions have the potential to forge therapeutic relationships with clients, enhanced patient–health professional autonomy, increased accountability in practice, and the opportunity to create change that really makes a difference in the lives of others.

Health educators' primary aims, then, should be to nourish clients, mentor staff, and serve as teachers and clinical instructors for health professional students. They must value their role in educating others and make it a priority for their clients, fellow colleagues, and the future members of the profession.

The Education Process Defined

The **education process** is a systematic, sequential, logical, scientifically based, planned course of action consisting of two major interdependent operations, teaching and learning. This process forms a continuous cycle that also involves two interdependent players, the teacher and the learner.

Together, they jointly perform teaching and learning activities, the outcome of which leads to mutually desired behavior changes. These changes foster growth in the learner and, it should be acknowledged, growth in the teacher as well. Thus, the education process is a framework for a participatory, shared approach to teaching and learning (Carpenter & Bell, 2002).

The education process is similar across the practice of many of the health professions. In fact, the educational process is often compared to the nursing process because the steps of each run parallel to one another. (See **Figure 1–1**.) The education process, like professional practice in nursing and most healthcare disciplines, consists of the basic elements of assessment, planning, implementation, and evaluation. Whereas the general practice of many of the health professions focuses on the planning and implementation of care based on the assessment and diagnosis of the physical and psychosocial needs of the patient, the education process, on the other hand, focuses on the planning and implementation of teaching based on an assessment and prioritization of the client's learning needs, readiness to learn, and learning styles (Carpenter & Bell, 2002). The outcomes of health professional practice are achieved when the physical and psychosocial needs of the client are met. The outcomes of the education process are achieved when changes in knowledge, attitudes, and skills occur. Both processes are ongoing, with assessment and evaluation perpetually redirecting the planning and implementation phases. If mutually agreed-on outcomes in either process are not achieved, as determined by evaluation, then the process can and should begin again through reassessment, replanning, and reimplementation.

Note that the actual act of **teaching** or **instruction** is merely one component of the education process. Teaching and instruction, terms often used interchangeably, are deliberate interventions that involve sharing information and experiences to meet intended learner outcomes in the cognitive, affective, and psychomotor domains according to an education plan. Teaching and instruction, both one and the same, are often formal, structured, organized activities prepared days in advance, but they can be performed informally on the spur of the moment during conversations or incidental encounters with the learner. Whether formal or informal, planned well in advance or spontaneous, teaching and instruction are nevertheless deliberate and conscious acts with the objective of producing learning (Carpenter & Bell, 2002).

The fact that teaching and instruction are intentional does not necessarily mean that they have to be lengthy and complex tasks, but it does mean that they comprise conscious actions on the part of the teacher in responding to an individual's need to learn. The cues that someone has a need to learn can be communicated in the form of a verbal request, a question, a puzzled or confused look, a blank stare, or a gesture of defeat or frus-

tration. In the broadest sense, then, teaching is a highly versatile strategy that can be applied in preventing, promoting, maintaining, or modifying a wide variety of behaviors in a learner who is receptive, motivated, and adequately informed (Duffy, 1998).

Learning is defined as a change in behavior (knowledge, attitudes, and/or skills) that can be observed or measured and that occurs at any time or in any place as a result of exposure to environmental stimuli. Learning is an action by which knowledge, skills, and attitudes are consciously or unconsciously acquired such that behavior is altered in some way (see Chapter 3). The success of the health professional educator's endeavors at teaching is measured not by how much content he or she imparts, but rather by how much the person learns (Musinski, 1999).

Specifically, **patient education** is a process of assisting people to learn health-related behaviors

Figure 1–1 Education Process Parallels Healthcare Practice

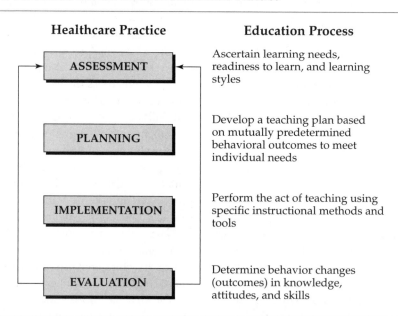

Healthcare Practice	Education Process
ASSESSMENT	Ascertain learning needs, readiness to learn, and learning styles
PLANNING	Develop a teaching plan based on mutually predetermined behavioral outcomes to meet individual needs
IMPLEMENTATION	Perform the act of teaching using specific instructional methods and tools
EVALUATION	Determine behavior changes (outcomes) in knowledge, attitudes, and skills

that they can incorporate into everyday life with the goal of optimal health and independence in self-care. **Staff education**, by contrast, is the process of influencing the behavior of colleagues by producing changes in their knowledge, attitudes, and skills to help them maintain and improve their competencies for the delivery of quality care to the consumer. Both patient and staff education involve forging a relationship between the learner and the educator so that the learner's information needs (cognitive, affective, and psychomotor) can be met through the process of education (see Chapter 10).

The ASSURE model is a useful paradigm originally developed to assist nurses to organize and carry out the education process (Rega, 1993). This model is appropriate for all health professional educators. The acronym stands for

- **A**nalyze the learner
- **S**tate the objectives
- **S**elect the instructional methods and materials
- **U**se the instructional methods and materials
- **R**equire learner performance
- **E**valuate the teaching plan and revise as necessary

Role of the Health Professional as Educator

Over the years, organizations governing and influencing the practice of various health professionals have identified teaching as an important responsibility. For health professionals to fulfill the role of educator, no matter whether their audience consists of patients, family members, students, staff, or other agency personnel, they must have a solid foundation in the principles of teaching and learning.

The role of educator is not primarily to teach, but to promote learning and provide for an environment conducive to learning—to create the teachable moment rather than just waiting for it to happen (Lawson & Flocke, 2009; Wagner & Ash, 1998). Also, the role of the health professional as teacher of clients, families, staff, and students certainly should stem from a partnership philosophy. A learner cannot be made to learn, but an effective approach in educating others is to actively involve learners in the education process (Bodenheimer et al., 2002).

Although health professionals are expected to teach, many lack formal preparation in the principles of teaching and learning. As you see in this textbook, a health professional needs a great deal of knowledge and skill to carry out the role as educator with efficiency and effectiveness. Although all health professionals are able to function as givers of information, they need to acquire the skills of being a facilitator of the learning process (Musinski, 1999). Consider the following questions:

- Is every health professional adequately prepared to assess for learning needs, readiness to learn, and learning styles?
- Can every health professional determine whether information given is received and understood?
- Are all health professionals capable of taking appropriate action to revise the approach to educating the client if the client does not comprehend the information provided?
- Do health professional educators realize they need to transition their role from being a content transmitter to being a process manager, from controlling the learner to releasing the learner, and from being a teacher to becoming a facilitator (Musinski, 1999)?

A growing body of evidence suggests that effective education and learner participation go hand in hand. The health professional should act as a facilitator, creating an environment conducive to learning that motivates individuals to want to learn and makes it possible for them to learn (Musinski,

1999). Both the educator and the learner should participate in the assessment of learning needs, the design of a teaching plan, the implementation of instructional methods and materials, and the evaluation of teaching and learning. Thus, the emphasis should be on the facilitation of learning from a nondirective rather than a didactic teaching approach (Donner, Levonian, & Slutsky, 2005; Knowles, Holton, & Swanson, 1998; Mangena & Chabeli, 2005; Musinski, 1999).

No longer should teachers see themselves as simply transmitters of content. Indeed, the role of the educator has shifted from the traditional position of being the giver of information to that of a process designer and coordinator. This role alteration from the traditional teacher-centered to the learner-centered approach is a paradigm shift that requires educators to possess skill in needs assessment as well as the ability to involve learners in planning, link learners to learning resources, and encourage learner initiative (Knowles et al., 1998; Mangena & Chabeli, 2005).

Instead of the teacher teaching, the new educational paradigm focuses on the learner learning. That is, the teacher becomes the guide on the side, assisting the learner in his or her effort to determine objectives and goals for learning, with both parties being active partners in decision making throughout the learning process. To increase comprehension, recall, and application of information, clients must be actively involved in the learning experience (Kessels, 2003; London, 1995). Glanville (2000) describes this move toward assisting learners to use their own abilities and resources as "a pivotal transfer of power" (p. 58).

Barriers to Teaching and Obstacles to Learning

It has been said by many educators that adult learning takes place not by the teacher's initiating and motivating the learning process, but rather by the teacher's removing or reducing obstacles to learning and enhancing the process after it has begun. The educator should not limit learning to the information that is intended but should clearly make possible the potential for informal, unintended learning that can occur each and every day with each and every teacher–learner encounter (Carpenter & Bell, 2002).

Unfortunately, health professionals must confront many barriers in carrying out their responsibilities for educating others. Also, learners face a variety of potential obstacles that can interfere with their learning. For the purposes of this textbook, **barriers to teaching** are defined as those factors that impede the health professional's ability to deliver educational services. **Obstacles to learning** are defined as those factors that negatively affect the ability of the learner to pay attention to and process information.

Factors Affecting the Ability to Teach

The following include the major barriers that interfere with the ability of health professionals to carry out their roles as educators (Carpenter & Bell, 2002; Casey, 1995; Chachkes & Christ, 1996; Duffy, 1998; Glanville, 2000; Honan, Krsnak, Petersen, & Torkelson, 1988) (see also **Figure 1–2**):

1. Lack of time to teach is a common barrier that prevents health professionals from being able to carry out their educator role effectively. Early discharge from inpatient and outpatient settings often results in health professionals and clients having fleeting contact with one another. In addition, the schedules and responsibilities of health professionals are very demanding. Finding time to allocate to teaching is very challenging in light of other work demands and expectations. In one survey by the Joint Commission, 28% of the nurses claimed that they were not able to provide patients and their

families with the necessary instruction because of lack of time during their shifts at work (Stolberg, 2002). Health professionals must know how to adopt an abbreviated, efficient, and effective approach to client and staff education by first adequately assessing the learner and then by using appropriate instructional methods and instructional tools at their disposal. Discharge planning plays an ever more important role in ensuring continuity of care across settings.

2. Many health professionals admit that they do not feel competent or confident with their teaching skills. As stated previously, although health professionals are expected to teach, few have ever taken a specific course on the principles of teaching and learning. The concepts of patient education are often integrated throughout health professional curricula rather than being offered as a specific course of study. Pohl (1965) compiled some interesting statistics re-

Figure 1–2 Barriers to Teaching

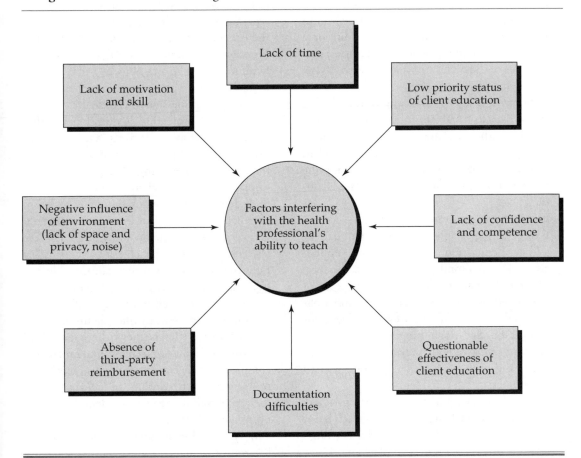

garding nursing, long considered one of the first health professions to have a strong teaching role. As early as the mid-1960s, Pohl found that one third of 1,500 nurses, when questioned, reported that they had no preparation for the teaching they were doing, while only one fifth felt they had adequate preparation. Almost 30 years later, Kruger (1991) surveyed 1,230 nurses in staff, administrative, and education positions regarding their perceptions of the extent of nurses' responsibility for and level of achievement of patient education. Although all three groups strongly believed that client and staff education is a primary responsibility of nurses, the vast majority of them rated their ability to perform educator role activities as unsatisfactory. Many of the other health professions share similar views. Few additional studies have been forthcoming on nurses' perceptions of their educator role (Trocino, Byers, & Peach, 1997).

3. Personal characteristics of the health professional educator play an important role in determining the outcome of a teaching–learning interaction. Motivation to teach and skill in teaching are prime factors in determining the success of any educational endeavor (see Chapter 11).

4. Until recently, administration and supervisory personnel assigned low priority to patient and staff education. With the strong emphasis on Joint Commission mandates, the level of attention paid to the educational needs of consumers as well as healthcare personnel has changed significantly. However, budget allocations for educational programs remain tight and can interfere with the adoption of innovative and time-saving teaching strategies and techniques.

5. The environment in the various settings where health professionals are expected to teach is not always conducive to carrying out the teaching–learning process. Lack of space, lack of privacy,

noise, and frequent interferences caused by client treatment schedules and staff work demands are just some of the factors that negatively affect the health professional's ability to concentrate and effectively interact with learners.

6. An absence of third-party reimbursement to support patient education relegates teaching and learning to less than high-priority status. Services of health professionals within healthcare facilities are subsumed under hospital room costs and, therefore, are not often specifically reimbursed by insurance payers. In fact, patient education in some settings, such as home care, often cannot be incorporated as a legitimate aspect of routine care delivery unless specifically ordered by a physician. Because there are no separate billing codes for patient education in the American Medical Association's Common Procedural Terminology (CPT) codes, it is difficult to make it an area of focus and it must be integrated into a therapeutic intervention for many health professionals (Hack, 1999).

7. Some health professionals question whether patient education is effective as a means to improve health outcomes. They view patients as impediments to teaching when patients do not display an interest in changing behavior, when they demonstrate an unwillingness to learn, or when their ability to learn is in question. Concerns about coercion and violation of free choice, based on the belief that patients have a right to choose and that they cannot be forced to comply, explain why some professionals feel frustrated in their efforts to teach. Unless all healthcare members buy into the utility of patient education (that is, they believe it can lead to significant behavioral changes and increased compliance to therapeutic regimens), then some professionals may continue to feel absolved of their responsibility to provide adequate and appropriate patient education.

8. The type of documentation system used by healthcare agencies has an effect on the quality

and quantity of patient teaching. Both formal and informal teaching are often done (Carpenter & Bell, 2002) but not written down because of insufficient time, inattention to detail, and inadequate forms on which to record the extent of teaching activities. Many of the forms used for documentation of teaching are designed to simply check off the areas addressed rather than allow for elaboration of what was actually accomplished. In addition, many health professionals do not recognize the scope and depth of teaching that they perform on a daily basis. Communication among healthcare providers regarding what has been taught needs to be coordinated and appropriately delegated so that teaching can proceed in a timely, smooth, organized, and thorough fashion.

Factors Affecting the Ability to Learn

The following are some of the major obstacles interfering with a learner's ability to attend to and process information (Glanville, 2000; Weiss, 2003) (see also **Figure 1–3**):

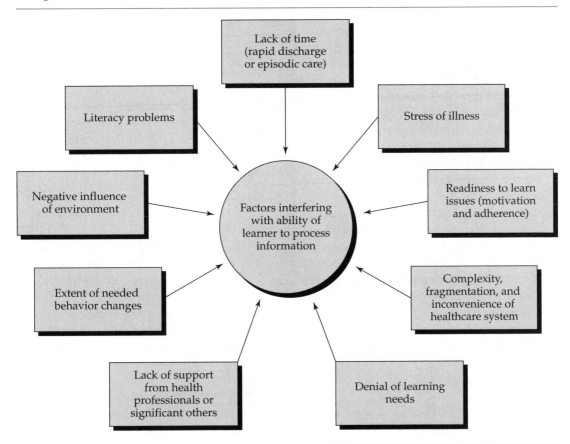

Figure 1–3 Obstacles to Learning

- Lack of time (rapid discharge or episodic care)
- Stress of illness
- Literacy problems
- Negative influence of environment
- Readiness to learn issues (motivation and adherence)
- Factors interfering with ability of learner to process information
- Extent of needed behavior changes
- Complexity, fragmentation, and inconvenience of healthcare system
- Lack of support from health professionals or significant others
- Denial of learning needs

1. Lack of time to learn resulting from rapid patient discharge from care and the amount of information a client is expected to learn can discourage and frustrate the learner, impeding his or her ability and willingness to learn.

2. The stress of acute and chronic illness, anxiety, and sensory deficits in patients are just a few problems that can diminish learner motivation and interfere with the process of learning. However, illness alone seldom acts as an impediment to learning. Rather, illness is often the impetus for patients to attend to learning, make contact with the healthcare professional, and take positive action to improve their health status.

3. Low literacy and functional health illiteracy have been found to be significant factors in the ability of clients to make use of the written and verbal instructions given to them by providers. Almost half of the American people read and comprehend at or below the eighth-grade level and an even higher percentage suffer from health illiteracy (see Chapter 7).

4. The negative influence of the hospital environment itself, resulting in loss of control, lack of privacy, and social isolation, can interfere with a patient's active role in health decision making and involvement in the teaching–learning process.

5. Personal characteristics of the learner have major effects on the degree to which behavioral outcomes are achieved. Readiness to learn, motivation and compliance, developmental-stage characteristics, and learning styles are some of the prime factors influencing the success of educational endeavors.

6. The extent of behavioral changes needed, both in number and in complexity, can overwhelm learners and dissuade them from attending to and accomplishing learning objectives and goals.

7. Lack of support and lack of ongoing positive reinforcement from health professionals and significant others serve to block the potential for learning.

8. Denial of learning needs, resentment of authority, and lack of willingness to take responsibility (locus of control) are some psychological obstacles to accomplishing behavioral change.

9. The inconvenience, complexity, inaccessibility, fragmentation, and dehumanization of the healthcare system often result in frustration and abandonment of efforts by the learner to participate in and comply with the goals and objectives for learning.

Questions to Be Asked About Teaching and Learning

To maximize the effectiveness of client, staff, and student education, the health professional must examine the elements of the education process and the role of the health professional as educator. Many questions arise related to the principles of teaching and learning. The following are some of the important questions that the chapters in this textbook address:

- How can members of the healthcare team work together more effectively to coordinate educational efforts?
- What are the ethical, legal, and economic issues involved in patient and staff education?
- Which theories and principles support the education process, and how can they be applied to change the behaviors of learners?
- What assessment methods and tools can health professionals as educators use to determine learning needs, readiness to learn, and learning styles?
- Which learner attributes negatively and positively affect an individual's ability and willingness to learn?

- What can be done about the inequities (in quantity and quality) in the delivery of education services?
- Which elements must the health professional as educator take into account when developing and implementing teaching plans?
- Which instructional methods and materials are available to support teaching efforts?
- Under which conditions should health professionals use certain teaching methods and materials?
- How can teaching be tailored to meet the needs of specific populations of learners?
- What common mistakes do health professionals make when teaching others?
- How can teaching and learning be best evaluated?

State of the Evidence

The literature on patient and staff education, from both a research- and non-research-based perspective, is particularly extensive in nursing. Much of it can be broadly applied to all the health professions. The nonresearch literature on patient education is prescriptive in nature and tends to give anecdotal tips on how to take individualized approaches to teaching and learning. A computer literature search, for example, reveals literally thousands of nursing and allied health articles and books on teaching and learning that are available from the general to the specific.

However, many research-based studies are being conducted on teaching specific population groups about a variety of topics, but only recently has the field focused attention on how to most effectively teach those with long-term chronic illnesses. Health professionals as educators must conduct much more research on the benefits of patient education as it relates to the potential for increasing quality of life, enabling patients to lead a

disability-free life and manage themselves independently at home, and decreasing the costs of health care through anticipatory teaching approaches. Studies from acute-care settings tend to focus on preparing a patient for a procedure, with emphasis on the benefits of information to alleviate anxiety and promote psychological coping. Evidence does suggest that patients cope much more effectively when taught exactly what to expect (Donovan & Ward, 2001; Duffy, 1998; Mason, 2001).

More research is definitely needed on the benefits of teaching methods and instructional tools that use the technologies of computer-assisted instruction, online and other distance learning modalities, cable television, podcasts, and Internet access to health information for both patient and staff education. These new approaches to information dissemination require a role change of the educator from one of teacher to resource facilitator as well as a shift in the role of the learner from being a passive to an active recipient. The rapid advances in technology for teaching and learning also require educators to have a better understanding of generational orientations and experiences of the learner (Billings & Kowalski, 2004). Also, the effectiveness of videotapes and audiotapes with different learners and in different situations must be further explored (Kessels, 2003). Given the significant incidence of low literacy rates among patients and their family members, much more investigation needs to be done on the impact of printed versus audiovisual materials as well as written versus verbal instruction on learner comprehension (Weiss, 2003).

Gender issues, the influence of socioeconomics on learning, and the strategies of teaching cultural groups and populations with disabilities need further exploration as well. Unfortunately, the findings from interdisciplinary research on the influence of gender on learning remain inconclusive.

Nevertheless, health professionals are expected to teach diverse populations with complex needs and a range of abilities in both traditional settings and nontraditional, unstructured settings. For more than 30 years, researchers have been studying how best to teach patients, but much more research is required (Mason, 2001). The health professions need to establish a stronger theoretical basis for intervening with clients throughout "all phases of the learning continuum, from information acquisition to behavioral change" (Donovan & Ward, 2001, p. 211).

In addition, health professionals as educators should further investigate the cost effectiveness of educational efforts in reducing hospital stays, decreasing readmissions, improving the personal quality of life, and minimizing complications of illness and therapies. Furthermore, given the number of variables that can potentially interfere with the teaching–learning process, additional studies must be conducted to examine the effects of environmental stimuli, the factors involved in readiness to learn, and the influences of learning styles on learner motivation, compliance, comprehension, and the ability to apply knowledge and skills once they are acquired. One particular void is the lack of information in the research database on how to assess motivation. The author of Chapter 6 proposes parameters to assess motivation but notes the paucity of information specifically addressing this issue.

More than 20 years ago, Oberst (1989) delineated the major issues in patient education studies related to the evaluation of the existing research base and the design of future studies. The following four broad problem categories that she identified remain pertinent today:

1. Selection and measurement of appropriate dependent variables (educational outcomes)
2. Design and control of independent variables (educational interventions)
3. Control of mediating and intervening variables

4. Development and refinement of the theoretical basis for education

Summary

Health professionals can be considered information brokers—educators who can make a significant difference in how patients and families cope with their illnesses and disabilities, how the public benefits from education directed at prevention of disease and promotion of health, and how colleagues and students gain competency and confidence in practice through education activities that are directed at continuous, lifelong learning. As this nation moves forward in the 21st century, many challenges and opportunities are ahead for health professional educators in the delivery of health care.

The teaching role is becoming even more important and more visible as health professionals respond to the social, economic, and political trends affecting health care today. The foremost challenge for health professionals is to be able to demonstrate, through research and action, that definite links exist between education and positive behavioral outcomes of the learner. In this era of cost containment, government regulations, and healthcare reform, the benefits of client, staff, and student education must be made clear to the public, to healthcare employers, to healthcare providers, and to payers of healthcare benefits. To be effective and efficient, health professionals must be willing and able to work collaboratively with each other to provide consistently high quality education to the audiences they serve.

Health professionals can demonstrate responsibility and accountability for the delivery of care to the consumer, in part, through education based on solid principles of teaching and learning. The key to effective education of the varied audiences of learners the health professional encounters is his or her understanding of and ongoing commitment to the role of educator.

REVIEW QUESTIONS

1. Which health profession historically has had the most significant impact on patient education?
2. What key factors influenced the growth of patient education during its formative period?
3. How did the concept of patient education change in the 1960s and 1970s?
4. What is the current focus and orientation of patient education?
5. What social, economic, and political trends today make it imperative that clients and health professional staff be adequately educated?
6. What are the similarities and differences between the education process and the general practice of health care?
7. What are three major barriers to teaching and three major obstacles to learning?
8. What common factor serves as both a barrier to education and as an obstacle to learning?
9. What is the current status of research- and non-research-based evidence pertaining to education?

CASE STUDY

As part of Lackney General Hospital's continuous quality improvement plan, and in preparation for the next Joint Commission accreditation visit, all departments in the hospital are in the process of assessing the quality and effectiveness of their patient and staff education efforts. When you solicit feedback from your staff regarding their feelings on this topic, you are surprised at the frustration they express. Liz states, "Although I am incredibly frustrated by the lack of administrative support for patient education, I do believe that patient education makes a difference." Jerimiah jumps in and says, "I am sick of all the boring, mandated continuing education programs we are required to complete." Finally, Jaipaul comments, "I have no idea how I am supposed to fit education in with all the other tasks I am supposed to complete." Because the staff obviously has some strong feelings about the department's education efforts, you feel a SWOT (strengths, weaknesses, opportunities, threats) analysis is a good place to begin to gather information from your colleagues.

1. As a prelude to the SWOT analysis, identify the goals of patient and staff education.
2. Use the section titled "Barriers to Teaching and Obstacles to Learning" as a beginning framework for the weaknesses and threats section of the SWOT analysis, and then describe five potential barriers to teaching and five potential obstacles to learning that your staff might identify.
3. Provide possible solutions to the issues you identified as barriers and obstacles that would serve to enhance patient and staff education.

References

American Dietetic Association. (1976). Position paper on recommended salaries and employment practice for members of The American Dietetic Association. *Journal of the American Dietetic Association, 69*(4), 412–419.

American Hospital Association. (1973). Statement on a patient's bill of rights. *Hospitals, 47*(4), 41.

American Hospital Association. (1976). Statement on the role and responsibilities of hospitals and other health care institutions in personal and community health education. *Health Education, 7*(4), 23.

American Medical Association. (1976). Statement on patient education. *Health Education, 7*(4), 22.

American Physical Therapy Association. (1978). *Standards for accreditation of Physical Therapy Education Programs (1978).* Alexandria, VA: Author.

American Society of Hospital Pharmacists. (1976). Statement on pharmacist-conducted patient counseling. *American Journal of Hospital Pharmacy, 33,* 644–645.

Bartlett, E. E. (1986). Historical glimpses of patient education in the United States. *Patient Education and Counseling, 8,* 135–149.

Berwick, D. (2006, December 12). IHI launches national campaign to reduce medical harm in U.S. hospitals: Building on its landmark 100,000 lives campaign. Retrieved December 21, 2006, from http://www.ihi.org

Billings, D., & Kowalski, K. (2004). Teaching learners from varied generations. *Journal of Continuing Education in Nursing, 35*(3), 104–105.

Birchenall, P. (2000). Nurse education in the year 2000: Reflection, speculation and challenge. *Nurse Education Today, 20,* 1–2.

Bodenheimer, T., Lorig, K., Holman, H., & Grumbach, K. (2002). Patient self-management of chronic disease in primary care. *JAMA, 288*(19), 2469–2475.

Breckon, D. J. (1982). *Hospital health education: A guide to program development.* Gaithersburg, MD: Aspen Publishers.

Breslow, L. (1985). Patient education in historical perspective. *Bulletin of the New York Academy of Medicine, 61*(2), 115–122.

Carpenter, J. A., & Bell, S. K. (2002). What do nurses know about teaching patients? *Journal for Nurses in Staff Development, 18*(3), 157–161.

Casey, F. S. (1995). Documenting patient education: A literature review. *Journal of Continuing Education in Nursing, 26*(6), 257–260.

Chachkes, E., & Christ, G. (1996). Cross cultural issues in patient education. *Patient Education and Counseling, 27,* 13–21.

Cipriano, P. F. (2007). Stop, look, and listen to your patients and their families. *American Nurse Today, 2*(6), 10.

Davidhizar, R. E., & Brownson, K. (1999). Literacy, cultural diversity, and client education. *Health Care Manager, 18*(1), 39–47.

DeSilets, L. D. (1995). Assessing registered nurses' reasons for participating in continuing education. *Journal of Continuing Education in Nursing, 26*(5), 202–208.

Donner, C. L., Levonian, C., & Slutsky, P. (2005). Move to the head of the class: Developing staff nurses as teachers. *Journal of Nurses in Staff Development, 21*(6), 277–283.

Donovan, H. S., & Ward, S. (2001, third quarter). A representational approach to patient education. *Journal of Nursing Scholarship,* 211–216.

Duffy, B. (1998). Get ready—Get set—Go teach. *Home Healthcare Nurse, 16*(9), 596–602.

Falvo, D. F. (2004). *Effective patient education: A guide to increased compliance* (3rd ed.). Sudbury, MA: Jones and Bartlett.

Gillespie, M., & McFetridge, B. (2006). Nursing education—The role of the nurse teacher. *Journal of Clinical Nursing, 15,* 639–644.

Glanville, I. K. (2000). Moving towards health oriented patient education (HOPE). *Holistic Nursing Practice, 14*(2), 57–66.

Grueninger, U. J. (1995). Arterial hypertension: Lessons from patient education. *Patient Education and Counseling, 26,* 37–55.

Hack, L. M., (1999). Health policy implications for patient education in physical therapy. *Journal of Physical Therapy Education, 13*(3), 57–61.

Health Services and Mental Health Administration. (1972). A model for planning patient education; an essential component of health care (DHEW publication no. (HSM) 72-4023). Rockville, MD: American Public Health Association. Committee on Educational Tasks in Chronic Illness.

Honan, S., Krsnak, G., Petersen, D., & Torkelson, R. (1988). The nurse as patient educator: Perceived responsibilities and factors enhancing role development. *Journal of Continuing Education in Nursing, 19*(1), 33–37.

Joint Commission on Accreditation of Healthcare Organizations. (1976). *Accreditation manual for hospitals.* Chicago: Author.

Joint Commission on Accreditation of Healthcare Organizations. (2001). *Patient and family education: The compliance guide to the JCAHO standards* (2nd ed.). Retrieved January 25, 2001, from http://www.accreditinfo.com/news/index.cfm?artid=2011

Kessels, R. P. C. (2003). Patients' memory for medical information. *Journal of the Royal Society of Medicine, 96,* 219–222.

Knowles, M. S., Holton, E. F., & Swanson, R. A. (1998). *The adult learner: The definitive classic in adult education and human resource development* (5th ed., pp. 198–201). Houston, TX: Gulf Publishing.

Kruger, S. (1991). The patient educator role in nursing. *Applied Nursing Research, 4*(1), 19–24.

Lawson, P. J. & Flocke, S. A. (2009). Teachable moments for health behavior change: A concept analysis. *Patient Education and Counseling, 76,* 25–39.

London, F. (1995). Teach your patients faster and better. *Nursing, 95,* 68, 70.

Mangena, A., & Chabeli, M. M. (2005). Strategies to overcome obstacles in the facilitation of critical thinking in nursing education. *Nurse Education Today, 25,* 291–298.

Mason, D. (2001). Promoting health literacy: Patient teaching is a vital nursing function. *American Journal of Nursing, 101*(2), 7.

May, B. J. (1999). Patient education: Past and present. *Journal of Physical Therapy Education, 13*(3), 3–7.

Monterio, L. A. (1985). Florence Nightingale on Public Health Nursing. *American Journal of Public Health, 75,* 181–186.

Musinski, B. (1999). The educator as facilitator: A new kind of leadership. *Nursing Forum, 34*(1), 23–29.

National League of Nursing Education. (1937). *A curriculum guide for schools of nursing.* New York: The League.

Nyswander, D. V. (1980). Public health education: Sources, growth and educational philosophy. *International Quarterly of Community Health Education, 1,* 5–18.

Oberst, M. T. (1989). Perspectives on research in patient teaching. *Nursing Clinics of North America, 24*(2), 621–627.

Orr, R. (1990). Illness as an educational opportunity. *Patient Education and Counseling, 15,* 47–48.

Pew Health Professions Commission. (1995). *Critical challenges: Revitalizing the health professions for the twenty-first century: The third report of the Pew Health Professions Commission.* San Francisco: University of California.

Pew Health Professions Commission. (1998). *Recreating health professional practice for a new century: The fourth report of the Pew Health Professions Commission, Center for the Health Professions.* San Francisco: University of California.

Pohl, M. L. (1965). Teaching activities of the nursing practitioner. *Nursing Research, 14*(1), 4–11.

Public Health Service. (1971). Public health then and now. *American Journal of Public Health, 61*(7), 1277–1279.

Rega, M. D. (1993). A model approach for patient education. *MEDSURG Nursing, 2*(6), 477–479, 495.

Reiser, S. J. (1978). *Medicine and the reign of technology.* Cambridge: Cambridge University Press.

Reising, D. L. (2007, February). Protecting yourself from malpractice claims. *American Nurse Today,* 39–44.

Rosen, G. (1977). *Preventive medicine in the United States, 1900–1995.* New York: Prodist.

Roter, D. L., Stashefsky-Margalit, R., & Rudd, R. (2001). Current perspectives on patient education in the U.S. *Patient Education and Counseling, 44,* 79–86.

Saad, L. (2008, November 24). Nurses shine, bankers slump in ethics ratings. Gallup Poll. Retrieved June 17, 2009, from http://www.gallup.com/poll/112264/Nurses-Shine-While-Bankers-Slump-Ethics-Ratings.aspx#

Starr, P. (1982). *The social transformation of medicine.* New York: Basic Books.

Stolberg, S. G. (2002, August 8). Patient deaths tied to lack of nurses. *New York Times.* Retrieved August 8, 2002, from http://www.nytimes.com/2002/08/08/health/08NURS.html?pagewanted=1

Sullivan, L. W., & Bristow, L. R. (2007, March 13). *Summary proceedings of the national leadership symposium on increasing diversity in the health professions.* Washington, DC: The Sullivan Alliance.

Trocino, L., Byers, J. F., & Peach, A. G. (1997). Nurses' attitudes toward patient and family education: Implications for clinical nurse specialists. *Clinical Nurse Specialist: A Journal for Advanced Nursing Practice, 11*(2), 77–84.

U.S. Department of Health and Human Services. (2000). *Healthy people 2010: Objectives for improving health* (Vol. II). Washington, DC: U.S. Government Printing Office.

U.S. Department of Health and Human Services, Office of Disease Prevention and Health Promotion. (2000). *Healthy People 2000.* Retrieved August 29, 2009, from http://odphp.osophs.dhhs.gov/pubs/hp2000/.

U.S. Department of Health and Human Services, Office of Disease Prevention and Health Promotion. (2010). *Healthy People 2010.* Retrieved August 28, 2009, from http://www.healthypeople.gov/

Veterans Administration. (1953). *Patient education and the hospital program* (TB 10–88). Washington, DC: Author.

Wagner, S. P., & Ash, K. L. (1998). Creating the teachable moment. *Journal of Nursing Education*, *37*(6), 278–280.

Weingarten, V. (1974). Report of the findings and recommendations of the president's committee on health education. *Health Education Monograph*, *1*, 11–19.

Weiss, B. D. (2003). *Health literacy: A manual for clinicians.* Chicago: American Medical Association and American Medical Association Foundation.

Zikmund-Fisher, B. J., Sarr, B., Fagerlin, S., & Ubel, P. A. (2006). A matter of perspective: Choosing for others differs from choosing for yourself in making treatment decisions. *Journal of General Internal Medicine*, *21*, 618–622.

Chapter 2

Ethical, Legal, and Economic Foundations of the Educational Process

M. Janice Nelson
Catherine V. Caldicott

CHAPTER HIGHLIGHTS

A Differentiated View of Ethics, Morality, and the Law

Evolution of Ethical and Legal Principles in Health Care

Application of Ethical Principles to Healthcare Education
- *Autonomy*
- *Veracity*
- *Confidentiality*
- *Nonmaleficence*
- *Beneficence*
- *Justice*

The Ethics of Education in Classroom and Practice Settings
- *The Student–Teacher Relationship*
- *The Client–Provider Relationship*

Legality in Healthcare Education and Information

Documentation

Economic Factors in Healthcare Education: Justice and Duty Revisited

Financial Terminology
- *Direct Costs*
- *Indirect Costs*

Cost Savings, Cost Benefit, and Cost Recovery

Program Planning and Implementation

Cost-Benefit Analysis and Cost-Effectiveness Analysis

State of the Evidence

KEY TERMS

- ❏ ethics
- ❏ practice acts
- ❏ code of ethics
- ❏ autonomy
- ❏ decision aids
- ❏ veracity
- ❏ confidentiality
- ❏ nonmaleficence
- ❏ negligence
- ❏ malpractice
- ❏ beneficence
- ❏ justice

❏ direct costs
❏ fixed costs
❏ variable costs
❏ indirect costs
❏ cost savings
❏ cost benefit

❏ cost recovery
❏ revenue generation
❏ cost-benefit analysis
❏ cost-benefit ratio
❏ cost-effectiveness analysis

OBJECTIVES

After completing this chapter, the reader will be able to

1. Identify major ethical principles related to education in health care.
2. Distinguish between ethical and legal dimensions of the healthcare delivery system with respect to patient and staff education.
3. Describe the importance of practice acts and codes of ethics on the conduct of health professionals.
4. Recognize the potential ethical consequences of power imbalances between the teacher and student or the health professional and patient in educational and practice settings.
5. Describe the legal and financial implications of documentation.
6. Delineate the ethical, legal, and economic importance of federal, state, and accrediting body regulations and standards in the delivery of healthcare services.
7. Differentiate among financial terms associated with the development, implementation, and evaluation of patient education programs.

Approximately 40 years ago, the field of modern Western bioethics arose in response to the increasing complexity of medical care and decision making. Novel challenges in health care continually stem from such influences as technological advances, changes in laws, and public awareness of scientific endeavors. The field of bioethics provides systematic theoretical and practical approaches for handling such complex issues and the dilemmas that ensue. As a result, programs of study for health professionals now provide formal ethics education, some by mandate. Healthcare providers who commit ethical infractions while in training or practice

may be referred for ethics remediation by their programs or specialty licensing boards—or risk professional sanctions.

In the popular media, bioethics translates into stem cell research, organ transplantation, genetic testing, and other sensational innovations. But every day, far from the spotlight, healthcare students and clinicians confront commonplace and vexing ethical dilemmas. Consider a patient who refuses a routine but life-saving blood transfusion. Should she be allowed to refuse, or should health professionals persuade her otherwise? Or when a medical imaging technologist wheels an obviously confused elderly patient into the fluoroscopy suite for a swallowing study, should she ask whether the patient had enough decisional capacity to consent to the procedure? Dilemmas also arise in educational contexts. Suppose a surgeon misleads a family that a surgical error was really a "complication." Should the cardiovascular perfusion student who observed the error speak up to a superior in the medical hierarchy? What about a physical therapy faculty member who habitually introduces a PT doctoral student to patients as "Dr." Smith, implying that Ms. Smith has completed her doctoral training? Should the PT student correct her faculty member and, if so, when, where, and how?

These scenarios describe not only medical problems, but moral problems. They arise so frequently that convening the ethics committee is impractical. Increasingly, health professionals and their students must be able to reason through both medical and ethical issues. However, knowledge of basic ethical principles and concepts does not always suffice. As the healthcare field has developed, so has a critical consciousness of individual rights stemming from both natural and constitutional law. Healthcare organizations are laden with laws and regulations ensuring clients' rights to a high-quality standard of care, to informed consent, and subsequently to self-determination. Further, in the interest of justice, it is worthwhile to acknowledge the relationship between costs to the healthcare facility and the provision of medical services. Consequently, it is crucial that the providers of care be equally proficient in educating both the public and health professions students—the practitioner educators of tomorrow.

This is an age of an enlightened public that is aware of and demands recognition of individual constitutional rights regarding freedom of choice and rights to self-determination. In fact, it may seem curious to some that federal and state governments, accrediting bodies, and professional organizations find it necessary to legislate, regulate,

or provide standards and guidelines to ensure the protection of human rights when it comes to matters of health care. The answer, of course, is that the federal government has abandoned its historical hands-off policy toward physicians and other health professionals in the wake of serious breaches of public confidence and shocking revelations of abuses of human rights in the name of biomedical research.

These issues of human rights are fundamental to the delivery of high-quality healthcare services. They are equally fundamental to the education process, in that the intent of the educator should be to empower the client to identify and articulate his or her values and preferences; acknowledge his or her role in a family, community, or other relationship; and to make well-informed choices, reasonably aware of the consequences of those choices. Thus, an explication of the role of the health professional in the teaching–learning process must include the ethical and legal foundations of that process. Teaching and learning principles, with their inherent legal and ethical dimensions, apply to any situation in which the educational process occurs.

The purpose of this chapter is to provide the ethical, legal, and economic foundations that underpin the patient education initiative, on the one hand, and the rights and responsibilities of the provider on the other. This chapter describes the differences between and among ethical, moral, and legal concepts. It explores the ethical and legal foundations of human rights, and it reviews the ethical and legal dimensions of health care. Furthermore, this chapter examines the importance of documentation of patient teaching while highlighting the economic factors that must be considered in the delivery of patient education in healthcare settings. An additional section provides a brief discussion of evidence-based practice and its relationship to quality and evaluation of patient education programs.

A Differentiated View of Ethics, Morality, and the Law

Although ethics as a branch of classical philosophy has been studied throughout the centuries, by and large these studies were left to the domains of philosophical and religious thinkers. More recently, because of the complexities of modern-day living and the heightened awareness of an educated public, ethical issues related to health care have surfaced as a major concern of both healthcare providers and recipients of these services. Thus, it is a widely held belief that the patient has the right to know his or her medical diagnosis, the treatments available, and the expected outcomes. This information is necessary so that patients can make informed choices relative to their respective diagnoses and treatments in concert with advice offered by health professionals.

Ethical principles that pertain to human rights are rooted in natural laws, which, in the absence of any other guidelines, are binding on human society. Inherent in these natural laws are, for example, the principles of respect for others, truth telling, honesty, and respect for life. Ethics as a discipline interprets these basic principles of behavior in broad terms that guide moral decision making in all realms of human activity (Tong, 2007).

Although multiple perspectives on the rightness or wrongness of human acts exist, among the most commonly referenced are the writings of the 16th-century German philosopher Immanuel Kant and those of the 19th-century English scholar and philosopher John Stuart Mill (Edward, 1967). Kant proposed that individual rights prevail and openly proclaimed the deontological notion of the "Golden Rule." Deontology (from the Greek word *deon*, which means duty) is the ethical belief system that stresses the importance of doing one's duty and following the rules. Thus, respect for individual rights is key, and one person should never be treated merely as a means to another person's benefit or a group's well-being (Tong, 2007). Mill, on the other hand, proposed the teleological notion or utilitarian approach to ethical decision making that allows for the sacrifice of one or more individuals so that a group of people can benefit in some important way. He believed that given the alternatives, choices should be made that result in the greatest good for the greatest number of people.

Likewise, the legal system and its laws are based on ethical and moral principles that, through experience and over time, society has accepted as behavioral norms (Hall, 1996; Lesnick & Anderson, 1962). In fact, the terms *ethical, moral,* and *legal* are often used in synchrony. It should be made clear, however, that although these terms are certainly interrelated, they are not necessarily synonymous.

Ethics refers to the guiding principles of behavior, and *ethical* refers to norms or standards of behavior. Although the terms *moral* and *morality* are generally used interchangeably with the terms *ethics* and *ethical*, health professionals can differentiate the notion of moral rights and duties from the notion of ethical rights and duties. *Moral* refers to an internal value system (the moral fabric of one's being) and this value system, defined as morality, is expressed externally through ethical behavior. Ethical principles deal with intangible moral values, so they are not enforceable by law, and neither are these principles laws in and of themselves. *Legal* rights and duties, on the other hand, refer to rules governing behavior or conduct that are enforceable under threat of punishment or penalty, such as a fine, imprisonment, or both.

The intricate relationship between ethics and the law explains why ethics terminology, such as informed consent, confidentiality, nonmaleficence, and justice, can be found within the language of the legal system. Health professionals may cite professional commitment or moral obligation to justify the education of clients as one dimension of their role. In reality, the legitimacy of this role may also stem from the practice acts that exist in the particular state where the health professional resides, is licensed, and is employed. **Practice acts** are documents that define a profession, describe that profession's scope of practice, and provide guidelines for state professional boards regarding entry into a profession via licensure and disciplinary actions that can be taken when necessary. Practice acts were developed to protect the public from unqualified practitioners and to protect the professional title (e.g., RN, OT, RT). A *model practice act* serves as a template for individual states to follow to minimize variability from state to state within a profession. From the model, a state or other jurisdiction can develop its own practice act that addresses its particular needs in addition to including the basic information regarding scope of practice, licensure requirements, and so forth (Flook, 2003). In essence, a professional practice act is not only legally binding, but it is also protected by the police authority of the state in the interest of protecting the public (Brent, 2001; Mikos, 2004). **Table 2–1** lists various health professions' ethics codes and practice acts.

Evolution of Ethical and Legal Principles in Health Care

In the past, ethics was relegated almost exclusively to the philosophical and religious domains. Likewise, from a historical vantage point, medical and nursing care was considered a humanitarian, if not charitable, endeavor. Often it was provided by members of religious communities and others considered to be generous of spirit, caring in nature, courageous, dedicated, and self-sacrificing in their service to others. Public sentiment was so strong in this regard that for many years healthcare organizations, which were considered to be charitable institutions, were largely immune from legal action "because it would compel the charity to divert its funds for a purpose never intended" (Lesnik & Anderson, 1962, p. 211). In the same manner, healthcare practitioners in the past—who were primarily physicians and nurses—were usually regarded as Good Samaritans who acted in good faith.

Although there are numerous court records of lawsuits involving hospitals, physicians, and nurses dating back to the early 1900s, those numbers pale in comparison with the volumes being generated on a daily basis in today's world (Reising & Allen, 2007). Further, despite the horror stories that have been handed down through the years regarding inhumane and often torturous treatment of prisoners, the mentally infirm, the disabled, and the poor, there was limited focus in the past on ethical aspects of that care. In turn, there was little thought of legal protection for the rights of such mentally, physically, or socioeconomically challenged people.

Clearly, this situation has changed dramatically. For example, informed consent—a basic tenet of the ethical practice of health care—was established in the courts as early as 1914 by Justice Benjamin Cardozo. Cardozo determined that every adult of sound mind has a right to protect his or her own body and to determine how it shall be treated (Hall, 1992; Schloendorff v. Society of New York Hospitals, 1914). Although the Cardozo decision was of considerable magnitude, governmental interest in the bioethical underpinnings of human rights in the delivery of healthcare services did not really surface until after World War II.

Over the years, legal authorities such as federal and state governments maintained a hands-off posture when it came to issues of biomedical research or physician–patient relationships. However, human atrocities committed by the Nazis in

Table 2–1 HEALTH PROFESSIONS CODES OF ETHICS AND PRACTICE ACTS

Codes of Ethics	Practice Acts
Cardiovascular perfusion http://abcp.org/code_of_ethics.htm	Practice acts for some states only
Cytotechnology and lab technology http://www.amt1.com/files/Standards%20of%20 Practice%20.pdf	Practice acts for some states only
Medical imaging http://www.medicalimaging.org/about/code.cfm	No practice act outside of medical practice act
Nursing http://nursingworld.org/ethics/code/protected_ nwcoe813.htm	Practice act by state: http://www.the-travel-nurse.com/nursepracticeacts.html
Nutrition http://www.iaacn.org/CCN%20Code%20of%20 Ethics%202005.pdf	Individual state practice acts and medical practice act
Occupational therapy http://www.aota.org/About/AboutOT/38527.aspx	Model practice act: http://www.aota.org/Practitioners/Advocacy/State/ Resources/PracticeAct/36445.aspx
Pharmacy http://www.pharmacist.com/AM/Template. cfm?Section=Search1&template=/CM/ HTMLDisplay.cfm&ContentID=2903	Model practice act: http://www.nabp.net/publications/assets/2009%20 Model%20Act.doc
Physical therapy http://www.ptboard.state.az.us/public/ptays/docs/ CodeofEthicsandGuide.pdf	Model Practice Act: https://www.fsbpt.org/RegulatoryTools/ ModelPracticeAct/index.asp
Radiation therapy https://www.asrt.org/content/RTs/CodeofEthics/ Therapy_CodeOfEthics.aspx	No practice act outside of medical practice act
Respiratory therapy http://www.aarc.org/resources/position_statements/ ethics.html	Model practice act: http://www.aarc.org/advocacy/state/licensure.html (only available to members)
Social work http://www.socialworkers.org/pubs/code/code.asp	Model practice act: http://www.aswb.org/pdfs/Model_law.pdf

the name of biomedical research during World War II shocked the world into critical awareness of gross violations of human rights. Unfortunately, such abuses were not confined to wartime Europe. On U.S. soil, for example, the nontreatment of syphilitic African Americans in Tuskegee, Ala-bama; the injection of live cancer cells into un-informed, nonconsenting older adults at the Brooklyn Chronic Disease Hospital; and the use of institutionalized mentally retarded children to study hepatitis at the Willowbrook State School on Staten Island, New York, shocked the nation and raised a public awareness of disturbing breaches in the physician–patient relationship (Brent, 2001; Centers for Disease Control and Prevention, 2005; Rivera, 1972; Thomas & Quinn, 1991; Weisbard & Arras, 1984).

Stirred to action by these disturbing phenomena, in 1974 Congress moved with all due deliberation to create the National Commission for the Protection of Human Subjects of Biomedical and Behavioral Research (U.S. Department of Health and Human Services [USDHHS], 1983). As an outcome of this unprecedented act, an institutional review board for the protection of human subjects (IRBPHS) was rapidly established at the local level by any hospital, academic medical center, agency, or organization where research on human subjects was being conducted. To this day, the primary function of these review boards is to safeguard all human study subjects by insisting that research protocols include voluntary participation and withdrawal, confidentiality, truth telling, and informed consent and address additional specific concerns for vulnerable populations such as infants, children, prisoners, and those with mental illnesses. Every proposal for biomedical research that involves human subjects must be submitted to a local IRBPHS for intensive review and approval before the proposed study proceeds (USDHHS, 1983). Further, in response to its concern about the range of ethical issues associated with medical practice and a perceived need to regulate biomedical research, Congress established in 1978 the President's Commission for the Study of Ethical Problems in Medicine and Biomedical and Behavioral Research (Brent, 2001; Thomas & Quinn, 1991; USDHHS, 1983).

In addition, in 1975, the American Hospital Association (AHA) followed suit by disseminating a document titled *A Patient's Bill of Rights*, which was revised in 1992 (Association of American Physicians and Surgeons, 1995). A copy of these patient rights is framed and posted in a public place in every healthcare facility across the United States. In addition, federal standards developed by the Center for Medicare and Medicaid Services (CMS)—an arm of the Health Care Financing Administration (HCFA)—require that the patient be provided with a personal copy of these rights either at the time of admission to the hospital or long-term care facility or prior to the initiation of care or treatment when admitted to a surgicenter, HMO, home care, or hospice. As a matter of fact, many states have adopted the statement of patient rights as part of their state health code. Thus, these rights fall under the jurisdiction of the law, rendering them legally enforceable by threat of penalty.

But did the professions themselves speak up in the face of the outrageous violations of human rights in the name of research? Indeed, two professional groups acted well before the 1970s to establish uniform standards for professional training and conduct. The first was the American Medical Association (AMA), which wrote and published its Code of Medical Ethics in 1847. Renamed *The Principles of Medical Ethics* in 1903, the code is currently in its fifth revision (AMA, 2001). All five versions address the precedence of patients' welfare and physicians' moral rectitude over scientific accomplishment and professional gain. Despite such regular attention to the values to which physicians commit themselves individually and collectively, the preceding historical examples attest to a disconnect between espoused values and actual practice, a failure of widespread individual and collective professional accountability.

In 1950, the American Nurses Association (ANA) developed and adopted an ethical code for professional practice that has since been revised and updated several times (ANA, 1976, 1985, 2001). The latest revision of the ANA's code, now titled the *Code of Ethics for Nurses With Interpretive Statements*, was released in 2001 for implementation in the new millennium. This **code of ethics** represents an articulation of professional values and moral obligations in relation to the nurse–patient relationship and in support of the profession and its mission. Although other health professions have adopted their own codes of ethics (as identified in Table 2–1), the nursing profession's code has been recognized as exemplary and has been used as a template by other health discipline organizations in the crafting of their own ethics documents.

Health professional organizations have accepted the responsibility for establishing standards of ethical behavior for members of their disciplines in the context of health care practice. In the end, however, it is up to the individual nurse, respiratory therapist, social worker, ultrasonographer, or other health professional to take his or her professional ethics code to heart. The following portion of this chapter addresses the application of ethical and legal principles and concepts by individual health professionals to their clients.

Application of Ethical Principles to Healthcare Education

Various theories and traditions can frame a health professional's understanding of the ethical dimensions in the healthcare setting. In considering the ethical and legal responsibilities inherent in the process of patient education, healthcare professionals and students can turn to a framework of six major ethical principles—including the so-called big four principles initially proposed by Beauchamp and Childress (1977)—that are intricately woven throughout the ANA's *Code of Ethics* (2001), the AHA's *A Patient's Bill of Rights* (1992), and similar documents promulgated by other healthcare organizations as well as the federal government. These principles, which encompass the very issues that precipitated federal intervention into healthcare affairs, are autonomy, veracity, confidentiality, nonmaleficence, beneficence, and justice.

Autonomy

The term **autonomy** is derived from the Greek words *auto* (self) and *nomos* (law) and refers to the right of self-determination (Tong, 2007). Laws have been enacted to protect the patient's right to make choices independently. Federal mandates, such as informed consent, must be evident in every application for federal funding to support biomedical research. The local IRBPHS assumes the role of judge and jury to ascertain adherence to this enforceable regulation (Dickey, 2006).

The Patient Self-Determination Act (PSDA), which was passed by Congress in 1991 (Ulrich, 1999), is a clear example of the principle of autonomy enacted into law. Any healthcare facility, such as acute- and long-term care institutions, surgicenters, HMOs, hospices, or home care, that receives Medicare and/or Medicaid funds must comply with the PSDA. The law requires, either at the time of hospital admission or prior to the initiation of care or treatment in a community health setting, "that every individual receiving health care be informed in writing of the right under state law to make decisions about his or her health care, including the right to refuse medical and surgical care and the right to initiate advance directives" (Mezey, Evans, Golob, Murphy, & White, 1994, p. 30). Although ultimate responsibility for discussing treatment options and a plan of care and obtaining informed consent rests with the physician, these authors readily acknowledge the nurse's responsibility to ensure informed decision making by patients, which includes but is certainly not limited to advance directives (e.g., living wills, durable power of attorney for health care, and designation of a healthcare agent). Evidence of such instruction must appear in the patient's record, which is the legal document validating that informed consent took place.

One principle worth noting in the ANA's *Code of Ethics* is that which addresses collaboration "with members of the health professions and other citizens in promoting community and national efforts to meet the health needs of the public" (New York State Nurses Association, 2001, p. 6). Similarly, the American Physical Therapy Association's *Code of Ethics* states in Principle 8, "A physical therapist shall provide and make available accurate and relevant information to patients/clients about their care and to the public about physical therapy services" (Federation of State Boards of Physical Therapy, 2006). These principles provide justification for patient education both within and outside the healthcare organization. Although health education, per se, is not an interpretive part of the principle of autonomy, it certainly lends credence to the ethical notion of assisting the public to attain greater autonomy when it comes to matters of health promotion and high-level wellness. In fact, the practice acts for nursing, occupational therapy, physical therapy, and respiratory care list patient education as within their scopes of practice. Even though other healthcare-related practice acts are not explicit on this point, many health professionals consider patient education a means of demonstrating their commitment to patient welfare, trustworthiness, and informed decision making.

An additional moral framework through which to view the practice of patient education is a framework of expansion of patient capabilities (Redman, 2008). The reason to view expansion of capabilities as a moral enterprise is that capabilities of, say, healthfulness, self-care, engaging in life, relationships, and pursuits, "have value in themselves and are of special importance in making possible any choice of a way of life" (p. 815).

Another example of autonomy is the development and use of patient decision aid interventions designed to assist clients to make informed treatment choices (Bekker, 2010). These patient **decision aids**, which include printed materials, videos, and interactive Web-based tutorials, provide clients with information about specific health issues, particular diagnoses, treatment risks and benefits, and questionnaires to determine whether clients need more information. "The emphasis on collaboration between providers and patients on decision making has, in turn, stimulated the development of tools to help patients and their families participate in clinical discussions and reach decisions that incorporate personal values and goals" (Wittmann-Price & Fisher, 2009).

Veracity

Veracity, or truth telling, is closely linked to informed decision making and informed consent. The early-20th-century landmark decision by Justice Benjamin Cardozo (Schloendorff v. Society of New York Hospitals, 1914) specifies an individual's fundamental right to make decisions about his or her own body. This ruling provides a basis in law for patient education or instruction regarding invasive medical procedures. Nurses are often confronted with issues of truth telling, as was exemplified in the *Tuma* case (Rankin & Stallings, 1990). In the interest of full disclosure of information, the nurse (Tuma) had advised a cancer patient of alternative treatments without consultation with the client's physician. Tuma was sued by the physician for interfering with the medical regimen that he had prescribed for care of this particular patient. Although Tuma was eventually exonerated from professional misconduct charges, the case emphasizes a significant point of law to be found in the New York State Nurse Practice Act (New York State Nurses Association, 1972), which states, "A nursing regimen shall be consistent with and shall not vary from any existing medical regimen." However, others insist that failure to instruct the patient properly relative to invasive procedures is tantamount to battery (Creighton, 1986). Therefore, in some instances, the health professional may find himself or herself in a double bind. If in such a dilemma, the health professional has a variety of actions available. Two possibilities would be to inform the physician of the professional double bind and engage with him or her in achieving a course of action that best meets the patient's medical needs while respecting the patient's autonomy; and to seek out the institutional ethics committee or an ethics consultant for assistance in negotiating interactions with both the physician and the patient.

Cisar and Bell (1995) address this concept of battery related to medical treatment and offer the following explanation of the four elements making up the notion of informed consent that are such vital aspects of patient education:

1. *Competence*, which refers to the capacity of the patient to make a reasonable decision.
2. *Disclosure of information*, which requires that sufficient information regarding risks and alternative treatments—including no treatment at all—be provided to the patient to enable him or her to make a rational decision.
3. *Comprehension*, which speaks to the individual's ability to understand or to grasp intellectually the information being provided. A child, for example, may not yet be of an age to understand any ramifications of medical treatment and must, therefore, depend on his or her parents to make a decision that will be in the child's best interest. Similarly, for an adequate informed consent conversation, all options must be expressed in a language the patient can understand and in lay terms.
4. *Voluntariness*, which indicates that the patient has made a decision without coercion or force from others.

Although all four of these elements might be satisfied, the patient might still choose to reject the regimen of care suggested by healthcare providers. This decision could be the result of the exorbitant cost of a treatment or certain personal or religious beliefs. Whatever the case, it must be recognized by all concerned that a competent, informed client cannot be forced to accept treatment as long as he or she is aware of the alternatives as well as the consequences of any decision (Cisar & Bell, 1995).

Finally, a dimension of the legality of truth telling relates to the role of the health professional as expert witness. Health professionals who are recognized for their skill or expertise in a particular area of practice may be called on to testify in court on behalf of either the plaintiff (the one who initiates the litigation) or the defendant (the one being sued). In any case, the concept of expert testimony speaks for itself. Regardless of the situation, the health professional must always tell the truth and the patient (or his or her healthcare agent) is always entitled to the truth (Hall, 1996).

Confidentiality

Confidentiality refers to personal information that is entrusted and protected as privileged information via a social contract, healthcare standard or code, or legal covenant. When acquired in a professional capacity from a patient, healthcare providers may not disclose such information without consent of that patient. If sensitive information were not to be protected, patients would lose trust in their providers and would be reluctant to openly share problems with them or even seek medical care at all.

A distinction must be made between the terms *anonymous* and *confidential*. Information is anonymous, for example, when researchers are unable to link any subject's identity in the medical record of that person. Information is confidential when identifying materials appear on subjects' records but can be accessed only by the researchers (Tong, 2007).

Only under special circumstances may secrecy be ethically broken, such as when a patient has been the victim or subject of a crime to which the health professional is a witness (Lesnick & Anderson, 1962). Other exceptions to confidentiality occur when health professionals suspect or are aware of child or elder abuse, narcotic use, legally reportable communicable diseases, gunshot or knife wounds, or the threat of violence toward someone. To protect others from bodily harm, health professionals are legally permitted to breach confidentiality.

In the case of communicable diseases, patients should not be forced or coerced to name their contacts, again because respecting confidentiality maintains trust between the patient and health professional. But is it fair to deprive a vulnerable spouse or contact of this important health information? Is it morally acceptable to put one person's rights above those of another? In some situations, yes, although these decisions are best considered after much deliberation with the patient and other trusted health professionals. Of course, if a patient discloses the identity of his or her contacts, health professionals are mandated to inform them in accordance with applicable state laws. But if a patient tests positive for HIV/AIDS, for example, and has no intention of telling his or her spouse about this diagnosis, the physician has an obligation to warn the spouse directly or indirectly (i.e., through anonymous lab reporting) of the risk of potential harm (Tong, 2007). Adequate deliberation with the patient and others can reveal circumstances in which the reality is even more complex. For example, if the physician or other primary healthcare provider explores the patient's rationale for not wanting to inform his or her spouse of the infectious disease status, it may be out of fear of inciting domestic violence. According to Brent (2001), "this area of legislation concerned with health care privacy and disclosure reveals the tension between what is good for the individual vis-à-vis what is good for society" (p. 141).

The 2003 updated Health Insurance Portability and Accountability Act (HIPAA) ensures nearly absolute confidentiality related to dissemination of client information, unless the client himself or herself authorizes release of such information (Kohlenberg, 2006). One goal of the HIPAA policy, first enacted by Congress in 1996, is to limit disclosure of patient healthcare information to third parties, such as insurance companies or employers. This law, which requires patients' prior written consent for release of their health information, was never meant to interfere with consultation between professionals, but is intended to prevent, for example, elevator conversations about private matters of individuals entrusted to the care of health professionals. In a technologically advanced society such as exists in the United States today, this law is a must to ensure confidentiality (Tong, 2007). Currently, in some states and under certain conditions, such as death or impending death, a spouse or members of the immediate family can be apprised of the patient's condition if this information was previously unknown to them. Despite federal and state legislation protecting the confidentiality rights of individuals, the issue of the ethical/moral obligation of the patient with HIV/AIDS or genetic disease, for example, to voluntarily divulge his or her condition to others who may be at risk remains largely unresolved (Legal Action Center, 2001).

Nonmaleficence

Nonmaleficence means "do no harm" and constitutes the ethical fabric of legal determinations encompassing negligence and/or malpractice. According to Brent (2001), **negligence** is defined as "conduct which falls below the standard established by law for the protection of others against unreasonable risk of harm" (p. 54). She further asserts that the concept of professional negligence "involves the conduct of professionals (e.g., nurses, physicians, dentists, and lawyers) that fall [*sic*] below a professional standard of due care" (p. 55). As clarified by Tong (2007), due care is "the kind of care healthcare professionals give patients when they treat them attentively and vigilantly so as to avoid mistakes" (p. 25). For negligence to exist, there must be a duty between the injured party and the person whose actions (or nonactions) caused the injury. A breach of that duty must have occurred, it must have been the immediate cause of the injury, and the injured party must have experienced damages from the injury (Brent, 2001).

The term **malpractice**, by comparison, still holds as defined by Lesnick and Anderson in 1962. Malpractice, these authors assert, "refers to a limited class of negligent activities committed within the scope of performance by those pursuing a particular profession involving highly skilled and technical services" (p. 234). More recently, malpractice has been specifically defined as "negligence, misconduct, or breach of duty by a professional person that results in injury or damage to a patient" (Reising & Allen, 2007). Thus, malpractice, per se, is limited in scope to those whose life work requires special education and training as dictated by specific educational standards. In contrast, negligence embraces all improper and wrongful conduct by anyone arising out of any activity. Reising and Allen (2007) describe the most common causes for malpractice claims specifically against nurses, but these causes are also relevant to the conduct of other health professionals within the scope of their practice responsibilities:

1. Failure to follow standards of care
2. Failure to use equipment in a responsible manner
3. Failure to communicate
4. Failure to document
5. Failure to assess and monitor
6. Failure to act as patient advocate
7. Failure to delegate tasks properly

The concept of duty is closely tied to the concepts of negligence and malpractice. Health professionals' duties are spelled out in job descriptions at their places of employment. Policy and procedure manuals of a particular facility exist certainly to protect the patient and ensure good quality care, but they also exist to protect the employee and the employer against litigation. Policies are more than

guidelines. Policies and procedures determine standards of behavior (duties) expected of employees of a particular institution and can be used in a court of law in the determination of negligence.

Health professionals' moral duties are the things that they ought to do or the way they ought to behave in a healthcare situation with ethical import. So, for example, imagine a laboratory technician notices a blood specimen labeled with a neighbor's name and birth date. The technician's duty is to respect or maintain patient confidentiality no matter how much he or she might want to look up the results of the tests (if a different technician ran them) or share the results with others. Even if the technician ran the test and is therefore privy to the results, and chooses to share the results only with the patient, the technician violates the standard practice regarding who has the right and responsibility to inform the patient of test results. In either case, the lab technician breaks confidentiality, violates his or her duty to maintain patient privacy, oversteps his or her professional role, and potentially erodes trust in the medical profession.

Expectations of healthcare providers' performance are also measured against each professional's level of education and concomitant skills, standing orders of the physician, institution-specific protocols, standards of care upheld by the profession, and standards of care adhered to by any subspecialty organizations of which the health professional may be a member. If, for example, a nurse is certified in a clinical specialty or is identified as a "specialist" although not certified, he or she will be held to the standards of that specialty (Yoder Wise, 1995).

In the instance of litigation, the key operational principle is that the health professional is not measured against the optimal or maximum of professional standards of performance; rather, the yardstick is laid against the prevailing practice of what a prudent and reasonable professional in that healthcare field would do under the same circumstances in a given community. Thus, a health professional's duty of patient education (or lack thereof) is measured against not only the prevailing policy of the employing institution, but also against prevailing practice in the community. For example, the social worker's, nutritionist's, or pharmacist's practice is measured against institutional policies for this level of worker as well as against the prevailing practice of these professionals performing at the same level in the community or in the same geographic region.

Beneficence

Beneficence is defined as "doing good" for the benefit of others. It is a concept that is legalized through adherence to critical tasks and duties contained in job descriptions; in policies, procedures, and protocols set forth by the healthcare facility; and in standards and codes of ethical behaviors established by health professional organizations. Adherence to these various professional performance criteria and principles, including adequate and current patient education, speaks to the health professional's commitment to acting in the best interest of the patient. Sometimes health professionals, such as radiation therapists and mammographers, are called upon to treat patients in ways that cause physical discomfort or harm. Although difficult, these professionals do their jobs because the patients believe that the treatments will, on balance, benefit them.

Unlike principles such as autonomy and veracity that are most directly applicable to health professionals who interact with patients, beneficence applies to the work of the full range of healthcare providers. Maintaining technical competence; attending to quality checks; being punctual, prepared, and attentive; and holding self and peers accountable to performance standards all demonstrate a commitment to benefiting the patient.

But in the clinical realm, a health professional's demonstration of beneficence is not always as simple as adherence to tasks, duties, and practice guidelines. Patients may not desire the recommended therapy or may introduce other considerations that make it difficult to follow protocols. The relationship between a health professional and a patient is described as *fiduciary*—characterized by trust. The client trusts that the health professional will act in the client's best interest and, if necessary, will subordinate self-interest. Should the X-ray technician go on a scheduled break when a backlog of patients waits to have their films taken? The X-ray technician may be tired or hungry, but patients' best interests nearly always trump the interests of others. If the technician is so overdue for a break that hunger or fatigue impair his or her ability to function competently, then of course patients' interests are better served if the technician goes on break. Patients trust that the healthcare provider will balance potential harms against benefits to make a decision about how to act ultimately in the patient's best interest.

But is it morally acceptable—or even expected—that health professionals put client benefit ahead of their own well-being? The effort to save lives and relieve human suffering is a duty to do good only within reasonable limits. For example, when AIDS first appeared, the cause and control of this fatal disease were unknown. Some health professionals protested that the duty of beneficence did not include caring for patients who put them at risk for this deadly, infectious, and untreatable disease. Others maintained that part of the decision to become a health professional involves the acceptance of certain personal risks: It is part of the job. Nevertheless, once it became clear that HIV transmission through occupational exposure was quite small, the majority of healthcare practitioners concurred with the opinion of the American Medical Association that they "may not ethically refuse to treat a patient whose condition is within [their] current realm of competence solely because the patient is seropositive" (Tong, 2007).

Justice

Justice speaks to fairness and the equitable distribution of goods and services. The law is the justice system. The focus of the law is the protection of society; the focus of health law is the protection of the consumer. It is unjust to treat a person better or worse than another person in a similar condition or circumstance, unless a difference in treatment can be justified with good reason. In today's healthcare climate, professionals must be as objective as possible in allocating scarce medical resources in a just manner. Decision making for the fair distribution of resources includes the following criteria as defined by Tong (2007):

1. To each, an equal share
2. To each, according to need
3. To each, according to effort
4. To each, according to contribution
5. To each, according to merit
6. To each, according to the ability to pay (p. 30)

According to Tong (2007), health professionals may have second thoughts about the application of these criteria in particular circumstances because one or more of the criteria could be at odds with the concept of justice. "To allocate scarce resources to patients on the basis of their social worth, moral goodness, or economic condition rather than on the basis of their medical condition is more often than not wrong" (p. 30).

As noted earlier, adherence to *A Patient's Bill of Rights* is legally enforced in most states. This means that any health professional can be subjected to penalty or to litigation for discrimination in provision of care. Regardless of his or her age, gender, physical disability, sexual orientation, or race, for example, the client has a right to proper instruction regarding risks and benefits of invasive medical procedures. She or he also has a right to proper instruction regarding self-care activities, such as home dialysis, for example, that are beyond normal activities of daily living for most people.

Furthermore, when a health professional is employed by a particular healthcare facility, she or he enters into a contract, written or tacit, to provide services in accordance with the policies of the facility. Failure to provide health care (including educational services) based on patient diagnosis or persistence in providing substandard care based on client age, diagnosis, culture, national origin, sexual preference, and the like can result in liability for breach of contract with the employing institution.

In 1986, it became illegal for virtually every U.S. hospital to deny emergency evaluation and treatment to patients solely based on their ability to pay. Called the Emergency Medical Treatment and Active Labor Act (EMTALA), this federal legislation prohibits hospitals from rejecting or "dumping" uninsured patients or those covered by Medicare or Medicaid on "charity" or county hospitals (Consolidated Omnibus Budget Reconciliation Act of 1985). In other words, all patients who present with an emergency medical condition (or in active labor) must be treated in the same way, regardless of insurance status.

But uninsured and Medicare and Medicaid patients are still subject to other, more subtle discrimination. Because many outpatient facilities do not accept these patients, this restriction on their right of access to health care extends to their right to access health education. Emanuel (2000) raises a critical point in asserting that "the diffuseness of decision making in the American health care system precludes a coherent process for allocating health care resources" (p. 8). Emanuel further contends that managed care organizations have systematically pursued drastic cost reductions by restructuring delivery systems and investing in expensive and elaborate information systems. HMOs have bought out physician practices and have become involved in a number of related activities with no substantial evidence that a high quality of health care will be achieved at lower prices.

These issues determine whether health educators can surmount the obstacles potentially blocking the patient education process. In the interest of cutting costs, HMOs have also succeeded in shortening lengths of hospital stays. This development, in turn, has had a tremendous effect on the delivery of education to the hospitalized patient and presents serious obstacles to the implementation of this mandate. Lack of time serves as a major barrier to the nurse's or other health professional's ability to give discharge instructions that contain sufficient information for self-care. Also, illness acuity level interferes with the patient's ability to process information necessary to meet his or her physical and emotional needs.

Nurses and occupational, physical, and respiratory therapists are mandated by organizational policy as well as by federal and state regulations (for example, practice acts) to provide client education. Thus, great care must be taken to ensure that the education justly due to the patient will be addressed post discharge, either in the ambulatory care setting, at home, or in the physician's office.

The Ethics of Education in Classroom and Practice Settings

The Student–Teacher Relationship

Many of the foundational principles and concepts of ethics that apply to client care also apply to questions of what ought to be done or how health professionals ought to behave in the education of students for the health professions. Students and teachers have their own perspectives, visions, values, and preferences that are unknown to each other. These two worldviews come together in the classroom. They must be negotiated and understood by each party for the process of education and training to proceed with trust and respect (Freedman, 2003).

A balance of power exists between the teacher (expert) and student (novice). The teacher possesses discipline-specific expertise, which is key to the student's academic success, career achievement, and competent care of patients. Students must be able to trust their teachers—even instantaneously—that the instruction will be accurate, appropriate, and up-to-date. Students have a right to assume their instructors are competent and employ that competence in the best interests of the students and the particular health profession.

Another area of ethical import inherent in student–teacher relationships is the potential blurring of professional-personal boundaries. Students experience personal difficulties that can interfere with their studies or with their goals in pursuing a degree in the health professions. If the nature of the student's concerns is outside pedagogic goals, how should the teacher respond? In such a case, the ethics of the situation applies not to the process of education itself but to two individuals who happen to know each other because of an educational context. This distinction is important. Whereas sometimes teachers are called upon to serve as advisors for students, typically the advice pertains to professional training matters. However, a teacher may be approached because he or she is known to the student and is trustworthy in a classroom context, but the issue at hand requires counseling of a noneducational nature. In such a case, the teacher is expected to address openly and honestly with the student the potential consequences to their student–teacher relationship of discussing personal issues (Ewashen & Lane, 2007).

Educators can use the following specific criteria to distinguish between interactions that are appropriate in the context of the educational process and those that are less appropriate or even frankly inappropriate (Martinez, 2000):

- Risk of harm to the student or to the student–teacher relationship
- Presence of coercion or exploitation

- Potential benefit to the student or to the student–teacher relationship
- Balance of student's interests and teacher's interests
- Presence of professional ideals

These five criteria can assist the teacher in being fully honest with him- or herself regarding the appropriateness of counseling the student and can serve as an extremely useful guide in uncertain situations.

Students are autonomous agents. If they choose to follow the prescribed course of study and are successful, they will develop professional autonomy, attain their professional goals, achieve professional competence, and be equipped to develop relationships with colleagues and patients. Students in disciplines such as cytotechnology or laboratory technology, who do not have direct patient care responsibilities but who will spend their careers in a laboratory, also have a fiduciary relationship to the patients whose diagnoses, treatments, and future lives depend on the accurate examination of tissues and other specimens.

Students are responsible for speaking up when they experience problems with or obstacles to their learning. Otherwise their teachers may make overly ambitious demands on and expectations for students in the learning process. Just as students have a right to expect honesty from their teachers, they have a reciprocal duty to be truthful as well—such as when they have not done an assignment or prepared for a class activity, or have made a mistake. In addition, truthfulness affects a vulnerable third party: the patient whose care is at the hands of the student. Taking responsibility for one's missteps as a student reveals the student's commitment to honesty, the primacy of patient welfare, and trustworthiness (Reiser, 1994).

Sometimes students in the health professions also decide to shield their instructors from the complexities of their patients' situations. Perhaps students want to help their patients appear as "good" as possible. Or, perhaps motivated by a desire to get a good evaluation themselves and avoid descriptors such as "difficult," "took up too much time with details," or "not a team player," students may select what they believe their instructors will want to deal with. One student who was following a postsurgical patient remarked, "[I]n bringing up my patient's [sore] throat, I was also wasting precious time . . . , and so I learned to keep quiet about his complaints" (Zucker, 2009). By acting in this way, students place their *perceptions* of their instructors' needs before the needs of their patients, at a time when the students are trying to learn exactly which bona fide medical needs should legitimately assume priority over others. Who else but instructors can most effectively assist students to learn how to prioritize among competing patient concerns? Yet how can instructors perform this important component of their jobs if they are hearing a censored rendition of those concerns?

By trying to appear "good" and restrict the range and depth of concerns patients bring to their health professionals, students may undermine the reciprocity of the healthcare provider–patient relationship. Without an explicitly bidirectional education model, patients may be reluctant to voice all their concerns, reservations, and questions about a proposed recommendation or treatment.

In addition, consider the ethical import of the transience of many student–teacher relationships (Christakis & Feudtner, 1997). The systems of health professions education create communities of relative strangers. For example, a respiratory therapy student may conflate trust with authority when a visiting professor teaches a core course in the curriculum. Although the visiting professor may be a renowned authority on lung mechanics, she may be authoritarian in the classroom, a poor exemplar of putting the student's educational needs foremost. The student may deferentially endure the class, knowing that sooner or later it will end and the professor will return to her home institution. The poor learning climate discourages any reciprocity of concern or trust, impedes the student's professional development, and deprives the professor of valuable opportunities to demonstrate humility before the students.

Students rely on their teachers to be role models and mentors. They observe how teachers hold themselves and other instructors accountable to honest and conscientious practice standards. They witness how teachers treat students and colleagues. Such teacher behaviors exemplify instruction in a relational context: Technical information is interwoven with role modeling. From these observations, students receive lessons that assist them in developing and establishing habits of interaction with coworkers, patients, and, if they become educators themselves, their own future students (Reiser, 1993).

The Client–Provider Relationship

Health professionals (and health professions students) and the clients they care for also have their own worldviews that come together in the practice setting. These perspectives must be negotiated and understood by each party for the process of patient education to occur with a sense of trust. Many types of health professionals have limited or no direct patient contact that would involve patient education, such as cardiovascular perfusion, laboratory, and medical imaging technologists. Nevertheless, the following discussion may be helpful to them as they reflect on their attitudes regarding patient responsibilities for self-care, disease prevention, and adhering to medical recommendations (i.e., compliance).

As with the student–teacher relationship, it is important to recognize the balance of power that exists between a health professional—and even a health professions student—and a patient. The health professional possesses medical expertise—keys to the patient's health, well-being, and ability to work, play, go to school, or engage in social relationships. For those reasons, the ethics of being a patient typically includes respecting health professionals and trusting them to have the patient's best interests at heart. Patients have a moral claim on the health professional's competence and on the use of that competence for the patient's welfare (Pellegrino, 1993).

The blurring of professional-personal boundaries is also an area of ethical import common to health professional (or health professions student)–patient relationships. The potential for blurred boundaries between professionals and clients is particularly evident because of the intimacies of the practice setting. Patient education can take place when patients are wearing little clothing, are lying down in a bed, are sharing personal information with the health professional, or are in the context of medically related physical contact. Again, the five criteria noted earlier in the students and teachers section (Martinez, 2000) are relevant. Simply substitute the word *patient* or *client* for *student* to see how these criteria can assist in distinguishing between interactions that are acceptable in the context of the practice setting and those that are less acceptable or even frankly unacceptable. Health professionals are obligated to remain mindful of the power imbalance between them and patients, to put the patient's welfare before their own concerns, and to reflect honestly on the consequences of blurred boundaries to the patient and to their relationship with the patient in the practice setting.

Out of a respect for patient autonomy, a model of medical decision making shared between health professional and patient has assumed primacy in various health communication curricula and practices (deBocanegra & Gany, 2004; Donetto, 2010; Visser, 1998). This model supports imparting health-related information selected by the health professional to the patient for the purposes of the patient making his or her choices and preferences known. Health professionals engaging in this process may be well-meaning. Nevertheless, the unidirectional nature of this model of patient education succeeds in reinforcing the power that health professionals have over patients by virtue of their technical knowledge.

Health professions students may be particularly inclined to rely on a largely information-dissemination method of educating patients. This is understandable during the formative years of their training when they are beginning to appreciate and employ their own technical knowledge. Inevitably, such a reductionistic conception of patient education will bump up against real practice situations in which the complexity of individual patients' circumstances will demand a more reciprocal model of education (Donetto, 2010).

Similar to students, patients are autonomous agents. They may choose to follow the recommended course of treatment because they trust their health professional and believe that what has been recommended will improve their condition. They may also follow recommendations because they understand the rationale for the treatment, they consider the treatment is acceptable or at least tolerable, the treatment fits into their lifestyle and worldview, they can afford it financially, and for many other reasons.

Furthermore, some patients believe that they should behave like "good" patients by taking all medications or doing all exercises as prescribed, adhering to a recommended diet, not complaining, and so forth, so that their health professional will like them, consider them worthy of their time, and want to continue to take care of them (Buckwalter, 2007; Freedman, 2003). This desire to be a "good" patient underscores how dependent and vulnerable patients can feel. Even when presenting for a screening mammogram or follow-up urine culture, patients are not at their best. At every medical encounter there exists the potential for discovering something that merits concern.

In the practice setting, it is plausible that a nurse providing discharge instructions to a patient may not necessarily give the patient a fair share of his or her time or be open to all the patient's questions if the nurse knows he or she will never see that patient again. Admittedly, the better the patient education, the longer he or she likely will remain out of the hospital. However, if the nurse is extremely busy with other competing priorities or is tired from having worked two shifts in a row, he or she may not reflect on how fatigue or work demands precipitate a failure to focus primarily on this particular patient's welfare. It may be easier for the nurse to assume a "let someone else deal with it" attitude. Similarly, a laboratory technician providing instructions to a patient about doing a 24-hour urine collection or an oral glucose tolerance test may not be inclined to hold himself or herself accountable to give the instructions clearly and carefully to someone he or she may never encounter again. Transient relationships facilitate a lack of focus on the welfare, time, and interests of each patient.

Legality in Healthcare Education and Information

The patient's right to adequate information regarding his or her physical condition, medications, risks, and access to information regarding alternative treatments is specifically spelled out in various renditions of *A Patient's Bill of Rights* (AHA, 1992; ANA, 2001; Association of American Physicians and Surgeons, 1995; President's Advisory Commission, 1998). As noted earlier, many states have adopted these rights as part of their health code, thus rendering them legal and enforceable by law. Patients' rights to education and information are also regulated through standards promulgated by accrediting bodies such as the Joint Commission (JC), formerly known as the Joint Commission on Accreditation of Healthcare Organizations (JCAHO). Although these standards are not enforceable in the same manner as law, lack of organizational conformity can lead to loss of accreditation, which in turn jeopardizes the facility's eligibility for third-party reimbursement, as well as loss of Medicare and Medicaid reimbursement. Lack of organizational conformity can also lead to loss of public confidence.

In addition, state regulations pertaining to patient education are published and enforced under threat of penalty (fine, citation, or both) by the department of health in many states. Federal regulations, enforceable as laws, also mandate patient education in those healthcare facilities receiving Medicare and Medicaid funding. And, as discussed earlier, the federal government also mandates full patient disclosure in cases of participation in biomedical research in any setting or for any federally funded project or experimental research involving human subjects.

It should be noted that the AHA's 1975 original draft rendition of *A Patient's Bill of Rights*, along with all the later renditions of these rights, is linked to or associated with every ethical principle. *A Patient's Bill of Rights* (AHA, 1992) is rooted in the conditions of participation in Medicare set forth under federal standards established by the Centers for Medicare and Medicaid Services (CMS). Corresponding accreditation standards promulgated by the JC further emphasize these standards. All these laws and professional standards serve to ensure the fundamental rights of every person as a consumer of healthcare services. **Table 2–2** is a visual representation of the relationship of ethical principles to the laws and professional standards applicable to each principle.

Federal authorities have generally tended to hold physicians responsible and accountable for proper patient education. However, often the nurse or some other physician-appointed designee carries out patient education. Physicians' responsibility notwithstanding, "patient education is central to the culture of nursing as well as to its legal practice" (Redman, 2008) by virtue of respective state nurse practice acts. The same can be said for the practice acts governing occupational, physical, and respiratory therapists, for example.

Documentation

The 89th Congress enacted the Comprehensive Health Planning Act in 1965, Public Law 89-97, 1965 (Boyd, Gleit, Graham, & Whitman, 1998). The entitlements of Medicare and Medicaid—which revolutionized the provision of health care for older adults and people who are socioeconomically deprived—were established through this act. One acknowledgment in the act was the importance of the preventive and rehabilitative dimensions of health care. Thus, to qualify for Medicare and Medicaid reimbursement, "a hospital has to show evidence that patient education has been a part of patient care" (Boyd et al., 1998, p. 26). Proper documentation provides written testimony that patient education has indeed occurred. For at least the past 20 years, the JC has reinforced the federal mandate by requiring documentation of patient and/or family education in the patient record.

Casey (1995) points out that of all lapses in documentation, patient teaching has been identified as "probably the most undocumented skilled service because nurses do not recognize the scope and depth of the teaching they do" (p. 257). Lack of documentation also reflects negligence in adhering to the mandates of the professional practice acts. This laxity is unfortunate because patient records can be subpoenaed for court evidence. Appropriate documentation can be the determining factor in the outcome of litigation. Pure and simple, if the instruction isn't documented, it didn't occur!

Furthermore, documentation is a vehicle of communication that provides critical information to other health professionals involved with the patient's care. Failure to document not only renders other staff potentially liable, but also renders the facility liable and in jeopardy of losing its JC accreditation. Concomitantly, the institution is also in danger of losing its appropriations for Medicare and Medicaid reimbursement. Thus, it behooves the health professional who provides pa-

Table 2–2 LINKAGES BETWEEN ETHICAL PRINCIPLES AND THE LAW

Ethical Principles	Legal Actions/Decisions and Standards of Practice
Autonomy (self-determination)	Cardozo decision regarding informed consent
	Institutional review boards
	Patient Self-Determination Act
	A Patient's Bill of Rights
	Joint Commission standards
	Centers for Medicare and Medicaid Services standards
Veracity (truth telling)	Cardozo decision regarding informed consent
	A Patient's Bill of Rights
	Health profession practice acts
	Tuma decision
	Joint Commission standards
	Centers for Medicare and Medicaid Services standards
Confidentiality (privileged information)	*A Patient's Bill of Rights*
	Health profession practice acts
	Joint Commission standards
	Centers for Medicare and Medicaid Services standards
	Health Insurance Portability and Accountability Act (HIPAA)
	State public health laws regarding reporting of communicable diseases and duty to warn
Nonmaleficence (do no harm)	Health profession practice acts
	Malpractice/negligence
	A Patient's Bill of Rights
	State health codes
	Joint Commission standards
	Centers for Medicare and Medicaid Services standards
Beneficence (do good)	*A Patient's Bill of Rights*
	State health codes
	Job descriptions
	Professional standards of practice
	Institutional policies and procedures
	Joint Commission standards
	Centers for Medicare and Medicaid Services standards
Justice (equitable distribution of benefits and burdens)	*A Patient's Bill of Rights*
	Antidiscrimination/affirmative action laws
	Americans with Disabilities Act
	Joint Commission standards
	Centers for Medicare and Medicaid Services standards

tient education to document it appropriately and be critically conscious of the legal and financial ramifications to the healthcare facility in which he or she is employed.

Snyder (1996) presents an invaluable description of an interdisciplinary method to document patient education. The method involves use of a flow sheet that fits into the client's chart. The flow sheet includes identification of client and family educational needs based on a number of variables; these include the following:

- Readiness to learn (based on admission assessment of the patient)
- Obstacles to learning, which might include language, lack of vision, or other challenges
- Referrals, which might include a patient advocate, the library, or an ethics committee

The form provides documentation space for who was taught (e.g., patient or family), what was taught (e.g., use of resistive exercise bands, proper inhaler technique), when it was taught, what strategies of teaching were used (instructional methods and materials), and how the patient responded to instruction (what outcomes were achieved).

Economic Factors in Healthcare Education: Justice and Duty Revisited

Some might consider the parameters of healthcare economics and finances as objective information that can be used for any number of purposes. Fiscal solvency and forecasting of economic growth of an organization are good examples of such purposes. Others would agree that in addition to the legal considerations that mandate adherence to regulations in health care regardless of the economics involved, there is also an ethical dimension that speaks certainly to quality of care and also to justice, which refers to the equitable distribution of goods and services.

In the interest of patient care, the patient as a human being has a right to good quality care regardless of his or her economic status, national origin, race, and the like. Furthermore, health professionals have a duty to see to it that such services are provided. In like manner, the healthcare organization has the right to expect that it will receive its fair share of reimbursable revenues for services rendered.

Thus, as employees of the provider organization, health professionals have the duty to carry out organizational policies and mandates by acting in an accountable and responsible manner. In an environment of shrinking healthcare dollars, continuous shortages of staff, and dramatically shortened lengths of stay yielding rapid patient turnover, organizations are challenged to ensure the competency of their professional staff to provide educational services, and to do so in the most efficient and cost-effective manner possible. This is an interesting dilemma considering that patient education is identified as a legal responsibility of nurses as well as occupational, physical, and respiratory therapists in their respective state practice acts. Prelicensure education programs are challenged to prepare students adequately for this critical function.

The principle of justice is a critical consideration within the discourse on patient education. The rapid changes and trends so evident in the contemporary healthcare arena are, for the most part, economically driven. Described as chaotic by some, the healthcare system in many ways defies the humanistic and charitable underpinnings that have characterized healthcare services in this country across the decades. Indeed, organizations that provide health care are caught between the proverbial horns of the dilemma of allocating scarce resources in a just yet economically feasible manner.

On the one hand, the realities of capitation and managed care result in shrinking revenues. This trend, in turn, dictates shorter patient stays in hospitals and doing more with less. Despite continued, severe shortages of healthcare personnel in most geographic areas of the country, healthcare facilities are concomitantly expanding their clinical expertise into satellite types of ambulatory and home care services. On the other hand, these same organizations are held to the exact standards of care that are underwritten by *A Patient's Bill of Rights* (AHA, 1992), which is regulated as a contingency of Medicare and Medicaid participation by the CMS and for agency accreditation by the JC. In turn, although there are some exceptions (e.g., home healthcare agencies), hospital accreditation in particular dictates eligibility for third-party reimbursement in both the public and private sectors. Thus, the regulated right of clients to health education carries a corresponding duty of healthcare organizations to provide that service.

Financial Terminology

Given the fact that the role of certain health professionals as educators is an essential aspect of care delivery, included is an overview of fiscal terminology that directly affects both staff and patient education. Such educational services are not provided without an accompanying cost of human and material resources. Thus, it is important to know that expenditures are essentially classified into two categories: direct and indirect costs.

Direct Costs

Direct costs are tangible, predictable expenditures, a substantial portion of which include personnel salaries, employment benefits, and equipment (Gift, 1994). This portion of an organizational budget is almost always the largest of the total budgetary outlay of any healthcare facility.

Because of the labor-intensive function of healthcare delivery, the costs of salaries and benefits usually account for at least 50%—if not more—of the total facility budget. Of course, the higher the

educational level of professional staff, the higher the salaries and benefits, and thus, the higher the institution's total direct costs.

Although the purpose of salary is to buy an employee's time and particular expertise, it is often difficult to predict how long it will take to plan, implement, and evaluate various educational programs being offered. For example, if planning and carrying out patient or staff education exceed the allocated time and the healthcare educator draws overtime pay, the extra cost may not have been anticipated in the budget planning process.

Time is also considered a direct cost and is a major factor included in a cost-benefit analysis. In other words, if the time it takes to prepare and offer patient or staff education programs is greater than the financial gain to the institution, the facility may seek other ways of providing this service, such as computerized programmed instruction or a patient television channel.

Also, equipment is classified as a direct cost. No organization can function without proper equipment and the need to replace it when necessary. Teaching requires written materials, audiovisual tools, and equipment for the delivery of instruction, such as handouts and brochures, models, closed-circuit televisions, computers, and copy machines. Although renting or leasing equipment may sometimes be less expensive than purchasing it, rental and leasing costs are still categorized as direct costs.

Direct costs are divided into two types: fixed and variable. **Fixed costs** are those that are predictable, remain the same over time, and can be controlled. Salaries, for example, are fixed costs because they remain relatively stable and can also be manipulated. The facility usually makes annual decisions to give employee raises, to freeze salaries, or to cut positions, thereby influencing the budgeted amount for direct cost expenditures. In addition, mortgages, loan repayments, and the like are included as fixed costs.

Variable costs are those costs that, in the case of healthcare organizations, depend on volume. The number of meals prepared, for example, depends on the patient census. From an educational perspective, the demand for patient teaching depends on the number and diagnostic types of patients. For example, if the volume of total hip replacement patients is low, educational costs may be high resulting from the fact that intensive one-to-one instruction must be offered to each patient admitted. Conversely, if the volume of total hip replacement surgeries is high, it is less expensive to provide standardized programs of instruction via group teaching sessions. As another example, if demand or turnover of health professions staff increases, the number of orientation sessions for new employees would also increase in volume. Supplies, also a direct, variable cost, can change depending on the amount and type needed. Variable costs can become fixed costs when volume remains consistently high or low over time.

Indirect Costs

Indirect costs are those costs not directly related to the actual delivery of an educational program. These include, but are not limited to, institutional overhead such as heating and air conditioning, lighting, space, and support services of maintenance, housekeeping, and security. Such services are necessary and ongoing whether or not an educational session is in progress.

Hidden costs, a type of indirect cost, can neither be anticipated nor accounted for until after the fact. Low employee productivity can produce hidden costs. Organizational budgets are prepared on the basis of what is known and predictable, with projections for variability in patient census included. Personnel budgets are based on levels of staff needed (e.g., number of radiographers, CT technicians, MRI technicians, and ultrasonographers) to accommodate the expected patient volume. This is determined by an annual projection of patient days and how many patients an employee can effectively care for on a daily basis. Low

productivity of one or two health professionals in a department or unit, for example, can have a significant impact on the workload of others, which, in turn, leads to low morale and employee turnover. Turnover increases recruitment and new employee orientation costs. In this respect, the costs are appropriately identified as hidden.

In a classic description of understanding costs, Gift (1994) makes a point of distinguishing between costs—direct or indirect—and charges. As just described, direct and indirect costs are those expenses incurred by the facility. Charges are set by the provider, but they are billed to the recipient of the services. There may or may not be equivalence between costs and charges. In the retail business, for example, if costs of raw materials are low, while charges for the items, goods, or services are high, the retailer yields a profit. In the healthcare arena, not-for-profit organizations are limited by federal law as to the amount they can charge in relation to the actual cost of a service. In many instances, particularly as it relates to pharmaceutical goods, the actual cost to the facility is what is charged. As such, the facility provides a service but realizes no financial profit (Kaiser Family Foundation, 2005).

Cost Savings, Cost Benefit, and Cost Recovery

Patient teaching is mandated by state laws, professional and institutional standards, accrediting body protocols, and regulations for participation in Medicare and Medicaid reimbursement programs. However, unless it is ordered by a physician, patient education costs are generally not recoverable as a separate entity under third-party reimbursement. Even though the costs of educational programs, for both patients and professional staff, are a legitimate expense to the facility, these costs usually are subsumed under hospital room rates and are, therefore, technically absorbed by the healthcare organization.

Hospitals realize **cost savings** when patient lengths of stay are shortened or fall within the allotted diagnostic related group (DRG) time frames. Patients who have fewer complications and use less expensive services will yield a cost savings for the institution. In an ambulatory care setting, cost savings may be realized when patient education keeps people healthy and independent for a longer period of time, thereby preventing high utilization of expensive diagnostic testing or inpatient services. However, and perhaps most important, patient education becomes even more essential when a pattern of early discharge is detected, resulting in frequent readmissions to a facility. The facility comes under scrutiny by HCFA/CMS and may be penalized either through citation or loss of payment—in which case any cost savings may be more than offset by the penalties incurred.

Cost benefit occurs when there is increased patient satisfaction with an institution as a result of the services it renders, including educational programs it provides such as childbirth classes, weight and stress reduction sessions, and cardiac fitness and rehabilitation programs. This is an opportunity for an institution to capture a patient population for lifetime coverage. Patient satisfaction is critical to individuals' return for future healthcare services.

Cost recovery results when either the patient or insurer pays a fee for educational services that are provided. Cost recovery can be realized through the marketing of health education programs offered for a fee. Also, under Medicare and Medicaid guidelines, reimbursement may be made for programs "furnished by providers of services to the extent that the programs are appropriate, integral parts in the rendition of covered services which are reasonable and necessary for the treatment of the individual's illness or injury" (Kaiser Family Foundation, 2005). The key to success in obtaining third-party reimbursement is the ability to demonstrate that as a result of education,

patients can manage self-care at home and consequently experience fewer hospitalizations.

To take advantage of cost recovery, hospitals and other healthcare agencies develop and market a cadre of health education programs that are open to all members of a community. If well attended, fee-for-service programs can result in revenues for the institution. The critical element, of course, is not only the recovery of costs but also revenue generation. **Revenue generation** (i.e., profit) refers to income realized over and above program costs.

To offset the dilemma of striving for cost containment and solvency in an environment of shrinking fiscal resources, healthcare organizations have developed alternative strategies for patient education to realize cost savings, cost benefit, cost recovery, or revenue generation. For example, a preoperative teaching program for surgical patients given prior to admission to the hospital has been found to lower patient anxiety, increase patient satisfaction, and decrease nursing hours during hospitalization (Wasson & Anderson, 1993).

Program Planning and Implementation

The key elements to consider when planning a patient education offering intended for generation of revenue include an accurate assessment of direct costs such as paper supplies, printing of program brochures, publicity, rental space, and time (based on an hourly rate) required of professional personnel to prepare and offer the service. If an hourly rate is unknown, a simple rule of thumb is to divide the annual base salary by 2,080, which is the standard number of hours for which people working full-time are paid in the course of one year.

If the program is to be offered on the premises of the facility, there may be no need to plan for a rental fee for space. However, indirect costs such as housekeeping and security should be prorated as a bona fide expense. Such a practice not only is good fiscal management, but also provides an accounting of the contributions of other departments to the educational efforts of the facility.

Fees for a program should be set at a level high enough to cover the aggregate costs of program preparation and delivery. If the intent of an education program is for cost savings to the facility, such as provision of education classes for diabetics in the community to reduce the number of costly hospital admissions, then the aim may be to break even on costs. The price is set by dividing the calculated cost by the number of anticipated attendees. If the goal is for cost benefit to the institution, success can be measured by increased patient satisfaction (as determined by questionnaires or evaluation forms) or by an increase in the use of the sponsor's services (as determined by record keeping). If the intent is to offer a series of classes for smoking cessation or childbirth to improve the wellness of the community and to generate income for the facility, then the fee is set higher than cost so as to realize a profit (cost recovery).

It is usually necessary for the health professionals providing the program to give an annual report to administration of time and money spent and whether such expenditures were profitable to the institution in terms of cost savings, cost benefit, or cost recovery.

Cost-Benefit Analysis and Cost-Effectiveness Analysis

In the majority of healthcare organizations, the education department bears the major responsibility for staff development, for in-service employee training, and for patient education programs that exceed the boundaries of bedside instruction. Total budget preparation for these departments is best explained by the experts in the field. Fisher, Hume, and Emerick (1998), for example, address the need for staff development departments to engage in responsibility-centered budgeting, which also is referred to as activity-based management. Given the shift away from providing at-will services and toward greater demand for cost accountability for educational programs, they propose a template for costing out programs that allows staff development departments to identify and recoup their true costs while responding to increased market competition.

There is no single best method for measuring the effectiveness of patient education programs. Most experts in the field tend to rely on determining actual costs or actual impact of programs in relationship to outcomes by employing one of two concepts: cost-benefit analysis or cost-effectiveness analysis (Abruzzese, 1992).

Cost-benefit analysis measures the relationship between costs and outcomes. Outcomes can be the actual amount of revenue generated as a result of an educational offering, or they can be expressed in terms of shorter patient stays or reduced hospitalizations for particular diagnostic groups of patients. If, under DRGs or capitation methods of reimbursement, the facility makes a profit, this can be expressed in monetary terms. If an analysis reveals that an educational program costs less than the revenue it generates, that expense can be recovered by third-party reimbursement. If savings exceed costs, then the program is considered to be a cost benefit for the facility. The measurement of costs against monetary gains is commonly referred to as the **cost-benefit ratio**.

Cost-effectiveness analysis measures the impact an educational offering has on patient behavior. If program objectives are achieved, as evidenced by positive and sustained changes in behavior of the participants over time, the program is said to be cost effective. Although behavioral changes are highly desirable, in many instances they are less observable, less tangible, and not easily measurable. For example, reduction in patient anxiety cannot be converted into a gain in real dollars. There-fore, it is wise to analyze the outcome of teaching interventions by comparing behavioral outcomes between two or more programs to identify the one that is most effective and efficient when actual costs cannot be determined.

A health professional as educator may be called upon to interpret the costs of behavioral changes (outcomes) to the institution by conducting a cost-effectiveness analysis between programs. This can be accomplished by first identifying and itemiz-ing for each program all direct and indirect costs, including any identifiable hidden costs. Second, it is necessary to identify and itemize any benefits derived from the program offering, such as revenue gained or decreased readmission rates that can be expressed in monetary values. Results of these find-ings can then be recorded on a grid so that each program's cost effectiveness is visually apparent (see **Figure 2–1**).

Figure 2–1 Cost-Effectiveness Grid

Program	I	II
Costs		
Direct	$	$
Indirect	$	$
Hidden	$	$
Benefits		
Decreased readmissions	$	$
Revenue generated	$	$
Total	$	$

Mitton and Donaldson (2004) suggest a non-vested team approach to an analysis of program effectiveness for the purpose of determining the allocation or reallocation of valuable resources between and among services or programs. This approach ensures the integrity of the total pro-cess of program evaluation. In addition to this recommendation, the International Council of Nurses published a position statement in 2001 that, among other things, obligates nurses to dem-onstrate their value in promoting cost-effective, quality care by playing a leadership role in pro-gram planning and evaluation, in policy setting, and in interactive networking on cost-effectiveness research, cost-saving strategies, and best practice standards (Ghebrehiwet, 2005).

State of the Evidence

Practice driven by evidence is defined as prac-tice "based on research, clinical expertise, and patient preferences that guide decisions about the health care of individual patients" (HPNA Position Paper, 2004, p. 66). Much evidence sug-gests that ethical principles and theories play a highly significant role in shaping contemporary healthcare delivery practices and decision making. Whereas complex and technological advances in health care have given rise to numerous questions about what is right or wrong—or more or less morally defensible—few situations yield clear-cut or perfectly right answers to solving a problem or need. Numerous case studies, books, and articles on how to deal with ethical dilemmas in health care abound. They attempt to provide evidence for how to deliver health care, including patient education, in the most equitable and beneficial manner possible. Our increasingly multicultural and pluralistic society is challenged to address the vast array of biomedical ethical issues confront-ing healthcare practitioners on a daily basis in a way that preserves an individual's rights but also protects the well-being of other persons, groups, and communities. Health professionals who deal directly with clients have many more resources to turn to than do those whose involvement with client care is more removed.

Laws and standards governing the role of certain health professionals as patient educators are firmly established and provide the legal foundations and professional expectations for the delivery of high-quality client care. Also well established is the importance of documenting client education interventions. More research must be conducted to provide evidence of the frequency and amount of informal patient education health professionals provide that never gets recorded in the chart. In addition, although strategies exist for analyzing the cost effectiveness and cost benefit of educational programming offered by health professionals, more research evidence is needed to substantiate the value of the educator's role in influencing overall costs of care.

Further comparative analysis research needs to be conducted to determine what types of patient education programs are the most equitable, beneficial, and cost effective for clients, professional staff, the institution, and the communities served. Evidence is scarce on the economics associated with various approaches to education and the value of the health professional's role as it affects behavioral outcomes related to cost savings, cost benefit, and cost recovery.

Summary

Ethical and legal dimensions of human rights provide the justification for client education, particularly as it relates to issues of self-determination and informed consent. These rights are enforced through federal and state regulations and through performance standards promulgated by accrediting bodies and professional organizations for implementation at the local level. The health professional's role as educator is legitimized through the definition of each discipline's practice as set forth by the prevailing laws and codes of ethics governing professional conduct in various employment settings. In this respect, client education is a duty that is grounded in justice; that is, the direct care providers have a responsibility to provide patient education and all clients, regardless of their age, gender, culture, race, ethnicity, literacy level, religious affiliation, or other defining attributes have a right to health education relevant to their physical and psychosocial needs. Justice also dictates that education programs should be designed to be consistent with organizational goals while meeting the needs of clients to be informed, self-directed, and in control of their own health, and ultimately of their own destiny.

REVIEW QUESTIONS

1. What are the definitions of the terms *ethical, moral,* and *legal,* and how are they distinct from one another?
2. Which national, state, professional, and private-sector organizations legislate, regulate, and provide standards to ensure the protection of human rights in matters of health care?
3. Which ethical viewpoint, deontological or teleological, refers to the decision-making approach that choices should be made for the common good of people?

4. With respect to ethical, moral, and legal obligations, how does the American Hospital Association's *A Patient's Bill of Rights* compare with the codes of ethics of the various health professions?
5. What are six ethical principles that dictate the actions of health professionals in delivering services to clients?
6. Why are practice acts useful to health professionals in carrying out their roles and responsibilities to educate the public they serve?
7. What is the difference between *negligence* and *malpractice*?
8. When was informed consent established as a basic tenet of ethics and which health professionals are accountable in situations involving informed consent?
9. How can ethical principles be applied specifically to the teaching of clients? Give an example for each of the principles described in this chapter.
10. How does ethics fit into the relationships between student and teacher and client and health professional in the classroom and practice setting, respectively?
11. Why is documentation of patient education efforts so important in the provision of care by health professionals?
12. What are four examples of direct costs and five examples of indirect costs in the provision of patient/staff education?
13. What are the definitions of the following terms: *fixed direct costs*, *variable direct costs*, *indirect costs*, *cost savings*, *cost benefit*, *cost recovery*, *cost-benefit analysis*, and *cost-effectiveness analysis*?

CASE STUDY*

Laura, a cytotechnology student, is practicing for an exam by reading slides from a study set from 5 years ago. On one slide of a cervical specimen, Laura believes she sees malignant cells. However, the slide had originally been read as normal by the cytotechnologist who, coincidentally, is now her instructor. She shows the slide to her instructor, who agrees with Laura—the cervical cells indeed show malignancy, and the specimen is not normal as originally read. Laura's instructor commends her on this "good pickup." When Laura asks if they should inform anyone about the error, her instructor says no. He reasons that if they were to point out his past mistake, others might lose their confidence in him and, besides, there would probably be no clinical impact because the specimen was already 5 years old.

1. What are plausible actions that Laura could take at this point?
2. What are the ethical reasons Laura would rely on to justify the plausible actions in question 1?
3. Which of her actions and associated justifications seem the most morally defensible to you? Why?

* This case is adapted from an actual student case.

References

Abruzzese, R. S. (1992). *Nursing staff development: Strategies for success.* St. Louis, MO: Mosby.

American Hospital Association. (1975). *Patient's bill of rights.* Chicago: Author.

American Hospital Association. (1992). *A patient's bill of rights.* Retrieved March 27, 2007, from http://www.patienttalk.info/AHA-Patient_Bill_of_Rights.htm

American Medical Association. (2001). *The principles of medical ethics.* Retrieved March 2, 2010, from http://www.ama-assn.org/ama/pub/physician-resources/medical-ethics.shtml

American Nurses Association. (1976). *Code of ethics for nurses with interpretive statements.* Kansas City, MO: Author.

American Nurses Association. (1985). *Code of ethics for nurses with interpretive statements.* Kansas City, MO: Author.

American Nurses Association. (2001). *Code of ethics for nurses with interpretive statements.* Washington, DC: American Nurses Publishing. Retrieved January 20, 2007, from http://www.nursingworld.org/MainMenuCategories/EthicsStandards/CodeofEthicsforNurses.aspx

Association of American Physicians and Surgeons. (1995). *Patients' bill of rights.* Retrieved March 27, 2007, from http://www.aapsonline.org/patients/billrts.htm

Beauchamp, T., & Childress, J. (1977). *Principles of biomedical ethics.* New York: Oxford University Press.

Bekker, H. L. (2010). The loss of reason in patient decision aid research: Do checklists damage the quality of informed choice interventions? *Patient Education and Counseling,* doi:10.1016/j.pec.2010.01.002.

Boyd, M. D., Gleit, C. J., Graham, B. A., & Whitman, N. I. (1998). *Health teaching in nursing practice: A professional model* (3rd ed.). Stamford, CT: Appleton & Lange.

Brent, N. J. (2001). *Nurses and the law* (2nd ed.). Philadelphia: Saunders.

Buckwalter, J. G. (2007). The good patient. *New England Journal of Medicine, 357*(25), 2534–2535.

Casey, F. S. (1995). Documenting patient education: A literature review. *Journal of Continuing Education in Nursing, 26*(6), 257–260.

Centers for Disease Control and Prevention. (2005). Tuskegee timeline. Retrieved March 27, 2007, from http://www.cdc.gov/nchstp/od/tuskegee/time.htm

Christakis, D. A., & Feudtner, C. (1997). Temporary matters: The ethical consequences of transient social relationships in medical training. *Journal of the American Medical Association, 278*(9), 739–743.

Cisar, N. S., & Bell, S. K. (1995). Informed consent: An ethical dilemma. *Nursing Forum, 30*(3), 20–28.

Consolidated Omnibus Budget Reconciliation Act (COBRA) of 1985, 42 U.S.C. 135dd§1867.

Creighton, H. (1986). Informed consent. *Nursing Management, 17*(10), 11–13.

deBocanegra, H. T., & Gany, F. (2004). Good provider, good patient: Changing behaviors to eliminate disparities in healthcare. *American Journal of Managed Care, 10,* SP20–SP28.

Dickey, S. B. (2006). Informed consent: Ethical issues. In V. D. Lachman (Ed.), *Applied ethics in nursing.* New York: Springer.

Donetto, S. (2010). Medical students' views of power in doctor–patient interactions: The value of teacher–learner relationships. *Medical Education, 44,* 187–196.

Edward, P. (1967). Kant, Immanuel. In *Encyclopedia of philosophy.* New York: Macmillan.

Emanuel, E. J. (2000). Justice and managed care: Four principles for the just allocation of health care resources. *Hastings Center Report, 30*(3), 8–16.

Ewashen, C., & Lane, A. (2007). Pedagogy, power and practice ethics: Clinical teaching in psychiatric/mental health settings. *Nursing Inquiry, 14*(3), 255–262.

Federation of State Boards of Physical Therapy. (2006). *The model practice act for physical therapy* (4th ed.). Retrieved March 8, 2010, from https://www.fsbpt.org/RegulatoryTools/ModelPracticeAct/index.asp

Fisher, M. L., Hume, R., & Emerick, R. (1998). Costing nursing education programs: It's as easy as 1-2-3. *Journal for Nurses in Staff Development, 14*(5), 227–285.

Flook, D. M. (2003). The professional nurse and regulation. *Journal of PeriAnesthesia Nursing, 18*(3),160–167.

Freedman, T. G. (2003). Prescriptions for health providers: From cancer patients. *Cancer Nursing, 26*(4), 323–330.

Ghebrehiwet, T. (2005). The ICN code of ethics for nurses. Helping nurses make ethical decisions. *Reflections on Nursing Leadership, 31*(3), 26–28. Retrieved January 18, 2007, from http://www.nursingsociety.org/RNL/3Q_2005/features/features6.html

Gift, A. G. (1994). Understanding costs. *Clinical Nurse Specialist, 8*(2), 90.

Hall, J. K. (1996). *Nursing ethics and the law.* Philadelphia: Saunders.

Hall, K. (1992). Cardozo, Benjamin N. In *The Oxford Companion to the Supreme Court of the United States* (pp. 126–127). New York: Oxford University Press.

HPNA position paper. (2004). Value of the professional nurse in end-of-life care. *Journal of Hospice and Palliative Nursing, 6*(1), 65–66.

International Council of Nursing. (2001). Position statement. Promoting the value and cost-effectiveness of nursing. Retrieved February 15, 2007, from http://www.icn.ch/psvalue.htm

Kaiser Family Foundation. (2005). Navigating Medicare and Medicaid, 2005. Retrieved March 27, 2007, from http://kff.org/medicare/7240.cfm

Kohlenberg, E. M. (2006). Patients' rights and ethical issues. In V. D. Lachman (Ed.), *Applied ethics in nursing* (pp. 39–46). New York: Springer.

Legal Action Center. (2001). *HIV/AIDS. Testing, confidentiality, and discrimination.* New York: Legal Action Center of the City of New York.

Lesnick, M. J., & Anderson, B. E. (1962). *Nursing practice and the law.* Philadelphia: Lippincott.

Martinez, R. (2000). A model for boundary dilemmas: Ethical decision-making in the patient–professional relationship. *Ethical Human Sciences and Services, 2*(1), 43–61.

Mezey, M., Evans, L. K., Golob, Z. D., Murphy, E., & White, G. B. (1994). The patient self-determination act: Sources of concern for nurses. *Nursing Outlook, 42*(1), 30–38.

Mikos, C. A. (2004). Inside the nurse practice act. *Nursing Management, 35*(9), 20, 22, 91.

Mitton, C., & Donaldson, C. (2004). Health care priority setting: Principles, practice and challenges. *Cost Effectiveness and Resource Allocation, 2*(3). Retrieved February 20, 2007, from http://www.resource-allocation.com/content/2/1/3

New York State Nurses Association. (1972). New York state nurse practice act. Retrieved March 4, 2007, from http://www.op.nysed.gov/nurse.htm

New York State Nurses Association. (2001). Code of ethics for nurses with interpretative statements. *NYSNA Report, 32*(7), 5–7.

Pellegrino, E. (1993). The metamorphosis of medical ethics: A thirty-year retrospective. *Journal of the American Medical Association, 269*, 1158–1162.

President's Advisory Commission on Consumer Protection and Quality in the Healthcare Industry. (1998). Consumer bill of rights and responsibilities. Retrieved January 20, 2007, from http://www.hcquality commission.gov/final/append_a.html

Rankin, S. H., & Stallings, K. D. (1990). *Patient education: Principles and practices.* Philadelphia: Lippincott.

Redman, B. K. (2008). When is patient education unethical? *Nursing Ethics, 15*(6), 813–820.

Reiser, S. J. (1993). Science, pedagogy, and the transformation of empathy in medicine. In H. Spiro, M. G. McCrea Curnen, E. Peschel, & D. St. James (Eds.), *Empathy and the practice of medicine.* New Haven, CT: Yale University Press.

Reiser, S. J. (1994). The ethics of learning and teaching in medicine. *Academic Medicine, 69*(11), 872–876.

Reising, D. L., & Allen, P. N. (2007). Protecting yourself from malpractice claims. *American Nurse Today, 2*(2), 39–44.

Rivera, G. (1972). *Willowbrook: A report on how it is and why it doesn't have to be that way.* New York: Vintage Books.

Schloendorff v. Society of New York Hospitals, 211 NY 125, 128, 105 N.E. 92, 93 (1914).

Snyder, B. (1996, March). An easy way to document patient ed. *RN,* 43–45.

Thomas, S. B., & Quinn, S. C. (1991). The Tuskegee Syphilis Study, 1932 to 1972: Implications for HIV education and AIDS risk education programs in the black community. *American Journal of Public Health, 81*(11), 1498–1505. Retrieved March 27, 2007, from http://ajph.aphapublications.org/cgi/content/abstract/81/11/1498

Tong, R. (2007). *New perspectives in health care ethics.* Upper Saddle River, NJ: Pearson Prentice Hall.

Ulrich, L. P. (1999). *The Patient Self-Determination Act: Meeting the challenges in patient care.* Washington, DC: Georgetown University Press.

U.S. Department of Health and Human Services. (1983). Protection of human subjects: Reports of the President's Commission for the Study of Ethical Problems in Medicine and Biomedical and Behavioral Research. *Federal Register, 48*(146), 34408–34412.

Visser, A. (1998). Ethical issues in patient education and counseling. *Patient Education and Counseling, 35*, 1–3.

Wasson, D., & Anderson, M. (1993). Hospital-patient education: Current status and future trends. *Journal of Nursing Staff Development, 10*(3), 147–151.

Weisbard, A. J., & Arras, J. D. (1984). Commissioning morality: An introduction to the symposium. *Cardozo Law Review, 6*(4), 223–241.

Wittmann-Price, R. A., & Fisher, K. M. (2009). Patient decision aids: Tools for patients and professionals. *American Journal of Nursing, 109*(12), 60–63.

Yoder Wise, P. S. (1995). *Leading and managing in nursing.* St. Louis, MO: Mosby.

Zucker, E. J. (2009). The good patient. *Academic Medicine, 84*(4), 524.

Chapter 3

Applying Learning Theories to Healthcare Practice

Margaret M. Braungart

Richard G. Braungart

Pamela R. Gramet

CHAPTER HIGHLIGHTS

Psychological Learning Theories
  Behaviorist Learning Theory
  Cognitive Learning Theory
  Social Learning Theory
  Psychodynamic Learning Theory
  Humanistic Learning Theory
Neuropsychology and Learning
Comparison of Learning Theories
Motor Learning

Stages of Motor Learning
Motor Learning Variables
Common Principles of Learning
  How Does Learning Occur?
  What Kinds of Experiences Facilitate or
    Hinder the Learning Process?
  What Helps Ensure That Learning Becomes
    Relatively Permanent?
State of the Evidence

KEY TERMS

- ❏ learning
- ❏ learning theory
- ❏ respondent conditioning
- ❏ systematic desensitization
- ❏ stimulus generalization
- ❏ discrimination learning
- ❏ spontaneous recovery
- ❏ operant conditioning
- ❏ escape conditioning
- ❏ avoidance conditioning
- ❏ metacognition
- ❏ gestalt perspective

- ❏ information processing
- ❏ cognitive development
- ❏ social constructivism
- ❏ social cognition
- ❏ cognitive-emotional perspective
- ❏ role modeling
- ❏ vicarious reinforcement
- ❏ defense mechanisms
- ❏ resistance
- ❏ transference
- ❏ hierarchy of needs
- ❏ therapeutic relationship

❏ motor learning
❏ motor performance
❏ contextual interference effects

❏ mental practice
❏ intrinsic feedback
❏ extrinsic feedback

OBJECTIVES

After completing this chapter, the reader will be able to

1. Define the principal constructs of each learning theory.
2. Differentiate among the basic approaches to learning for each of the five psychological learning theories.
3. Give an example applying each psychological theory to changing the attitudes and behaviors of learners in a specific situation.
4. Outline alternative strategies for learning in a given situation using at least two different psychological learning theories.
5. Identify the differences and similarities in the psychological learning theories specific to (a) the basic procedures of learning, (b) the assumptions made about the learning, (c) the task of the educator, (d) the sources of motivation, and (e) the way in which the transfer of learning is facilitated.
6. Discuss how neuroscience research has contributed to a better understanding of learning and learning theories.
7. Identify specific teaching strategies for each stage of Fitts and Posner's three stages of motor learning.
8. Explain how different types of practice and feedback variables in motor learning can be applied to client teaching.

Learning is defined in this chapter as a relatively permanent change in mental processing, emotional functioning, skill, and/or behavior as a result of experience. It is the lifelong, dynamic process by which individuals acquire new knowledge or skills and alter their thoughts, feelings, attitudes, and actions.

Learning enables individuals to adapt to demands and changing circumstances and is crucial in health care—whether for patients and families grappling with ways to improve their health and adjust to their medical conditions, students acquiring the information and skills necessary to become health professionals, or healthcare staff devising and learning more effective approaches to educating and treating patients and each other in partnership. Despite the significance of learning to each individual's development, functioning, health, and well-being, debate continues about how learning occurs, what kinds of experiences facilitate or hinder the learning process, and what ensures that learning becomes relatively permanent.

Until the late 19th century, most of the discussions and debates about learning were grounded in philosophy, school administration, and conventional wisdom (Hilgard, 1996). Around the dawn of the 20th century, the new field of educational psychology emerged and became a defining force for the scientific study of learning, teaching, and assessment (Woolfolk, 2001). As a science, educational psychology rests on the systematic gathering of evidence or data to test theories and hypotheses about learning.

A **learning theory** is a coherent framework of integrated constructs and principles that describe, explain, or predict how people learn. Psychological learning theories and motor learning are discussed in this chapter, each of which has direct applicability to health care. Rather than offering a single theory of learning, psychology provides alternative theories and perspectives on how learning occurs and what motivates people to learn and change (Hilgard & Bower, 1966; Ormrod, 2004; Snowman & Biehler, 2006). Motor learning evolved as a branch of experimental psychology and can be differentiated from "verbal" learning (Newell, 1991). By the middle of the 20th century, it was established as a specialized area of study and it has been influenced by behavioral theory, cybernetics, and information processing (VanSant, 2003). Psychological learning theories are useful in acquiring information and in situations involving human thought, emotions, and social interaction. Motor learning is of particular interest to health professionals who try to help their clients and students learn or relearn skills.

The construction and testing of learning theories over the past century have contributed much to the understanding of how individuals acquire knowledge and change their ways of thinking, feeling, and behaving. Reflecting an evidence-based approach to learning, the accumulated body of research information can be used to guide the educational process and has challenged a number of popular notions and myths about learning (e.g., "Spare the rod and spoil the child," "Males are more intelligent than females," "You can't teach an old dog new tricks," "The more feedback, the better"). In addition, the major learning theories have wide applicability and form the foundation of not only the field of education but also psycho-

logical counseling, sports, workplace organization and human resource management, and marketing and advertising.

Whether used singly or in combination, learning theories have much to offer the practice of health care. Increasingly, health professionals must demonstrate that they regularly employ sound methods and a clear rationale in their education efforts, patient and client interactions, staff management and training, and continuing education and health promotion programs (Ferguson & Day, 2005).

Given the current structure of health care in the United States, health professionals are often responsible for designing and implementing plans and procedures for improving health education and encouraging wellness. Beyond one's profession, however, knowledge of the learning process relates to nearly every aspect of daily life. Health professionals can apply learning theories at the individual, group, and community levels not only to comprehend and teach new material and tasks, but also to solve problems, change unhealthy habits, build constructive relationships, manage emotions, and develop effective behavior.

This chapter reviews the principal psychological and motor learning theories that are useful to health education and clinical practice. Behaviorist, cognitive, and social learning theories are most often applied to patient education as an aspect of professional healthcare practice. This chapter argues that emotions and feelings also need explicit focus in relation to learning in general (Goleman, 1995) and to health care in particular (Halpern, 2001). Why? Emotional reactions are often learned as a result of experience, they play a significant role in the learning process, and they are a vital consideration when dealing with health, disease, prevention, wellness, medical treatment, recovery, healing, and relapse prevention. To address this concern, this chapter treats psychodynamic and humanistic perspectives as learning theories because they encourage a patient-centered approach to care and add much to our understanding of human motivation and emotions in the learning process. The review includes motor learning because it provides a framework for health professionals teaching motor tasks to clients and students.

The chapter is organized as follows. First, the basic psychological principles of learning advocated by behaviorist, cognitive, social learning, psychodynamic, and humanistic theories are summarized and illustrated with examples from psychology and healthcare research. With the current upsurge and interest in neuroscience research, brief mention is made of the contributions of neuropsychology to understanding the dynamics of learning and sorting out the claims of learning theories. Then, the psychological learning theories are compared with regard to the following aspects:

- Their fundamental procedures for changing behavior
- The assumptions made about the learner
- The role of the educator in encouraging learning
- The sources of motivation for learning
- The ways in which learning is transferred to new situations and problems

Next, motor learning theories and variables, as well as their application for teaching skills to patients and clients, are addressed. Finally, the theories are compared and then synthesized by identifying their common features and addressing three questions: (1) How does learning occur? (2) What kinds of experiences facilitate or hinder the learning process? (3) What helps ensure that learning becomes relatively permanent? While surveying this chapter, readers are encouraged to think of ways to apply the learning theories to both their professional and personal lives.

The goals of this chapter are to provide a conceptual framework for subsequent chapters in this book and to offer a toolbox of approaches that health professionals can use to enhance learning

and change in clients, students, staff, and themselves. Although there is a trend toward integrating learning theories in education, it is argued that knowledge of each theory's basic principles, advantages, and shortcomings allows health professionals to select, combine, and apply the most useful components of learning theories to specific patients and situations in health care. After completing the chapter, readers should be able to identify the essential principles of learning, describe various ways in which the learning process can be approached, and develop alternative strategies to change attitudes, behaviors, and skills in different settings.

Psychological Learning Theories

This section summarizes the basic principles and related concepts of the behaviorist, cognitive, social learning, psychodynamic, and humanistic learning theories. While reviewing each theory, readers are asked to consider the following questions:

- How do the environment and the internal dynamics of the individual influence learning?
- Is the learner viewed as relatively passive or more active?
- What is the educator's task in the learning process?
- What motivates individuals to learn?
- What encourages the transfer of learning to new situations?
- What are the contributions and criticisms of each learning theory?

Behaviorist Learning Theory

Focusing mainly on what is directly observable, behaviorists view learning as the product of the stimulus conditions (S) and the responses (R) that follow—sometimes termed the S-R model of learning. Whether dealing with animals or people, the learning process is relatively simple. Generally ignoring what goes on inside the individual—which, of course, is always difficult to ascertain—behaviorists closely observe responses and then manipulate the environment to bring about the intended change. Currently in education and clinical psychology, behaviorist theories are more likely to be used in combination with other learning theories, especially cognitive theory (Bush, 2006; Dai & Sternberg, 2004). Behaviorist theory continues to be considered useful in health care.

To modify people's attitudes and responses, behaviorists either alter the stimulus conditions in the environment or change what happens after a response occurs. Motivation is explained as the desire to reduce some drive (drive reduction); hence, satisfied, complacent, or satiated individuals have little motivation to learn and change. Getting behavior to transfer from the initial learning situation to other settings is largely a matter of practice (strengthening habits). Transfer is aided by a similarity in the stimuli and responses in the learning situation relative to future situations where the response is to be performed. Much of behaviorist learning is based on respondent conditioning and operant conditioning procedures.

Respondent conditioning (also termed *classical* or *Pavlovian conditioning*) emphasizes the importance of stimulus conditions and the associations formed in the learning process (Ormrod, 2004). In this basic model of learning, a neutral stimulus (NS)—a stimulus that has no particular value or meaning to the learner—is paired with a naturally occurring unconditioned or unlearned stimulus (UCS) and unconditioned response (UCR) (**Figure 3–1**). After a few such pairings, the neutral stimulus alone, without the unconditioned stimulus, elicits the same unconditioned response. Thus, learning takes place when the newly conditioned stimulus (CS) becomes associated with the conditioned response (CR)—a process that may well occur without conscious thought or awareness.

Consider an example from health care. Someone without much experience with hospitals (NS) may visit a relative who is ill. While in the relative's room, the visitor may smell offensive odors (UCS) and feel queasy and light-headed (UCR). After this initial visit and later repeated visits, hospitals (now the CS) may become associated with feeling anxious and nauseated (CR), especially if the visitor smells odors similar to those encountered during the first experience (see Figure 3–1). Respondent conditioning highlights the importance of the atmosphere and its effects on staff morale in health care. Often without thinking or reflection, patients and visitors formulate these associations as a result of their hospital experiences, providing the basis for long-lasting attitudes toward medicine, healthcare facilities, and health professionals.

Besides influencing the acquisition of new responses to environmental stimuli, principles of respondent conditioning may be used to extinguish a previously learned response. Responses decrease if the presentation of the conditioned stimulus is not accompanied by the unconditioned stimulus over time. Thus, if the visitor who became dizzy in one hospital subsequently goes to other hospitals to see relatives or friends without smelling offensive odors, then her discomfort and anxiety about hospitals may lessen after several such experiences.

Systematic desensitization is a technique based on respondent conditioning that is used by psychologists to reduce fear and anxiety in their clients (Wolpe, 1982). The assumption is that fear of a particular stimulus or situation is learned, so it can, therefore, be unlearned or extinguished. Fearful individuals are first taught relaxation techniques. While they are in a state of relaxation, the fear-producing stimulus is gradually introduced at a nonthreatening level so that anxiety and emotions are not aroused. After repeated pairings of the stimulus under relaxed, nonfrightening conditions, the individual learns that no harm will come to him from the once fear-inducing stimulus. Fi-

Figure 3–1 Respondent Conditioning Model of Learning

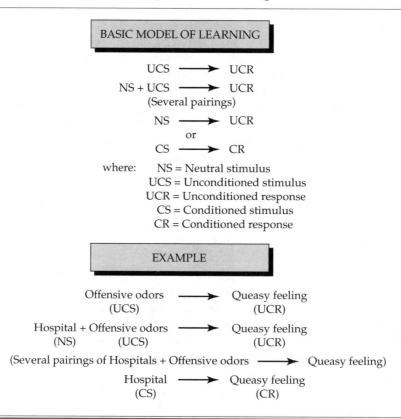

nally, the client is able to confront the stimulus without being anxious and afraid.

In healthcare research, respondent conditioning has been used to extinguish chemotherapy patients' anticipatory nausea and vomiting (Stockhurst, Steingrueber, Enck, & Klosterhalfen, 2006), while systematic desensitization has been used to treat drug addiction (Piane, 2000), phobias (McCullough & Andrews, 2001), tension headaches (Deyl & Kaliappan, 1997), and to teach children with attention deficit hyperactivity disorder (ADHD) or autism to swallow pills (Beck, Cataldo, Slifer, Pulbrook, & Guhman, 2005). As

another illustration, prescription drug advertisers regularly employ conditioning principles to encourage consumers to associate a brand name medication with happy and improved lifestyles; once conditioned, consumers will likely favor the advertised drug over competitors' medications and the much less expensive generic form. As a third example, taking the time to help patients relax and reduce their stress when applying some medical intervention—even a painful procedure—lessens the likelihood that patients will build up negative and anxious associations about medicine and health care.

Certain respondent conditioning concepts are especially useful in the healthcare setting. **Stimulus generalization** is the tendency of initial learning experiences to be easily applied to other similar stimuli. For example, when listening to friends and relatives describe a hospital experience, it becomes apparent that a highly positive or negative personal encounter may color patients' evaluations of their hospital stays as well as their subsequent feelings about having to be hospitalized again. With more and varied experiences, individuals learn to differentiate among similar stimuli, and then **discrimination learning** has occurred. As an illustration, patients who have been hospitalized a number of times often have learned a lot about hospitalization. As a result of their experiences, they make sophisticated distinctions and can discriminate among stimuli (e.g., what the various noises mean and what the various health professionals do) that novice patients cannot. Much of professional education and clinical practice involves moving from being able to make generalizations to discrimination learning.

Spontaneous recovery is a useful respondent conditioning concept that needs to be given careful consideration in relapse prevention programs. The principle of the concept operates as follows: Although a response may appear to be extinguished, it may recover and reappear at any time (even years later), especially when stimulus conditions are similar to those in the initial learning experience. Spontaneous recovery helps us understand why it is so difficult to completely eliminate unhealthy habits and addictive behaviors such as smoking, alcoholism, or drug abuse.

Another widely recognized approach to learning is **operant conditioning**, which was developed largely by B. F. Skinner (1974, 1989). Operant conditioning focuses on the behavior of the organism and the reinforcement that occurs after the response. A reinforcer is a stimulus or event applied after a response that strengthens the probability that the response will be performed again. When specific responses are reinforced on the proper schedule, behaviors can be either increased or decreased.

Table 3–1 summarizes the principal ways to increase and decrease responses by applying the contingencies of operant conditioning. Understanding the dynamics of learning presented in this table

---

Table 3–1 OPERANT CONDITIONING MODEL: CONTINGENCIES TO INCREASE AND DECREASE THE PROBABILITY OF AN ORGANISM'S RESPONSE

I. To *increase* the probability of a response:	II. To *decrease* or extinguish the probability of a response:
A. *Positive reinforcement:* application of a pleasant stimulus *Reward conditioning:* a pleasant stimulus is applied following an organism's response	A. *Nonreinforcement:* an organism's conditioned response is not followed by any kind of reinforcement (positive, negative, or punishment)
B. *Negative reinforcement:* removal of an aversive or unpleasant stimulus *Escape conditioning:* as an aversive stimulus is applied, the organism makes a response that causes the unpleasant stimulus to cease *Avoidance conditioning:* an aversive stimulus is anticipated by the organism, which makes a response to avoid the unpleasant event	B. *Punishment:* following a response, an aversive stimulus that the organism cannot escape or avoid is applied

can prove useful to health professionals in assessing and identifying ways to change individuals' behaviors in the healthcare setting. The key is to carefully observe individuals' responses to specific stimuli and then decide the best reinforcement procedures to use to change a behavior.

Two methods to *increase* the probability of a response are to apply positive or negative reinforcement after a response occurs. According to Skinner (1974), giving positive reinforcement (i.e., reward) greatly enhances the likelihood that a response will be repeated in similar circumstances. As an illustration, although a patient moans and groans as he attempts to get up and walk for the first time after an operation, praise and encouragement (reward) for his efforts at walking (response) will improve the chances that he will continue struggling toward independence.

A second way to increase a behavior is by applying negative reinforcement after a response is made. This form of reinforcement involves the removal of an unpleasant stimulus through either escape conditioning or avoidance conditioning. The difference between the two types of negative reinforcement relates to timing.

In **escape conditioning**, as an unpleasant stimulus is being applied, the individual responds in some way that causes the uncomfortable stimulation to cease. Suppose, for example, that when a member of the healthcare team is being chastised in front of the group for being late and missing meetings, she says something humorous. The head of the team stops criticizing her and laughs. Because the use of humor has allowed the team member to escape an unpleasant situation, chances are that she will employ humor again to alleviate a stressful encounter and thereby deflect attention from her problem behavior.

In **avoidance conditioning**, the unpleasant stimulus is anticipated rather than being applied directly. Avoidance conditioning has been used to explain some people's tendency to become ill so as to avoid doing something they do not want to

do. For example, a child fearing a teacher or test may tell his mother that he has a stomachache. If allowed to stay home from school, the child increasingly may complain of sickness to avoid unpleasant situations. Thus, when fearful events are anticipated, sickness, in this case, is the behavior that has been increased through negative reinforcement.

According to operant conditioning principles, behaviors also may be *decreased* through either nonreinforcement or punishment. Skinner (1974) maintained that the simplest way to extinguish a response is not to provide any kind of reinforcement for some action. For example, offensive jokes in the workplace may be handled by showing no reaction; after several such experiences, the joke teller, who more than likely wants attention—and negative attention is preferable to no attention—may curtail his use of offensive humor. Keep in mind, too, that desirable behavior that is ignored may lessen as well.

If nonreinforcement proves ineffective, then punishment may be employed as a way to decrease responses, although there are many risks in using this approach. Under punishment conditions, the individual cannot escape or avoid an unpleasant stimulus. Suppose, for example, a health professional student is continually late for class and noisily disrupts the class, annoying other students and the instructor when she arrives. The instructor discovered there is no valid reason for the student's lateness—the student says she overslept, did not allow sufficient time to find a parking place, and other factors she should have more control over. The instructor tried praising the student the few times she came to class on time (positive reinforcement) and tried not paying attention to her when she arrived late (nonreinforcement), but the student continues to be late to class more often than on time. The student appears to enjoy the attention she receives. As a last resort, the instructor may try punishment, which involves applying a negative reinforcer and removing a positive reinforcer. The positive reinforcers to be removed are the attention the student receives and that she really does not need to change her behavior to conform to classroom expectations. The instructor might tell the student that if she is late, she must come in the back door and sit in back of the class, making sure not to disturb anyone (removal of the positive reinforcer of attention). Each time the student is late, the instructor will make note in her grade book (negative reinforcer of not doing well in the course). The problem with using punishment as a technique for teaching is that the learner may become highly emotional and may well divert attention away from the behavior that needs to be changed. Some people who are being punished become so emotional (sad or angry) that they do not remember the behavior for which they are being punished. One of the cardinal rules of operant conditioning is to "punish the behavior, not the person." In this example, the instructor must make it clear that she is punishing being late and disruptive in class rather than convey that she does not like the student.

If punishment is employed, it should be administered immediately after the response with no distractions or means of escape. Punishment must also be consistent and at the highest reasonable level (e.g., health professionals who apologize and smile as they admonish the behavior of a staff member or client are sending out mixed messages and are not likely to be taken seriously or to decrease the behavior they intend). Moreover, punishment should not be prolonged (bringing up old grievances or complaining about a misbehavior at every opportunity), but there should be a time-out following punishment to eliminate the opportunity for positive reinforcement. The purpose of punishment is not to do harm or to serve as a release for anger; rather, the goal is to decrease a specific behavior and to instill self-discipline. Operant conditioning and discussions of punishment were more popular during the mid-20th century than they are currently. However, it is important

for health professionals to be aware of the many cautions about punishment because punishment continues to be used more than it should in the healthcare setting, and all too often in damaging ways.

The use of reinforcement is central to the success of operant conditioning procedures. For operant conditioning to be effective, it is necessary to assess what kinds of reinforcement are likely to increase or decrease behaviors for each individual. Not every client, for example, finds health practitioners' terms of endearment rewarding. Comments such as, "Very nice job, dear," may be presumptuous or offensive to some clients. A second issue involves the timing of reinforcement. Through experimentation with animals and humans, it has been demonstrated that the success of operant conditioning procedures partially depends on the schedule of reinforcement. Initial learning requires a continuous schedule, reinforcing the behavior quickly every time it occurs. If the desired behavior does not occur, then responses that approximate or resemble it can be reinforced, gradually shaping behavior in the direction of the goal for learning. As an illustration, for geriatric patients who appear lethargic and unresponsive, health professionals might begin by rewarding small gestures such as eye contact or a hand that reaches out, and then build on these friendly behaviors toward greater human contact and connection with reality. Once a response is well established, however, it becomes ineffective and inefficient to continually reinforce the behavior; reinforcement then can be administered on a fixed (predictable) or variable (unpredictable) schedule after a given number of responses have been emitted or after the passage of time.

Operant conditioning techniques provide relatively quick and effective ways to change behavior. Carefully planned programs using behavior modification procedures can readily be applied to health care. For example, computerized instruction and tutorials for patients and staff rely heavily on operant conditioning principles in structuring learning programs. In the clinical setting, the families of patients with chronic back pain have been taught to minimize their attention to the patients whenever they complain and behave in dependent, helpless ways, but to pay a lot of attention when the patients attempt to function independently, express a positive attitude, and try to live as normal a life as possible. Some patients respond so well to operant conditioning that they report experiencing less pain as they become more active and involved. Operant conditioning and behavior modification techniques also have been found to work well with some nursing home and long-term care residents, especially those who are losing their cognitive skills (Proctor, Burns, Powell, & Tarrier, 1999).

The behaviorist theory is simple and easy to use, and it encourages clear, objective analysis of observable environmental stimulus conditions, learner responses, and the effects of reinforcements on people's actions. There are, however, some criticisms and cautions to consider. First, this is a teacher-centered model in which learners are assumed to be relatively passive and easily manipulated, which raises a crucial ethical question: Who is to decide what the desirable behavior should be? Too often the desired response is conformity and cooperation to make someone's job easier or more profitable. Second, the theory's emphasis on extrinsic rewards and external incentives reinforces and promotes materialism rather than self-initiative, a love of learning, and intrinsic satisfaction. Third, research evidence supporting behaviorist theory is often based on animal studies, the results of which may not be applicable to human behavior. A fourth shortcoming of behavior modification programs is that clients' changed behavior may deteriorate over time, especially once they are back in their former environment—an environment with a system of rewards and punishments that may have fostered their problems in the first place.

The next section moves from focusing on responses and behavior to the role of mental processes in learning.

Cognitive Learning Theory

Whereas behaviorists generally ignore the internal dynamics of learning, cognitive learning theorists stress the importance of what goes on inside the learner. Cognitive theory is assumed to comprise a number of subtheories and is widely used in education and counseling. The key to learning and changing is the individual's cognition (perception, thought, memory, and ways of processing and structuring information). Cognitive learning, a highly active process largely directed by the individual, involves perceiving the information, interpreting it based on what is already known, and then reorganizing the information into new insights or understanding (Bandura, 2001; Hunt, Ellis, & Ellis, 2004).

Cognitive theorists, unlike behaviorists, maintain that reward is not necessary for learning. More important are learners' goals and expectations, which create disequilibrium, imbalance, and tension that motivate learners to act. Educators trying to influence the learning process must recognize the variety of past experiences, perceptions, ways of incorporating and thinking about information, and diverse aspirations, expectations, and social influences that affect any learning situation. A learner's **metacognition**, or understanding of her way of learning, influences the process as well. To promote transfer of learning, the learner must mediate or act on the information in some way. Similar patterns in the initial learning situation and subsequent situations facilitate this transfer.

Cognitive learning theory includes several well-known perspectives, such as gestalt, information processing, human development, social constructivism, and social cognition theory. More recently, attempts have been made to incorporate considerations related to emotions within cognitive theory. Each of these perspectives emphasizes a particular feature of cognition, which, when pieced together, indicates much about what goes on inside the learner. As the various cognitive perspectives are briefly summarized here, readers are encouraged to think of their potential applications in the healthcare setting. In keeping with cognitive principles of learning, being mentally active with information encourages memory and retention.

One of the oldest psychological theories is the **gestalt perspective**, which emphasizes the importance of perception in learning and lays the groundwork for the various other cognitive perspectives that followed (Kohler, 1947, 1969; Murray, 1995). Rather than focusing on discrete stimuli, gestalt refers to the configuration or patterned organization of cognitive elements, reflecting the maxim that the whole is greater than the sum of the parts. A principal assumption is that each person perceives, interprets, and responds to any situation in his or her own way. Whereas there are many gestalt principles worth knowing (Hilgard & Bower, 1966), several are discussed here as they relate to health care.

A basic gestalt principle is that psychological organization is directed toward simplicity, equilibrium, and regularity. For example, study the bewildered faces of some patients listening to a complex, detailed explanation about their disease, when what they desire most is a simple, clear explanation that settles their uncertainty and relates directly to them and their familiar experiences.

Another central gestalt principle that has several ramifications is that perception is selective. First, because no one can attend to all the surrounding stimuli at any given time, individuals orient themselves to certain features of an experience while screening out or ignoring other features. Patients in severe pain or worried about their hospital bills may not attend to well-intentioned patient education information. Second, what individuals pay attention to and what they ignore are influenced by a host of factors: past experiences, needs, personal motives and attitudes, reference groups, and the particular structure of the stimulus or situation (Sherif & Sherif, 1969). Assessing these internal and external dynamics has a direct bearing on how a health educator approaches any learning situation with an individual or group. Moreover, because individuals vary widely with regard to these and other characteristics, they will perceive, interpret, and respond to the same event in different ways, perhaps distorting reality to fit their goals and expectations. This tendency helps explain why an approach that is effective with one client may not work with another client. People with chronic illnesses—even different people with the same illness—are not alike, and helping any patient with disease or disability includes recognizing each person's unique perceptions and subjective experience (Imes, Clance, Gailis, & Atkeson, 2002).

Information processing is a cognitive perspective that emphasizes thinking processes: thought, reasoning, the way information is encountered and stored, and memory functioning (Gagné, 1985; Sternberg, 2006). How information is incorporated and retrieved is useful for health professionals to know, especially in relation to older people's learning (Hooyman & Kiyak, 2005; Kessels, 2003).

Figure 3–2 illustrates an information-processing model of memory functioning. Tracking learning through the various stages is helpful in assessing what happens to information as each learner perceives, interprets, and remembers it, which, in turn, may suggest ways of improving the structure of the learning situation as well as how to correct misconceptions, distortions, and errors in learning.

The first stage in the memory process involves paying attention to environmental stimuli; attention, then, is the key to learning. Thus, if a client is not attending to what the educator is saying,

Figure 3–2 Information-Processing Model of Memory

perhaps because the client is weary or distracted, it would be prudent for the educator to try the explanation at another time when the client is more receptive and attentive.

In the second stage, the information is processed by the senses. Here it becomes important to consider the client's preferred mode of sensory processing (visual, auditory, or motor manipulation) and to ascertain whether there are sensory deficits.

In the third stage, the information is transformed and incorporated (encoded) briefly into short-term memory, after which it is either disregarded and forgotten or stored in long-term memory. Long-term memory involves the organization of information by using a preferred strategy for storage (e.g., imagery, association, rehearsal, or breaking the information into units). Although long-term memories are enduring, a central problem is retrieving the stored information at a later time.

The last stage involves the action or response that the individual makes on the basis of how information was processed and stored. Education involves assessing how a learner attends to, processes, and stores the information that is presented as well as finding ways to encourage the retention and retrieval processes. Errors are corrected by helping learners reprocess what needs to be learned (Kessels, 2003).

In general, cognitive psychologists note that memory processing and the retrieval of information are enhanced by organizing information and making it meaningful. A widely used descriptive model has been provided by Robert Gagné (1985). Subsequently, Gagné and his colleagues outlined nine events and their corresponding cognitive processes that activate effective learning (Gagné, Briggs, & Wagner, 1992):

- Gain the learner's attention (reception)
- Inform the learner of the objectives and expectations (expectancy)
- Stimulate the learner's recall of prior learning (retrieval)
- Present information (selective perception)

- Provide guidance to facilitate the learner's understanding (semantic encoding)
- Have the learner demonstrate the information or skill (responding)
- Give feedback to the learner (reinforcement)
- Assess the learner's performance (retrieval)
- Work to enhance retention and transfer through application and varied practice (generalization)

In employing this model, instructors must carefully analyze the requirements of the activity, design and sequence the instructional events, and select appropriate media to achieve the outcomes.

Within the information-processing perspective, Sternberg (1996) reminds educators to consider styles of thinking, which he defines as "a preference for using abilities in certain ways" (p. 347). Thinking styles concern differences, he notes, and not judgments of better or worse. In education, the instructor's task is to get in touch with the learner's way of processing information and thinking. Some implications for health care are the need to carefully match jobs with styles of thinking, to recognize that people may shift from preferring one style of thinking to another, and, most important, to appreciate and respect the different styles of thinking reflected among the many players in the healthcare setting (see Chapter 4 on learning styles). Yet striving for a match in styles is not always necessary or desirable. Tennant (2006) notes that adult learners may actually benefit from grappling with views and styles of learning unlike their own, which may promote maturity, creativity, and a greater tolerance for differences. Because health professionals are expected to instruct a variety of people with diverse styles of learning, Tennant's suggestion has interesting implications for professional education programs.

The information-processing perspective is particularly helpful for assessing problems in acquiring, remembering, and recalling information. Some strategies include the following: (1) have learners indicate how they believe they learn (metacognition); (2) ask them to describe what they are thinking as they are learning; (3) evaluate learners' mistakes; and (4) give close attention to their inability to remember or demonstrate information. For example, forgetting or having difficulty in retrieving information from long-term memory is a major stumbling block in learning. This problem may occur because the information has faded from lack of use, other information interferes with its retrieval (what comes before or after a learning session may well confound storage and retrieval), or individuals are motivated to forget for a variety of conscious and unconscious reasons. This material on memory processing and functioning is highly pertinent to healthcare practice—whether in developing health education brochures, engaging in one-to-one patient education, delivering a staff development workshop, preparing community health lectures, or studying for courses and examinations. Focusing on attention, storage, and memory is essential in the patient education of older adults, including the identification of fatigue, medications, and anxieties that may interfere with learning and remembering (Kessels, 2003).

Heavily influenced by gestalt psychology, **cognitive development** is a third perspective on learning that focuses on qualitative changes in perceiving, thinking, and reasoning as individuals grow and mature (Santrock, 2006; Vander Zanden, Crandell, & Crandell, 2007). Cognitions are based on how external events are conceptualized, organized, and represented within each person's mental framework or schema, which is partially dependent on the individual's stage of development in perception, reasoning, and readiness to learn.

Much of the theory and research in this area has been concerned with identifying the characteristics and advances in the thought processes of children and adolescents. A principal assumption is that learning is a developmental, sequential, and active process that transpires as the child interacts with the environment, makes discoveries about how the world operates, and interprets these discoveries in keeping with what she knows (schema).

Jean Piaget is the best known of the cognitive developmental theorists. His observations of children's perceptions and thought processes at different ages have contributed much to our recognition of the unique, changing abilities of youngsters to reason, conceptualize, communicate, and perform (Piaget & Inhelder, 1969). By watching, asking questions, and listening to children, Piaget identified and described four sequential stages of cognitive development (sensorimotor, preoperational, concrete operations, and formal operations). These stages become evident over the course of infancy, early childhood, middle childhood, and adolescence, respectively (see Chapter 5 on developmental stages). According to Piaget's theory of cognitive learning, children take in information as they interact with people and the environment. They either make their experiences fit with what they already know (assimilation) or change their perceptions and interpretations in keeping with the new information (accommodation). Health professionals and family members need to determine what children are perceiving and thinking in a given situation. As an illustration, young children usually do not comprehend fully that death is final. They respond to the death of a loved one in their own way, perhaps asking God to give back the dead person or believing that if they act like a good person, the deceased loved one will return to them (Gardner, 1978).

Within the cognitive development perspective are some differences worth considering. For example, while Piaget stresses the importance of perception in learning and views children as little scientists exploring, interacting, and discovering the world in a relative solitary manner, Russian psychologist Lev Vygotsky (1986) emphasizes the significance of language, social interaction, and adult guidance in the learning process. When teaching children, Vygotsky says the job of adults is to interpret, respond, and give meaning to children's actions. Rather than the discovery method favored by Piaget, Vygotsky advocates clear, well-designed instruction that is carefully structured to advance each person's thinking and learning.

In practice, some children may learn more effectively by discovering and putting pieces together on their own, whereas other children benefit from a more social and directive approach. It is the health educator's responsibility to identify the child's or teenager's stage of thinking, to provide experiences at an appropriate level for children to actively discover and participate in the learning process, and to determine whether a child learns best through language and social interaction or through perceiving and experimenting in his or her own way. Research suggests that young children's learning is often more solitary, whereas older children may learn more readily through social interaction (Palincsar, 1998).

What do cognitive developmental theorists say about adult learning? First, although the cognitive stages develop sequentially, some adults never reach the formal operations stage. These adults may learn better from explicitly concrete approaches to health education. Second, adult developmental psychologists and gerontologists have proposed advanced stages of reasoning in adulthood beyond formal operations. For example, it is not until the adult years that people become better able to deal with contradictions, synthesize information, and more effectively integrate what they have learned—characteristics that differentiate adult thought from adolescent thinking (Kramer, 1983). Third, older adults may demonstrate an advanced level of reasoning derived from their wisdom and life experiences, or they may reflect lower stages of thinking resulting from lack of education, disease, depression, extraordinary stress, or medications (Hooyman & Kiyak, 2005).

Research indicates that adults generally do better with self-directed learning (emphasizing learner control, autonomy, and initiative), an explicit rationale for learning, a problem-oriented rather than subject-oriented approach, and the opportunity to use their experiences and skills to help others (Tennant, 2006). Also, educators must keep in mind that anxiety, the demands of adult life, and childhood experiences may interfere with learning in adulthood.

Because cognitive theory was criticized for neglecting the social context, the effects of social factors on perception, thought, and motivation are receiving increased attention. **Social constructivism** and **social cognition** are two increasingly popular perspectives within cognitive theory. Drawing heavily from gestalt psychology and developmental psychology, social constructivists take issue with some of the highly rational assumptions of the information-processing view and build on the works of John Dewey, Jean Piaget, and Lev Vygotsky (Palincsar, 1998). Social constructivists posit that individuals formulate or construct their own versions of reality and that learning and human development are richly colored by the social and cultural context in which people find themselves. A central tenet of this approach is that ethnicity, social class, gender, family life, past history, self-concept, and the learning situation itself all influence an individual's perceptions, thoughts, emotions, interpretations, and responses to information and experiences. A second principle is that effective learning occurs through social interaction, collaboration, and negotiation (Shapiro, 2002).

According to this view, the players in any healthcare setting may have differing perceptions of external reality, including distorted perceptions and interpretations. Every person operates on the basis of her unique representations and interpretations of a situation, all of which have been heavily influenced by that individual's social and cultural experiences. The impact of culture cannot be ignored, and learning is facilitated by sharing beliefs, by acknowledging and challenging differing conceptions, and by negotiating new levels of conceptual understanding (Marshall, 1998). Cooperative learning and self-help groups are examples of social constructivism in action. With the rapidly changing age and ethnic composition in the United States, the social constructivist perspective has much to contribute to health education and health promotion efforts.

Rooted in social psychology, the social cognition perspective reflects a constructivist orientation and highlights the influence of social factors on perception, thought, and motivation. A host of scattered explanations can be found under the rubric of social cognition (Fiske & Taylor, 1991; Moskowitz, 2005), which, when applied to learning, emphasizes the need for instructors to consider the dynamics of the social environment and groups on both interpersonal and intrapersonal behavior. As an illustration, attribution theory concerns the cause-and-effect relationships and explanations that individuals formulate to account for their own and others' behavior and the way in which the world operates. Many of these explanations are unique to the individual and tend to be strongly colored by cultural values and beliefs. For example, patients with certain religious views or a particular parental upbringing may believe that their disease is a punishment for their sins (internalizing blame); other patients may attribute their disease to the actions of others (externalizing blame). From this perspective, patients' attributions may or may not promote wellness and well-being. The route to changing health behaviors is to change distorted attributions. The medical staff's prejudices, biases (positive and negative), and attributions need to be considered as well in the healing process.

Cognitive theory has been criticized for neglecting emotions, and recent efforts have been made to incorporate considerations related to emotions within a cognitive framework, known as the **cognitive-emotional perspective**. As Eccles and Wigfield (2002) comment, " 'Cold' cognitive models cannot adequately capture conceptual change; there is a need to consider affect as well" (p. 127).

Several slightly different cognitive orientations to emotions have been proposed and are briefly summarized in the following list:

- Empathy and the moral emotions (e.g., guilt, shame, distress, moral outrage) play a significant role in influencing children's moral development and in motivating people's prosocial behavior and ethical responses (Hoffman, 2000).
- Memory storage and retrieval, as well as moral decision making, involve both cognitive and emotional brain processing, especially in response to situations that directly involve the self and are stressful (Greene, Sommerville, Nystrom, Darley, & Cohen, 2001).
- Emotional intelligence (EI) entails an individual managing his emotions, motivating himself, reading the emotions of others, and working effectively in interpersonal relationships, which some argue is more important to leadership, social judgment, and moral behavior than cognitive intelligence is (Goleman, 1995).
- Self-regulation includes monitoring cognitive processes, emotions, and the individual's surroundings to achieve goals, which is considered a key factor to successful living and effective social behavior (Eccles & Wigfield, 2002).

The implications are that health professional education programs would do well to exhibit and encourage empathy and emotional intelligence in working with patients, family, and staff and to attend to the dynamics of self-regulation as a way to promote positive personal growth and effective leadership. Research indicates that the development of these attributes in self and patients is associated with a greater likelihood of healthy behavior, psychological well-being, optimism, and meaningful social interactions (Brackett, Lopes, Ivcevic, Mayer, & Salovey, 2004).

A significant benefit of the cognitive theory to health care is its encouragement of recognizing and appreciating individuality and diversity in how people learn and process experiences. When applied to health care, cognitive theory has been useful in formulating exercise programs for breast cancer patients (Rogers et al., 2004), understanding individual differences in bereavement (Stroebe, Folkman, Hansson, & Schut, 2006), and dealing with adolescent depression in girls (Papadakis, Prince, Jones, & Strauman, 2006). Cognitive theory highlights the wide variation in how learners actively structure their perceptions; confront a learning situation; encode, process, store, and retrieve information; and manage their emotions, all of which are affected by social and cultural influences. The challenge to educators is to identify each learner's level of cognitive development and the social influences that affect learning, and then find ways to foster insight, creativity, and problem solving. Difficulties lie in ascertaining exactly what is transpiring inside the mind of each individual and in designing learning activities that encourage people to restructure their perceptions, reorganize their thinking, regulate their emotions, change their attributions and behavior, and create solutions.

The next learning theory combines principles from both the behaviorist and cognitive theories.

Social Learning Theory

Social learning theory is largely the work of Albert Bandura (1977, 2001), who mapped out a perspective on learning that includes consideration of the personal characteristics of the learner, behavior patterns, and the environment. The theory has gone through several "paradigm shifts" (Bandura, 2001, p. 2). In early formulations, Bandura emphasized behaviorist features and the imitation of role models; next the focus shifted to cognitive considerations, such as the attributes of the self and the internal processing of the learner. More recently, Bandura's attention turned to the impact of social factors and the social context within which learning and behavior occur. As the model has evolved, the learner has become viewed as central (what Bandura calls a "human agency"), which suggests the need to identify what learners are perceiving and how they are interpreting and responding to social situations. As such, careful consideration needs to be given to the healthcare environment as a social situation.

One of Bandura's early observations was that individuals need not have direct experiences to learn; considerable learning occurs by taking note of other people's behavior and what happens to them. Thus, learning is often a social process, and other individuals, especially significant others, provide compelling examples or role models for how to think, feel, and act. **Role modeling** is a central concept of the theory. As an example, a more experienced healthcare provider who demonstrates desirable professional attitudes and behaviors sometimes is used as a mentor for a less experienced colleague. When asked what qualities make an "exceptional" clinical practice educator in occupational therapy, students identified being a role model as an important characteristic (Mulholland, Derdall, & Roy, 2006). Research indicates that nurse managers' attitudes and actions—ensuring safety, integrating knowledge with practice, sharing feelings, challenging staff nurses and students, and demonstrating competence and willingness to provide guidance to others—influence the outcomes of the clinical supervision process (Berggren & Severinsson, 2006). How nurse mentors perceive their role is an important consideration in the leadership selection process (Neary, 2000).

Vicarious reinforcement is another concept from the social learning theory and involves determining whether role models are perceived as rewarded or punished for their behavior. Reward is not always necessary, however, and a learner may

imitate the behavior of a role model even when no reward is involved for either the role model or the learner. In many cases, however, whether the model is viewed by the observer as rewarded or punished may have a direct influence on learning. This relationship may be one reason why it is difficult to attract health professionals to geriatric care. Although some highly impressive role models work in the field, geriatric health care is often accorded lower status with less pay in comparison to other specialty areas.

Although social learning theory is based partially on behaviorist principles, the self-regulation and control that the individual exerts in the process of acquiring knowledge and changing behavior are considered more critical and are more reflective of cognitive principles. Bandura (1977) outlines a four-step, largely internal process that directs social learning, as can be seen in **Figure 3–3**. Although some components are similar to the information-processing model described previously, a principal difference is the inclusion of a motivational component in the social learning theory model.

First is the attentional phase, a necessary condition for any learning to occur. Research indicates that role models with high status and competence are more likely to be observed, although the learner's own characteristics (needs, self-esteem, competence) may be the more significant determiner of attention. Second is the retention phase, which involves the storage and retrieval of what was observed. Third is the reproduction phase, where the learner copies the observed behavior. Mental rehearsal, immediate enactment, and corrective feedback strengthen the reproduction of behavior. Fourth is the motivational phase, which focuses on whether the learner is motivated to perform a certain type of behavior. Reinforcement or punishment for a role model's behavior, the learning situation, and the appropriateness of subsequent situations where the behavior is to be displayed all affect a learner's performance (Bandura, 1977; Gage

Figure 3–3 Social Learning Theory

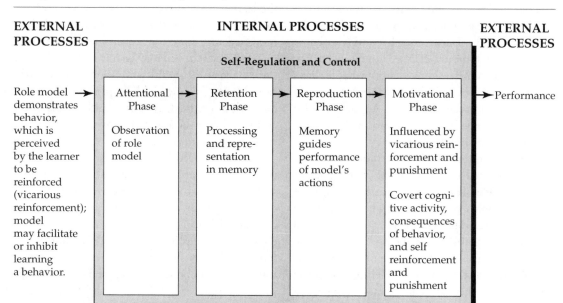

& Berliner, 1998). Well suited to conducting health education and staff development training, this organized approach to learning requires attention to the social environment, the behavior to be performed, and the individual learner (Bahn, 2001).

Reflecting a constructivist orientation, Bandura (2001) shifts his focus to sociocultural influences, viewing the learner as the agent through which learning experiences are filtered. As he argues, the human mind is not just reactive; it is generative, creative, and reflective. Essentially, the individual engages in a transactional relationship between the social environment and the self, where sociocultural factors are mediated by "psychological mechanisms of the self-system to produce behavioral effects" (p. 4). In his model, Bandura stresses the internal dynamics of personal selection, intentionality, self-regulation, self-efficacy, and self-evaluation in the learning process. Culture and self-efficacy play a

key role, with Bandura noting that individualistic cultures interpret self-efficacy differently from how group-oriented cultures interpret it. However defined, a low sense of self-efficacy in either kind of culture produces stress. This perspective applies particularly well to the acquisition of health behaviors and partially explains why some people select positive role models and effectively regulate their attitudes, emotions, and actions, whereas other people choose negative role models and engage in unhealthy and destructive behaviors. Health professionals need to find ways to encourage patients' feelings of competency and to promote wellness rather than fostering dependency, helplessness, and feelings of low self-worth.

The social learning theory extends the learning process beyond the educator–learner relationship to the larger social world. The theory helps explain the socialization process as well as the breakdown of behavior in society. Responsibility is placed on the educator or leader to act as an exemplary role model and to choose socially healthy experiences for individuals to observe and repeat (requiring the careful evaluation of learning materials for stereotypes, mixed or hidden messages, and negative effects). Yet simple exposure to role models correctly performing a behavior that is rewarded (or performing some undesirable behavior that is punished) does not ensure learning. Attention to the learner's self-system and the dynamics of self-regulation may help sort out the varying effects of the social learning experience.

In health care, social learning theory has been applied to health professional education, to community mental health settings, to addressing psychosocial problems, and to maximizing the use of support groups. For example, research indicates that those managers who are aware of their roles and responsibilities in promoting a positive work environment enhance learning, competence, and satisfaction; dissatisfaction, of course, has a detrimental effect and is a significant cause of staff turnover (Kane-Urrabazo, 2006). Nurses have applied social learning principles successfully when working with teenage mothers (Stiles, 2005) and in addressing alcoholism among older adults (Akers, 1989). Mental health providers used a social learning theory paradigm to organize training and changes within their system to make employment a higher priority among community mental health services (Waynor, Pratt, Dolce, Bates, & Roberts, 2005). A major difficulty is that this theory is complex and not easily operationalized, measured, and assessed.

The final two theories reviewed in this chapter focus on the importance of emotions and feelings in the learning process.

Psychodynamic Learning Theory

Although not typically treated as a learning theory, some of the constructs from the psychodynamic theory (based on the work of Sigmund Freud and his followers) have significant implications for learning and changing behavior (Hilgard & Bower, 1966; Slipp, 2000). Largely a theory of motivation stressing emotions rather than cognition or responses, the psychodynamic perspective emphasizes the importance of conscious and unconscious forces in guiding behavior, personality conflicts, and the enduring effects of childhood experiences. As Pullen (2002) points out, negative emotions are important to recognize and assess in nurse–patient–doctor–family interactions, and the psychodynamic theory can be helpful in this regard.

A central principle of the theory is that behavior may be conscious or unconscious—that is, individuals may or may not be aware of their motivations and why they feel, think, and act as they do. According to the psychodynamic view, the most primitive source of motivation comes from the id and is based on libidinal energy (the basic instincts, impulses, and desires humans are born with), which includes eros (the desire for pleasure and sex, sometimes called the "life force") and thanatos (aggressive and destructive impulses, or death wish). Patients who survive or die despite all predictions to the contrary provide illustrations of such primitive motivations. The id, according to Freud, operates on the basis of the pleasure principle—to seek pleasure and avoid pain. For example, dry, dull lectures given by health professional educators who go through the motions of the presentation without much enthusiasm or emotion inspire few people (clients, staff, or students) to listen to the information or heed the advice being given. This does not mean, however, that only pleasurable presentations are acceptable.

The id (primitive drives) and superego (internalized societal values and standards, or the conscience) are mediated by the ego, which operates on the basis of the reality principle—rather than insisting on immediate gratification, people learn to take the long road to pleasure and to weigh the choices or dilemmas in the conflict between the id and superego. Healthy ego (self) development, as emphasized by Freud's followers, is an important consideration in the health fields. For example, patients with ego strength can cope with painful medical treatments because they recognize the long-term value of enduring discomfort and pain to achieve a positive outcome. Clients with weak ego development, in contrast, may miss their appointments and treatments or engage in short-term pleasurable activities that work against their healing and recovery. Helping clients develop ego strength and adjust realistically to a changed body image or lifestyle brought about by disease and medical interventions is a significant aspect of the learning and healing processes. Health professionals, too, require personal ego strength to cope with the numerous predicaments in the everyday practice of delivering care as they face conflicting values, ethics, and demands. Professional burnout, for example, is rooted in an overly idealized concept of the healthcare role and unrealistic expectations for the self in performing the role. Malach-Pines

(2000) notes that burnout may stem from nurses' childhood experiences with lack of control.

When the ego is threatened, as can easily occur in the healthcare setting, **defense mechanisms** may be employed to protect the self. The short-term use of defense mechanisms is a way of coming to grips with reality. The danger comes in the overuse or long-term reliance on defense mechanisms, which allows individuals to avoid reality and may act as a barrier to learning and transfer. **Table 3–2** describes some of the more commonly used defense mechanisms. Because of the stresses involved in health care, knowledge of defense mechanisms is useful, whether students are grappling with the challenges of health professional education, staff are dealing with the strains of working in hospitals and long-term care facilities, or clients and their families are learning to cope with illness.

As an example of defense mechanisms in health care, Kübler-Ross (1969) points out that many terminally ill patients' initial reaction to being told they have a serious threat to their health and well-being is to employ the defense mechanism

---

Table 3–2 EGO DEFENSE MECHANISMS: WAYS OF PROTECTING THE SELF FROM PERCEIVED THREAT

Denial: Ignoring or refusing to acknowledge the reality of a threat

Rationalization: Excusing or explaining away a threat

Displacement: Taking out hostility and aggression on other individuals rather than directing anger at the source of the threat

Depression: Keeping unacceptable thoughts, feelings, or actions from conscious awareness

Regression: Returning to an earlier (less mature, more primitive) stage of behavior as a way of coping with a threat

Intellectualization: Minimizing anxiety by responding to a threat in a detached, abstract manner without feeling or emotion

Projection: Seeing one's own unacceptable characteristics or desires in other people

Reaction formation: Expressing or behaving the opposite of what is really felt

Sublimation: Converting repressed feelings into socially acceptable action

Compensation: Making up for weaknesses by excelling in other areas of denial. It is too overwhelming for patients to process the information that they are likely to die. Although most patients gradually accept the reality of their illness, the dangers are that if they remain in a state of denial, they may not seek treatment and care, and if their illness is contagious, they may not protect others against infection. In turn, a common defense mechanism employed by healthcare staff is to intellectualize rather than deal realistically at an emotional level with the significance of disease and death. This defense mechanism may contribute to the reported tendency of oncologists to often ignore, rather than address, the emotion that patients express during communication (Friedrichsen & Strang, 2003; Friedrichsen, Strang, & Carlsson, 2000; Pollak et al., 2007). One study in particular found that oncologists responding to patients expressing fear more often addressed the topic causing the fear, rather than addressing the emotion itself (Kennifer et al., 2009). Telford, Kralik, and Koch (2006) report that nurses may strive too quickly to classify terminally ill patients within a denial–acceptance framework and, as a result, may not listen to patients attempting to tell their stories and interpret their illness experiences. Protecting the self (ego) by dehumanizing patients and treating them as diseases and body parts rather than as whole individuals (with spiritual, emotional, and physical needs) are occupational hazards for health professionals.

Another central assumption of the psychodynamic theory is that personality development occurs in stages, with much of adult behavior derived from earlier childhood experiences and conflicts. One of the most widely used models of personality development is Erikson's (1968) eight stages of life, organized around a psychosocial crisis to be resolved at each stage (see Chapter 5). Treatment regimens, communication, and health education need to include considerations of the patient's stage of personality development. For example, in working with 4- and 5-year-old patients, where the crisis is

initiative versus guilt, health professionals should encourage the children to offer their ideas and to make and do things themselves. Staff also must be careful not to make these children feel guilty for their illness or misfortune. As a second example, the adolescent's psychosocial developmental needs to have friends and to find an identity require special attention in health care. Adolescent patients may benefit from help and support in adjusting to a changed body image and in addressing their fears of weakness, lack of activity, and social isolation. One danger is that young people may treat their illness or impairment as a significant dimension of their identity and self-concept—well described in poet Lucy Grealy's (1994) personal account in *Anatomy of a Face.*

According to the psychodynamic view, personal difficulties arise and learning is limited when individuals become fixated or stuck at an earlier stage of personality development. They then must work through their previously unresolved crises to develop and mature emotionally. For example, some staff members and clients feel an inordinate need to control the self, other people, and certain social situations. This behavior may be rooted in their inability to resolve the crisis of trust versus mistrust at the earliest stage of life. In working with these individuals, it is essential to build a trusting relationship and to encourage them gradually to relinquish some control.

Past conflicts, especially during childhood, may interfere with the ability to learn or to transfer learning. What people resist talking about or learning, termed **resistance**, is an indicator of underlying emotional difficulties, which must be dealt with for them to move ahead emotionally and behaviorally. For instance, a young, pregnant teenager who refuses to engage in a serious conversation about sexuality (e.g., changes the subject, giggles, looks out into space, expresses anger) indicates that she has underlying emotional conflicts that need to be addressed. One study explored psychodynamic sources of resistance among nursing students and how they engaged with or resisted the learning process. A number of factors requiring consideration surfaced, including childhood struggles, a history of overadaptation, self-image, and learning climate (Gilmartin, 2000).

Serious problems in miscommunication can occur in health care as a result of childhood learning experiences. For example, some health professionals may have had the childhood experience of standing helplessly by watching someone they loved and once depended on endure disease, suffering, and death. Although they could do little as children to improve the situation, they may be compensating for their childhood feelings of helplessness and dependency as adults by devoting their careers to fending off and fighting disease and death. These motivations, however, may not serve them well as they attempt to cope, communicate, and educate patients who are dying and their families.

Emotional conflicts are not always caused by internal forces; society exerts pressures on individuals that promote emotional difficulties as well. The reluctance of health professionals to be open and honest with a terminally ill patient partially may be derived from American culture, which encourages medical personnel to fix their patients and extend life. Staff members may or may not be conscious of these pressures, but either way they are likely to feel guilty and that they are failures when dealing with a patient who is dying.

The concept of transfer has special meaning to psychodynamic theorists. **Transference** occurs when individuals project their feelings, conflicts, and reactions—especially those developed during childhood with significant others such as parents—onto authority figures and other individuals in their lives. The danger is that the relationship between the health professional and the patient may become distorted and unrealistic because of the biases inherent in the transference reaction. For example, because patients are sick, they may feel helpless and dependent and then regress to

an earlier stage in life when they relied on their parents for help and support. Their childhood feelings and relationship with a parent—for better or worse—may be transferred to a health professional taking care of them. While sometimes flattering, the love and dependency that patients feel may operate against the autonomy and independence they need to get back on their feet. A particular patient may also remind a health professional of someone from his past, creating a situation of countertransference.

The psychodynamic approach reminds health professionals to pay attention to emotions, unconscious motivations, and the psychological growth and development of all those involved in health care and learning. Health care rests on both interpersonal and intrapersonal processes involved in the therapeutic use of the self in carrying out patient care (Gallop & O'Brien, 2003). Psychodynamic theory is well suited to understanding patient and family noncompliance (Menahern & Halasz, 2000), trauma and loss (Duberstein & Masling, 2000), palliative care and the deeply emotional issues of terminal illness (Chochinov & Breitbart, 2000), and the anxieties of working with long-term psychiatric residents (Goodwin & Gore, 2000).

The psychodynamic approach has been criticized because much of the analysis is speculative and subjective, and the theory is difficult to operationalize and measure. Psychodynamic theory also can be used inappropriately; it is not the job of health professionals with little clinical psychology or psychiatric training to probe into the private lives and feelings of patients so as to uncover deep, unconscious conflicts. Another danger is that health professionals may depend on the many psychodynamic constructs as a way of intellectualizing or explaining away, rather than dealing with, people as individuals who need emotional care. The psychodynamic perspective is helpful in more fully understanding learning and teaching because it highlights a number of underlying considerations and subtleties in the process, such as motivations, emotional development and conflicts in learning, and identifying problems in learning or with the teacher–learner relationship.

Humanistic Learning Theory

Underlying the humanistic perspective on learning is the assumption that each individual is unique and that all individuals have a desire to grow in a positive way. Unfortunately, positive psychological growth may be damaged by some of society's values and expectations (e.g., males are less emotional than females, some ethnic groups are inferior to others, making money is more important than caring for people) and by adults' mistreatment of their children and each other (e.g., inconsistent or harsh discipline, humiliation and belittling, abuse and neglect). Spontaneity, the importance of emotions and feelings, the right of individuals to make their own choices, and human creativity are the cornerstones of a humanistic approach to learning (Rogers, 1994; Snowman & Biehler, 2006). Humanistic theory is especially compatible with health care's focus on caring and patient centeredness—an orientation that is increasingly challenged by the emphasis on science, technology, cost efficiency, for-profit medicine, bureaucratic organization, and time pressures.

Like the psychodynamic theory, the humanistic perspective is largely a motivational theory. From a humanistic perspective, motivation is derived from each person's needs, subjective feelings about the self, and the desire to grow. The transfer of learning is facilitated by curiosity, a positive self-concept, and open situations in which people respect individuality and promote freedom of choice. Under such conditions, transfer is likely to be widespread, enhancing flexibility and creativity.

Maslow (1954, 1987), a major contributor to humanistic theory, is perhaps best known for identifying the **hierarchy of needs (Figure 3–4)**, which he says plays an important role in human

motivation. At the bottom of the hierarchy are physiological needs (food, warmth, sleep); then come safety needs; then the need for belonging and love; followed by self-esteem. At the top of the hierarchy are self-actualization needs (maximizing one's potential). Additional considerations include cognitive needs (to know and understand) and, for some individuals, aesthetic needs (the desire for beauty). An assumption is that basic-level needs must be met before individuals can be concerned with learning and self-actualizing. Thus, clients who are hungry, tired, and in pain are motivated to get these biological needs met before being interested in learning about their illness, rules for self-care, and health education. Although intuitively appealing, research has not been able to support Maslow's hierarchy of needs with much consistency. For example, although some people's basic needs may not be met, they may nonetheless engage in creative activities, extend themselves to other people, and enjoy learning (Pfeffer, 1985).

Besides personal needs, humanists contend that self-concept and self-esteem are necessary considerations in any learning situation. The therapist Carl Rogers (1961, 1994) argues that what people want is unconditional positive self-regard (the feeling of being loved without strings attached). Experiences that are threatening, coercive, and judgmental undermine the ability and enthusiasm of individuals to learn. It is essential that those in positions of authority convey a fundamental respect for the people with whom they work. If a health professional is prejudiced against patients with AIDS, then little will be healing or therapeutic in her relationship with them until she is genuinely able to feel respect for the patient as an individual.

Rather than acting as an authority, say humanists, the role of any educator or leader is to be a facilitator (Rogers, 1994). Listening—rather than talking—is the skill needed. Because the uniqueness of the individual is fundamental to the humanistic perspective, much of the learning experience requires a direct relationship between

Figure 3–4 Maslow's Hierarchy of Needs

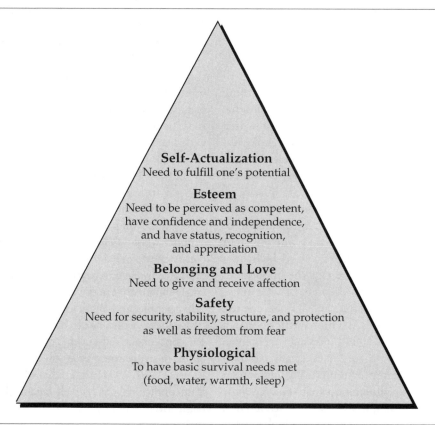

the educator and the learner, with instruction tailored to the needs, self-esteem, and positive growth of each learner. Learners, not educators, choose what is to be learned, and within this framework educators serve as resource persons whose job is to encourage learners to make wise choices. Because the central focus is on learners' perceptions, desires, and decision making, the humanistic orientation is referred to as a learner-directed approach (Snowman & Biehler, 2006).

Mastering information and facts is not the central purpose of the humanistic model of learning. Instead, fostering curiosity, enthusiasm, initiative,

and responsibility is much more important and enduring and should be the primary goal of any educator. Rather than inserting health education videos into television sets for clients in hospitals to view or routinely distributing lots of pamphlets and pages of small-print instructions, the humanistic perspective would suggest establishing rapport and becoming emotionally attuned to patients and their family members. In professional education, the goal is to provide psychologically safe classrooms and clinical environments, where humanistic principles can be taught through caring, role modeling, small-group discussion, case discussions, attention to self-awareness and feelings, role-playing, and videotaping students in the clinical setting followed by feedback and reflection (Biderman, 2003). Providing time for student reflection is essential, and instructor feedback must be given sensitively and thoughtfully (Fryer-Edwards et al., 2006).

Humanistic psychology contends that feelings and emotions are the keys to learning, communication, and understanding. Humanists worry that in today's stressful society, people can easily lose touch with their feelings, which sets the stage for emotional problems and difficulties in learning (Rogers, 1961). To humanists, "tell me how you feel" is a much more important instruction than "tell me what you think" because thoughts and admonitions (the latter of which Rogers calls "the shoulds") may be at odds with true feelings. Consider the implications of the following statements: (1) a young person who says, "I know I should go to medical school and become a doctor because I am smart and that is what my parents want, but I don't feel comfortable with people who are sick—I don't even like them!" or (2) the patient who is dying who says, "I realize that I am going to die and should be brave, but I feel so sad that I am losing my family, my friends, and my self; frankly, I am afraid of dying—all the pain and suffering, being a burden—I'm scared!" In both cases, humanists would argue, the overriding factor that will affect the behavior of the young person and the patient who is dying is their feelings, not their cognitions.

The humanistic learning theory has modified the approach to education and changing behavior by giving primary focus to the subjective needs and feelings of the learner and by redefining the role of the educator. Humanistic principles have been a cornerstone of self-help groups, wellness programs, and palliative care. Humanistic theory has also been found to be well suited to working with children and young patients undergoing separation anxiety caused by illness, surgery,

and recovery (Holyoake, 1998) and for working in the areas of mental health and palliative care (Barnard, Hollingum, & Hartfiel, 2006). Similar to psychodynamic theory, a principal emphasis is on the healing nature of the **therapeutic relationship** (Pearson, 2006) and the need for students and health professionals to grow emotionally from their healthcare experiences (Block & Billings, 1998).

The humanistic theory has its weaknesses as well. Research has not been able to substantiate some of its strongest claims, and the theory has been criticized for promoting self-centered learners who cannot take criticism or compromise their deeply felt positions. Charged with being more of a philosophy—or a cult—than a science, the touchy-feely approach of humanists makes some learners and educators feel truly uncomfortable. Moreover, information, facts, memorization, drill, practice, and the tedious work sometimes required to master knowledge, which humanists minimize and sometimes disdain, have been found to contribute to significant learning, knowledge building, and skill development (Gage & Berliner, 1992).

Neuropsychology and Learning

One of the newest and most rapidly growing areas of psychology research involves investigations into the physiological and neurological bases of thinking, learning, and behavior. Neuroscience research has implications for learning in several ways: (1) by documenting the dynamics of brain and central nervous system processing of information; (2) by understanding and working with children and adults who have neurological conditions, face mental health issues, or have learning disabilities; (3) by answering questions about the relationship between stress and learning; and (4) by providing evidence to support the assumptions of various learning theories or the integration of these theories.

Much of the information in these areas has been gained through advances in neuroimaging techniques such as functional magnetic resonance imaging (fMRI) and positron emission tomography (PET). Other methodologies include animal studies based on surgery, electrical recordings (EEG and ERP), and case studies of children and adults with head trauma, brain lesions, and neurological abnormalities (Byrnes, 2001). Although the research findings highlight some of the underlying biological mechanisms of learning and provide evidence to support some of the principal constructs and dynamics of existing learning theories, there is as yet no coherent physiological or neuropsychological theory of learning.

In synthesizing neuropsychology research, some generalizations about learning can be made (Anderson, 1997; Gazzaniga, 2000; Page, 2006; Phelps, 2006; Shors, 2006; Silverstein & Uhlhaas, 2004). Each of the following generalizations has implications for health education in the clinical setting, and readers are encouraged to formulate applications to health care:

- Emotions have been found to play a key role in Pavlovian conditioning, information processing, memory, and motivation. Emotions are considered to interact with cognitive factors in any learning situation, suggesting that they cannot be ignored when teaching, learning, reasoning, or making decisions.
- Neuropsychology studies of learning confirm a number of learning theories and constructs, including gestalt principles, constructivism, Piaget's notions of assimilation and accommodation, and Freud's conceptualization of conscious and unconscious processes. Neurological studies also document physiological arousal and track attention, perception, and the organization of experience while learning.
- Learning is a function of physiological and neurological developmental changes that are ongoing and dynamic; the brain is less fixed than

once thought, and it changes with learning and experience (called "plasticity").
- Brain processing is different for each learner; thus, methods of gaining the learner's attention, controlling the pace of learning, and identifying the specific mechanisms for enhancing learning are unique for each person.
- Learning is an active, multifaceted, complex process that involves preferred and interacting sensory modes, is colored by the past and present social context, and is regulated largely by the learner on the basis of his or her development, experiences, and sense of self.
- Meaningful practice strengthens learning connections, which may fade from lack of use; thus, one-shot patient education efforts are not likely to be effective in changing behavior.
- Stress can interfere with or stimulate learning, although the responses to stress may change with age and differ for males and females and for those who have experienced traumatic events.

Neurophysiological aspects of learning become all the more germane for children and adults with physiological disorders; for those with mental, emotional, and behavioral problems; and for those facing the stresses of trauma, disease, disability, and socioeconomic hardship. Despite numerous neuroscientific studies related to learning, the research is in its early stages and remains fragmented, scattered, and lacking in integration. In addition, neuropsychological studies are often based on animal research or on highly specialized and restricted human samples, so few generalizations can be made about most people. Although addressing the various biological connections to learning is currently a popular and relatively well-funded area of research, there is a risk of reducing human behavior to mere biology while ignoring the individual as a person as well as the significance and complexity of psychological and social processes in any learning situation.

Comparison of Learning Theories

Table 3–3 provides a comparative summary of the five psychological learning theories outlined in this chapter. Health educators can make generalizations about both the differences and the similarities in what the theories say about acquiring knowledge and changing feelings, attitudes, and behavior. With regard to some of the differences among the theories, each theory has its own assumptions, vocabulary, and way of conceptualizing the learning process. The theories differ in their emphasis on the relative influence of external or internal factors in learning, the view of the learner as more passive or active, the task of the educator, the explanation of motivation, and the way in which the transfer of learning is accomplished.

A logical question is which of these five theories best describes or explains learning—which theory, in other words, would be the most helpful to health professionals interested in increasing knowledge or changing the behavior of patients, clients, staff, or themselves? The answer to this question is that each theory contributes to understanding various aspects of the learning process and can be used singly or in combination to help practitioners acquire new information and alter existing thoughts, feelings, and behavior.

Each theory gives focus to important considerations in any learning situation, involving the consideration of external social factors and internal psychological processing. For example, behaviorists urge health professionals as educators to pay attention to and change stimulus conditions and to provide reinforcement to alter behavior. Although criticized for being reductionistic, behaviorists' emphasis on manipulating the environment and reinforcements is admittedly simpler and easier than trying to undertake a massive overhaul of an individual's internal dynamics (perceptions, cognition, memory, feelings, and personality history

and conflicts). Moreover, asking someone first to behave in a more appropriate way (abstaining from bad habits and engaging in healthy behavior) may not be as threatening or daunting to the learner as it is to suggest the need for internal personality changes. Desired responses are modified and strengthened through practice; the new learned responses, in turn, may lead to more fundamental changes in attitudes and emotions. The social learning perspective is another relatively simple theory to use, stressing the importance of effective role models, who, by their example, demonstrate exactly what behavior is expected.

Cognitive, social learning, psychodynamic, and humanistic theories remind health practitioners to consider internal factors—perceptions, thoughts, ways of processing information, feelings, and emotions. Educators cannot ignore these factors because, ultimately, the learner controls and regulates learning: how information is perceived, interpreted, and remembered, and whether the new knowledge is expressed or performed.

In practice, psychological learning theories should not be considered to be mutually exclusive but rather to operate together to change attitudes and behavior. For example, patients undergoing painful procedures are first taught systematic desensitization (behaviorist) and while experiencing pain or discomfort are encouraged to employ imagery, such as thinking about a favorite, beautiful place or imagining the healthy cells gobbling up the unhealthy cells (cognitive). Staff members are highly respectful, upbeat, and emotionally supportive of each patient (humanistic) and create the time and opportunity to listen to clients discuss some of their deepest fears and concerns (psychodynamic). Waiting rooms and lounge areas for patients and their families are designed to be comfortable, friendly, and pleasant to facilitate conversation and interaction, while support groups may help patients and family members learn from each other about how to cope with illness or disability and how to regulate their emotions so that

Table 3–3 SUMMARY OF LEARNING THEORIES

Learning Procedures	Assumptions About the Learner	Educator's Task	Sources of Motivation	Transfer of Learning
BEHAVIORIST				
Environmental stimulus conditions and reinforcement promote changes in responses. To change behavior, change the environment.	Passive, reactive learner responds to environmental conditions (stimuli and reinforcement).	Active educator manipulates stimuli and reinforcement to direct learning and change.	Drive reduction	Practice; similarity in stimulus conditions and responses between learning and new situations.
COGNITIVE				
Internal perception and thought processing within context of human development promote learning and change. To change behavior, change cognitions.	Active learner determines patterning of experiences, is strongly influenced by attributions.	Active educator structures experiences (through organization and meaningfulness) to encourage the reorganization of cognitions.	Goals Expectations Disequilibrium	Mental and physical activity. Common patterns. Understanding. Learning to learn.
SOCIAL LEARNING				
External role models and their perceived reinforcement along with learner's internal influences. To change behavior, change role models, perceived reinforcement, and the learner's self-regulating mechanisms.	Active learner observes others and regulates decision to reproduce behavior.	Active educator models behavior, encourages perception of reinforcement, carefully evaluates learning materials for social messages, and attempts to influence learner's self-regulation.	Socialization experiences, role models, and self-reactive influences (observe self, set goals, and reinforce performance)	Similarity of setting and role models' behavior.

PSYCHODYNAMIC

Internal forces such as developmental stage, childhood experiences, emotional conflicts, and ego strength influence learning and change. To change behavior, change interpretations and make unconscious motivations conscious.	Active learner's lifestyle, past experiences, and current emotional conflicts influence what is learned and how it is remembered and performed.	Educator as a reflective interpreter makes sense of learner's personality and motivation by listening and posing questions to stimulate conscious awareness, insight, and ego strength.	Pleasure principle and reality principle Imbalance Conscious and unconscious influence of conflict, development, and defense mechanisms	Personality conflict, resistance, and transference associated with learning situations may act as barrier.

HUMANISTIC

Internal feelings about self, ability to make wise choices, and needs affect learning and change. To change behavior, change feelings, self-concept, and needs.	Active learner attempts to actualize potential for positive self-growth and confirm self-concept; is spontaneous, creative, and playful.	Facilitative educator encourages positive self-growth, listens empathetically, allows freedom of choice, and respects learner.	Needs, desire for positive self-growth, and confirmation of self-concept	Positive or negative feelings about self and freedom to learn promote or inhibit transfer.

their health is not further compromised (social learning).

Another generalization from this discussion is that some psychological learning theories are better suited to certain kinds of individuals than to others. Theoretical assumptions about the learner range from passive to highly active. Passive individuals may learn more effectively from behaviorist techniques, whereas curious, highly active, and self-directed persons may do better with cognitive and humanistic approaches. Also, educators must keep in mind that some learners require external reinforcement and incentives, whereas other learners do not seem to need—and may even resent—attempts to manipulate and reinforce them.

Individuals who are well educated, verbal, and reflective may be better candidates for cognitive and psychodynamic approaches, whereas behaviorist approaches may be more suitable for persons whose cognitive processes are impaired or who are uncomfortable dealing with abstractions or scrutinizing and communicating their thoughts and emotions.

In addition, each individual's preferred modes of learning and processing may help determine the selection of suitable theoretical approaches. That is, although some individuals learn by acting and responding (behaviorist), the route to learning for others may be through perceptions and thoughts (cognitive) or through feelings and emotions (humanistic and psychodynamic). Most people appear to benefit from demonstration and example (social learning).

Motor Learning

Because the majority of health professionals teach motor skills to clients and students at one time or another, it is important for them to explore theories and applications of **motor learning** in addition to theories of psychological learning. Theories and variables of motor learning are useful when teaching skilled movement-related activities in a variety of settings that range from acute care to rehabilitation to sports. The client learning to walk with crutches, the student learning to perform a spinal mobilization, and the athlete perfecting a tennis serve can all benefit from the application of motor learning principles. The objective of this section is to provide a summary of selected aspects of this topic that are relevant and applicable to a wide variety of teaching and learning situations involving health professionals, clients, and students; it is not to provide an exhaustive review of the vast topic of motor learning.

Health professionals teach clients and students an assortment of skills that can range from putting on a colostomy bag, to walking, to operating sophisticated medical equipment. Using theory and evidence to support and guide them as they teach motor skills can help health professionals make their instruction more effective and efficient. *Motor learning* is defined as "a set of processes associated with practice or experience leading to relatively permanent changes in the capability for movement" (Schmidt & Lee, 2005, p. 302). Motor learning differs from **motor performance**, the latter of which involves acquisition of a skill but not necessarily retention of the skill (Schmidt & Wrisberg, 2004). Often, health professionals tend erroneously to equate *performance* of a skill with *learning*. As an illustration, a health professional may demonstrate a skill to the client, such as changing a sterile dressing, and then ask the client to "teach back" the skill. If the client is able to do so relatively accurately, it is assumed the skill has been "learned." Yet when the client is asked to carry out the skill 2 days later during a home visit, the client cannot perform the skill. He may struggle with the order of the steps of changing the dressing, or forget how to keep the field sterile, or not be able to manipulate the bandages. Performance is not always an accurate reflection of learning because it can be influenced by a number of variables, and the changes observed in the skill may only be temporary. Retention, which involves demonstrating a skill over time and after a period of no practice, indicates that learning has occurred (O'Sullivan, 2007).

There are multiple theories of motor learning (Adams, 1971; Newell, 1991; Schmidt, 1975) as well as theories related to stages of learning motor skills (Fitts & Posner, 1967; Gentile, 1972). Each theory has its clinical implications and limitations (Shumway-Cook & Woollacott, 2007). Applying different aspects of these theories to patient care and education is challenging because so many variables affect the desired outcome and research in this area is often contradictory. Different individual characteristics, different types of tasks and skills, and different environments all affect the client's or student's ability to learn a motor skill.

Stages of Motor Learning

Similar to Cronbach's concept of the learning curve (see Chapter 10), Fitts and Posner's (1967) three-stage sequential model of motor learning is a classic model that provides a framework that health professionals can use as they organize learning strategies for clients and students. Three phases of skill learning are identified as follows:

1. The cognitive stage
2. The associative stage
3. The autonomous stage

In the first (cognitive) stage, the learner works to develop an overall understanding of the skill, called the *cognitive map* or *cognitive plan*—basically solving the problem of "what is to be done." Learners must focus and pay attention in this stage. During this stage of learning, the use of specific teaching techniques and strategies is probably the most beneficial (Nicholson, 2002). Instructional strategies for health professionals during this stage include the following:

- Emphasizing the purpose of the skill in a context that is functionally relevant to the learner

- Pointing out similarities to other learned motor skills
- Minimizing distractions
- Using clear and concise instructions
- Demonstrating ideal performance of the skill
- Breaking down complex movements into parts, where appropriate
- Encouraging the learner to verbalize the instructions and watch the movement
- Providing some manual guidance but also allowing for errors in performance (Kisner & Colby, 2007; O'Sullivan, 2007)

Initially, health practitioners can expect irregular performance with many errors. Learners eventually can process sensory cues and organize their perceptual-motor system to carry out reasonable approximations of the skill (O'Sullivan, 2007). Rapid improvement but variable performance characterizes this stage.

The second (associative) stage of learning entails more consistent performance, slower gains, and fewer errors (Schmidt & Lee, 2005). The client or student focuses on "how to do" the skill. The goal in this stage is to fine-tune the skill through continued practice. During this stage, better organization is evident, and the movement becomes coordinated and more accurate (O'Sullivan, 2007). Dependence on visual cues decreases and movement feedback becomes more important. In this stage, health professionals can continue to provide opportunities for practice, emphasizing how the movement feels and assisting learners in finding the safest and most efficient ways to carry out the skills. Helpful instructional strategies for this stage include the following:

- Increasing the complexity of the task
- Increasing the level of distraction in the environment
- Encouraging learners to practice independently
- Emphasizing problem solving
- Decreasing guidance and feedback

- Avoiding manual guidance (Kisner & Colby, 2007)

Clients and students must be encouraged to self-evaluate and self-correct their performance, and health professionals should only intervene when errors appear to be consistent (O'Sullivan, 2007).

The third and final (autonomous) stage is described as the automatic stage where speed and efficiency of performance gradually improve and require little attention and conscious information processing (Nicholson, 2002). An advanced level of skill is achieved and the learner can perform different tasks simultaneously and in changeable environments. In this stage, learners no longer have to "think about" the skill. Health professionals can set up progressively more difficult activities in this stage and provide more challenging environments (Kisner & Colby, 2007). Some clients with disabilities never reach this stage, and the majority of clients are discharged from healthcare facilities prior to reaching this stage.

Motor Learning Variables

It is clear from review of motor learning research that the variables of practice and feedback have widespread clinical applications for health professionals. Gaining an understanding of these variables can assist health professionals in optimizing their motor-skill teaching with clients and students.

Prepractice

Certain variables can influence motor learning even before the learner begins to practice the skill. Health professionals must be concerned with prepractice variables that include motivation, attention, goal setting, understanding of the task goals, modeling, and demonstrations (Kisner & Colby, 2007; Nicholson, 2002). These variables are particularly important when health professionals work with clients who have illnesses or disabilities that may impair their ability to focus on a task. As discussed in Chapter 10, goals should be measurable and achievable and should focus on a functional task. Family members and clients should have input into the goals, and the task should be meaningful to the learner. It is important to determine whether the learner understands the goals and the strategies for achieving a task and is able to pay attention to the task.

Modeling and/or demonstration should always be part of teaching any task. For example, a therapist working in the home care setting with a client who is recovering from a stroke may believe the most important goal for the client is to be independent in toileting activities. The client, on the other hand, believes that carrying firewood into the house from the garage is all he wants to work on. He claims this is something his wife cannot do because of her back problems and he wants to be able to resume his previous role of carrying out this task. The client states he has no interest in toileting activities because his wife helps him when needed. He is highly motivated and focused on carrying wood into the house. For the therapist to take advantage of his drive and enthusiasm, it makes sense to set this task as an initial goal and work on toileting at a later time. Other important skills such as walking, stair climbing, and use of his involved extremity can all be worked into the functional task of carrying wood. Before teaching the task, the therapist makes sure the client pays close attention as she explains the activities that are involved with carrying wood into the house, and she confirms that he demonstrates an understanding of those activities. The stage is now set for the therapist to demonstrate and then practice the task with the client.

Practice

Practice is the most important factor in retraining motor skills. The amount, type, and variability of practice all affect how well a target skill is acquired and retained (Schmidt & Lee, 2005). Because it is generally true that skill in performance increases as a direct function of practice, staff and family members need to continuously reinforce the skills taught by therapists, nurses, and other health professionals. The emphasis on reinforcement reflects behaviorist theory, as discussed previously in this chapter.

Types of practice variables include massed versus distributed practice (see Chapter 10); variability of practice; whole versus part practice; random versus blocked practice; guidance versus discovery learning; and mental practice. Each type of practice has advantages and disadvantages and specific populations for which it is better suited.

Massed practice is a sequence of practice and rest times in which the rest time is much less than the practice time (Schmidt & Lee, 2005). For example, health professionals may use massed practice in an outpatient setting when working with a relatively healthy client who is a tennis player recovering from a wrist injury. The practitioner asks the client to practice hitting a tennis ball against a target in sets of 20 with only a short period of rest between sets. Massed practice can lead to fatigue and possible injury, so it must be used with caution in treating at-risk populations. This type of practice has been shown to markedly decrease motor performance in continuous tasks (such as walking, which involves repetitive, uninterrupted movements); however, massed practice seems to affect learning only slightly when learning is measured on a transfer task in distributed conditions (Shumway-Cook & Woollacott, 2007). Thus, the decrease in performance that occurs with massed practice does not seem to affect retention negatively. This finding may be due to the result of fatigue masking the original learning effects during the massed practice. Massed practice is useful when working with individuals with high levels of motivation and skill who exhibit good endurance, attention, and concentration (O'Sullivan, 2007).

Distributed practice is spaced practice intervals in which the amount of rest between practice times is equal to or greater than the amount of time within each practice trial (Schmidt & Lee, 2005). This is more typical of the type of practice health professionals might use in a hospital setting where, because of the severity of their conditions, patients need frequent rest periods as they learn to manipulate necessary medical equipment, walk, or climb stairs. This type of practice results in the most learning in relation to training time, but the total training time is increased as compared to massed practice (Schmidt & Lee, 2005). It is the preferred mode of practice for individuals with limited endurance or those who are at risk of injury, as are many of the clients seen in the healthcare environment (O'Sullivan, 2007).

An important goal for learning new motor skills is that clients and students are able to transfer the learning to new situations or new tasks. For example, health professionals often teach patients how to get in and out of the chair next to their hospital bed. The goal is that clients can transfer the learning to the new situations they face at home when they try to get in and out of their own kitchen and living room chairs. Researchers find that the more closely the processing demands in the practice environment resemble those in the actual environment, the better the transfer of learning will be (Schmidt & Lee, 2005; Winstein, 1991a). Therefore, it is important to use a variety of chairs in the hospital that resemble chairs at home when teaching this task and not to limit practice to the chair next to the bed.

Variable practice conditions also appear to increase the client's ability to generalize learning to new situations and seem to be particularly effective for children and adult females (Schmidt & Lee, 2005). Research in which subjects practiced a timing task showed that those who practiced at variable speeds were more successful than those who practiced at constant speeds in transferring the learning to a novel speed situation (Catalano

& Kleiner, 1984). According to Shumway-Cook and Woollacott (2007), using variable practice conditions may be most important when teaching tasks that the client will perform in diverse conditions. For example, clients need to practice walking under as many different conditions as possible (in a busy corridor, in a narrow hallway, on different surfaces) to help them generalize the skill to the novel conditions and environments they face when they return home. In regard to self-care tasks such as self-catheterization, clients need to practice these types of tasks in a variety of settings such as in bed, on a commode, and in a public restroom.

Health professionals often break down tasks into component parts for easier learning. The effectiveness of this type of teaching depends on the type of task they are trying to teach the client or the student. Breaking tasks into smaller units is an effective way to teach tasks that can be naturally divided into segments that reflect the inherent goals of the task or that require information processing versus coordination (Nicholson, 2002; Winstein, 1991a). For example, the tasks of preparing a meal or setting up sterile fields both have many components that clients need to perform in an orderly fashion. Some components of the tasks, such as using the stove, measuring the ingredients, or opening packages of bandages, are more difficult than are others. Breaking these types of tasks into their component parts is an effective way to teach the tasks. On the other hand, when the task to be learned involves timing between segments and coordinated movements, such as in a continuous task like walking, practice should focus on the whole task (Nicholson, 2002).

An interesting and counterintuitive finding of motor learning research is that factors that make the initial performance of a task more difficult often make learning more effective (Shumway-Cook & Woollacott, 2007). These factors, first identified by Battig (1966) in verbal learning studies, are called **contextual interference effects** (Brady, 2008). It is natural to assume that practicing several different tasks in blocked order (practicing one specific task repeatedly and uninterruptedly in a block, and then the next task in a block, and then the third task in a block) would make for more effective learning than practicing them in random order (defined as high contextual interference). However, this is not necessarily the case. Although blocked practice makes acquisition of the skill easier, some research shows that it is not as effective as random practice for application of the skill to other environments and for retention of the task (Shumway-Cook & Woollacott, 2007; Wulf & Schmidt, 1997). In random practice, it is hypothesized that more depth of cognitive processing develops in retrieving information from memory stores (O'Sullivan, 2007). As an illustration, the concept of contextual interference effect can be applied to the earlier example of the client in the hospital learning how to get into the chair from the hospital bed. Once the client understands what to do, it may be better for the health professional to vary the practice routine and have the client work on all the different skills he would like her to achieve in random order. Rather than just practicing getting in the chair for a set number of trials, and then performing breathing exercises, and then walking, the health professional can vary the order of the activities in the training session: The client can practice getting in the chair, and then perform breathing exercises, go back to the task of getting up from the chair again for several trials, walk for a while, do breathing exercises again, repeat getting in the chair, and continue the activities in random order.

It is important to note that the health professional must consider characteristics of both the task and the learner when deciding whether to use blocked or random practice. Individual characteristics such as intellectual ability and experience levels may influence the outcome of random practice (Rose, 1997). In fact, random practice has not been found to be superior to blocked practice in adolescents with Down syndrome (Edwards, Elliott, & Lee, 1986) or in a pilot study of adults with Parkinson disease (Lin, Sullivan, Wu, Kantak, & Winstein, 2007). Clients who need a high degree of consistency and structure for learning may benefit most from blocked practice (O'Sullivan, 2007). In a comprehensive review of the subject, Brady (2008) suggests that the contextual interference effect may actually be weaker in application than it is in basic research.

Health professionals routinely give verbal and physical (manual) guidance to assist the client or student in performing tasks. Guidance seems to be most effective at the initial stages of teaching a task when the task is unfamiliar to the learner and for tasks that are slow in time (Schmidt & Lee, 2005). Too much guidance, however, can actually interfere with learning because it does not allow the learner to problem solve. Therefore, it is important for health professionals to resist the common urge to give continual direction and assistance to clients and students, especially once the learners are familiar with the task.

The opposite of guidance is trial and error or *discovery learning*—a cornerstone of cognitive and humanistic theories. This type of teaching presents learners with challenging, yet achievable problems and encourages them to discover their own solutions. Discovery learning seems to be less effective for the speed of initial skill acquisition, but more effective for later transfer and retention of the skill (Schmidt & Wulf, 1997; Singer, 1980). For example, a respiratory therapy instructor introduces new students to an unfamiliar piece of equipment, tells them to figure out how the equipment works, and then leaves the classroom for about 15 to 20 minutes. The instructor contends that many students learn how to operate equipment more effectively by having time initially to discover for themselves before being formally taught how to use medical equipment. Discovery learning is important, the instructor maintains, because respiratory therapists are faced throughout their careers with having to learn for themselves how to use new and updated equipment in a variety of different practice settings.

Whereas physical practice is best for learning a motor skill, **mental practice** (imagining or visualizing the skill without body movement) can have positive effects on the performance of the skill (Dickstein & Deutsch, 2007). In fact, Allami, Paulignan, and Brovelli (2008) found high rates of imagery even led to similar performance as physical practice in an object-slot task. Research indicates that when mental practice is used together with physical practice, motor skill acquisition is enhanced (Gentili, Papaxanthis, & Pozzo, 2006; Hamel & Lajoie, 2005) and occurs at a faster rate than with physical practice alone (Malouin, Richards, Doyon, Desrosiers, & Belleville, 2004; Page, Levine, Sisto, & Johnston, 2001). Several researchers assert that familiarity with the task is necessary for mental imagery practice to be successful (Mulder, Zijlstra, Zijlstra, & Hochstenbach, 2004; Mutsaarts, Steenbergen, & Bekkering, 2006). Nevertheless, clients who cannot carry out physical practice of motor skills as a result of fatigue, pain, or impairments are often good candidates for the technique of mental practice alone. Clients who are too ill to exercise or get out of bed can gain a head start on learning by mentally "practicing" these activities. They can do this by reviewing the steps to getting out of bed with the health professional, and then imagining themselves carrying out those steps, one after the other. Mental practice can also help to increase self-efficacy (Callow, Hardy, & Hall, 2001; Martin, Moritz, & Hall, 1999) and can decrease anxiety in clients who are apprehensive about making the initial movement, perhaps because of fear of falling or pain (O'Sullivan, 2007). When possible, mental practice should be combined with physical practice to increase the rate and quality of skill learning.

Feedback

Feedback plays a critical role in promoting motor learning and is considered the second most important element involved with learning a skill after practice (Bilodeau, 1966; Newell, 1976). Feedback can be either intrinsic or extrinsic. **Intrinsic (inherent) feedback** is the sensory and perceptual information that occurs when a movement is produced and can include both visual and somatosensory information. **Extrinsic (augmented or enhanced) feedback** is information provided to the learner from an outside source (Schmidt & Wrisberg, 2004). The outside source can be the health professional, or it can be some type of instrumentation, such as biofeedback.

Extrinsic feedback supplements intrinsic feedback. Variables to consider when giving extrinsic feedback include the type, timing, and frequency of feedback. Types of extrinsic feedback include knowledge of results (KR) and knowledge of performance (KP). Knowledge of results (KR) is terminal feedback about the outcome of the movement relative to the movement's goal, whereas knowledge of performance (KP) is feedback about the movement pattern used to achieve the goal (Schmidt & Lee, 2005). For example, a therapist working with a client who is learning to tie his shoes gives the client KR feedback when he says, "You tied a nice, tight bow." A little later in the session, the therapist gives KP feedback to the client when he says, "You kept your balance really well as you leaned forward to reach for your feet—can you tell what that feels like?" Extrinsic feedback can be given at the same time as the task (concurrently) or immediately after the task, or it can be delayed for a specified period of time. It can also be given continuously or intermittently.

Some types of skills, such as tracking tasks, depend more on KP, whereas KR is more important in other types of tasks such as transfers where information is needed about how to shape the general movements for the next attempt at the task (O'Sullivan, 2007). Research by Wulf, Hob, and Prinz (1998) demonstrates that focusing a person's attention on the outcomes of movements (KR) enhances learning more than when the person focuses on the details of the movements. Health professionals need to adjust the timing of feedback during the learning process. Initially, concurrent, continuous feedback may be necessary in the early stages of teaching a skill to ensure safety and understanding; however, continuous feedback can interfere with learning. For example, the nurse teaches a patient how to give herself an injection. Initially, the nurse must show the patient how to hold the needle, often physically guiding the placement of the patient's hands on the needle. He also tells the patient step by step how to proceed with the injection, giving praise along the way when the patient is successful. If he continues to give this level of extensive feedback each time the patient practices, it may actually retard the patient from learning the skill. For retention and longer-term learning, learners need to self-detect and self-correct errors, so educators should use the least amount of concurrent feedback for the shortest time possible (Gentile, 2000). Health professionals can often find this challenging because many view giving large amounts of concurrent feedback as a way of positively supporting the client or student. Intermittent feedback during practice promotes learning more effectively than does continuous feedback. Immediate, postresponse feedback, in which the health professional provides knowledge of the outcome of the task right after each trial, is often used in the early stages of learning. Although this type of feedback may enhance early skill performance, it delays learning (Kisner & Colby, 2007).

Effective learning includes retention. Providing continuous feedback interferes with learners developing the ability to problem solve and self-detect errors (Kisner & Colby, 2007). Conversely, feedback that is not given after every trial (summary feedback) slows initial skill acquisition but improves performance on retention tests (Winstein & Schmidt, 1990). Winstein (1987, 1991b) demonstrates that progressively decreasing the rate at which feedback is given, called fading of feedback, appears to be most effective in promoting learning. Fading feedback and using summary feedback (allowing several repetitions of a task before providing feedback) are good ways of reducing the amount of feedback the health professional provides. For example, the health professional teaching a client to use an incentive spirometer first explains and demonstrates its use. He then allows the client to practice using the spirometer two or three times (as long as no harmful errors occur) before giving feedback about how good a seal the client made around the device, how deeply she inhaled, and how well she held her breath. Eventually, the health professional "fades" the feedback and gives it after four or five trials rather than after two or three, hoping the client will self-correct any errors. The extensive use of any type of augmented feedback can create dependence on the feedback, so health professionals need to develop a comfort level that balances safety and support with allowing clients and students to problem solve, self-monitor, and self-correct when learning new motor skills. See **Table 3–4** to review practice variables and feedback variables in motor learning.

Including motor learning principles in their repertoire adds depth and breadth to the teaching skills of health professionals. Although different areas of the brain are involved in motor learning as compared to psychological learning, there is considerable overlap and the integration and application of both sets of principles are necessary for optimal teaching and learning of motor skills. Selective aspects of some of the psychological theories, such as reinforcement from behaviorist theory, the gestalt and information-processing perspective from cognitive theory, modeling from social learning theory, and focusing on subjective needs and feelings of the learner from humanistic theory, are seminal to the teaching of motor skills.

Although there is a large body of complex research in the area of motor learning, following several simple guidelines can help health professionals be more effective when they teach motor skills to clients or to students. Health professionals should remember to do the following:

1. Practice motor skills with clients and students as much as possible and encourage other staff and family members to also practice skills with clients.
2. Encourage mental practice prior to or along with motor practice.
3. Make sure clients and students understand the purpose of the skill and give clear guidance and assistance in the initial stages of learning.
4. Vary the conditions of learning as much as possible.
5. Within the limits of safety, decrease the amount of guidance and feedback to allow learners to problem solve, make mistakes, and self-correct errors.

Health professionals who consistently apply knowledge of the three stages of motor learning and the variables of practice and feedback when teaching motor skills to clients give themselves the best chances for successful teaching outcomes.

The next section discusses common principles of learning integrating information from all the learning theories presented in this chapter.

Common Principles of Learning

Taken together, the theories discussed in this chapter indicate that learning is a more complicated process than any one theory implies. Besides the distinct considerations for learning suggested by each theory, the similarities among the perspectives

Table 3–4 PRACTICE AND FEEDBACK VARIABLES IN MOTOR LEARNING

PRACTICE VARIABLES IN MOTOR LEARNING

- *Massed practice:* Practice time is more than rest time.
- *Distributed practice:* Rest time is the same as or greater than practice time.
- *Variability of practice:* The task is practiced under a variety of conditions.
- *Whole-task practice:* The entire task is practiced at once.
- *Part-task practice:* The task is divided into its component parts and each part is practiced separately.
- *Random practice:* Randomly practicing a variety of tasks over different trials.
- *Blocked practice:* Practicing one task continuously without interruption.
- *Guidance practice/learning:* Providing physical and verbal guidance while practicing the task.
- *Discovery practice/learning:* Practicing a task by encouraging the learner to find a solution to a challenging yet attainable problem.
- *Mental practice:* Cognitively rehearsing a motor task without any body movement.

FEEDBACK VARIABLES IN MOTOR LEARNING

- *Intrinsic (inherent) feedback:* Sensory and perceptual information originating from the learner when movement is produced
- *Extrinsic (augmented or enhanced) feedback:* Supplemental information provided from an outside source such as the teacher or instrumentation when movement is produced
  - *Knowledge of results (KR) feedback:* Terminal feedback about the outcome of the movement relative to the movement goal
  - *Knowledge of performance (KP) feedback:* Feedback about the movement pattern used to achieve the goal
  - *Continuous feedback:* Is ongoing during performance of the movement
  - *Intermittent feedback:* Occurs randomly and irregularly during performance of the movement
  - *Concurrent feedback:* Occurs during performance of the movement
  - *Postresponse (terminal) feedback:* Occurs after completion of the movement and may be:
    - Immediate: Occurs directly after the movement is completed
    - Delayed: Occurs after a period of time to allow reflection by the learner
    - Summary: Occurs after several repetitions of the movement and describes average performance

Sources: Dickstein and Deutsch (2007); Kisner and Colby (2007); O'Sullivan (2007); Schmidt and Lee (2005); Schmidt and Wrisberg (2004); Shumway-Cook and Woollacott (2007).

point to some core features of learning. The issues raised at the beginning of the chapter can be addressed by synthesizing the learning theories and identifying their common principles.

How Does Learning Occur?

Learning is an active process that takes place as individuals interact with their environment and incorporate new information or experiences with what they already know or have learned. Factors in the environment that affect learning include the society and culture, the structure or pattern of stimuli, the effectiveness of role models and reinforcements, feedback for correct and incorrect responses, and opportunities to process and apply learning to new situations.

Furthermore, the individual exerts significant control over learning, often involving considerations of his or her developmental stage, past history (habits, cultural conditioning, socialization, childhood experiences, and conflicts), cognitive style, dynamics of self-regulation, conscious and unconscious motivations, personality (stage, conflicts, and self-concept), and emotions. Also, learners often have a preferred mode for taking in information (visual, motor, auditory, or symbolic), and, although some individuals may learn best on their own, others benefit from expert guidance, social interaction, and cooperative learning.

Learning is an individual matter. Neuropsychology research is beginning to document the uniqueness of each person's way of actively perceiving and processing information, his or her flexibility and reactions to stress, and the impact of culture and emotions on how and what is learned.

A critical influence on whether learning occurs is motivation (see Chapter 6). The learning theories reviewed here suggest that to learn, the individual must want to gain something (receive rewards and pleasure, meet goals and needs, master a new skill, confirm expectations, grow in positive ways, or resolve conflicts), which, in turn, arouses

the learner by creating tension (drives to be reduced, disequilibrium, and imbalance) and the propensity to act or change behavior.

The relative success or failure of the learner's performance may affect subsequent learning experiences. In some cases, an inappropriate, maladaptive, or harmful previously learned behavior may need to be extinguished and then replaced with a more positive response. It is, of course, easier to instill new learning than to correct faulty learning.

What Kinds of Experiences Facilitate or Hinder the Learning Process?

The educator exerts a critical influence on learning through role modeling, the selection of learning theories, and how the learning experience is structured for each learner. To be effective, educators must have knowledge (of the material or skill to be learned, the learner, the social context, and educational psychology), and they must be competent (be imaginative, flexible, and able to employ teaching methods; display solid communication skills; and have the ability to motivate others).

All the learning theories discussed in this chapter acknowledge the need to recognize and relate the new information to the learner's past experiences (old habits, previous skills, culture, familiar patterns, childhood memories, feelings about the self, and what is valued, normative, and perceived as successful or rewarded in society). The ultimate control over learning rests with the learner, but effective educators influence and guide the process so that learners advance in their knowledge, skills, perceptions, thoughts, emotional maturity, or behavior.

Ignoring these considerations, of course, may hinder learning. Other impediments to learning may involve a lack of clarity and meaningfulness in what is to be learned, neglect or harsh punishment, fear, and negative or ineffective role models. Providing inappropriate materials for the individual's ability, readiness to learn, or stage of life-cycle development is another obstacle to learning. Moreover, individuals are unlikely to want to learn if they have had detrimental socialization experiences, are deprived of stimulating environments, or are without goals and realistic expectations for themselves.

What Helps Ensure That Learning Becomes Relatively Permanent?

Four considerations assist learning in becoming permanent. First, the likelihood of learning is enhanced by organizing the learning experience, making it meaningful and pleasurable, recognizing the role of emotions in learning, and by pacing the teaching session in keeping with the learner's ability to process information. Second, practicing (mentally and physically) new knowledge or skills under varied conditions strengthens learning. The third issue concerns reinforcement. Although reinforcement may or may not be necessary, some theorists have argued that it may be helpful because it serves as a signal to the individual that learning has occurred.

A fourth consideration involves whether learning transfers beyond the initial educational setting. Learning cannot be assumed to be relatively lasting or permanent; it must be assessed and evaluated by the educator soon after the learning experience has occurred as well as by follow-up measurements at later times. Research skills, knowledge of evaluation procedures, and the willingness and resources to engage in assessment are now considered essential responsibilities of the educator in carrying out the teaching–learning process. Evaluation feedback can then be used by the health professional educator to revamp and revitalize learning experiences.

State of the Evidence

The study of learning in educational psychology is based on evidence from research similar to that advocated in health care. Rather than assuming the instructor knows best, researchers gather evidence and test learning theories, teaching methods, and what is believed to be true about learners, teachers, and the environment. The research results are then evaluated for the purpose of modifying the theories, methods, and assumptions about learning.

Ideally in health education, existing research is used to design learning experiences for patients, clients, families, and communities. The same is true for developing, implementing, and evaluating teaching and learning experiences for health professional students and staff. On the basis of the research findings, what does not work is eliminated, modifications are made grounded in additional research, and new programs are attempted and assessed. Educational accountability is stressed, and decisions about how to educate must be justified on the basis of data and research.

The applications of the learning theories and principles discussed in this chapter are illustrated by a number of research studies in psychology, education, sports, and health care. Because of the research, health professionals can feel confident about their ability to choose the most appropriate theories and principles for each educational experience and hone their approach to teaching and learning in the healthcare setting. Educational research confirms many of the constructs and principles from the various learning perspectives. It also provides evidence to dispute some of the conventional wisdom and myths about learning—helping health professionals as educators realize that punishment is not generally effective and may inhibit learning; males are not necessarily more intelligent than females are; more feedback is not always better; and when teaching people, there are a number of strongly held realities that may or may not be rational that strongly influence each learner's processing of the educational experience. The research on learning in general and health care in particular clearly demonstrates there is no one-size-fits-all approach to educating patients, clients, health professional students, or staff. To be effective, educational experiences need to be refined and tailored to each individual learner.

Though many advancements have been made in understanding the learning process over the past century, much remains unknown and requires careful research, such as why some patients and health professional students are so much more eager to learn than are others, what can be done to encourage reluctant learners to change their attitudes or behavior, how the various learning theories and principles can work together for every learner, and how the healthcare setting changes the teaching–learning situation. In the future, more interdisciplinary efforts between psychologists and health professionals are needed to move toward a more sophisticated level of research and understanding that can be applied to the healthcare setting.

Research is not a panacea, however. Critics charge that the widely promoted research-based evidence approach to education and health care is jargonistic, places the emphasis on outcomes rather than on the process of learning, and oversimplifies the complexity of learning in any attempt to measure and evaluate it. The challenges of measurement are immense and require a highly sophisticated knowledge of research methods and their weaknesses. Another problem is the lack of resources, support, and well-trained personnel needed to truly implement and sustain a research-based approach to teaching and learning (Ferguson & Day, 2005).

Summary

This chapter demonstrates that learning is complex. Readers may feel overwhelmed by the diverse theories, sets of learning principles, and cautions associated with employing the various approaches. Yet, like the blind men exploring the elephant, each theory highlights an important dimension that affects the overall learning process, and together the theories provide a wealth of complementary strate-

gies and alternative options. There is, of course, no single best way to approach learning, although all the theories indicate the need to be sensitive to the unique characteristics and motivations of each learner. For additional sources of information about psychological theories of learning and health care, see **Table 3–5**.

Educators in the health professions cannot be expected to know everything about the teaching and learning process. More important, perhaps, is that they can determine what needs to be known, where to find the necessary information, and how to help individuals, groups, and themselves benefit directly from a learning situation. Psychology and health care work well together. Psychology has much to contribute to healthcare practice, and the health professions are in a strategic position to apply and test psychological and motor learning principles, constructs, and theories in both educational and clinical settings.

Table 3–5 PSYCHOLOGICAL THEORIES OF LEARNING AND HEALTH CARE: LINKS

McMaster University: Evidence-based medicine links:
http://www.mlanet.org/education/telecon/ebhc/resource.html

American Psychological Association (search for learning topics):
http://www.apa.org

National Institutes of Health (search for patient education topics):
http://www.nih.gov

Learning Theory links (emTech.net):
http://www.emtech.net/learning_theories.htm

Nursing Patient Education resources (about.com):
http://nursing.about.com/od/patienteducation/Patient_Education_Tools_and_Information_for_Nurses.htm

---

REVIEW QUESTIONS

1. What are the six major learning theories discussed in this chapter?
2. What are the principal constructs and contributions of each of the six learning theories?
3. According to the concept of operant conditioning, what are three techniques to increase the probability of a response, and what are two techniques to decrease or extinguish the probability of a response?
4. What are some ways the behaviorist theory (which focuses on the environment and responses to it) and the cognitive perspective (which emphasizes the individual's internal processing) could be combined to facilitate knowledge acquisition or change a health behavior?
5. What is meant by the term *gestalt*, and with which major learning theory is it associated?
6. Which learning theory is a combination of the principles from both the behaviorist and cognitive perspectives?
7. Which perspective is based primarily on the theory of motivation and stresses emotions rather than cognition and stimulus–response connections?
8. How do the major psychological learning theories compare to one another with regard to their similarities and differences?
9. How does motivation serve as the critical influence on whether learning occurs or not?
10. What types of experiences can facilitate or hinder the learning process?
11. Which factors help ensure that learning becomes relatively permanent?
12. What are some ways that emotions might be given more explicit consideration in health professionals' education and in patient education?
13. How has neuroscience research contributed to the understanding of learning and learning theories?
14. In motor learning, how do the instructional strategies used during the associative stage of learning differ from those used during the cognitive stage?
15. What is the difference between performance and learning?
16. What variables make initial skill acquisition more difficult but strengthen retention and learning?
17. How do the different types of practice and feedback variables affect learning?

CASE STUDY

You are designing an education session for your colleagues on transitioning from a paper-based documentation system to an electronic medical record (EMR) system. Time is of the essence, and you have three 1-hour sessions planned to cover the information they need to incorporate the new EMR system into their daily practice. Several of your colleagues are concerned about their ability to master the new system. Jack, the department supervisor, confides, "I am terrified. Learning a whole new system of documentation is overwhelming to my staff, given all of their other responsibilities. I worry that this new EMR system will have a negative impact on morale, just at the time when we are feeling pressure to increase the amount of work that we do."

1. Describe how you will structure the educational sessions using two of the psychological learning theories discussed in this chapter. Explain why you chose each theory.
2. Judge which learning theory can best assist you in addressing the issues your colleagues raise about their ability to master the new system and feelings of being overwhelmed. Why did you choose this theory?
3. What can you do to ensure that learning will become relatively permanent?

References

Adams, J. A. (1971). A closed-loop theory of motor learning. *Journal of Motor Behavior, 3*, 111–150.

Akers, R. L. (1989). Social learning theory and alcohol behavior among the elderly. *Sociological Quarterly, 30*, 625–638.

Allami, N., Paulignan, Y., & Brovelli, A. (2008). Visuo-motor learning with combination of different rates of motor imagery and physical practice. *Experimental Brain Research, 184*, 105–113.

Anderson, O. R. (1997). A neurocognitive perspective on current learning theory and science instructional strategies. *Science Education, 81*, 67–89.

Bahn, D. (2001). Social learning theory: Its application to the context of nurse education. *Nurse Education Today, 21*, 110–117.

Bandura, A. (1977). *Social learning theory.* Englewood Cliffs, NJ: Prentice Hall.

Bandura, A. (2001). Social cognitive theory: An agentic perspective. *Annual Review of Psychology, 52*, 1–26.

Barnard, A., Hollingum, C., & Hartfiel, B. (2006). Going on a journey: Understanding palliative care nursing. *International Journal of Palliative Nursing, 12*, 6–12.

Battig, W. F. (1966). Facilitation and interference. In E. A. Bilodeau (Ed.), *Acquisition of skill* (pp. 215–244). New York: Academic Press.

Beck, M. H., Cataldo, M., Slifer, K. J., Pulbrook, V., & Guhman, J. K. (2005). Teaching children with attention deficit hyperactivity disorder (ADHD) and autistic disorder (AD) how to swallow pills. *Clinical Pediatrics, 44*, 515–526.

Berggren, I., & Severinsson, E. (2006). The significance of nurse supervisors' different ethical decision-making styles. *Journal of Nursing Management, 14*, 637–643.

Biderman, A. (2003). Family medicine as a frame for humanized medicine in education and clinical practice. *Public Health Review, 31*, 23–26.

Bilodeau, E. A. (1966). Information feedback. In E. A. Bilodeau (Ed.), *Acquisition of skill* (pp. 255–296). New York: Academic Press.

Block, S., & Billings, J. A. (1998). Nurturing humanism through teaching palliative care. *Academic Medicine, 73*, 763–765.

Brackett, M. A., Lopes, P. N., Ivcevic, Z., Mayer, J. D., & Salovey, P. (2004). Integrating emotion and cognition: The role of emotional intelligence. In D. Y. Dai & R. J. Sternberg (Eds.), *Motivation, emotion, and cognition: Integrative perspectives on intellectual functioning and development* (pp. 175–194). Mahwah, NJ: Erlbaum.

Brady, F. (2008). The contextual interference effect and sport skills. *Perceptual and Motor Skills, 106*, 461–472.

Bush, G. (2006). Learning about learning: From theories to trends. *Teacher Librarian, 34*, 14–18.

Byrnes, J. P. (2001). *Minds, brains, and learning: Understanding the psychological and educational relevance of neuroscientific research.* New York: Guilford.

Callow, N., Hardy, L., & Hall, C. (2001). The effects of a motivational general-mastery imagery intervention on the sport confidence of high-level badminton players. *Research Quarterly for Exercise and Sport, 72*, 389–400.

Catalano, J. F., & Kleiner, B. M. (1984). Distant transfer and practice variability. *Perceptual Motor Skills, 58*, 851–856.

Chochinov, H. M., & Breitbart, W. (Eds.). (2000). *Handbook of psychiatry in palliative medicine.* New York: Oxford University Press.

Dai, D. Y., & Sternberg, R. J. (Eds.). (2004). *Motivation, emotion, and cognition: Integrative perspectives on intellectual functioning and development.* Mahwah, NJ: Erlbaum.

Deyl, S. G., & Kaliappan, K. V. (1997). Improvement of psychosomatic disorders among tension headache subjects using behaviour therapy and somatic inkblot series. *Journal of Projective Psychology and Mental Health, 4*, 113–120.

Dickstein, R., & Deutsch, J. E. (2007). Motor imagery in physical therapist practice. *Physical Therapy, 87*(7), 942–953.

Duberstein, P. R., & Masling, J. M. (Eds.). (2000). *Psychodynamic perspectives on sickness and health.* Washington, DC: American Psychological Association.

Eccles, J. S., & Wigfield, A. (2002). Motivational beliefs, values, and goals. *Annual Review of Psychology, 53*, 109–132.

Edwards, J. M., Elliott, D., & Lee, T. D. (1986). Contextual interference effects during skill acquisition and transfer in Down's syndrome adolescents. *Adapted Physical Activity Quarterly, 3*, 250–258.

Erikson, E. (1968). *Identity: Youth and crisis.* New York: Norton.

Ferguson, L., & Day, R. A. (2005). Evidence-based nursing education: Myth or reality? *Journal of Nursing Education, 44*, 107–115.

Fiske, S. T., & Taylor, S. E. (1991). *Social cognition.* New York: McGraw-Hill.

Fitts, P. M., & Posner, M. I. (1967). *Human performance.* Belmont, CA: Brooks/Cole.

Friedrichsen, M. J., & Strang, P. M. (2003). Doctors' strategies when breaking bad news to terminally ill patients. *Journal of Palliative Medicine, 6*, 565–574.

Friedrichsen, M. J., Strang, P. M. & Carlsson, M. E. (2000). Breaking bad news in the transition from curative to palliative cancer care—patient's view of the doctor giving the information. *Support Care Cancer, 8*, 472–478.

Fryer-Edwards, K., Arnold, R. M., Baile, W., Tulsky, J. A., Petracca, F., & Back, A. (2006). Reflective teaching practices: An approach to teaching communication skills in a small-group setting. *Academic Medicine, 81*, 638–644.

Gage, N. L., & Berliner, D. C. (1992). *Educational psychology* (5th ed.). Boston: Houghton Mifflin.

Gage, N. L., & Berliner, D. C. (1998). *Educational psychology* (6th ed.). Boston: Houghton Mifflin.

Gagné, R. M. (1985). *The conditions of learning* (4th ed.). New York: Holt, Rinehart & Winston.

Gagné, R. M., Briggs, L. J., & Wagner, W. W. (1992). *Principles of instructional design* (4th ed.). Fort Worth, TX: HBJ College Publishers.

Gallop, R., & O'Brien, L. (2003). Re-establishing psychodynamic theory as foundational knowledge for psychiatric/mental health nursing. *Issues in Mental Health Nursing, 24*, 213–227.

Gardner, H. (1978). *Developmental psychology: An introduction.* Boston: Little, Brown.

Gazzaniga, M. S. (Ed.). (2000). *The new cognitive neurosciences* (2nd ed.). Cambridge, MA: MIT Press.

Gentile, A. M. (1972). A working model of skill acquisition with application to teaching. *Quest, 17*, 3–23.

Gentile, A. M. (2000). Skill acquisition: Action, movement and neuromotor processes. In J. Carr & R. Shepherd (Eds.), *Movement science: Foundations for physical therapy in rehabilitation* (pp. 111–187). Gaithersburg, MD: Aspen Publishers.

Gentili, R., Papaxanthis, C., & Pozzo, T. (2006). Improvement and generalization of arm motor performance through motor imagery practice. *Neuroscience, 137*, 761–772.

Gilmartin, J. (2000). Psychodynamic sources of resistance among student nurses: Some observations in a human relations context. *Journal of Advanced Nursing, 32*, 1533–1541.

Goleman, D. (1995). *Emotional intelligence.* New York: Bantam Books.

Goodwin, A. M., & Gore, V. (2000). Managing the stresses of nursing people with severe and enduring mental illness: A psychodynamic observation study of a long-stay psychiatric ward. *British Journal of Medical Psychology, 73*, 311–325.

Grealy, L. (1994). *Anatomy of a face.* Boston: Houghton Mifflin.

Greene, J. D., Sommerville, R. B., Nystrom, L. E., Darley, J. M., & Cohen, J. D. (2001). An fMRI investigation of emotional engagement in moral judgment. *Science, 293*, 2105–2108.

Halpern, J. (2001). *From detached concern to empathy: Humanizing medical practice.* New York: Oxford University Press.

Hamel, M. F., & Lajoie, Y. (2005). Mental imagery: Effects on static balance and attentional demands of the elderly. *Aging Clinical Experimental Research, 17*, 223–228.

Hilgard, E. R. (1996). History of educational psychology. In D. C. Berliner & R. C. Calfee (Eds.), *Handbook of educational psychology* (pp. 990–1004). New York: Simon & Schuster Macmillan.

Hilgard, E. R., & Bower, G. H. (1966). *Theories of learning* (3rd ed.). New York: Appleton-Century-Crofts.

Hoffman, M. L. (2000). *Empathy and moral development: Implications for caring and justice.* New York: Cambridge University Press.

Holyoake, D. D. (1998). A little lady called Pandora: An exploration of philosophical traditions of humanism and existentialism in nursing ill children. *Child Care, Health and Development, 24*, 325–336.

Hooyman, N., & Kiyak, H. A. (2005). *Social gerontology* (7th ed.). Boston: Allyn & Bacon.

Hunt, R. R., Ellis, H. C., & Ellis, H. (2004). *Fundamentals of cognitive psychology* (7th ed.). New York: McGraw-Hill.

Imes, S. A., Clance, P. R., Gailis, A. T., & Atkeson, E. (2002). Mind's response to the body's betrayal: Gestalt/existential therapy for clients with chronic or life-threatening illnesses. *Journal of Clinical Psychology, 58,* 1361–1373.

Kane-Urrabazo, C. (2006). Management's role in shaping organizational culture. *Journal of Nursing Management, 14,* 188–194.

Kennifer, S. L., Alexander, S. C., Pollak, K. I., Jeffreys, A. S., Olsen, M. K., Rodriguez, K. L., Arnold, R. M., & Tulsky, J. A. (2009). Negative emotions in cancer care: Do oncologists' responses depend on severity and type of emotion? *Patient Education and Counseling, 76,* 51–56.

Kessels, R. P. C. (2003). Patients' memory of medical information. *Journal of the Royal Society of Medicine, 96,* 219–222.

Kisner, C., & Colby, L. A. (2007). *Therapeutic exercise* (5th ed.). Philadelphia: F. A. Davis.

Kohler, W. (1947). *Gestalt psychology.* New York: Mentor Books.

Kohler, W. (1969). *The task of gestalt psychology.* Princeton, NJ: Princeton University Press.

Kramer, D. A. (1983). Post-formal operations? A need for further conceptualization. *Human Development, 26,* 91–105.

Kübler-Ross, E. (1969). *On death and dying.* New York: Macmillan.

Lin, C. H. J., Sullivan, K. J., Wu, A. D., Kantak, S., & Winstein, C. J. (2007). Effects of task practice on motor skill learning in adults with Parkinson disease: A pilot study. *Physical Therapy, 87*(9) 1120–1131.

Malach-Pines, A. (2000). Nurses' burnout: An existential psychodynamic perspective. *Journal of Psychosocial Nursing and Mental Health Services, 38,* 23–31.

Malouin, F., Richards, C. L., Doyon, J., Desrosiers, J., & Belleville, S. (2004). Training mobility tasks after stroke with combined mental and physical practice: A feasibility study. *Neurorehabilitation & Neural Repair, 18,* 66–75.

Marshall, H. H. (1998). Teaching educational psychology: Learner-centered constructivist perspectives. In N. M. Lambert & B. L. McCombs (Eds.), *How students learn: Reforming schools through learner-centered education* (pp. 449–473). Washington, DC: American Psychological Association.

Martin, K., Moritz, S., & Hall, C. (1999). Imagery use in sport: A literature review and applied model. *Sport Psychologist, 13,* 245–268.

Maslow, A. (1954). *Motivation and personality.* New York: Harper & Row.

Maslow, A. (1987). *Motivation and personality* (3rd ed.). New York: Harper & Row.

McCullough, L., & Andrews, S. (2001). Assimilative integration: Short-term dynamic psychotherapy for treating affect phobias. *Clinical Psychology Science and Practice, 8,* 82–97.

Menahern, S., & Halasz, G. (2000). Parental noncompliance—a paediatric dilemma: A medical and psychodynamic perspective. *Child Care, Health and Development, 26,* 61–72.

Moskowitz, G. B. (2005). *Social cognition: Understanding self and others.* New York: Guilford.

Mulder, T., Zijlstra, S., Zijlstra, W., & Hochstenbach, J. (2004). The role of motor imagery in learning a totally novel movement. *Experimental Brain Research, 154,* 211–217.

Mulholland, S., Derdall, M., & Roy, B. (2006) The student's perspective on what makes an exceptional practice placement educator. *British Journal of Occupational Therapy, 69,* 567–571.

Murray, D. J. (1995). *Gestalt psychology and the cognitive revolution.* New York: Harvester Wheatsheaf.

Mutsaarts, M., Steenbergen, B., & Bekkering, H. (2006). Anticipatory planning and task context effects in hemiparetic cerebral palsy. *Experimental Brain Research, 172,* 151–162.

Neary, M. (2000). Supporting students' learning and professional development through the process of continuous assessment and mentorship. *Nurse Education Today, 20,* 463–474.

Newell, K. M. (1976). Knowledge of results and motor learning. *Exercise Sport Science Review, 4,* 195–228.

Newell, K. M. (1991). Motor skill acquisition. *Annual Review of Psychology, 42,* 213–237.

Nicholson, D. E. (2002). Teaching psychomotor skills. In K. F. Shepard & G. M. Jensen (Eds.), *Handbook of teaching for physical therapists* (2nd ed., pp. 387–418). Woburn, MA: Butterworth-Heinemann.

Ormrod, J. E. (2004). *Human learning* (4th ed.). Upper Saddle River, NJ: Prentice Hall.

O'Sullivan, S. B. (2007). Strategies to improve motor function. In S. B. O'Sullivan & T. J. Schmitz (Eds.), *Physical rehabilitation* (5th ed., pp. 471–522). Philadelphia: F. A. Davis.

Page, M. P. A. (2006). What can't functional neuroimaging tell the cognitive psychologist? *Cortex, 42,* 428–443.

Page, S. J., Levine, P., Sisto, S. A., & Johnston, M. V. (2001). Mental practice combined with physical practice for upper-limb motor deficit in subacute stroke. *Physical Therapy, 81,* 1455–1462.

Palincsar, A. S. (1998). Social constructivist perspectives on teaching and learning. *Annual Review of Psychology, 49,* 345–375.

Papadakis, A. A., Prince, R. P. O., Jones, N. P., & Strauman, T. J. (2006). Self-regulation, rumination, and vulnerability to depression in adolescent girls. *Developmental Psychopathology, 18,* 815–829.

Pearson, A. (2006). Powerful caring. *Nursing Standard, 20*(48), 20–22.

Pfeffer, J. (1985). Organizations and organizational theory. In G. Lindzey & E. Aronson (Eds.), *Handbook of social psychology: Vol. 1. Theory and method* (3rd ed., pp. 379–440). New York: Random House.

Phelps, E. Z. (2006). Emotion and cognition: Insights from studies of the human amygdala. *Annual Review of Psychology, 57,* 27–53.

Piaget, J., & Inhelder, B. (1969). *The psychology of the child* (H. Weaver, Trans.). New York: Basic Books.

Piane, G. (2000). Contingency contracting and systematic desensitization for heroin addicts in methadone maintenance programs. *Journal of Psychoactive Drugs, 32,* 311–319.

Pollak, K. I., Arnold, R. M., Jeffreys, A. S., Alexander, S. C., Olsen, M. K., Abernathy, A. P, Skinner, C. S., Rodriguez, K. L., & Ja, T. (2007). Oncologist communication about emotions during visits with patients with advanced cancer. *Journal of Clinical Oncology, 25,* 5748–5752.

Proctor, R., Burns, A., Powell, H. S., & Tarrier, N. (1999). Behavioural management in nursing and residential homes: A randomized controlled trial. *Lancet, 354,* 26–29.

Pullen, M. L. (2002). Joe's story: Reflection on a difficult interaction between a nurse and a patient's wife. *International Journal of Palliative Nursing, 8,* 481–488.

Rogers, C. (1961). *On becoming a person.* Boston: Houghton Mifflin.

Rogers, C. (1994). *Freedom to learn* (3rd ed.). New York: Merrill.

Rogers, L. Q., Matevey, C., Hopkins-Price, P., Shah, P., Dunnington, G., & Courneya, K. S. (2004). Exploring social cognitive theory constructs for promoting exercise among breast cancer patients. *Cancer Nursing, 27,* 462–473.

Rose, D. J. (1997). *A multilevel approach to the study of motor control and learning.* Needham Heights, MA: Allyn & Bacon.

Santrock, J. W. (2006). *Life-span development* (10th ed.). Boston: McGraw-Hill.

Schmidt, R. A. (1975). A schema theory of discrete motor skill learning. *Psychological Review, 82,* 225–260.

Schmidt, R. A. & Lee, T. D. (2005). *Motor control and learning: A behavioral emphasis* (4th ed.). Champaign, IL: Human Kinetics.

Schmidt, R. A., & Wrisberg, C. A. (2004). *Motor learning and performance: A problem-based learning approach* (3rd ed.). Champaign, IL: Human Kinetics.

Schmidt, R. A. & Wulf, G. (1997). Continuous concurrent feedback degrades skill learning: Implications for training and simulation. *Human Factors, 39,* 509–525.

Shapiro, A. (2002). The latest dope on research (about constructivism): Part I: Different approaches to constructivism—What it's all about. *International Journal of Education Reform, 12,* 62–77.

Sherif, M., & Sherif, C. W. (1969). *Social psychology.* New York: Harper & Row.

Shors, T. J. (2006). Stressful experience and learning across the lifespan. *Annual Review of Psychology, 57,* 55–85.

Shumway-Cook, A. S., & Woollacott, M. H. (2007). *Motor control: Translating research into clinical practice* (3rd ed.). Philadelphia: Lippincott Williams & Wilkins.

Singer, R. N. (1980). *Motor learning and human performance* (3rd ed.). New York: Macmillan.

Silverstein, S. M., & Uhlhaas, P. J. (2004). Gestalt psychology: The forgotten paradigm in abnormal psychology. *American Journal of Psychology, 117,* 259–277.

Skinner, B. F. (1974). *About behaviorism.* New York: Vintage Books.

Skinner, B. F. (1989). *Recent issues in the analysis of behavior.* Columbus, OH: Merrill.

Slipp, S. (2000). Subliminal stimulation research and its implications for psychoanalytic theory and treatment. *Journal of the American Academy of Psychoanalysis, 28,* 305–320.

Snowman, J., & Biehler, R. (2006). *Psychology applied to teaching* (11th ed.). Boston: Houghton Mifflin.

Sternberg, R. J. (1996). Styles of thinking. In P. B. Baltes & U. M. Staudinger (Eds.), *Interactive minds: Life-span perspectives on the social foundation of cognition* (pp. 347–365). New York: Cambridge University Press.

Sternberg, R. J. (2006). *Cognitive psychology* (4th ed.). Belmont, CA: Thomson/Wadsworth.

Stiles, A. S. (2005). Parenting needs, goals, and strategies of adolescent mothers. *MCN American Journal of Maternal/Child Nursing, 30,* 327–333.

Stockhurst, U., Steingrueber, H. J., Enck, P., & Klosterhalfen, S. (2006). Pavlovian conditioning of nausea and vomiting. *Autonomic Neuroscience, 129,* 50–57.

Stroebe, M. S., Folkman, S., Hansson, R. O., & Schut, H. (2006). The prediction of bereavement outcome: Development of an integrative risk factor framework. *Social Science and Medicine, 63,* 2440–2451.

Telford, K., Kralik, D., & Koch, T. (2006). Acceptance and denial: Implications for people adapting to chronic illness. Literature review. *Journal of Advanced Nursing, 55,* 457–464.

Tennant, M. (2006). *Psychology and adult learning* (3rd ed.). New York: Routledge.

Vander Zanden, J. W., Crandell, T. L., & Crandell, C. H. (2007). *Human development* (8th ed.). Boston: McGraw-Hill.

VanSant, A. F. (2003). Motor control, motor learning and motor development. In P. C. Montogomery & B. H. Connolly (Eds.), *Clinical applications for motor control* (pp. 25–52). Thorofare, NJ: Slack.

Vygotsky, L. S. (1986). *Thought and language.* Cambridge, MA: MIT Press.

Waynor, W. R., Pratt, C. W. Dolce, J., Bates, F. M., & Roberts, M. (2005). Making employment a priority in community mental health: Benefits of demonstrating direct employment practice. *American Journal of Psychiatric Rehabilitation, 8,* 103–112.

Winstein, C. J. (1987). Motor learning considerations in stroke rehabilitation. In P. W. Duncan & M. B. Badke (Eds.), *Stroke rehabilitation: The recovery of motor control* (pp. 109–134). Chicago, IL: Yearbook.

Winstein, C. J. (1991a). Designing practice for motor learning: Clinical applications. In M. J. Lister (Ed.), *Contemporary management of motor control problems:* *Proceedings of the II STEP conference* (pp. 65–76). Alexandria, VA: Foundation for Physical Therapy.

Winstein, C. J. (1991b). Knowledge of results and motor learning—implications for physical therapy. *Physical Therapy, 71,* 140–149.

Winstein, C. J., & Schmidt, R. A. (1990). Reduced frequency of knowledge of results enhances motor skill learning. *Journal of Experimental Psychology: Learning, Memory & Cognition, 16,* 677–691.

Wolpe, J. (1982). *The practice of behavior therapy* (3rd ed.). New York: Pergamon.

Woolfolk, A. E. (2001). *Educational psychology.* Boston: Allyn & Bacon.

Wulf, G., Hob, M., & Prinz, W. (1998). Instructions for motor learning: Differential effects of internal vs. external focus of attention. *Journal of Motor Behavior, 30,* 169–180.

Wulf, G., & Schmidt, R. A. (1997). Variability of practice and implicit motor learning. *Journal of Experimental Psychology: Learning, Memory & Cognition, 23,* 987–1006.

Part Two

Characteristics of the Learner

Chapter 4

Determinants
of Learning

Sharon Kitchie

CHAPTER HIGHLIGHTS

KEY TERMS

- determinants of learning
- learning needs
- readiness to learn
- learning styles

OBJECTIVES

After completing this chapter, the reader will be able to

1. Explain the health professional educator's role in the learning process.
2. Identify the three components of what are known as determinants of learning.
3. Describe the steps involved in the assessment of learning needs.
4. Explain methods that can be used to assess learner needs.
5. Discuss the factors that need to be assessed in each of the four types of readiness to learn.
6. Describe what is meant by learning styles.
7. Discriminate between the major learning style models and instruments identified.
8. Discuss ways to assess learning styles.
9. Identify the evidence that supports assessment of learning needs, readiness to learn, and learning styles.

In a variety of settings, health professionals are responsible for the education of clients, families, staff, and students. Numerous factors make the health professional educator's role particularly challenging in meeting the information needs of these various groups of learners. For example, short lengths of stay have compressed patient and family contact with the health professional, making it difficult to capture the teachable moments. In the case of staff, educational and experiential levels differ widely and time constraints are ever present in the practice arena. Staffing patterns such as 10- or 12-hour days, part-time employment, and various job functions can put the educator's ability to complete an accurate education assessment of staff to the test. In addition, many students are entering the health professions at an older age, bringing with them diverse life experiences and the demands of working and raising families while furthering their education. These and other changing healthcare trends and population demographics mean that health professional educators must constantly assess the **determinants of learning** for the varied audiences of learners they teach.

To meet these challenges, the health professional educator must be aware of the factors that influence how well an individual learns. The three determinants of learning that require assessment are (1) the needs of the learner, (2) the state of readiness to learn, and (3) the preferred learning styles for processing information. This chapter addresses these three determinants of learning as they affect the effective and efficient delivery of patient, client, student, and staff education.

The Educator's Role in Learning

The role of educating others is of paramount importance in the health professions. To do it well, the health professional must identify the information learners need, as well as consider their readiness to learn and their styles of learning. The learner, not the teacher, is the single most important person in the education process. Educators can greatly enhance learning when they serve as facilitators helping the learner become aware of what needs to be known, the value of knowing, and how to be actively involved in acquiring information (Musinski, 1999). Just providing information to the learner, however, does not ensure that learning will occur. There is no guarantee that the learner will learn the information given, although there is more of an opportunity to learn if the educator assesses the determinants of learning.

Assessment permits the health professional educator to facilitate the process of learning by arranging experiences within the environment that assist the learner to find the purpose, the will, and the most suitable approaches for learning. An assessment of the three determinants of learning enables the educator to identify information and present it in a variety of ways, which a learner cannot do alone. Manipulating the environment allows learners to experience meaningful parts and wholes to reach their individual potentials.

The educator plays a crucial role in the learning process by doing the following:

- Assessing problems or deficits
- Providing important information and presenting it in unique and appropriate ways
- Identifying progress being made
- Giving feedback and follow-up
- Reinforcing learning in the acquisition of new knowledge, skills, and attitudes
- Evaluating learners' abilities

The educator is vital in giving support, encouragement, and direction during the process of learning. Learners may make self-choices without the assistance of an educator, but these choices may be limited or inappropriate. For example, the health professional facilitates necessary changes in the home environment, such as minimizing distractions by having family members turn off the television to provide a quiet environment conducive for concentrating on a learning activity. The educator assists in identifying optimal learning approaches and activities that can both support and challenge

the learner based on his or her individual learning needs, readiness to learn, and learning style.

Assessment of the Learner

Assessment of learners' needs, readiness, and styles of learning is the first and most important step in instructional design—but it is also the step most likely to be neglected. The importance of assessment of the learner may seem self-evident, yet often only lip service is given to this initial phase of the educational process. Frequently, the health professional delves into teaching before addressing all of the determinants of learning. It is not unusual that patients with the same condition are taught with the same materials in the same way (Haggard, 1989). The result is that information given to the patient is neither individualized nor based on an adequate educational assessment. Recent evidence suggests, however, that individualizing teaching based on prior assessment improves patient outcomes (Corbett, 2003; Kim et al., 2004; Miaskowski et al., 2004). For example, Corbett's research demonstrates that providing individualized education to home care patients with diabetes significantly improves their foot care practices.

Health professionals are taught that any intervention should be preceded by an assessment. Few would deny that this is the correct approach, no matter whether planning for giving treatments, meeting the psychosocial needs of a client, or teaching someone to be independent in self-care or in the delivery of care. The effectiveness of care clearly depends on the scope, accuracy, and comprehensiveness of assessment prior to interventions.

What is it about assessment that is so significant and fundamental to the educational process? This initial step in the process validates the need for learning and the approaches to be used in designing learning experiences. Clients who desire or require information to maintain optimal health or health professional colleagues who must have a greater scope or depth of knowledge to deliver quality care to clients deserve to have an assessment done by the educator so that their needs as learners are appropriately addressed.

Assessments do more than simply identify and prioritize information for purposes of setting behavioral goals and objectives, planning instructional interventions, and being able to evaluate in the long run whether the learner has achieved the desired goals and objectives. Good assessments ensure that optimal learning can occur with the least amount of stress and anxiety for the learner. Assessment prevents needless repetition of known material, saves time and energy on the part of both the learner and the educator, and helps to establish rapport between the two parties (Haggard, 1989). Furthermore, it increases the motivation to learn by focusing on what the patient or health professional feels is most important to know or to be able to do.

Why, then, is this first step in the education process so overlooked or only partially carried out? Lack of time is the number one reason for health professional educators to shortchange the assessment phase. Such factors as shortened hospital stays and limited contact with clients and families in other settings as well as tighter schedules of staff resulting from increased practice demands have reduced the amount of time available for instruction. Because time constraints are a major concern when carrying out patient or staff education, health professionals must become skilled in accurately conducting assessments of the three determinants of learning so as to have reserve time for actual teaching. In addition, many health professionals, although expected and required by their practice acts to instruct others, are unfamiliar with the principles of teaching and learning. The health professional in the role of educator must become more acquainted and comfortable with all the elements of instructional design, but particularly with

the assessment phase because it provides the foundation for the rest of the educational process.

Assessment of the learner includes attending to the following three determinants (Haggard, 1989):

1. Learning needs—what the learner needs and wants to learn
2. Readiness to learn—when the learner is receptive to learning
3. Learning style—how the learner best learns

Assessing Learning Needs

Learning needs are defined as gaps in knowledge that exist between a desired level of performance and the actual level of performance (Healthcare Education Association, 1985). A learning need is the gap between what someone knows and what someone needs or wants to know. Such gaps exist because of a lack of knowledge, attitude, or skill.

Of the three determinants, health professional educators must identify learning needs first so that they can design an instructional plan to address any deficits in the cognitive, affective, or psychomotor domains. Once the educator discovers what needs to be taught, he can determine when and how learning can optimally occur.

Not every individual perceives a need for education. Often, learners are not aware of what they don't know or want to know. Consequently, it is up to the educator to assist them in identifying, clarifying, and prioritizing their needs and interests. Once these are determined, the information gathered can, in turn, be used to set objectives and plan appropriate and effective teaching and learning approaches for education to begin at a point suitable to the learner rather than from an unknown or inappropriate place.

Differences often exist between the perception of needs identified by patients versus the needs identified by the health professionals caring for them. In one early study, there was only a 20% nurse–patient agreement score with respect to congruency on needs/problems identified (Roberts, 1982). Mordiffi, Tan, and Wong (2003) cite more recent evidence from their research that the preoperative information provided by nurses and doctors was considered insufficient by the majority (66.7%) of patients who rated knowledge about anesthesia before scheduled surgery to be very or extremely important to them. Findings from a comprehensive review of preference-match strategies in physician–patient communication by Kiesler and Auerbach (2006) indicate that a large number (median 52%) of patients' preferences for medical information were "mismatched" with what they received. In these situations, the patients were dissatisfied with the medical information they were given, felt they had not been given adequate information about their condition, and reported a desire for more information. An interesting finding by Sandberg, Sharma, Wiklund, and Sandberg (2008) is that the information given to patients by anesthesiologists and nurse practitioners during preoperative teaching vastly exceeded patients' short-term memory capacity. Other authors also substantiate comparative incongruence in the perception of learning needs by patients and providers (Burkhart, 2008; Carlson, Ivnik, Dierkhising, O'Byrne, & Vickers, 2006; Suhonen, Nenonen, Laukka, & Valimaki, 2005; Timmins, 2005).

According to the estimates of many cognitive experts in behavior and social sciences (Bloom, 1968; Bruner, 1966; Carroll, 1963; Kessels, 2003; Ley, 1979; Skinner, 1954), most learners—90–95% of them—can master a subject with a high degree of success if given sufficient time and appropriate support. It is the educator's task to facilitate the determination of what exactly needs to be learned and identify approaches for presenting information in a way that the learner will best understand.

The following are important steps in the assessment of learning needs:

1. *Identify the learner.* Who is the audience? If the audience is one individual, is there a single need or do many needs have to be fulfilled? Is there more than one learner? If so, are their needs congruent or diverse? The development of formal and informal education programs for patients and their families, staff, or students must be based on accurate identification of the learner. For example, an educator may believe that all parents of children with asthma need a formal class on potential hazards in the home. This perception may be based on the educator's interaction with a few clients and may not be true of all families. Or the manager of a healthcare agency might request an in-service workshop for all staff on documentation of infection control because of an isolated incident involving one staff member's failing to appropriately follow established infection control procedures. This break in protocol may or may not indicate that everyone needs to have an update on policies and procedures.

2. *Choose the right setting.* Establishing a trusting environment helps learners feel a sense of security in confiding information, believe their concerns are taken seriously and are considered important, and feel respected. Ensuring privacy and confidentiality is recognized as essential to establishing a trusting relationship.

3. *Collect data about the learner.* Once the learner is identified, the educator can determine characteristic needs of the population by exploring typical health problems or issues of interest to that population. Subsequently, a literature search can assist the educator in identifying the type and extent of content to be included in teaching sessions as well as the educational strategies for teaching a specific population based on the analysis of needs. For example, Bibb (2001) collected data about a targeted patient population at one military treatment facility and found that education programs did not

provide adequate support for the growing number of participants who were older and more chronically ill. Rutten, Arora, Bakos, Aziz, and Rowland (2005) studied patients with cancer to determine the characteristic learning needs of that population.

4. *Collect data from the learner.* Learners are usually the most important source of needs assessment data about themselves. Allow clients and/or family members to identify what is important to them, what they perceive their needs to be, what types of social support systems are available, and what assistance these supports can provide. If the audience for teaching consists of staff members or students, solicit them for information as to those areas of practice in which they feel they need new or additional information. Actively engaging learners in defining their own problems and needs motivates them to learn because they have an investment in planning for a program specifically tailored to their unique circumstances. Also, the learner is important to include as a source of information because, as noted previously, the educator may not always perceive the same learning needs as the learner.

5. *Involve members of the healthcare team.* Other health professionals likely have insight into patient or family needs or the educational needs of the staff or students as a result of their frequent contacts with consumers as well as caregivers. Educators must remember to collaborate with other members of the healthcare team for a richer assessment of learning needs. In addition, associations such as the American Heart Association, the American Diabetes Association, and the American Cancer Society are excellent sources of health information.

6. *Prioritize needs.* A list of identified needs can become endless and seemingly impossible to accomplish. Maslow's (1970) hierarchy of human needs (see Figure 3–4 in Chapter 3) can help the educator prioritize so that the learner's basic needs are attended to first and foremost before higher needs can be met. For example, learning about energy conservation techniques cannot occur if a client faces problems with basic physiological needs such as pain and discomfort. These latter needs must be addressed before any other higher-order learning can occur.

Setting priorities for learning is often difficult when the educator is faced with many learning needs in several areas. Prioritizing the identified needs helps the client or staff to set realistic and achievable learning goals. Choosing what information to cover is imperative, and educators must make choices deliberately. Educators should prioritize learning needs based on the criteria in **Table 4–1** (Healthcare Education Association, 1985, p. 23) to foster maximum learning.

Without good assessment, a common mistake is to provide more information than the client wants or needs. It is important for the health professional to discriminate between information that clients need to know versus information that is nice for them to know. Often, highly technical information serves only to confuse and distract clients from the essential information they need to carry out their regimen (Hansen & Fischer, 1998; Kessels, 2003).

Education in and of itself is not always the answer to a problem. Often, healthcare providers believe that more education is necessary when something goes wrong, when something is not being done, when a patient is not following a prescribed regimen, or when a staff member does not adhere to a protocol. In such instances, always look for other nonlearning needs. For example, the health professional may discover that the client is not taking his medication and may begin a teaching plan without adequate assessment. The client may already understand the importance of taking a prescribed medication, know how to administer it, and be willing to follow the regimen, but he may not have the finances necessary to purchase the medication. In this case, the client does not have a learning need but rather requires social or financial support to obtain the medication.

7. *Determine availability of educational resources.* The educator may identify a need, but it may be useless to proceed with interventions if the proper educational resources are not available, are unrealistic to obtain, or do not match the learner's needs. In this case, it may be better to focus on other identified needs. For example, a patient who has asthma needs to learn how to use an inhaler and peak-flow meter. The educator may determine that this patient learns best if the health professional first gives a demonstration on the use of the inhaler and peak-flow meter and then allows the patient the opportunity to do a return demonstration. If the proper equipment is not available for demonstration/return demonstration at that moment, it might be better for the educator to concentrate on teaching the signs and symptoms the patient might experience when hav-

ing poor air exchange than it is to cancel the encounter altogether. Thereafter, the educator would work immediately on obtaining the necessary equipment for future encounters.

8. *Assess demands of the organization.* This assessment yields information that reflects the climate of the organization. What are the organization's philosophy, mission, strategic plan, and goals? The educator should be familiar with standards of performance required in various employee categories, along with job descriptions and hospital, professional, and agency regulations. If, for example, the organization is focused on health promotion versus trauma care, then there likely will be a different educational focus or emphasis that dictates learning needs of both consumers and employees.

9. *Take time-management issues into account.* Because time constraints are a major impediment to the assessment process, Rankin and Stallings (2005) suggest the educator should emphasize the following important points with respect to time-management issues:

Table 4–1 CRITERIA FOR PRIORITIZING LEARNING NEEDS

Mandatory: Needs that must be learned for survival or situations in which the learner's life or safety is threatened. Learning needs in this category must be met immediately. For example, a patient who has experienced a recent heart attack needs to know the signs and symptoms and when to get immediate help. The health professional who works in a hospital must learn how to do cardiopulmonary resuscitation or be able to carry out correct isolation techniques for self-protection.

Desirable: Needs that are not life dependent but that are related to well-being or the overall ability to provide quality care in situations involving changes in institutional procedure. For example, it is important for clients who have cardiovascular disease to understand the effects of a high-fat diet on their condition. It is desirable for health professionals to update their knowledge by attending an in-service program when hospital management decides to focus more attention on the appropriateness of patient education materials in relation to the patient populations being served.

Possible: Needs for information that are nice to know but not essential or required or situations in which the learning need is not directly related to daily activities. The patient who is newly diagnosed as having diabetes mellitus most likely does not need to know about traveling across time zones or staying in a foreign country because this information does not relate to the patient's everyday activities.

- Although close observation and active listening take time, it is much more efficient and effective to take the time to do a good initial assessment up front than to waste time having to go back to uncover information that should have been obtained before beginning instruction.
- Learners must be given time to offer their own perceptions of their learning needs if the educator expects them to take charge and become actively involved in the learning process.
- Assessment can be conducted anytime and anywhere the educator has formal or informal contact with learners. Data collection does not have to be restricted to a specific, predetermined schedule. With patients, many potential opportunities arise, such as when administering a treatment, dropping off a piece of equipment, making rounds, distributing medications, and so forth. For staff, assessments can be made when stopping to talk in the hallway or while enjoying lunch or break time together.
- Informing a client ahead of time that the educator wishes to spend time discussing problems or needs gives the person advanced notice to sort out his or her thoughts and feelings.
- Minimizing interruptions and distractions during planned assessment interviews maximizes productivity such that the educator might accomplish in 15 minutes what otherwise might have taken an hour in less directed, more frequently interrupted circumstances.

Methods to Assess Learning Needs

The health professional in the role of educator must obtain objective data about the learner as well as subjective data from the learner. The following are various methods that educators can use to assess learner needs and should be used in conjunction with one another to yield the most reliable information (Haggard, 1989).

Informal Conversations

Often learning needs are discovered during impromptu conversations that take place with other healthcare team members involved in the care of the client and between the health professional and the client or his or her family. The educator must rely on active listening to pick up cues and information regarding learning needs. Staff can provide valuable input about their learning needs by responding to open-ended questions.

Structured Interviews

The structured interview is perhaps the most common form of needs assessment to solicit the learner's point of view. The health professional educator asks the learner direct and often predetermined questions to gather information about learning needs. As with the gathering of any information from a learner in the assessment phase, the educator should strive to establish a trusting environment, use open-ended questions, choose a setting that is free of distractions, and allow the learner to state what are believed to be the learning needs.

It is important to remain nonjudgmental when collecting information about the learner's strengths, beliefs, and motivations. Educators should take notes with the learner's permission so that important information is not lost. The telephone is a good tool to use for an interview if it is impossible to ask questions in person. The major drawback of a telephone interview, however, is the inability on the part of the educator to perceive nonverbal cues from the learner.

Interviews yield answers that may reveal uncertainties, conflicts, inconsistencies, unexpected problems, anxieties, fears, and present knowledge base. Examples of questions that health professional educators can ask patients as learners are as follows:

- What do you think caused your problem?
- How severe is your illness?
- What does your illness/health mean to you?
- What do you do to stay healthy?
- What results do you hope to obtain from treatments?
- What are your strengths and weaknesses as a learner?
- How do you learn best?

If the learner is a staff member or student, the following questions could be asked:

- What do you think are your biggest challenges to learning?
- Which skill(s) do you need help in performing?
- What obstacles have you encountered in the past when you were learning new information?
- What do you see as your strengths and weaknesses as a learner?

These types of questions help to determine the needs of the learner and serve as a foundation for beginning to plan for an educational intervention.

Focus Groups

Focus groups involve getting together a small number (4 to 12) of potential learners (Breitrose, 1988) to determine areas of educational need by using group discussion to identify points of view or knowledge about a certain topic. A facilitator leads the discussion by asking questions that are open ended to encourage detailed discussion. These groups of potential learners in most cases should be homogeneous, with similar characteristics such as age, gender, and past experience with the topic

under discussion. However, if the purpose of the focus group is to solicit attitudes about a particular subject or to discuss ethical issues, for example, it may not be necessary or recommended to have a homogeneous group. Focus groups are ideal during the initial stage of information gathering to provide qualitative data for a complete assessment of learning needs.

Self-Administered Questionnaires

Educators can obtain the learner's written responses to questions about learning needs by using survey instruments. Checklists are one of the most common forms of questionnaires. They are easy to administer, provide more privacy than do interviews, and yield easy-to-tabulate data. Learners seldom object to this method of obtaining information about their learning needs. Sometimes learners may have difficulty rating themselves and may need the educator to clarify terms or provide additional information to help them understand what is being assessed. The educator's role is to encourage learners to make as honest a self-assessment as possible. Because checklists usually reflect what the health professional educator perceives as needs, there should also be a space for the learner to add any other items of interest or concern.

One example of a highly reliable and valid self-assessment tool is the Patient Learning Needs Scale (Redman, 2003). This instrument is designed to measure patients' perceptions of learning needs to manage their health care at home following a medical or surgical illness (Bubela et al., 2000).

Tests

Giving written pretests before teaching is planned can help identify the knowledge levels of potential learners regarding a particular subject and assist in identifying their specific learning needs. Also, this approach prevents the educator from repeating already known material in the teaching plan.

Furthermore, pretest results are useful to the educator after the completion of teaching: Educators can compare pretest scores to posttest scores to determine whether learning has taken place.

The Diabetes Knowledge Test is an example of a tool available to assess learning needs for self-management of diabetes (Panja, Starr, & Colleran, 2005). These researchers compared patients' diabetes knowledge with their glycemic control. Their findings demonstrate that an inverse linear relationship exists between performance on this diabetes test and HbA1c values. This test is available at the Michigan Diabetes Research and Training Center (www.med.umich.edu/mdrtc/survey/index.html). Redman (2003) describes this and many other measurement instruments for patient education that measure knowledge and learning assessment/design/delivery.

The educator must always consider the reported characteristics of the self-administered questionnaire or test before using it. The criteria to consider are the purpose of the tool (i.e., if it is relevant to what the health professional educator plans to assess), whether the results will be meaningful, whether each of the measured constructs is well defined, whether adequate testing of the instrument has been conducted, whether the instrument has been used in a similar setting, and whether the instrument has been used with a population similar to the educator's. The educator needs to consider the purpose, conceptual basis, development, and psychometric properties when evaluating the adequacy of any questionnaire or test (Waltz, Strickland, & Lenz, 2005).

Observations

Observing health behaviors in several different time periods can help to determine conclusions about established patterns of behavior that cannot and should not be drawn from a single observation. Actually watching the learner perform a skill

more than once is an excellent way of assessing a psychomotor need. Are all steps performed correctly? Does the learner have any difficulty with manipulating various pieces of equipment? Does the learner require prompting? Learners may believe they can accurately perform a skill or task (e.g., walking with crutches, changing a dressing, transferring in and out of a car), but by observing the skill performance the educator can best determine whether additional learning may be needed.

Learners who can observe a videotape of themselves performing a skill can more easily identify their learning needs. This process is known as reflection on action (Grant, 2002). The learner identifies what was done well and what could have been done better in his or her actual performance. Landry, Smith, and Swank (2006) provide evidence to support this method of assessing learning needs in their study measuring mothers' critiques of their own videotaped responsive behaviors in the home setting that would facilitate their infants' development.

Documentations

Initial assessments, progress notes, care plans, staff notes, and discharge planning forms can provide information on the learning needs of clients. Health professional educators need to follow a consistent format for reviewing charts so that they review each chart in the same manner to identify learning needs based on the same information. Also, documentation by members of the healthcare team outside of the health professional's discipline can yield valuable insights with respect to the needs of the learner.

Assessing Learning Needs of Staff

Williams (1998) specifically addresses the importance of identifying the learning needs of staff nurses using the following methods, which also apply to all health professional staff.

WRITTEN JOB DESCRIPTIONS

A written description of what is required to effectively carry out job responsibilities can reflect the potential learning needs of staff. This information forms the basis for establishing content in an orientation program for new staff or for designing continuing education opportunities for experienced staff members.

FORMAL AND INFORMAL REQUESTS

Often staff are asked for ideas for educational programs, and these ideas reflect what they perceive as needs. When conducting a formal educational program, the educator must verify that these requests are congruent with the needs of other staff members.

QUALITY ASSURANCE REPORTS

Trends found in incident reports indicating safety violations or errors in procedures are a source for establishing learning needs of staff that education can address.

CHART AUDITS

Educators can identify trends in practice through chart auditing. Does the staff have a learning need in terms of the actual charting? Is a new intervention being implemented? Does the record indicate some inconsistency with implementation of an intervention?

RULES AND REGULATIONS

A thorough knowledge of hospital, professional, and healthcare requirements helps to identify possible learning needs of staff. The educator should monitor new rules of practice arising from changes occurring within an institution or external to the organization that may have implications for the delivery of care.

FOUR-STEP APPRAISAL OF NEEDS

Panno (1992), expanding on Knox's (1974, 1977, 1986) interest in teaching related to adult development and learning, describes a systematic approach for assessing learning needs of caregivers and the organizations in which they practice. Knox's interpretation of how adults learn has led to information for the development and coordination of education programs that are responsive to the backgrounds and aspirations of various adult learners. Panno's four steps in assessing learning needs are as follows:

1. Defining the target population
2. Analyzing learner and organizational needs
3. Analyzing the perceived needs of the learner and comparing these to the actual needs
4. Using data to prioritize learning needs identified

Educators can use this organizing framework to assess staff at multiple levels, from aides and assistants to licensed professionals, who are typically the target audiences for in-service programs in an institution. Panno (1992) points out that often plans for educational activities are based on personal preference, mandates from administration, intuition, or trends in the profession, which may meet the sponsor's needs but not necessarily the needs of the learner. This systematic approach is useful because it benefits all involved and is a process that justifies the resources required for the assessment process.

Readiness to Learn

Once the educator has identified learning needs, the next step is to determine the learner's readiness to receive information. **Readiness to learn** can be defined as the time when the learner demonstrates an interest in learning the information necessary to maintain optimal health or to become more skillful in a job. Often, educators have noted that when a client or staff member asks a question, the time is prime for learning. Readiness to learn occurs when the learner is receptive, willing, and able to participate in the learning process. It is the responsibility of the educator to discover through assessment exactly when patients or staff are ready to learn, what they need or want to learn, and how to adapt the content to fit each learner.

To assess readiness to learn, the educator must first understand what needs to be taught, collect and validate that information, and then apply the same methods used previously to assess learning needs, including making observations, conducting interviews, gathering information from the learner as well as other healthcare team members, and reviewing documentation. The educator must do this prior to the time when actual learning is to occur.

No matter how important the information is or how much the educator feels the recipient of teaching needs the information, if the learner is not ready, the information will not be absorbed. The educator, in conjunction with the learner, must determine what needs to be learned and what the learning objectives should be to establish which domain and at what level these objectives should be classified (see Chapter 10). Otherwise, both the educator's and the learner's time could very well be wasted because the established objectives may be beyond the readiness of the learner.

Timing—that is, the point at which teaching should take place—is very important. Anything that affects physical or psychological comfort can affect a learner's ability and willingness to learn. A learner who is not receptive to information at one time may be more receptive to the same information at another time. Because the health professional often has limited contact with patients and family members as a result of short hospital stays

or short visits in the outpatient setting, teaching must be brief and basic. Timing also is an important factor when working with staff. Readiness to learn is based on current demands of practice and needs to correspond to the ever constant changes in health care. Adults, whether they are patients, family, staff, or students, are eager to learn when the subject of teaching is relevant and applicable to their everyday concerns.

Before teaching can begin, the educator must find the time to first take a PEEK (Lichtenthal, 1990) at the four types of readiness to learn—physical readiness, emotional readiness, experiential readiness, and knowledge readiness. The educator must take into consideration these four types of readiness to learn, which may be obstacles or enhancers to learning (**Table 4–2**).

Physical Readiness

The educator must consider five major components of physical readiness—measures of ability, complexity of task, environmental effects, health status, and gender—because they affect the degree or extent to which learning will occur.

MEASURES OF ABILITY

Ability to perform a task requires fine and/or gross motor movements, sensory acuity, adequate strength, flexibility, coordination, and endurance. Each developmental stage in life is characterized by physical and sensory abilities or is affected by individual disabilities. For example, walking on crutches is a psychomotor skill for which a patient must have the physical ability to be ready to learn. If a person has a visual deficit, the educator can make available eyeglasses or a magnifying glass so that the client can, for example, see the lines on a piece of equipment such as a spirometer. If the educator is conducting an in-service workshop on lifting and transfer activities, staff must have the endurance level required to return demonstrate this skill. Creating a stimulating and accepting

Table 4–2 Take Time to Take a PEEK at the Four Types of Readiness to Learn

P = PHYSICAL READINESS
- Measures of ability
- Complexity of task
- Environmental effects
- Health status
- Gender

E = EMOTIONAL READINESS
- Anxiety level
- Support system
- Motivation
- Risk-taking behavior
- Frame of mind
- Developmental stage

E = EXPERIENTIAL READINESS
- Level of aspiration
- Past coping mechanisms
- Cultural background
- Locus of control
- Orientation

K = KNOWLEDGE READINESS
- Present knowledge base
- Cognitive ability
- Learning disabilities
- Learning styles

Source: From Lichtenthal, C. (1990, August). *A self-study model on readiness to learn.* Reprinted with permission from Cheryl Lichtenthal. Unpublished manuscript.

environment by using instructional tools to match learners' physical and sensory abilities can encourage readiness to learn.

Complexity of Task

Variations in the complexity of the task affect the extent to which the learner can master the behavioral changes in the cognitive, affective, and psychomotor domains. The more complex the task, the more difficult it is to achieve. Psychomotor skills, once acquired, are usually retained better and longer than learning in the other domains

(Greer, Hitt, Sitterly, & Slebodnick, 1972). Once ingrained, psychomotor, cognitive, and affective behaviors become habitual and may be difficult to alter. For example, if the learner has been performing a psychomotor skill over a long period of time and then the procedural steps of the task change, the learner must unlearn those steps and relearn the new way. This requirement may increase the complexity of the task and put additional physical demands on the learner by lengthening the time the learner needs to adjust to doing something in a new way. Older adults, in particular, develop elaborate cognitive schemas over the years, and when they are faced with information contrary to their preexisting knowledge and beliefs, they find the effort to change difficult, confusing, and time consuming (Kessels, 2003).

Environmental Effects

An environment conducive to learning helps to keep the learner's attention and stimulate interest in learning. Unfavorable conditions, such as extremely high levels of noise or frequent interruptions, can interfere with a learner's accuracy and precision in performing cognitive and manual dexterity tasks. Intermittent noise tends to have greater disruptive effects on learning than the more rapidly habituated steady-state noise. McDonald, Wiczorek, and Walker (2004) examined background noise and interruption for these effects on college students learning health information. The results of their research suggest that distraction, including noise, during health teaching adversely affects readiness to learn.

Older adults, in particular, need more time to react and respond to stimuli. Increased inability to receive, process, and transmit information is a characteristic of aging. Environmental demands that make older persons feel rushed or like they must perform tasks in a short time frame can overwhelm them. When an activity is self-paced, older learners respond more favorably.

Health Status

The amounts of energy available, as well as an individual's present comfort level, are factors that significantly influence that individual's readiness to learn. Energy-reducing demands caused by the body's response to illness require the learner to expend large amounts of physical and psychic energy, with little reserve left for actual learning. Health professional educators must seriously consider a person's health status, whether well, acutely ill, or chronically ill, when assessing for readiness.

Healthy learners have energy available for learning. Readiness to learn about health-promoting behaviors is based on their perception of self-responsibility. (See Chapter 6 on the Health Belief Model.) The extent to which an individual perceives illness to potentially affect future well-being influences that person's desire to learn preventive and promotion measures. If learners perceive a threat to their quality of life, they likely will seek more information in an attempt to control the negative effects of an illness (Bubela & Galloway, 1990).

Learners who are acutely ill tend to focus their energies on the physiological and psychological demands of their illness. Learning is at a minimum because most of these individuals' energy is needed for the demands of the illness and gaining immediate relief. Any learning that may occur should be related to treatments, tests, and minimizing pain or other discomforts. As these patients improve and the acute phase of illness diminishes, they can then focus on learning follow-up management and the avoidance of complications.

Educators must assess acutely ill persons' readiness to learn by observing their energy levels and comfort status. Improvement in physical status usually results in more receptivity to learning. However, medications that induce side effects such as drowsiness, mental depression, impaired depth perception, decreased ability to concentrate, and learner fatigue also reduce task-handling capacity.

For example, giving a patient a sedative prior to a learning experience may result in less apprehension, but cognitive and psychomotor abilities may be impaired.

Chronic illness, on the other hand, has no time limits and is of long-term duration. Models of how people deal with chronic illness also are useful as frameworks for understanding readiness to learn in chronically ill people (Lubkin & Larsen, 2006). The physiological and psychological demands vary in chronic illness and are not always predictable. Patients may go through different stages in dealing with their illness similar to the adjustment stages of a person experiencing a loss (Boyd, Gleit, Graham, & Whitman, 1998). If the learner is in the avoidance stage, readiness to learn likely is limited to simple explanations because the patient's energy is concentrated on denial. Energy levels stabilize and become redirected as awareness of the realities of the situation increase. Readiness to learn may be indicated by the questions the patient asks. Exploring another perspective, Telford, Kralik, and Koch (2006) encourage health professionals to listen carefully to their patients' stories of how they actually experience the illness, rather than attempt to categorize patients into specific stages. Listening to patient stories may provide clues as to individuals' readiness to learn.

Burton (2000) describes the Corbin and Strauss (1991) chronic illness trajectory framework. This framework reflects the continual nature of adaptation required in living with chronic illness. Unlike the Corbin and Strauss model, Patterson (2001) describes a shifting perspectives model that suggests that living with chronic illness is an ongoing and continually dynamic process. This model provides an explanation of chronically ill persons' variations in attention to symptoms over time. Individuals' perspectives shift in the degree to which illness is in the foreground or background of their world. It is important for educators to understand this cycle when assessing readiness to learn because educators cannot assume that an approach that worked at one time will be just as effective at another time. A chronically ill person's receptivity to learning and practicing self-care measures is not static and fluctuates over time.

GENDER

Research indicates that women are generally more receptive to medical care and take fewer risks with their health than do men (Ashton, 1999; Bertakis, Rahman, Helms, Callahan, & Robbins, 2000; Rosen, Tsai, & Downs, 2003; Stein & Nyamathi, 2000). This difference may arise because women traditionally have taken the role of caregivers and therefore are more open to health promotion teaching. In addition, women have more frequent contacts with health providers while bearing and raising children. Men, on the other hand, tend to be less receptive to healthcare interventions and are more likely to be risk takers. A good deal of this behavior is thought to be socially induced. Changes are beginning to be seen in the health-seeking behavior of men and women as a result of the increased focus on healthier lifestyles and the blending of gender roles in the home and workplace.

Emotional Readiness

Learners must be emotionally ready to learn. Like physical readiness, emotional readiness includes several factors that need to be assessed. These factors include anxiety level, support system, motivation, risk-taking behavior, frame of mind, and developmental stage.

ANXIETY LEVEL

Anxiety influences a person's ability to perform at cognitive, affective, and psychomotor levels. Anxiety affects patients' ability to concentrate and retain information (Kessels, 2003; Stephenson, 2006). The level of anxiety may or may not be a hindrance to the learning of new skills: Some degree of anxiety is a motivator to learn, but anxiety

that is too low or too high interferes with readiness to learn. On either end of the continuum, mild or severe anxiety may lead to inaction on the part of the learner. If anxiety is low, the individual is not driven to take steps to promote his or her health or prevent diseases. Moderate anxiety, on the other hand, drives someone to take action. As the level of anxiety increases, emotional readiness peaks and then begins to decrease in an inversely U-shaped curvilinear manner based on the Yerkes–Dodson law (Ley, 1979), as shown in **Figure 4–1**. A moderate level of anxiety is best for success in learning and is considered the optimal time for teaching.

Fear is a major contributor to anxiety and thus negatively affects readiness to learn in any of the learning domains. The performance of a task in and of itself may be fear inducing to a patient because of its very nature or meaning. For example, learning to cook on a gas stove may produce fear for the client because of the perceived danger of starting a fire or sustaining a burn. A staff member or student, on the other hand, may have real

Figure 4–1 Effect of Anxiety on Emotional Readiness to Learn

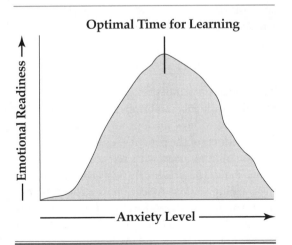

difficulty mastering a skill because of the fear of harming a patient or failing to do a procedure correctly.

Fear may also lead clients to deny their illness or disability, which interferes with their ability to learn. If a situation is life threatening or overwhelming, anxiety will be high and readiness to learn will be diminished. Although teaching may be imperative for survival, learning usually can take place only if instructions are simple and are repeated over and over again. In such circumstances, families and support persons also should be educated to reinforce information and assist with caregiving responsibilities. In later stages of adaptation, acceptance of illness or disability allows the individual to be more receptive to learning because anxiety levels are less acute.

Discovering what stressful events or major life changes the learner is experiencing gives the educator clues about that person's emotional readiness to learn. The health professional must first identify the source and level of anxiety. High stress levels can be moderated by encouraging the person to participate in such activities as support groups and use of relaxation techniques such as imagery and yoga (Stephenson, 2006). After anxiety levels have been moderated and anxiety has been lessened, education is an excellent intervention to spur someone to take action when dealing with a stressful life event.

Support System

The availability and strength of a support system also influence emotional readiness and are closely tied to how anxious an individual might feel. Members of the patient's support system who are available to assist with self-care activities at home should be present during at least some of the teaching sessions to learn how to help the patient if the need arises. Kitchie's (2003) descriptive correlational study suggests that families and friends are important for medication adherence among older adults who experience chronic illness. Although the educator should not draw any conclusions about causal relationships from this type of study, the educator's assessment benefits from incorporating questions about the learner's social network. Social support is important in buffering the effects of stressful events (Gavan, 2003; Kitchie, 2003). A strong positive support system can decrease anxiety, whereas the lack of one can increase anxiety levels.

Health professionals often act as sources of social and emotional support to clients. Epstein and Street (2007) describe the significance of fostering healing relationships with patients and responding to patients' emotions as fundamental functions of patient–clinician communication in cancer care. Street, Makoul, Arora, and Epstein (2009) identify the importance of clinicians enhancing patients' abilities to manage emotions in one of their several recommended pathways to improved health outcomes. Beddoe (1999) describes the unique opportunity that nurses have to provide emotional support to patients. She labels this opportunity as the reachable moment—the time when a nurse truly connects with clients by directly meeting them on mutual terms. The reachable moment allows for the mutual exchange of concerns and a sharing of possible intervention options without the nurse being inhibited by prejudice or bias. When the client feels emotionally supported, the stage is set for the teachable moment, when the client is most receptive to learning.

Motivation

Emotional readiness is strongly associated with motivation, which is a willingness to take action. Knowing the motivational level of the learner assists the educator in determining when that person is ready to learn. Assessment of emotional readiness involves ascertaining the level of motivation, not necessarily the reasons for the motivation. A learner may be motivated to learn for many reasons, and almost any reason to learn is a valid one.

The level of motivation is related to what learners perceive as an expectation of themselves or others. Interest in informal or formal teacher–learner interactions is a cue to motivation. The learner who is ready to learn shows an interest in what the health professional educator is doing by demonstrating a willingness to participate or to ask questions. Prior learning experiences, whether they be past accomplishments or failures, are reflected in the current level of motivation demonstrated by the learner for accomplishing the task at hand (see Chapter 6).

RISK-TAKING BEHAVIOR

Taking risks is intrinsic in the activities people perform daily. Many activities are done without thinking about the outcome. According to Joseph (1993), some patients, by the very nature of their personalities, take more risks than others do. The educator can assist patients to develop strategies that help reduce the risk of their choices. If patients participate in activities that may shorten their life span rather than complying with a recommended treatment plan, the educator must be willing to teach these patients how to recognize certain body symptoms and then what to do if they have them.

Understanding staff willingness to take risks helps the health professional educator understand why some learners may be hesitant to try new approaches to delivering care. Wolfe (1994) states that taking risks can be threatening when the outcomes are not guaranteed. Educators can, however, help individuals learn how to take risks. First, the person must decide to take the risk. The next step is to develop strategies to minimize the risk. Then, the learner needs to develop a worst-, best-, and most probable case scenario. Last, the learner must decide whether the worst-case scenario developed is acceptable.

FRAME OF MIND

Frame of mind involves concern about the here and now versus the future. If survival is of primary concern, readiness to learn will be focused on the present to meet basic human needs. According to Maslow (1970), physical needs such as food, warmth, comfort, and safety as well as psychosocial needs of feeling accepted and secure must be met before someone can focus on higher-order learning. People from lower socioeconomic levels tend to concentrate on immediate, current concerns because they are trying to satisfy everyday needs.

Ramanadhan and Viswanath (2006) use national data from the 2003 Health Information National Trends survey to examine information-seeking behaviors of adults. They found that a significant percentage of those diagnosed with a serious disease, such as cancer, report that they do not seek or receive health information beyond that given by healthcare providers. Furthermore, compared to seekers of health information, non-seeker patients were more likely to come from the lowest income and education groups and were less attentive about getting health information from the media. These findings have implications for educators when deciding on the best method for reaching various segments of the population.

Children regard life in the here and now because they are developmentally focused on what makes them happy and satisfied. This affects their willingness to learn health information. In addition, their thinking is concrete rather than abstract. Adults who have reached self-actualization and those whose basic needs are met are more ready to learn health promotion tasks and are said to have a more futuristic orientation.

DEVELOPMENTAL STAGE

Each task associated with human development produces a peak time for readiness to learn, known as a teachable moment (Hansen & Fisher, 1998; Hotelling, 2005; Tanner, 1989; Wagner & Ash,

1998). Unlike children, adults can build on meaningful past experiences and are strongly driven to learn information that helps them to cope better with real-life tasks. They see learning as relevant when they can apply new knowledge to help them solve immediate problems. Children, on the other hand, desire to learn for learning's sake and actively seek out experiences that give them pleasure and comfort. Erickson's well-accepted theory on the eight stages of psychosocial learning is most relevant to an individual's emotional readiness (see Chapter 5).

Experiential Readiness

Experiential readiness refers to the learner's past experiences with learning and includes five elements. The educator should assess whether previous learning experiences have been positive or negative in overcoming problems or accomplishing new tasks. Someone who has had negative experiences with learning is not likely to be motivated or willing to take a risk to change behavior or acquire new behaviors.

LEVEL OF ASPIRATION

The extent to which someone is driven to achieve is related to the type of short- and long-term goals established—not by the educator, but by the learner. Previous failures and past successes influence the goals learners set for themselves. Early successes are important motivators in learning subsequent skills. Satisfaction, once achieved, elevates the level of aspiration, which, in turn, increases the probability of continued performance output in undertaking future endeavors to change behavior.

PAST COPING MECHANISMS

Educators must explore the coping mechanisms learners have been using to understand how they have dealt with previous problems. Once these mechanisms are identified, the educator must determine whether past coping strategies have been effective and, if so, whether they work well in the present learning situation.

CULTURAL BACKGROUND

The educator's knowledge about other cultures and sensitivity to behavioral differences between cultures are important so that the educator can avoid teaching in opposition to cultural beliefs (see Chapter 8). Assessment of what an illness means to the patient from the patient's cultural perspective is imperative in determining readiness to learn. Remaining sensitive to cultural influences allows the educator to bridge the gap, when necessary, between the medical healthcare culture and the patient's culture. Building on the learner's knowledge base or belief system (unless it is dangerous to well-being), rather than attempting to change it or claim it is wrong, encourages rather than dampens readiness to learn.

Language is also a part of culture and may prove to be a significant obstacle to learning if the educator and the learner do not speak the same language fluently. Assessing whether the learner understands English well enough to be able to express herself so that others understand is the first step. A qualified interpreter is necessary if the learner and health professional do not speak the same language fluently. Enlisting the help of someone other than a trained interpreter to bridge language differences may negatively influence learning. This effect depends on such issues as the sensitivity of the topic and the need for privacy. In some instances, the patient may not want family members or associates to know about a health concern or illness.

Medical terminology in and of itself may be a foreign language to many patients, whether or not they are from another culture or their primary language is the same or different from that of the educator. In addition, sometimes a native language does not have an equivalent word to describe the terms that are being used in the teaching situation. Differences in language compound cultural barriers. Educators should not start teaching unless they have determined that the learner understands and that they understand the learner's culture (see Chapter 8).

Locus of Control

Educators can determine whether readiness to learn comes from internal or external stimuli by ascertaining the learner's previous life patterns of responsibility and assertiveness. When patients are internally motivated to learn, they have what is called an internal locus of control. They are ready to learn when they feel a need to know about something. This drive to learn comes from within the learner. Usually, this type of learner indicates a need to know by asking questions. Remember that when someone asks a question, the time is prime for learning. If patients have an external locus of control—that is, they are externally motivated—then someone other than themselves must encourage in them a feeling of wanting to know something. The responsibility often falls on the educator to motivate the client to want to learn.

Orientation

The tendency to adhere to a parochial or cosmopolitan point of view is known as orientation. Patients with a parochial orientation tend to be more close-minded in their thinking, are more conservative in their approach to situations, are less willing to learn new material, and place the most trust in traditional authority figures such as the physician. This type of orientation is seen most often in people who have been raised in a small-town atmosphere or who come from cohesive neighborhoods or protective family environments. Conversely, people who exhibit a cosmopolitan orientation most likely have a more worldly perspective on life as a result of broader experiences outside their

immediate spheres of influence. These individuals are more likely to be receptive to new ideas and to opportunities to learn new ways of doing things. Educators must be careful not to stereotype individuals unfairly, but learners usually possess representative characteristics of one or the other of these two opposing orientations.

Knowledge Readiness

Knowledge readiness refers to the learner's present knowledge base, the level of learning capability, and the preferred style of learning. Health professional educators must assess these components to determine readiness to learn and should plan teaching accordingly.

Present Knowledge Base

How much someone already knows about a particular subject or how proficient that person is at performing a task is an important factor to determine before designing and implementing instruction. If educators make the mistake of teaching subject material that has already been learned, they risk at the very least creating boredom and disinterest in the learner or at the extreme insulting the learner, which could produce resistance to further learning. The health professional educator must always find out what the learner knows prior to teaching and build on this knowledge base to encourage readiness to learn. In teaching clients, the educator also must consider how much information the client wants to receive. Some clients want to know the details to make informed decisions about their care, whereas others prefer a more general and less in-depth approach and can be overwhelmed with too much information.

Cognitive Ability

The extent to which information can be processed is indicative of the learner's capabilities. The educator must match the level of behavioral objectives to the cognitive ability of the learner. The learner who is capable of understanding, memorizing, recalling, or recognizing subject material is functioning at a lower level in the cognitive domain than the learner who demonstrates problem solving, concept formation, or application of information. For example, staff or students who can answer questions about cardiopulmonary resuscitation (CPR) on a written test demonstrate an understanding of the subject, but this does not necessarily mean that they can transfer this knowledge to perform CPR in the clinical setting. Clients who can identify risk factors of hypertension (a low level of functioning in the cognitive domain) may struggle with generalizing this information to incorporate a low-salt diet in their lifestyle.

Individuals with cognitive impairment present a special challenge to the educator and require simple explanations and step-by-step instruction with frequent repetition. Health educators should be sure to make information meaningful to those with cognitive impairments by teaching at their level and communicating in ways that learners can understand (see Chapter 9). Enlisting the help of members of the client's support system by teaching them requisite skills allows them to contribute positively to the reinforcement of self-care activities.

LEARNING AND READING DISABILITIES

Learning disabilities, which may be accompanied by low-level reading skills, are not necessarily indicative of an individual's intellectual abilities but require educators to use special or innovative approaches to instruction to sustain or bolster readiness to learn. Individuals with low literacy skills and learning disabilities become easily discouraged unless the educator recognizes their special needs and seeks ways to help them accommodate or overcome their problems with encoding words and comprehending information (see Chapters 7 and 9).

LEARNING STYLES

A variety of preferred styles of learning exists, and assessing how someone learns best and likes to learn helps the educator to select teaching approaches accordingly. Knowing the teaching methods and materials with which a learner is most comfortable or, conversely, those that the learner does not tolerate well helps the educator to tailor teaching to meet the needs of individuals with different styles of learning, thereby increasing their readiness to learn. For more information on learning styles, see the following discussion.

Learning Styles

Learning styles refer to the ways in which and conditions under which learners most efficiently and most effectively perceive, process, store, and recall what they are attempting to learn (James & Gardner, 1995) and how they prefer to approach different learning tasks (Cassidy, 2004). Keefe (1979) further defines learning style as the way the learners learn, taking into account cognitive, affective, and physiological factors that affect how learners perceive, interact with, and respond to the learning environment.

Learning style models are based on the premise that certain characteristics of learning are biological in origin, whereas others are sociologically developed as a result of environmental influences. Recognizing that people have different approaches to learning helps the health professional educator understand the differences in educational interests and needs of diverse populations. Accepting diversity of style can help educators create an atmosphere for learning that offers experiences that encourage each individual to reach his or her full potential. Understanding learning styles also can help educators make deliberate decisions about program development and instructional design (Arndt & Underwood, 1990; Churchill, 2008; Coffield, Moseley, Hall, & Ecclestone, 2004b;

Jessee, O'Neill, & Dosch, 2006; Morse, Oberer, Dobbins, & Mitchell, 1998; Vaughn & Baker, 2008).

No learning style is better or worse than another. Given the same content, most learners can assimilate information with equal success, but how they go about mastering the content is determined by their individual style. The more flexible the educator is in using teaching methodologies and tools related to individual learning styles, the greater the likelihood that learning will occur.

Six Learning Style Principles

Six principles have emerged from research about learning styles. To develop these six principles, Friedman and Alley (1984) reviewed an enormous volume of literature, which included more than 30 different learning style instruments. The six principles remain valid and are summarized as follows:

1. Both the style by which the educator prefers to teach and the style by which the learner prefers to learn can be identified. Identification of different styles offers specific clues as to the way a person learns. By understanding their own learning style, educators can appreciate why it may be easier to help one style of learner to master information but more difficult to work with another learner who needs an entirely different approach to learning.
2. Educators need to guard against relying on teaching methods and tools that match their own preferred learning styles. Health professional educators need to realize that just because they gravitate to learning in a certain way, it does not mean that everyone else can or wants to learn this way. It is much easier for an educator to incorporate a variety of teaching approaches than for learners to adapt to the educator's style.
3. Educators are most helpful when they assist learners in identifying and learning according to

the learners' own style preferences. Each learner is unique and complex, with a distinct learning style preference that distinguishes him or her from other learners. Making learners aware of their individual style preferences leads to an understanding of which teaching–learning approaches work best for them. Also, an awareness of their preference for a particular learning style sensitizes learners to the fact that whichever style is most comfortable for them may not be the best approach for others.

4. Learners should initially have the opportunity to learn through their preferred style. The health professional educator can provide the means by which each learner can experience successful learning. Visual learners, for example, should be given reading materials, videos, computer simulations, models, and diagrams from which to learn rather than insisting that they listen to a lecture or audiotape or become involved in role-playing. As another example, to capitalize on their strengths concrete thinkers need facts, whereas abstract thinkers need theories.
5. Learners should be encouraged to diversify their style preferences. Today, learners are constantly faced with learning situations in which one approach to learning does not suffice if they are to reach their fullest potential. Without encouragement, learners tend to gravitate automatically to using their preferred style of learning. The more frequently learners are exposed to different methods of learning, the less stressful those methods are in future learning situations.
6. Educators can develop specific learning activities that reinforce each modality or style. Awareness of various methods and materials available is the key to addressing and augmenting different learning styles. Using only a limited number of educational strategies selectively excludes many learners.

Three mechanisms to determine learning style are observation, interviews, and administration of learning style instruments. By observing the learner in action, the educator can ascertain how the learner grasps information and problem solves. For example, when doing a math calculation, does the learner write down every step or only the answer? In an interview, the educator can ask the learner about preferred ways of learning as well as the environment most comfortable for learning. Is group discussion or self-instruction preferable? Is a warm or cold room more conducive to concentration? Simply asking the question, "How do you learn best?" yields valuable information. Finally, the educator can administer learning style instruments such as those described in the next section.

Educators should use all three techniques to determine learning style. Assessment is foremost in the educational process. Once data are gathered through interview, observation, and instrument administration, the educator can validate learning style and choose methods and materials for instruction to match learner preferences and direct clients, students, or staff toward those ways they best can learn.

Using the learning style approach to instruction has enormous and exciting implications. Understanding and recognizing various styles can influence decision making about planning, implementing, and evaluating educational programs.

Learning Style Models and Instruments

The identification and application of information about learning styles continues to be an emerging movement, but it is just beginning to be applied to the health education field. To date, researchers have defined learning styles differently, although the concepts in each definition are often overlapping. No single framework for instructional design is forthcoming, yet each proposed framework provides the educator with a more profound view of

the learner than previously known (Knowles, 1990; Morse et al., 1998; Villejo & Meyers, 1991).

This chapter does not attempt to include all the instruments that are available, but rather highlights those commonly cited in recent reviews and in health sciences research literature that refer to the psychometric properties of each. These instruments are believed to be the most useful to health professional educators for assessment purposes.

Before using any learning style instrument, it is important to determine its reliability and validity and to realize that a totally inclusive instrument that measures all domains of learning—cognitive, affective, and psychomotor—does not exist. Therefore, it is best to use more than one measurement tool for assessment. Also, the educator should not rely heavily on these instruments because they are intended not for diagnosis but rather to validate what the learner perceives in comparison to what the educator perceives. These instruments will help the health professional in developing a more personalized form of instruction.

Right-Brain/Left-Brain and Whole-Brain Thinking

Although not technically a model, right-brain/left-brain thinking along with whole-brain thinking adds to the understanding of brain functions that are associated with learning. More than 30 years ago, Dr. Roger Sperry and his research team established that in many ways the brain operates as two brains (Herrmann, 1988; Sperry, 1977), with each hemisphere having separate and complementary functions. The left hemisphere of the brain was found to be the vocal and analytical side, which is used for verbalization and for reality-based and logical thinking. The right hemisphere was found to be the emotional, visual-spatial, and nonverbal side, with thinking processes that are intuitive, subjective, relational, holistic, and time free. Sperry and his colleagues discovered that learners are able to use both sides of the brain because of a connector between the two hemispheres called the corpus callosum.

There is no correct or wrong side of the brain. Each hemisphere gathers in the same sensory information but handles the information in different ways. One hemisphere may take over and inhibit the other in processing information, or the task may be divided between the two sides, with each handling the part best suited to its way of processing information. Recognizing that one side of the brain is better equipped for certain kinds of tasks than for others, educators can find the most effective way to present information to learners who may have a dominant brain hemisphere (**Table 4–3**). Brain hemisphericity is linked to cognitive learning style or the way individuals perceive and gather information to problem solve, complete assigned tasks, relate to others, and meet the daily challenges of life.

Neuroimaging methods, such as positron emission tomography (PET) and functional magnetic resonance imaging (fMRI), provide information on how the brain works. This information adds to the relevance of learning styles and brain hemisphere performance. McIntosh (1998) proposes a general hypothesis that learning and memory are emergent properties of network interactions. Sylvester (1995, 1998) reports on the research that has led to a better understanding of the functions of the brain and individual learning differences. Iaccino (1993) provides more detailed accounts of the clinical evidence that has contributed to the left–right dichotomy of the brain. These advances in technology have confirmed many of the assumptions about the functioning of the brain, which educators can apply to assessing learning styles, choosing education techniques (Caulfield, Kidd, & Kocher, 2000; Stover, 2001), and identifying strengths and weaknesses in their own teaching approaches.

Most individuals have a dominant side of the brain. Gondringer (1989) reports that most learners have left-brain dominance and that only ap-

---

Table 4–3 EXAMPLES OF HEMISPHERE FUNCTIONS

Left-Hemisphere Functions	Right-Hemisphere Functions
Thinking is critical, logical, convergent, focal	Thinking is creative, intuitive, divergent, diffuse
Analytical	Synthesizing
Prefers talking and writing	Prefers drawing and manipulating objects
Responds to verbal instructions and explanations	Responds to written instructions and explanations
Recognizes/remembers names	Recognizes/remembers faces
Relies on language in thinking and remembering	Relies on images in thinking and remembering
Solves problems by breaking them into parts, then approaches the problem sequentially, using logic	Solves problems by looking at the whole, the configurations, then approaches the problem through patterns, using hunches
Good organizational skills, neat	Loose organizational skills, sloppy
Likes stability, willing to adhere to rules	Likes change, uncertainty
Conscious of time and schedules	Frequently loses contact with time and schedules
Algebra is the preferred math	Geometry is the preferred math
Not as good at interpreting body language	Good at interpreting body language
Controls emotions	Free with emotions

proximately 30% have right-brain dominance. This may be because the Western world is geared toward rewarding left-brain skills to the extent that right-brain skills go undeveloped. However, educators need to employ teaching methods that enable the learner to use both sides of the brain. For example, to stimulate the development of left-brain thinking, the health professional educator should provide a structured environment by relying on specific objectives and a course outline. To stimulate the development of the right brain, the educator should provide a more unstructured, free-flowing environment that allows for creative opportunities. By employing teaching strategies aimed at helping the learner use both brain hemispheres, the educator facilitates more effective and efficient learning. Whole-brain thinking allows the learner to get the best of both worlds in developing his or her thought processes. Duality of thinking is what educators should strive to teach to encourage learners to reach their full learning potential.

As Gardner (1999a) points out, the brain does not exist in isolation but rather is connected to the entire body. He argues that for the brain to be more than an organ, consideration must be given to a number of variables, such as mental processes, feelings, desires, and cultural influences, that are important in the development and expression of a learner's learning style. What learners choose to learn is influenced by the set of values both educators and learners bring to the teaching–learning situation.

INSTRUMENTS TO MEASURE RIGHT-BRAIN/LEFT-BRAIN AND WHOLE-BRAIN THINKING

Two instruments are used to measure right- and left-brain dominance. The first is called the brain preference indicator (BPI). It consists of a set of questions used to determine hemispheric functioning. The BPI instrument reveals a general style of thought that results in a consistent pattern of be-

havior in all areas of the individual's life. Although there is no reported reliability or validity of this instrument, it does provide a starting point for the educator to understand his or her own right- or left-brain preferences. More information about the BPI can be found in *Whole-Brain Thinking* by Wonder and Donovan (1984).

The other instrument available with widespread commercial use is the Herrmann Brain Dominance Instrument (HBDI). Herrmann's (1988) model incorporates theories on growth and development and considers learning styles as learned patterns of behavior. The HBDI classifies learners in terms of the following four modes, with each quadrant corresponding to a brain structure and different preferences for thinking:

Quadrant A (left brain, cerebral)—Logical, analytical, quantitative, factual, critical

Quadrant B (left brain, limbic)—Sequential, organized, planned, detailed, structured

Quadrant C (right brain, limbic)—Emotional, interpersonal, sensory, kinesthetic, symbolic

Quadrant D (right brain, cerebral)—Visual, holistic, innovative

The author suggests that his HBDI is psychometrically sound, although there are very few independent studies of its reliability and validity (Coffield et al., 2004b). The HBDI mostly has been used in the business world with minimal validation in the health sciences. More information about the model is available at Herrmann International's Web site, www.hbdi.com.

Field-Independent/Field-Dependent Perception

An extensive series of studies by Witkin, Oltman, Raskin, and Karp (1971b) identify two styles of learning in the cognitive domain, which are based on the bipolar distribution of characteristics of how learners process and structure information in their environment. They hypothesize that learners have preference styles for certain environmental cues. A field-independent person perceives items as separate or differentiated from the surrounding field; a field-dependent person's perception is influenced by or immersed in the surrounding field.

Field-independent individuals have internalized frames of reference such that they experience themselves as separate or differentiated from others and the environment. They are less sensitive to social cues, are not affected by criticism, favor an active participant role, and are eager to test out their ideas or opinions in a group.

Field-dependent individuals, on the other hand, are more externally focused and as such are socially oriented, more aware of social cues, able to reveal their feelings, and are more dependent on others for reinforcement. They have a need for extrinsic motivation and externally defined objectives and learn better if the material has a social context. They are more easily affected by criticism, take a passive, spectator role, and change their opinions in the face of peer pressure.

Field independence/dependence is thought to be related to hemispheric brain processes (Chall & Mirsky, 1978). The studies in *Sex and the Brain* (Durden-Smith & deSimone, 1983) reveal that the right hemisphere in males tends to be more dominant than their left hemisphere; the opposite is true for females. Males tend to have better visual-spatial abilities, and females tend to have better linguistic skills. Although females generally do not do as well as males on tests of spatial ability, men should be measured only against other men, and women against women, to reduce the differential test effect on the sexes. To date, sex-related differences in behavior have been documented in the literature (Speck et al., 2000), but the neuroanatomic processes remain unclear (Gur et al., 1999) and significance of these research findings for the educator is difficult to gauge. Garity (1985) suggests that these individual differences in characteristics and interpersonal behavior can be used as a basis for understanding different learning styles and can facilitate the way educators work with learners, structure the learning task, and structure the environment (**Table 4–4**).

Table 4–4 CHARACTERISTICS OF FIELD-INDEPENDENT AND FIELD-DEPENDENT LEARNERS

Field-Independent Learners	Field-Dependent Learners
Are not affected by criticism	Are easily affected by criticism
Will not conform to peer pressure	Will conform to peer pressure
Are less influenced by external feedback	Are influenced by feedback (grades and evaluations)
Learn best by organizing their own material	Learn best when material is organized
Have an impersonal orientation to the world	Have a social orientation to the world
Place emphasis on applying principles	Place emphasis on facts
Are interested in new ideas or concepts for own sake	Prefer learning to be relevant to own experience
Provide self-directed goals, objectives, and reinforcement	Need external goals, objectives, and reinforcements
Prefer lecture method	Prefer discussion method

INSTRUMENT TO MEASURE FIELD INDEPENDENCE/FIELD DEPENDENCE

Witkin, Oltman, Raskin, and Karp (1971a) devised a tool called the Group Embedded Figures Test (GEFT) to measure field independence/dependence—how a person's perception of an item is influenced by the context in which it appears. Bonham (1988) notes that the GEFT, which takes approximately 30 minutes to complete, is designed to determine a person's ability to find simple geometric figures within complex drawings. Witkin's work is based on 35 years of psychological research on more than 2,000 individuals. Educators must keep in mind that the GEFT is based on psychological research when they attempt to apply findings broadly to the educational setting (Witkin, Moore, & Oltman, 1977). Bonham (1988) points out in her analysis of learning style instruments that the GEFT measures the ability to do something, not the manner (style) in which it is done. There is no way to tell whether a person could choose which style is most effective in a given situation (Shipman & Shipman, 1985; Witkin & Goodenough, 1981). Older adults generally do not do well on tests in which speed is important (Botwinick, 1978), but this assessment tool is a timed test, so age bias is a concern (Santrock, 2006).

The best time to use the GEFT seems to be when the educator wants to measure field independence, not field dependence, in determining the extent to which learners are able to ignore distractions from other persons who may offer incorrect information or ideas. The results could help individuals understand why they may have trouble with a particular learning experience (Bonham, 1988). For example, Deture (2004) designed a study to identify those learner attributes that can be used to predict student success in Web-based distance education courses. He administered the GEFT and the Online Technologies Self-Efficacy Scale (OTSES) to community college students to determine their entry-level confidence with computer skills for online learning. His findings show a significant positive correlation between the GEFT and the OTSES scores, supporting the notion that field-independent students tend to be more confident with online technologies. Thus, field-dependent students may need more assistance with Web-based courses, and the educator may need to find other methods of instruction for their learning to be more successful and less anxiety producing.

Flynn and associates (1999) found a significant association between the number of interruptions and distractions in an ambulatory care pharmacy and dispensing errors (incorrect label information). As the distractions (field background elements) increased, more errors occurred. Field-dependent pharmacists tend to get more distracted and to fill prescriptions inaccurately. Consideration of field independence/dependence can be useful for the educator who is involved with teaching in a clinical setting characterized by constant distractions.

Also, the educator can use this instrument to determine whether a learner sees the whole first (global, field independent) and then the individual parts (specific, field dependent), or vice versa. The field-independent person wants to know the end result of teaching and learning prior to concentrating on the individual parts of the process, whereas the field-dependent person wants to know the individual parts in sequence prior to looking at the expected overall outcome of teaching–learning efforts. The GEFT has been reasonably well validated in predicting academic performance (Oltman, Raskin, Witkin, & Karp, 1978). This instrument is available for purchase at Mind Garden, which can be accessed at www.mindgarden.com.

Dunn and Dunn Learning Styles

In 1967, Rita Dunn and Kenneth Dunn set out to develop a user-friendly model that would assist educators in identifying characteristics that allow individuals to learn in different ways (Dunn &

Dunn, 1978). The model includes motivational factors, social interaction, and physiological and environmental elements. These researchers identified the following five basic stimuli (as shown in **Figure 4–2**) that affect a person's ability to learn:

1. Environmental elements (such as sound, light, temperature, and design), which are biological in nature
2. Emotional elements (such as motivation, persistence, responsibility, and structure), which are developmental and emerge over time as an outgrowth of experiences that have happened at home, school, play, or work
3. Sociological patterns (such as the desire to work alone or in groups or a combination of these

two approaches), which are thought to be socioculturally based
4. Physical elements (such as perceptual strength, intake, time of day, and mobility), which are also biological in nature and relate to the way learners function physically
5. Psychological elements (such as the way learners process and react to information), which are also biological in nature

THE ENVIRONMENTAL ELEMENTS

SOUND   Individuals react to sound in different ways. Some learners need complete silence, others are able to block out sounds around them, and

Figure 4–2 Dunn and Dunn's Learning Style Elements

Stimuli	Elements			
Environmental	SOUND	LIGHT	TEMPERATURE	DESIGN
Emotional	MOTIVATION	PERSISTENCE	RESPONSIBILITY	STRUCTURE M T W TH F
Sociological	PEERS SELF	PAIR	TEAM ADULT	VARIED
Physical	PERCEPTUAL	INTAKE	TIME	MOBILITY
Psychological	ANALYTIC GLOBAL	HEMISPHERIC PREFERENCE	IMPULSIVE	REFLECTIVE

still others require sound in their environment for learning. Cognizant of the effect of sound on learning, the educator should permit learners to study either in silent areas or with music from headsets to prevent interfering with those who need quiet.

Light   Some learners work best under bright lights, whereas others need dim or low lighting. The educator should provide lighting conducive to learning by moving furniture around to establish both well- and dimly lit areas and permitting learners to sit where they are most comfortable.

Temperature   Some learners have difficulty thinking or concentrating if a room is too hot or, conversely, if it is too cold. The educator needs to make learners aware of the temperature of the environment and encourage them to wear lighter or heavier clothing. If windows are available, they should be opened to permit variable degrees of temperature in the room to accommodate different comfort levels.

Design   Dunn and Dunn established that when learners are seated on wooden, steel, or plastic chairs, 75% of the total body weight is supported on only four square inches of bone. This results in fatigue, discomfort, and the need for frequent body position changes (Dunn & Dunn, 1987). Also, some learners are more relaxed and can learn better in an informal environment by being able to position themselves in a lounge chair, on the floor, on pillows, or on carpeting. Others cannot learn in an informal environment because it makes them drowsy. If possible, the educator should vary the furniture in the classroom to allow some to sit more formally or informally while learning.

The Emotional Elements

Motivation   Motivation, or the desire to achieve, increases when learning success increases. Unmotivated learners need short learning assign-

ments that enhance their strengths. Motivated learners, by comparison, are eager to learn and should be told exactly what they are required to do, with resources available so that they can self-pace their learning.

Persistence   Learners differ in their preference to complete tasks in one sitting or to take periodic breaks and return to the task at a later time. By giving learners objectives and a time interval for completion of a task ahead of time, those with long attention spans can get the job done in a block of time, while those whose attention span is short can take the opportunity for breaks without feeling guilty or rushed.

Responsibility   Responsibility involves the desire to do what the learner thinks is expected. It is related to the concept of conformity or following through on what an educator asks or tells the learner to do. Learners with low responsibility scores usually are nonconforming. They do not like to do something because someone asks them to do it. Knowing this, the educator should give them choices and allow learners to select different ways to complete the assignment. When given appropriate choices, the nonconformist will likely be more willing to meet expectations set forth.

Structure   Structure refers to either the preference for specific directions, guidance, or rules prior to carrying out an assignment or the preference for doing an assignment without structure in the learner's own way. Structure should vary in the amount and kind that is provided, depending on the learner's ability to make responsible decisions and the requirements of the task.

The Sociological Elements

Learning Alone   Some learners prefer to study by themselves, whereas others prefer to learn with a friend or colleague. When learners prefer to be with others, group discussion and role-playing can facilitate learning. For learners who do not do well learning with others because they tend to socialize or are unable to concentrate, self-instruction, one-to-one interaction, or lecture-type methods are the best approaches.

PRESENCE OF AN AUTHORITY FIGURE   Some learners feel more comfortable when someone with authority or recognized expertise is present during learning. Others become nervous, feel stifled, and have trouble concentrating. Depending on the style of the learner, either one-to-one interaction or self-study may be the appropriate approach.

VARIETY OF WAYS   Some learners are flexible and can learn as well alone as they can with authority figures and peer groups. These learners are versatile in their style of learning and would benefit from having different opportunities as opposed to routine approaches.

THE PHYSICAL ELEMENTS

PERCEPTUAL STRENGTHS   Four types of learners are distinguished in this category: (1) those with auditory preferences, who learn best while listening to verbal instruction; (2) those with visual preferences, who learn best from reading or observation; (3) those with tactile preferences, who learn best when they can underline as they read, take notes when they listen, and otherwise keep their hands busy; and (4) those with kinesthetic preferences, who absorb and retain information best when allowed to perform whole-body movement or participate in simulated or real-life experiences.

Auditory learners should be introduced to new information first by hearing about it, followed by verbal feedback for reinforcement of the information. Lecture and group discussion are instructional methods best suited to their style. Visual learners learn more easily by viewing, watching, and observing. Simulation and demonstration

methods of instruction are therefore most beneficial to their learning. Tactile learners learn through touching, manipulating, and handling objects, so they remember more when they write, doodle, draw, or move their fingers. The use of models and computer-assisted instruction is most suitable for their learning style. Kinesthetic learners learn more easily by doing and experiencing. They profit most from opportunities for field trips, role-playing, interviewing, and participating in return demonstration.

INTAKE   Some learners need to eat, drink, chew, or bite objects while concentrating. Others prefer no intake until after they have finished studying. A list of rules needs to be established to satisfy the oral needs of those who prefer intake while learning so that their behavior does not disturb others or interfere with building rules and regulations of the agency.

TIME OF DAY   Some learners perform better at one time of day than another. The four time-of-day preferences are on a continuum, and the educator needs to identify these preferences with an effort toward structuring teaching and learning to occur during the times that are most suitable for the learner:

Early-morning learners—Their ability to concentrate and focus energies on learning is high in the early hours of the day and wanes as the day progresses.

Late-morning learners—Their concentration and energy curve peaks around noontime, when their ability to perform is at its height.

Afternoon learners—Their concentration and energy curve is highest in the mid- to late afternoon, when performance is at its peak.

Evening learners—Their ability to concentrate and focus energies is greatest at the end of the day.

Dunn (1995) contends that among adults, the majority fall on the two extremes of the continuum: 55% are morning people and 28% work best in the evening. Many adults experience energy lows in the afternoon. School-aged children, on the other hand, have high energy levels in the late morning and early afternoon. About 13% of high school students work best in the evening. This time sensitivity means that it may be easier or more difficult for a person to learn a new skill or behavior at certain times of the day than at other times. To enhance learning potential, the educator should try to schedule teaching during the learner's best time of day.

MOBILITY   Mobility refers to how still the learner can sit and for how long a period of time. Some learners need to move about, whereas others can sit for hours engaged in learning. For those who require mobility, it is necessary to provide opportunity for movement by assigning them to less restrictive sections of the room. During workshops or any type of group learning, health professional educators should give frequent 30- to 60-second breaks during which participants can stand. This is a good time to have the participants turn to one another and share one thing that they have learned during that time.

THE PSYCHOLOGICAL ELEMENTS

GLOBAL VERSUS ANALYTIC   Some learners are global in their thinking and learn best by obtaining meaning from a broad, overall concept before focusing on the details in the surrounding environment. Other learners are analytic in their thinking and learn sequentially in a step-by-step process.

HEMISPHERIC PREFERENCE   Learners who possess right-brain preference tend to learn best in environments that have low illumination, background music, casual seating, and tactile instructional resources. Learners with left-brain preference

require an opposite environment of bright lighting, quiet setting, formal seating, and visual or auditory instructional resources.

IMPULSIVITY VERSUS REFLECTIVITY   Impulsive learners prefer opportunities to participate verbally in groups and tend to answer questions spontaneously and without consciously processing their thinking. Reflective learners seldom volunteer information unless they are asked to do so, prefer to contemplate information, and tend to be uncomfortable participating in group discussions (Dunn, 1984).

INSTRUMENT TO MEASURE THE DUNN AND DUNN LEARNING STYLE INVENTORY

The Dunn and Dunn learning style inventory is a self-reporting instrument that is widely used in the identification of how individuals prefer to function, learn, concentrate, and perform in their educational activities. It is available in three different forms: for grades 3–5; for grades 6–12; and in an adult version, called the Productivity Environmental Preference Survey (PEPS). Dunn and Dunn stress that the PEPS is not intended to be used as an indicator of underlying psychological factors, value systems, or the quality of attitudes. This instrument yields information concerned with the patterns through which learning occurs but does not assess the finer aspects of an individual's skills, such as the ability to outline procedures and to organize, classify, or analyze new material. It indicates how people prefer to learn, not the abilities they possess.

What has evolved since the model was first developed is a highly tested and continuously revised instrument that is valid and reliable as reported by those who like and use the instrument (Dunn & Griggs, 2003). However, others highlight major problems with the design and reliability of the instrument (Coffield et al., 2004b).

Jung and Myers-Briggs Typology

Carl G. Jung (1921/1971), a Swiss psychiatrist, developed a theory that explains personality similarities and differences by identifying attitudes of people (extraverts and introverts) along with opposite mental functions, which are the ways people perceive or prefer to take in and make use of information from the world around them. Jung proposed that people are likely to operate in a variety of ways depending on the circumstances. Despite these situational adaptations, each individual tends to develop comfortable patterns, which dictate behavior in certain predictable ways. Jung used the word *type* to identify these styles of personality.

Jung said that everyone uses these opposing perceptions to some degree when dealing with people and situations, but each person has a preference for one way of looking at the world. Individuals become more skilled in arriving at a decision in either a thinking or feeling way and can function as extraverts at one time and as introverts at another time, but they tend to develop patterns that are most typical and comfortable.

Isabel Myers and her mother, Katherine Briggs, became convinced that Jung's theories had an application for increasing human understanding (Myers, 1980). In addition to Jung's dichotomies, Myers and Briggs discovered another dichotomy (Myers, 1987) and thus made explicit one underdeveloped aspect of Jung's model (**Figure 4–3**). According to Myers and Briggs, an individual comes to a conclusion about or becomes aware of something through a preference of judging or perceiving.

By combining the different preferences, Myers and Briggs identified 16 personality types, each with its own strengths and interests (**Figure 4–4**). People can be classified into the 16 personality types by using the following four constructs:

1. Extraversion–introversion (E–I) reflects an orientation to either the outside world of people and things or to the inner world of concepts

Figure 4–3 Myers-Briggs Dichotomous Dimensions or Preferences

Extraversion (E) ⟷ Introversion (I)

Sensing (S) ⟷ Intuition (N)

Thinking (T) ⟷ Feeling (F)

Judgment (J) ⟷ Perception (P)

Figure 4–4 Myers-Briggs Types

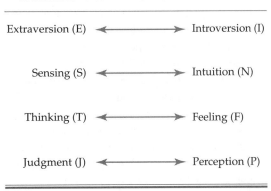

ISTJ	ISFJ	INFJ	INTJ
ISTP	ISFP	INFP	INTP
ESTP	ESFP	ENFP	ENTP
ESTJ	ESFJ	ENFJ	ENTJ

and ideas. This pair of opposite preferences describes the extent to which behavior is determined by attitudes toward the world. Jung invented the terms from Latin words meaning outward turning (*extraversion*) and inward turning (*introversion*).

Individuals who prefer extraversion operate comfortably and successfully by interacting with things external to themselves, such as other people, experiences, and situations. They like to clarify thoughts and ideas through talking and doing. Those who operate more comfortably in an extraverted way think aloud.

Those with a preference for introversion, on the other hand, are more interested in the internal world of their minds, hearts, and souls. They like to brew over thoughts and actions, reflecting on them until they become more personally meaningful. Those who operate more comfortably in an introverted way are often thoughtful, reflective, and slow to act because they need time to translate internal thoughts to the external world. Their thoughts are well formulated before they are willing to share them with others.

2. Sensing–intuition (S–N) describes perception as coming directly through the five senses or indirectly by way of the unconscious. This pair of opposite preferences explains how people understand what is experienced. People who prefer sensing experience the world through their senses—vision, hearing, touch, taste, and smell. They observe what is real, what is factual, and what is actually happening. Seeing or experiencing is believing. These sensory functions allow the individual to observe carefully, gather facts, and focus on practical actions.

Conversely, those people who prefer intuition tend to read between the lines, focus on meaning, and attend to what might be. Those with intuition preferences view the world through possibilities and relationships and are tuned into subtleties of body language and tones of voice. This kind of perception leads them to examine problems and issues in creative and original ways.

3. Thinking–feeling (T–F) is the approach used by individuals to arrive at judgments through objective versus subjective processes. Think-

ing types analyze information, data, situations, and people and make decisions based on logic. They are careful and slow in the analysis of the data because accuracy and thoroughness are important to them. They trust objectivity and put faith in logical predictions and rational arguments. Thinking types explore and weigh all alternatives, and the final decision is reached impersonally, unemotionally, and carefully.

In the feeling preference, on the other hand, the approach to decision making takes place through a subjective, perceptive, empathetic, and emotional perspective. Individuals who prefer feeling search for the effect of a decision on themselves and others. They consider alternatives and examine evidence to develop a personal reaction and commitment. They believe the decision-making process is complex and not totally objective. Circumstantial evidence is extremely important, and these individuals see the world as gray rather than black and white.

4. Judging–perceiving (J–P) According to Myers and Briggs, an individual comes to a conclusion about or becomes aware of something through a preference of judging, which is the desire to regulate and bring closure to circumstances in life, or through their preference of perceiving, which is the desire to be open-minded and understanding.

INSTRUMENT TO MEASURE THE MYERS-BRIGGS PERSONALITY TYPES

Myers and Briggs developed an instrument called the Myers-Briggs Type Indicator (MBTI) that permits people to learn about their own type of behavior and thus understand themselves better with respect to the way in which they interact with others. Although the MBTI is not a learning style instrument per se, it does measure differences in personality types, which are combinations of the four dichotomous preferences. The MBTI is a forced-choice, self-report inventory.

The Myers-Briggs Type Indicator can be useful for the educator to understand the many different ways in which learners perceive and judge information and how they prefer to learn. Logical, detailed individuals (Sensing–Thinking type) may have difficulty communicating with those who are more holistically oriented (Intuitive–Feeling type). What each party values and believes most and the ways to go about learning or dealing with information are different and may lead to misunderstandings and conflicts (Bargar & Hoover, 1984). Findings of significant differences between medical graduates and the general U.K. adult population in three of the four basic personality dimensions of the MBTI as well as in combinations of perception and judgment suggest potential points for miscommunication between physicians and patients (Clack, Allen, Cooper, & O'Head, 2004). Another example of how these two preferences function is that the Sensing–Thinking learner's preferred learning style emphasizes hands-on experience, demonstration, and application of concepts, whereas Intuition–Feeling learners prefer emphasis on the theoretical concerns before they can concentrate on the practical applications. Examples are listed in **Table 4–5**.

Since its development in the 1920s, this instrument has undergone several revisions, with mixed reviews on its reliability and validity (Capraro & Capraro, 2002; Coffield et al., 2004b). Schoessler,

Table 4–5 MYERS-BRIGGS TYPES: EXAMPLES OF LEARNING

Extraversion	Introversion
Likes group work	Likes quiet space
Dislikes slow-paced learning	Dislikes interruptions
Likes action and to experience things so as to learn	Likes learning that deals with thoughts, ideas
Offers opinions without being asked	Offers opinions only when asked
Asks questions to check on the expectations of educator	Asks questions to allow understanding of learning activity
Sensing	**Intuition**
Practical	Always likes something new
Realistic	Imaginative
Observant	Sees possibilities
Learns from orderly sequence of details	Prefers the whole concept versus details
Thinking	**Feeling**
Low need for harmony	Values harmony
Finds ideas and things more interesting than people	More interested in people than things or ideas
Analytical	Sympathetic
Fair	Accepting
Judging	**Perceiving**
Organized	Open ended
Methodical	Flexible
Work oriented	Play oriented
Controls the environment	Adapts to the environment

Conedera, Bell, Marshall, and Gilson (1993) discuss the use of the MBTI to develop a continuing education department for nursing, and Hardy and Smith (2001) explain how they restructured their orientation program to match preceptor and orientee relative to teaching and learning traits as a result of individual MBTI scores. Stilwell, Wallick, Thal, and Burlescon (2000) identify how the MBTI is useful for understanding how some aspects of personality relate to medical graduates' choice of medical specialty areas. The MBTI instrument and MBTI products are available at CPP, which can be accessed at www.cpp. com/products/mbti/index.asp.

Kolb's Experiential Learning Model

David Kolb (1984), a management expert from Case Western Reserve University, developed his learning style model in the early 1970s. He believed that knowledge is acquired through a transformational process, which is continuously created and re-created. The learner is not a blank slate, but he or she approaches a topic to be learned with preconceived ideas. Kolb's theory on learning style is that it is a cumulative result of past experiences, heredity, and the demands of the present environment. These factors combine to produce different individual orientations to learning.

Kolb's model, known as the cycle of learning, includes four modes of learning that reflect two major dimensions: perception and processing. He hypothesizes that learning results from the way learners perceive as well as how they process what they perceive. The dimension of perception involves two opposite perceptual viewpoints. Some learners perceive through concrete experience (CE mode), whereas others perceive through abstract conceptualization (AC mode).

At the CE stage of the learning cycle, learners tend to rely more on feelings than on a systematic approach to problems and situations. Learners who fall into this category like relating with

people, benefit from specific experiences, and are sensitive to others. They learn from feeling.

At the AC stage, on the other hand, learners rely on logic and ideas rather than on feelings to deal with problems or situations. People who fall into this category use systematic planning and logical analysis to solve problems. They learn by thinking.

The process dimension also has two opposing orientations. Some learners process information through reflective observation (RO mode), whereas others process information through active experimentation (AE mode).

At the RO stage of the learning cycle, learners rely on objectivity, careful judgment, personal thoughts, and feelings to form opinions. People who fall into this category look for the meaning of things by viewing them from different perspectives. They learn by watching and listening.

At the AE stage of the learning cycle, learning is active, and learners like to experiment to get things done. They prefer to influence or change situations and see the results of their actions. They enjoy involvement and are risk takers. They learn by doing.

Kolb describes each learning style as a combination of the four basic learning modes (CE, AC, RO, and AE), identifying separate learning style types that best define the strengths and weaknesses of a learner. The learner predominantly demonstrates characteristics of one of four style types: (1) diverger, (2) assimilator, (3) converger, or (4) accommodator, which are discussed as they appear in clockwise order in **Figure 4–5**, starting with the diverger.

The diverger combines the learning modes of CE and RO. People with this learning style are good at viewing concrete situations from many points of view. They like to observe, gather information, and gain insights rather than take action. Working in groups to generate ideas appeals to them. They place a high value on understanding for knowledge's sake and like to personalize learn-

---

Figure 4–5 Kolb's Learning Style Inventory

Concrete Experience (CE)
"Feeling"

	Diverger
Accommodator	Diverger
Converger	Assimilator

Active Experimentation (AE)
"Doing"

Reflective Observation (RO)
"Watching"

Abstract Conceptualization (AC)
"Thinking"

Source: Kolb, D. (1984). *Experiental learning: Experience as a source of learning and development* © 1984, Figures 3.1, 4.2. Reprinted with permission of Prentice-Hall, Inc., Upper Saddle River, NJ.

---

ing by connecting information with something familiar in their experiences. They have active imaginations, enjoy being involved, and are sensitive to feelings. Divergent thinkers learn best, for example, through group discussions and participating in brainstorming sessions.

The assimilator combines the learning modes of RO and AC. People with this learning style demonstrate the ability to understand large amounts of information by putting it into concise and logical form. They are less interested in people and more focused on abstract ideas and concepts. They are good at inductive reasoning, value theory over practical application of ideas, and need time to reflect on what has been learned and how information can be integrated into their past experiences. They rely on knowledge from experts. Assimilative thinkers learn best, for example, through lecture, one-to-one instruction, and self-instruction methods with ample reading materials to support their learning.

The converger combines the learning modes of AC and AE. People with this learning style type find practical application for ideas and theories and have the ability to use deductive reasoning to solve problems. They like structure and factual information, and they look for specific solutions to problems. Learners with this style prefer technical tasks rather than dealing with social and interpersonal issues. Kolb postulates that individuals with this learning style have skills that are important for specialist and technology careers. The convergent thinker learns best, for example, through demonstration/return demonstration methods of teaching accompanied by handouts and diagrams.

The accommodator combines the learning modes of AE and CE. People with this learning style learn best by hands-on experience and enjoy new and challenging situations. They act on intuition and gut feelings rather than on logic. These risk takers like to explore all possibilities and learn by experimenting with materials and objects. Accommodative thinkers are perhaps the most challenging to educators because they demand new and exciting experiences and are willing to take risks that might endanger their safety. Role-playing, gaming, and computer simulations, for example, are methods of teaching most preferred by this style of learner.

For every group of learners, about 25% will fall into each of the four categories. Kolb believes that understanding a person's learning style, including its strengths and weaknesses, represents a major step toward increasing learning power and helping learners to get the most from their learning experiences. By using different teaching strategies to address these four learning styles, particular modes of learning can be matched, at least some of the time, with the educator's methods of teaching. If the educator predominantly uses only one method of teaching, such as the lecture to promote learning, then 75% of all learners will be selectively excluded.

When teaching groups of learners, the instructor may want to begin with activities best suited to the divergent thinker and progress sequentially to include activities for the assimilator, converger, and accommodator, respectively (Arndt & Underwood, 1990). This pattern works because learners must first have foundational knowledge of a subject before they can test out information. Otherwise, they operate from a level of ignorance. They must first have familiarity with facts and ideas before they can explore and test concepts.

INSTRUMENT TO MEASURE KOLB'S EXPERIENTIAL LEARNING STYLE

The Learning Style Inventory (LSI) is a self-report questionnaire that requires respondents on each of the 12 items to rank four sentence endings corresponding to each of the four learning styles. A scoring process reduces the ranking evidence to four mode scores (CE, RO, AC, and AE), which are further reduced to two dimension scores (concrete-abstract and reflective-active). Two combinations of dimension scores measure the learner's preference for abstractness versus concreteness (AC–CE) and for action versus reflection (AE–RO). The predominant score indicates the learner's style (diverger, assimilator, converger, or accommodator).

The Kolb model is popular in the healthcare field and has been the subject of many studies. Some scholars believe that the model's validity has not been demonstrated (Coffield et al., 2004b). Kolb argues otherwise and states that the LSI has considerable construct validity (Delahoussaye, 2002). Version 3 of the LSI significantly improves psychometric properties, especially test-retest reliability (Castro, 2006). A considerable body of research positively reports on Kolb's Learning Style Instrument. The LSI (version 3.1) can be obtained from Hay Resources Direct (www.haygroup.com/TL/).

4MAT System

McCarthy (1981) developed a model based on previous research on learning styles and brain functioning. In particular, she used Kolb's model combined with right-brain/left-brain research findings to create the 4MAT system (**Figure 4–6**).

McCarthy's model describes four types of learners:

Type 1/Imaginative: Learners who demand to know why. These learners like to listen, speak, interact, and brainstorm.

Type 2/Analytic: Learners who want to know what to learn. These learners are most comfortable observing, analyzing, classifying, and theorizing.

Type 3/Common sense: Learners who want to know how to apply the new learning. These

Figure 4–6 McCarthy's 4MAT System

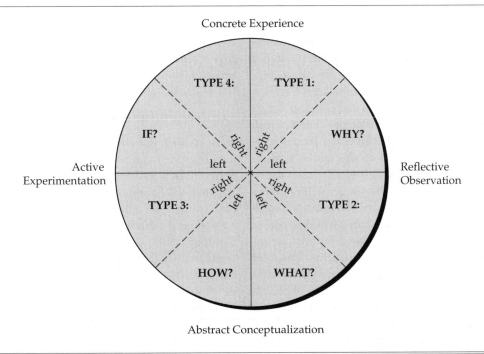

Concrete Experience

TYPE 4:   TYPE 1:

IF?   WHY?

right   *right*

left   left

Active Experimentation   Reflective Observation

right   *right*

left   *left*

TYPE 3:   TYPE 2:

HOW?   WHAT?

Abstract Conceptualization

Source: From Guild, P. B., & Garger, S. (1998). *Marching to different drummers*. Alexandria, VA: Association for Supervision and Curriculum Development. Reprinted with permission.

learners are happiest when experimenting, manipulating, improving, and tinkering.

Type 4/Dynamic: Learners who ask, what if? These learners enjoy modifying, adapting, taking risks, and creating.

McCarthy defines the learning process as a natural sequence from Type 1 to Type 4. Educators can address all four learning styles by teaching sequentially, thus attending to all types of learners. Learners are then able to work with their own strongest learning style, while at the same time developing the ability through exposure to work in the other quadrants.

To use this sequence, learners begin in the first quadrant, known as Type 1, and engage the right

brain by sensing and feeling their way through an experience. Eventually, they move to the left brain to analyze what they have experienced. They ask, "Why is this important? Why should I try to learn this?"

The next quadrant is Type 2, in which learning also begins with the right brain to make observations and integrate data with present knowledge. Learners then engage the left brain to think about new theories and concepts relative to these observations. They ask, "What is it I am supposed to be learning? What is the relationship?"

In the third quadrant, Type 3 learners begin with the left brain by working with defined concepts, and then shift to the right brain to experiment with what has to be learned. They ask, "How does this work? How can I figure this out?"

Finally, Type 4 learners also begin with the left brain by analyzing the practicality of what has been learned. They then move to the right brain to show mastery through application and the sharing of findings with others. They ask, "If I learn this, what can I do with it? Can I apply it?"

The learning sequence is circular and cyclic, beginning at Type 1 and moving to Type 4, which is characteristic of a higher level and greater complexity of learning. Based on this model, it is important for the educator to begin Type 1 learning by including personal meaning for the learner to make the learning experience relevant and to answer the why question. Next, it is essential to introduce new knowledge based on accurate information to answer the what question. The third step in sequential learning is to deal with reality in a practical manner through application of knowledge to enable learners to answer the how question. Finally, in the fourth step, the learning experience must allow the learner to be innovative and inspiring and to create new dynamic possibilities so that the if question is answered.

By using this sequential approach to learning, the educator can instill personal meaning and motivation for what is to be learned (Type 1), assist the learner in the acquisition of the new knowledge and concepts (Type 2), allow for active experimentation (Type 3), and provide the opportunity for more complex synthesis and extension through practical application (Type 4). Through use of the 4MAT system, each learning style has an opportunity to exert itself at least part of the time.

INSTRUMENT TO MEASURE THE 4MAT SYSTEM

McCarthy's consulting and publishing company has its own Web site at www.aboutlearning.com. The 4MAT instructional design and the learning type measure instrument is a 26-point, self-report questionnaire. Although there is little published information on the psychometric properties of the 4MAT system, including the learning type measure, it appears to have face validity. There seems to be no direct criticism of the 4MAT model, and it is accepted by many educators as a useful approach for presenting new information.

Gardner's Eight Types of Intelligence

Most models and measurement instruments on learning style focus on the adult as learner. However, children also have their own way of learning that can be assessed from the standpoint of each individual's unique pattern of growth and neurological functioning. Psychologist Howard Gardner (1983) developed a theory focused on seven kinds of intelligence in children. Gardner based his theory on findings from brain research, developmental work, and psychological testing. He identified seven kinds of intelligence located in different parts of the brain: (1) linguistic, (2) logical-mathematical, (3) spatial, (4) musical, (5) bodily kinesthetic, (6) interpersonal, and (7) intrapersonal. Also, Gardner (1999b) identified an eighth kind of intelligence called naturalistic. Each learner has all the eight kinds of intelligence but in different proportions.

Linguistic intelligence seems to be in the Broca's area of the left side of the brain. Children with a tendency for this type of intelligence have highly developed auditory skills and think in words. They like writing, telling stories, spelling words, and reading, and they can recall names, places, and dates. These children learn best by verbalizing, hearing, or seeing words. Word games or crossword puzzles are an excellent method for helping these children to learn new material.

Logical-mathematical intelligence involves both sides of the brain. The right side deals with concepts, and the left side remembers symbols. The children who are strong in this intelligence explore patterns, categories, and relationships. In the adolescent years, they have the ability for logical thinking with a high degree of abstraction. As learners, they question many things and ask where, what, and when. A question such a learner might ask is, "If people are always supposed to be good to each other, then why do people always say they are sorry?" They can do arithmetic problems quickly in their heads, like to learn by computers, and do experiments to test concepts they do not understand. They enjoy strategy board games such as chess and checkers.

Spatial intelligence is related to the right side of the brain. Children with high spatial intelligence learn by images and pictures. They enjoy such things as building blocks, jigsaw puzzles, and daydreaming. They like to draw or do other art activities, can read charts and diagrams, and learn with visual methods such as videos or photographs.

Musical intelligence is also related to the right side of the brain. Musically intelligent children can be found singing a tune, indicating when a note is off key, playing musical instruments with ease, dancing to music, and keeping time rhythmically. They are also sensitive to sounds in the environment, such as the sound of walking on snow on a cold winter morning. Often, musically intelligent children learn best with music playing in the background.

Bodily kinesthetic intelligence includes the basal ganglia and cerebellum of the brain in addition to other brain structures. Children with this type of intelligence learn by processing knowledge through bodily sensations, such as moving around or acting things out. It is difficult for these learners to sit still for long periods of time. They are good at athletic sports and have highly developed fine-motor coordination. Use of body language to communicate and copying people's behaviors or movements come easily for this group of learners.

Interpersonal intelligence involves the prefrontal lobes of the brain. Children with high interpersonal intelligence understand people, are able to notice others' feelings, tend to have many friends, and are gifted in social skills. They learn best in groups and gravitate toward activities that involve others in problem solving.

Intrapersonal intelligence also involves the prefrontal lobes of the brain. Children with this type of intelligence have strong personalities, prefer the inner world of feelings and ideas, and like being alone. They are very private individuals, desire a quiet area to learn, and prefer to be by themselves to learn. They tend to be self-directed and self-confident. They learn well with independent, self-paced instruction.

Naturalistic intelligence refers to sensing abilities in making patterns and connections to elements in nature. Children with high naturalistic intelligence can distinguish and categorize objects or phenomena in nature. They enjoy subjects, shows, and stories that deal with animals or naturally occurring phenomena and are keenly aware of their surroundings and subtle changes in their environment.

Educators should always approach children from the perspective of these different intelligences (Armstrong, 1987). Often it can be difficult to assess the preferred learning style of a child when he or she is facing an illness or surgery. Asking some key questions of the child or parents may give the educator some clues. What subjects does the child excel in or like best? What kinds of hobbies does the child have? What excites this child? What kinds of toys does the child play with? What inner qualities does the child possess, such as courage, playfulness, curiosity, friendliness, or creativity? What talents does the child possess?

By using Gardner's theory of the eight intelligences, the educator can assess each child's style of learning and tailor teaching accordingly. For example, if the educator wants to assist a child in learning about exercise, the educator can use one of these following eight approaches, depending on the child's style of learning:

Linguistic—Practice quizzing the child orally on the different parts of the body that need exercise, the outcomes of exercise, and different ways to get exercise.

Spatial—Have a diagram or chart that allows the child to associate different colors or shapes with concepts. Storytelling illustrating a child doing exercise can be used.

Kinesthetic—Have a model of the body or a doll available that can be felt, taken apart, and manipulated. Have the child identify tactile features of the body or demonstrate different exercises.

Logical-mathematical—Group concepts into categories, starting with simple generalizations about exercise or health behaviors. Reasoning works well in showing the child the consequences of actions.

Musical—Have the child "dance" to music as a form of exercise. Soft music also serves as a relaxing influence on the child.

Interpersonal—Have a group of children play a card game such as a version of Old Maid that matches health information with pictures of exercises or have the children play a game together where they all have to repeat the exercise that the person next to them just performed.

Intrapersonal—Suggest that the child become active by teaching classmates the importance of exercise. Such learners need to research the facts, and then convey these findings to others.

Naturalist—Allow the child to engage in outside activities that are a form of exercise such as gardening or nature walks, or offer videos about exercise where nature, science, or animals are featured.

Although this theory on multiple intelligences was originally designed for use with children, several recent articles address its application with adults. For example, this theory was implemented with nursing students for classroom learning (Amerson, 2006). Many educators see the theory as simple common sense—that children (and adults) have varied talents and learn in different ways even though there is no empirical evidence supporting multiple intelligences theory (Gardner, 2004; Waterhouse, 2006). Additional information about Gardner's theory is available for purchase at his Web site (www.howardgardner.com).

VARK Learning Styles

Fleming and Mills (1992) suggest four categories or preferences—visual, aural, read/write, and kinesthetic—that seem to reflect learning style experiences of their students. VARK is technically about a person's preference for taking in and putting out information. According to Fleming and Mills, an individual learns most effectively and comfortably by one of the following ways:

Visual learners—Like graphical representations such as flowcharts with step-by-step directions

Aural learners—Enjoy listening to lectures, often need directions read aloud, and prefer to discuss topics and form study groups

Read/write learners—Like the written word by reading or writing with references to additional sources of information

Kinesthetic learners—Enjoy doing hands-on activities, such as role-playing and return demonstration

INSTRUMENT TO MEASURE THE VARK

The VARK questionnaire provides users with a profile of their learning preferences for taking in and giving out information. VARK's modalities are a part of the Myers-Briggs personality type indicator and Gardner's multiple intelligences theory.

The VARK consists of 16 questions with four options, and the learner can select more than one option for each question. This instrument, recently updated, is free either as an online or printable version (www.vark-learn.com). There is some evidence of the validity of the VARK scores that supports its use as a low-stakes diagnostic tool by students and teachers, but, at this time, it is not recommended as a research tool until other sources of evidence of the validity of its scores are collected (Leite, Syinicki, & Shi, in press). Educators may find it to be an excellent way to help open a dialogue with learners on the differences that exist in the way individuals prefer to learn. The VARK questionnaire is easy to use and can readily be applied in the healthcare setting.

Interpretation of the Use of Learning Style Models and Instruments

Learning style is an important concept, but educators must exercise caution in assessing styles so as not to ignore other factors that are equally important to teaching and learning, such as readiness and capabilities to learn, educational background, and rates of learning. Styles, which vary from person to person, also differ from capabilities. The style by which someone learns describes how that individual processes stimuli as opposed to capabilities that define how much and how well the person processes the information (Thompson & Crutchlow, 1993). Another caution to keep in mind is that much of the advice offered with regard to using learning styles often consists of "logical deductions from the various theories of learning style, rather than conclusions drawn from empirical research" (Coffield et al., 2004a, p. 125).

Some learning theorists advocate that learning style be matched with a similar teaching style

for learners to attain an optimal level of achievement. However, research in this area is clouded by inconsistent findings (Coffield et al., 2004b). It may be that learning occurs not so much as a result of matching teacher and learner styles, but that when the educator uses a variety of teaching approaches rather than relying on just one, learners feel less stressed and more confident. As a result, they are more satisfied overall with their learning experience and hence more motivated to learn. Application of learning style theory to facilitate the education process allows the educator to approach each learner holistically by recognizing that not all learners process information in the same way (Arndt & Underwood, 1990).

Research indicates that learning style preferences prevail over time, although they may fluctuate depending on the context in which learners are operating at any given moment. The concept of matching styles implies that individuals are static, which contradicts the purpose of education. Learners need to experience some discomfort before they can grow. Educators need to generate dynamic disequilibrium rather than create an environment that is too harmonious (Joyce, 1984).

When selecting a learning style instrument, the educator must first evaluate the instrument for validity, reliability, and the population for which it is intended. In addition, the ease of administering the instrument as well as analyzing the results need to be taken into consideration. Also, educators must adhere to copyright laws, which means that they must buy the instrument or obtain the author's permission before using the tool.

For purposes of assessment, the health professional educator is encouraged to use multiple learning style models and instruments. If the educator focuses on only one model, the possibility arises of trying to make learners fit into a particular style type that does not suit them—a forced choice with no options. Given the teaching–learning situation, the educator may find certain learning style models and instruments to be more appropriate than others in providing strategies for dealing with needs, problems, or unique circumstances.

Of course, it may not always be practical to administer learning style instruments because of cost, time, accessibility, or appropriateness for a specific population. Therefore, educators should follow these general guidelines when assessing individual learning styles:

- Become familiar with the different models and instruments available and the various ways in which styles are classified so that they are easier to recognize.
- Identify key elements of an individual's learning style by observing and asking questions to verify observations. Then, initially match instructional methods and materials to those unique qualities. For example, the following questions could elicit valuable information: Do you prefer to attend lectures or group discussions? Which do you like best, reading or viewing a film? Would you like me to demonstrate this skill first, or would you rather learn by doing while I talk you through the procedure?
- Always allow learners the opportunity to say when a teaching method or instructional material is not working for them.
- Encourage learners to become aware of their learning styles as a way to increase understanding both from the educator's and the learner's perspectives. Everyone should realize that a variety of learning modalities exist and that no one style is better than another.
- Be cautious about saying that certain instructional methods are always more effective for certain styles. Remember that everyone is unique, circumstances may alter preferences, and there are many different ways to influence learning.
- Prompt learners to expand their style ranges rather than to seek only comfortable experiences.

- Provide learning choices that enable learners to operate, at least some of the time, in the style by which they prefer to learn.
- When possible, use a team of educators who have varied teaching styles to present new and complex information in different ways to ensure mastery of information.

Educators must exercise caution when using any of these instruments to assess learning style. They must remember not to place too much emphasis or reliance on these tools to categorize learners. The goal should not be to stereotype learners as to style but rather to ensure that each learner is given an equal opportunity to learn in the best or most comfortable way. Understanding how someone prefers to learn assists the educator in choosing diverse teaching methods and materials to meet the needs of that learner and all learners.

State of the Evidence

Interwoven into each section of this chapter are examples of specific published research about the determinants of learning. This chapter's framework for assessing the evidence to be included in support of the three determinants of learning is based on the framework suggested by Lohr (2004). She cites four dimensions of evidence that health professional educators need to consider when deciding about the available evidence:

1. Level of evidence (study design)
2. Quality of evidence (concern with bias)
3. Relevance of evidence (implying applicability)
4. Strength of evidence (precision, reproducibility, and attributability)

For this chapter, using this framework was helpful in deciding what is considered appropriate evidence, where the evidence comes from (refereed journals as opposed to Internet commercial sites), and whether all the evidence counts (or counts in the same way when there are several articles from which to choose). Most of the literature about the determinants of learning is descriptive in nature or expert opinion, and many lack the scientific rigor needed as evidence of strength. These studies were not included in this chapter.

The research included in this chapter gives support to the importance of conducting an educational assessment. However, a deficit of evidence on the process and criteria for assessment is striking when compared to the number of studies that provide evidence for the effectiveness of different teaching methodologies. Many of the current scientifically designed studies do not take into account all the determinants of learning before examining the benefits of various teaching interventions. Every learner has different learning needs, readiness to learn, and learning styles, which may account for the paucity of experimental research. Even though very few systemic reviews that pertained to learning styles were found, the evidence suggests that learning style instruments should be used with caution.

The lack of research-based evidence about the three determinants of learning suggests that educational assessment is not an easy area in which to conduct research. It is essential to acknowledge this limitation and to remember that research in the health professions in this area in comparison to other sciences is still young. In addition, research in the health professions is supported by a much smaller number of investigators.

Even though much more evidence is needed, the available evidence on conducting an educational assessment substantiates its importance and provides direction for the health professional educator. Conducting a needs assessment on all three determinants is essential before any educational intervention is performed.

Summary

This chapter stresses the importance of the assessment phase of learning because the educator must be aware of and know how to determine learning needs, readiness to learn, and individual learning styles prior to planning for any educational encounter.

Learning is a complex concept that is not directly seen but that can be inferred from permanent changes that occur in the learner's behavior in the cognitive, psychomotor, and affective domains. Educators should not set behavioral objectives for these three domains until they establish what the needs of the learner are, when the learner is ready to learn, and how the learner best learns. Based on the findings from assessment of these determinants, the educator can choose the teaching approaches and learning activities most suited for each individual.

Identifying and prioritizing learning needs require the educator to discover what the learner feels is important and the educator knows to be important. Once needs are established and agreed upon, the educator must assess the learner's readiness to learn based on the physical, emotional, experiential, and knowledge components particular to each learner. Assessing learning styles by way of interviewing, observing, and using instrument measurement can reveal how individuals best learn as well as how they prefer to learn.

By accepting the diversity of needs, readiness levels, and styles among learners, the educator can create a versatile atmosphere and facilitate optimal experiences that encourage all learners to reach their full potential. Whoever the audience may be, health professionals should select teaching interventions and learning activities most beneficial for the learner based on the three determinants of learning.

REVIEW QUESTIONS

1. How would you define the term *determinants of learning*?
2. What are four of the seven methods to assess patient learning needs?
3. What is meant by the term *readiness to learn*?
4. What are the four types of readiness to learn?
5. What are the components of each type of readiness to learn?
6. What is the definition of the term *learning style*?
7. What are the six learning style principles that should guide the health professional educator in teaching any audience of learners?
8. Which models and instruments are available to determine someone's learning style?
9. What does each of the eight learning style models and instruments measure?
10. What evidence is available to support the determinants of learning?

CASE STUDY

You are a member of the interdisciplinary team working with Barbara Lund, a 36-year-old woman recovering from a recent surgical resection of a malignant thoracic spinal cord tumor. Mrs. Lund has a supportive husband and a 2-year-old son. Mrs. Lund's husband, James, states, "I am really worried about Barbara because she was quite distressed for about 6 months prior to this surgery over the death of her father. I fear the surgery may have pushed her over the edge." Currently, 2 weeks status post resection, Mrs. Lund is beginning to ask team members questions about her prognosis and potential functional abilities. She says, "I remember my surgeon trying to explain the surgery to me, but honestly, I didn't really understand much of what he told me. I am a bit naive when it comes to anything medical." Mrs. Lund appears quite anxious about the cancer diagnosis and about how she will be able to continue caring for her son.

1. What are two methods you might use to assess Mrs. Lund's learning needs? List the advantages and disadvantages of each method.
2. Describe the criteria your team and the client will use to prioritize her learning needs. Give examples of specific learning needs that will likely be a priority.
3. What major clues indicate Mrs. Lund's readiness to learn? Using the PEEK model, identify potential obstacles that might interfere with her readiness to learn.
4. According to the VARK model, how will knowledge of Mrs. Lund's learning preference(s) affect your team's instructional approach? Choose one VARK learning preference for Mrs. Lund and describe the instructional approach your team will use to support this preference.

References

Amerson, R. (2006). Energizing the nursing lecture: Application of the theory of multiple intelligence learning. *Nursing Education Perspectives, 27*(4), 194–196.

Armstrong, T. (1987). *In their own way*. New York: St. Martin's.

Arndt, M. J., & Underwood, B. (1990). Learning style theory and patient understanding. *Journal of Continuing Education in Nursing, 21*(1), 28–31.

Ashton, K. C. (1999). How men and women with heart disease seek care: The delay experience. *Progress in Cardiovascular Nursing, 14*(2), 53–60.

Bargar, R., & Hoover, R. (1984). Psychological type and the matching of cognitive styles. *Theory into Practice, 23*(1), 56–63.

Beddoe, S. S. (1999). Reachable moment. *Image: Journal of Nursing Scholarship, 31*(3), 248.

Bertakis, K. D., Rahman, A., Helms, L. J., Callahan, E. J., & Robbins, J. A. (2000). Gender differences in the utilization of health care services. *Journal of Family Practice, 49*(2), 147–152.

Bibb, S. C. (2001). Population based needs assessment in the design of patient education programs. *Military Medicine, 166*(4), 297–300.

Bloom, B. (1968). *Learning for mastery*. Instruction and Curriculum, Topical Papers and Reprints No. 1. Durham, NC: National Laboratory for Higher Education.

Bonham, L. A. (1988). Learning style instruments: Let the buyer beware. *Lifelong Learning, 11*(6), 14–17.

Botwinick, J. (1978). *Aging and behavior* (2nd ed.). New York: Springer.

Boyd, M. D., Gleit, C. J., Graham, B. A., & Whitman, N. I. (1998). *Health teaching in nursing practice: A professional model* (3rd ed.). Stamford, CT: Appleton & Lange.

Breitrose, P. (1988). *Focus groups—When and how to use them: A practical guide*. Palo Alto, CA: Health Promotion Resource.

Bruner, J. (1966). *Toward a theory of instruction*. Cambridge, MA: Harvard University Press.

Bubela, N., & Galloway, S. (1990). Factors influencing patients' informational needs at time of hospital discharge. *Patient Education and Counseling, 16*, 21–28.

Bubela, N., Galloway, S., McCay, E., McKibbon, A., Nagle, L., Pringle, D., et al. (2000). Patient learning needs scale. Informational needs of surgical patients following discharge. *Applied Nursing Research, 13*, 12–18.

Burkhart, J. A. (2008). Training nurses to be teachers. *The Journal of Continuing Education in Nursing, 39*(11), 503–510.

Burton, C. (2000). Re-thinking stroke rehabilitation: The Corbin and Strauss chronic illness trajectory framework. *Journal of Advanced Nursing, 32*(3), 595–602.

Capraro, R. M., & Capraro, M. M. (2002). Myers-Briggs Type Indicator score reliability across studies: A meta-analytic approach. *Educational and Psychological Measurement, 62*, 590–602.

Carlson, M. L., Ivnik, M. A., Dierkhising, R. A., O'Byrne, M. M., & Vickers, K. S. (2006). A learning needs assessment of patients with COPD. MEDSURG *Nursing, 15*(4), 204–212.

Carroll, I. (1963). A model of school learning. *Teachers College Record, 64*, 723–733.

Cassidy, S. (2004). Learning styles: An overview of theories, models, and measures. *Educational Psychology, 24*(4), 419–444.

Castro, O. (2006). Learning styles—How making too many "wrong mistakes" is the right thing to do: A response to Sparks. *Foreign Language Annals, 39*(3), 529–535.

Caulfield, J., Kidd, S., & Kocher, T. (2000). Brain-based instruction in action. *Educational Leadership, 58*(3), 62–65.

Chall, J., & Mirsky, A. (Eds.). (1978). *Education and the brain. Seventy-seventh yearbook of the National Society for the Study of Education* [Part 2]. Chicago: University of Chicago Press.

Churchill, J. (2008). Teaching nutrition to the left and right brain: An overview of learning styles. *Journal of Veterinary Medical Education, 35*(2), 275–280.

Clack, G., Allen, J., Cooper, D., & O'Head, J. (2004). Personality differences between doctors and their patients: Implications for the teaching of communication skills. *Medical Education, 38*, 177–186.

Coffield, F., Moseley. D., Hall, E., & Ecclestone, K. (2004a). *Learning styles and pedagogy in post-16 learning: A systematic and critical review*. London: Learning and Skills Research Centre.

Coffield, F., Moseley, D., Hall, E., & Ecclestone, K. (2004b). *Should we be using learning styles? What research has to say about practice*. London: Learning and Skills Research Centre.

Corbett, C. F. (2003). A randomized pilot study of improving foot care in home health patients with diabetes. *Diabetes Educator, 29*(2), 273–282.

Corbin, J. M., & Strauss, A. (1991). A nursing model for chronic illness management based upon the trajectory framework. *Scholarly Inquiry for Nursing Practice: An International Journal, 5*(3), 155–174.

Delahoussaye, M. (2002). The perfect learner: An expert debate on learning styles. *Training, 39*(5), 28–36.

Deture, M. L. (2004). Investigating the predictive value of cognitive style and online technologies self-efficacy in predicting student success in online distance education courses. *Dissertation Abstracts International Section A: Humanities and Social Sciences, 64*(8-A), 2761.

Dunn, K., & Dunn, R. (1987). Dispelling outmoded beliefs about student learning. *Educational Leadership, 44*(6), 55–62.

Dunn, R. (1984). Learning style: State of the science. *Theory into Practice, 23*(1), 10–19.

Dunn, R. (1995). *Strategies for educating diverse learners.* Bloomington, IN: Phi Delta Kappa.

Dunn, R., & Dunn, K. (1978). *Teaching students through their individual learning styles: A practical approach.* Reston, VA: National Association of Secondary School Principals.

Dunn, R., & Griggs, S. (2003). *Synthesis of the Dunn and Dunn learning styles model research: Who, what, when, where and so what: The Dunn and Dunn learning styles model and its theoretical cornerstone.* New York: St. John's University.

Durden-Smith, J., & deSimone, D. (1983). *Sex and the brain.* New York: Arbor House.

Epstein, R., & Street, R., Jr. (2007). *Patient-centered communication in cancer care: Promoting healing and reducing suffering.* Bethesda, MD: National Cancer Institute. Publication No. 07-6225.

Fleming, N. D., & Mills, C. (1992). Not another inventory, rather a catalyst for reflection. *To Improve the Academy, 11*, 137–144.

Flynn, E. A., Barker, K. N., Gibson, J. T., Pearson, R. E., Berger, B. A., & Smith, L. A. (1999). Impact of interruptions and distractions on dispensing errors in an ambulatory care pharmacy. *American Journal of Health-System Pharmacy, 56*(13), 1319–1325.

Friedman, P., & Alley, R. (1984). Learning/teaching styles: Applying the principles. *Theory into Practice, 23*(1), 77–81.

Gardner, H. (1983). *Frames of mind.* New York: Basic Books.

Gardner, H. (1999a). *The disciplined mind: What all students should understand.* New York: Simon and Schuster.

Gardner, H. (1999b). *Intelligence reframed: Multiple intelligences for the 21st century.* New York: Basic Books.

Gardner, H. (2004). *Changing minds: The art and science of changing our own and other people's minds.* Boston: Harvard Business School Press.

Garity, J. (1985). Learning styles: Basis for creative teaching and learning. *Nurse Educator, 10*(2), 12–16.

Gavan, C. S. (2003). Successful aging families—a challenge for nurses. *Holistic Nursing Practice, 17*(1), 11–18.

Gondringer, N. (1989). Whole brain thinking: A potential link to successful learning. *Journal of the American Association of Nurse Anesthetists, 57*(3), 217–219.

Grant, J. (2002). Learning needs assessment: Assessing the need. *British Medical Journal, 324*, 156–159.

Greer, G., Hitt, J. D., Sitterly, T. E., & Slebodnick, E. B. (1972). An examination of four factors impacting on psychomotor performance effectiveness. In D. P. Ely (Ed.), *Psychomotor domain: A resource book for media specialists.* Washington, DC: Gryphon House.

Gur, R. C., Turetsky, B. I., Matsui, M., Yan, M., Bilker, W., Hughett, P., et al. (1999). Sex differences in brain gray and white matter in healthy young adults: Correlations with cognitive performance. *Journal of Neuroscience, 19*(10), 4065–4072.

Haggard, A. (1989). *Handbook of patient education.* Rockland, MD: Aspen.

Hansen, M., & Fisher, J. C. (1998). Patient-centered teaching: From theory to practice. *American Journal of Nursing, 98*(1), 56–60.

Hardy, R., & Smith, R. (2001). Enhancing staff development with a structured preceptor program. *Journal of Nursing Quality Assurance, 15*(2), 9–17.

Healthcare Education Association. (1985). *Managing hospital education.* Laguna Niguel, CA: Author.

Herrmann, N. (1988). *The creative brain.* Lake Lure, NC: Brain Books.

Hotelling, B. A. (2005). Promoting wellness in Lamaze classes. *Journal of Perinatal Education, 14*(3), 45–50.

Iaccino, J. F. (1993). *Left-brain–right-brain differences: Inquiries, evidence and new approaches.* Hillsdale, NJ: Erlbaum.

James, W. B., & Gardner, D. L. (1995). Learning styles: Implications for distance learning. *New Directions for Adult and Continuing Education, 67*(1), 19–32.

Jessee, S, O'Neill, P., & Dosch, R. (2006). Matching student personality types and learning preferences to teaching methodologies. *Journal of Dental Education, 70*(6), 644–651.

Joseph, D. H. (1993). Risk: A concept worthy of attention. *Nursing Forum, 28*(1), 12–16.

Joyce, B. (1984). Dynamic disequilibrium: The intelligence of growth. *Theory into Practice, 23*(1), 26–34.

Jung, C. G. (1971). Psychological types. In *Collected works* (Vol. 6, R. F. C. Hull, Trans.). Princeton, NJ: Princeton University Press. (Originally published in German as *Psychologische Typen.* Zurich: Rasher Verlag, 1921).

Keefe, J. W. (1979). *Student learning styles: Diagnosing and prescribing programs.* Reston, VA: National Association of Secondary School Principals.

Kessels, R. P. C. (2003). Patients' memory for medical information. *Journal of the Royal Society of Medicine, 96*(5), 219–222.

Kiesler, D. J., & Auerbach, S. M. (2006). Optimal matches of patient preferences for information, decision making and interpersonal behavior: Evidence, models and interventions. *Patient Education and Counseling, 61*(3), 319–341.

Kim, J., Dodd, M., West, C., Paul, S., Facione, N., Schumacher, K., et al. (2004). The PRO-SELF Pain Control Program improves patients' knowledge of cancer pain management. *Oncology Nursing Forum, 31*(6), 1137–1143.

Kitchie, S. (2003). *Rural elders with chronic disease: Place of residence, social network, social support, and medication adherence.* (Doctoral dissertation, Binghamton University, 2003). Dissertation Abstracts International–B [Online], 64(08), 3745. (UMI No. 3102848).

Knowles, M. (1990). The application of brain dominance technology to the training profession. In M. Knowles (Ed.), *The adult learner: A neglected species* (4th ed.). Houston, TX: Gulf Publishing Company.

Knox, A. B. (1974). *Life-long self-directed education.* San Francisco: Jossey-Bass.

Knox, A. B. (1977). *Adult development and learning.* San Francisco: Jossey-Bass.

Knox, A. B. (1986). *Helping adults learn.* San Francisco: Jossey-Bass.

Kolb, D. A. (1984). *Experiential learning: Experience as the source of learning and development.* Englewood Cliffs, NJ: Prentice Hall.

Landry, S. H., Smith, K. E., & Swank, P. R. (2006). Responsive parenting: Establishing early foundations for social, communication, and independent problem-solving skills. *Developmental Psychology, 42*(4), 627–642.

Leite, W. L., Syinicki, M., & Shi, Y. (in press). Attempted validation of the scores of the VARK learning styles inventory with multitrait-multimethod confirmatory factor analysis models. *Educational and Psychological Measurement.*

Ley, P. (1979). Memory for medical information. *British Journal of Social & Clinical Psychology, 18*(2), 245–255.

Lichtenthal, C. (1990). A self-study model on readiness to learn. Unpublished manuscript.

Lohr, N. K. (2004). Rating the strength of scientific evidence: Relevance for quality improvement programs. *International Journal for Quality in Health Care, 16*(1), 9–18.

Lubkin, I. M., & Larsen, P. D. (2006). *Chronic illness: Impact and interventions* (6th ed.). Sudbury, MA: Jones and Bartlett.

Maslow, A. (1970). *Motivation and personality.* New York: Harper & Row.

McCarthy, B. (1981). *The 4MAT system: Teaching to learning styles with right/left mode techniques.* Barrington, IL: Excel.

McDonald, D. D., Wiczorek, M., & Walker, C. (2004). Factors affecting learning during health education sessions. *Clinical Nursing Research, 132*, 156–167.

McIntosh, A. R. (1998). Understanding neural interactions in learning and memory using functional neuroimaging. *Annals of the New York Academy of Sciences. Olfaction and Taste XII: An International Symposium, 855,* 556–571.

Miaskowski, C., Dodd, M., West, C., Schumacher, K., Paul, S. M., Tripathy, D., et al. (2004). Randomized clinical trial of the effectiveness of a self-care intervention to improve cancer pain management. *Journal of Clinical Oncology, 22*(9), 1713–1720.

Mordiffi, S. Z., Tan, S. P., & Wong, M. K. (2003). Information provided to surgical patients versus information needed. *Association of Operating Room Nurses, 77*(3), 546–562.

Morse, J. S., Oberer, J., Dobbins, J. A., & Mitchell, D. (1998). Understanding learning styles. Implications for staff development educators. *Journal of Nursing Staff Development, 14*(1), 41–46.

Musinski, B. (1999). The educator as facilitator: A new kind of leadership. *Nursing Forum, 34*(1), 23–29.

Myers, I. B. (1980). *Gifts differing.* Palo Alto, CA: Consulting Psychologists Press.

Myers, I. B. (1987). *Introduction to type.* Palo Alto, CA: Consulting Psychologists Press.

Oltman, P. K., Raskin, E., Witkin, H. A., & Karp, S. A. (1978). Group embedded figures test. In O. K. Buros (Ed.), *The eighth mental measurements yearbook* (Vol. 1). Lincoln: University of Nebraska Press.

Panja, S., Starr, B., & Colleran, K. M. (2005). Patient knowledge improves glycemic control: Is it time to go back to the classroom? *Journal of Investigative Medicine, 53*(5), 264–266.

Panno, J. M. (1992). A systematic approach for assessing learning needs. *Journal of Nursing Staff Development, 8*(6), 267–273.

Patterson, B. L. (2001). The shifting perspectives model of chronic illness. *Journal of Nursing Scholarship, 33*(1), 21–26.

Ramanadhan, S., & Viswanath, K. (2006). Health and the information nonseeker: A profile. *Health Communication, 20*(2), 131–139.

Rankin, S. H., & Stallings, L. D. (2005). *Patient education in health and illness* (5th ed.). Philadelphia: Lippincott, Williams & Wilkins.

Redman, B. K. (2003). *Measurement tools in patient education.* New York: Springer.

Roberts, C. (1982). Identifying the real patient problems. *Nursing Clinics of North America, 17*(3), 484–485.

Rosen, A., Tsai, J., & Downs, S. (2003). Variations in risk

attitude across race, gender and education. *Medical Decision Making, 23,* 511–517.

Rutten, L. J., Arora, N. K., Bakos, A. D., Aziz, N., & Rowland, J. (2005). Information needs and sources of information among cancer patients: A systematic review of research (1980–2003). *Patient Education and Counseling, 57*(3), 250–261.

Sandberg, E. H., Sharma, R., Wiklund, R., & Sandberg, W. S. (2008). Clinicians consistently exceed a typical person's short-term memory during preoperative teaching. *Anesthesia & Analgesia, 107*(3), 972–977.

Santrock, J. W. (2006). *Life-span development* (10th ed.). Boston: McGraw-Hill.

Schoessler, M., Conedera, F., Bell, L. F., Marshall, D., & Gilson, M. (1993). Use of the Myers-Briggs Type Indicator to develop a continuing education department. *Journal of Nursing Staff Development, 9*(1), 8–13.

Shipman, S., & Shipman, V. C. (1985). Cognitive styles: Some conceptual, methodological, and applied issues. In E. W. Gordon (Ed.), *Review of research in education* (12th ed.). Washington, DC: American Educational Research Associates.

Skinner, B. F. (1954). The science of learning and the art of teaching. *Harvard Educational Review, 24,* 86–97.

Speck, O., Ernst, T., Braun, J., Koch, C., Miller, E., & Chang, L. (2000). Gender differences in the functional organization of the brain for working memory. *Neuroreport, 11*(11), 2581–2585.

Sperry, R. W. (1977). Bridging science and values: A unifying view of mind and brain. *American Psychologist, 32*(4), 237–245.

Stein, J. A., & Nyamathi, A. (2000). Gender differences in behavioural and psychosocial predictors of HIV testing and return for test results in a high-risk population. *AIDS Care, 12*(3), 343–356.

Stephenson, P. L. (2006). Before the teaching begins: Managing patient anxiety prior to providing education. *Clinical Journal of Oncology Nursing, 10*(2), 241–245.

Stilwell, N., Wallick, M., Thal, S., & Burleson, J. (2000). Myers-Briggs type and medical specialty choice: A new look at an old question. *Teaching and Learning in Medicine, 12*(1), 14–20.

Stover, D. (2001). Applying brain research in the classroom is not a no-brainer. *Education Digest, 66*(8), 26–29.

Street, R., Jr., Makoul, G., Arora, N., & Epstein, R. (2009). How does communication heal? Pathways linking clinician–patient communication to health outcomes. *Patient Education and Counseling, 74,* 295–301.

Suhonen, R., Nenonen, A., Laukka, A., & Valimaki, M. (2005). Patients' informational needs and information received do not correspond in hospital. *Journal of Clinical Nursing, 14,* 1167–1176.

Sylvester, R. (1995). *A celebration of neurons: An educator's guide to the human brain.* Alexandria, VA: Association for Supervision and Curriculum Development.

Sylvester, R. (1998). The brain revolution. *School Administrator, 55*(1), 6.

Tanner, G. (1989). A need to know. *Nursing Times, 85*(31), 54–56.

Telford, K., Kralik, D., & Koch, T. (2006). Acceptance and denial: Implications for people adapting to chronic illness. *Journal of Advanced Nursing, 55*(4), 457–464.

Thompson, C., & Crutchlow, E. (1993). Learning style research: A critical review of the literature and implications for nursing education. *Journal of Professional Nursing, 9*(1), 34–40.

Timmins, F. (2005). A review of the information needs of patients with acute coronary syndromes. *Nursing in Critical Care, 10*(4), 174–183.

Vaughn, L., & Baker, R. (2008). Do different pairings of teaching styles and learning styles make a difference? Preceptor and resident perceptions. *Teaching and Learning in Medicine, 20*(3), 239–247.

Villejo, L., & Meyers, C. (1991). Brain function, learning styles, and cancer patient education. *Seminars in Oncology Nursing, 7*(2), 97–104.

Wagner, P. S., & Ash, K. L. (1998). Creating the teachable moment. *Journal of Nursing Education, 37*(6), 278–280.

Waltz, C. F., Strickland, O. L., & Lenz, E. L. (2005). *Measurement in nursing and health research* (3rd ed.). New York: Springer.

Waterhouse, L. (2006). Multiple intelligences, the Mozart effect, and emotional intelligence: A critical review. *Educational Psychologist, 41*(4), 207–225.

Williams, M. L. (1998). Making the most of learning needs assessments. *Journal for Nurses in Staff Development, 14*(3), 137–142.

Witkin, H., & Goodenough, D. R. (1981). *Cognitive styles: Essence and origins.* New York: International Universities Press.

Witkin, H., Moore, C. A., & Oltman, P. K. (1977). Cognitive styles and their educational implications. *Review of Educational Research, 47,* 1–64.

Witkin, H., Oltman, P. K., Raskin, E., & Karp, S. (1971a). *Group embedded figures test.* Palo Alto, CA: Consulting Psychologists Press.

Witkin, H., Oltman, P. K., Raskin, E., & Karp, S. (1971b). *A manual for the embedded figures test.* Palo Alto, CA: Consulting Psychologists Press.

Wolfe, P. (1994). Risk taking: Nursing's comfort zone. *Holistic Nurse Practice, 8*(2), 43–52.

Wonder, J., & Donovan, M. (1984). *Whole-brain thinking.* New York: Ballantine.

Chapter 5

Developmental Stages of the Learner

Susan B. Bastable

Michelle A. Dart

CHAPTER HIGHLIGHTS

KEY TERMS

- ❏ pedagogy
- ❏ object permanence
- ❏ causality
- ❏ animistic thinking
- ❏ syllogistic reasoning
- ❏ conservation
- ❏ imaginary audience
- ❏ personal fable
- ❏ andragogy
- ❏ dialectical thinking
- ❏ ageism
- ❏ gerogogy
- ❏ crystallized intelligence
- ❏ fluid intelligence

OBJECTIVES

After completing this chapter, the reader will be able to

1. Identify the physical, cognitive, and psychosocial characteristics of learners that influence learning at various stages of growth and development.
2. Recognize the role of the health professional in assessing stage-specific learner needs according to maturational levels.
3. Determine the role of the family in patient education.
4. Discuss appropriate teaching strategies effective for learners at different developmental stages.

When planning, designing, implementing, and evaluating an educational program, the health professional must carefully consider the characteristics of learners with respect to their developmental stage in life. The more heterogeneous the target audience, the more complex the development of an educational program to meet the diverse needs of the population. Conversely, the more homogeneous the population of learners, the more straightforward the approach to teaching.

An individual's developmental stage significantly influences the ability to learn. Pedagogy, andragogy, and gerogogy are three different orientations to learning in childhood, young and middle adulthood, and older adulthood, respectively. To meet the health-related educational needs of learners, a developmental approach must be used. Three major stage-range factors associated with learner readiness—physical, cognitive, and psychosocial maturation—must be taken into account at each developmental period throughout the life cycle.

Developmental psychologists have for years explored the various patterns of behavior particular to stages of development. Educators, more than ever before, acknowledge the effects of growth and development on an individual's willingness and ability to make use of instruction.

This chapter has specific implications for health professional educators because of the recent man-

dates by the Joint Commission (formerly known as JCAHO—the Joint Commission on Accreditation of Healthcare Organizations). For healthcare agencies to meet Joint Commission accreditation requirements, teaching plans must address stage-specific competencies of the learner. In this chapter, the distinct life stages of learners are examined from the perspective of physical, cognitive, and psychosocial development; the role of the health professional in assessment of stage-specific learner needs; the role of the family in the teaching–learning process; and the teaching strategies specific to meeting the needs of learners at various developmental stages of life.

A deliberate attempt has been made to minimize reference to age as the criterion for categorization of learners. Research on life-span development shows that chronological age per se is not the only predictor of learning ability (Santrock, 2006; Vander Zanden, Crandell, & Crandell, 2007; Whitener, Cox, & Maglich, 1998). At any given age, one finds a wide variation in the acquisition of abilities related to the three fundamental domains of development: physical (biological), cognitive, and psychosocial (emotional-social) maturation. Age ranges, included after each developmental stage heading in this chapter, are intended only to be used as approximate age-strata reference points or general guidelines; they do not imply that chronological ages necessarily correspond perfectly to the various stages of development. Thus, the term *developmental stage* is the perspective used based on the confirmation by psychologists that human growth and development are sequential but not always specifically age related.

Recently it has become clear that development is contextual. Even though the passage of time has traditionally been synonymous with chronological age, social and behavioral psychologists have begun to consider the many other changes occurring over time that affect the dynamic relationship between a human being's biological makeup and the environment. It is now understood that three important contextual influences act on and interact with the individual to produce development (Santrock, 2006; Vander Zanden et al., 2007):

1. Normative age-graded influences are strongly related to chronological age and are similar for individuals in a particular age group, such as the biological processes of puberty and menopause, and the sociocultural processes of transitioning to different levels of formal education or to retirement.
2. Normative history-graded influences are common to people in a particular age cohort or generation because they have been uniquely exposed to similar historical circumstances, such as the Vietnam War, the age of computers, or the terrorist event of September 11, 2001.
3. Normative life events are the unusual or unique circumstances, positive or negative, that are turning points in individuals' lives that cause them to change direction, such as a house fire, serious injury in an accident, winning the lottery, divorce, or an unexpected career opportunity.

Although this chapter focuses on the client as the learner throughout the life span, health professional educators can apply the stage-specific characteristics of adulthood and the associated principles of adult learning presented herein to any audience of young, middle, or older adult learners, whether the health professional is instructing the general public in the community, preparing students in an education program, or teaching continuing education to colleagues.

Developmental Characteristics

As noted, actual chronological age is only a relative indicator of someone's physical, cognitive, and psychosocial stage of development. Unique as each individual is, however, some typical developmental trends have been identified as milestones of normal progression through the life cycle. When dealing with the teaching–learning process, it is imperative to examine the developmental phases as individuals progress from infancy to senescence so as to fully appreciate the behavioral changes that occur in the cognitive, affective, and psychomotor domains.

As influential as age can be to learning readiness, it should never be examined in isolation. Growth and development interact with experiential background, physical and emotional health status, and personal motivation, as well as numerous environmental factors such as stress, the surrounding conditions, and the available support systems, to affect a person's ability and readiness to learn.

Musinski (1999) describes three phases of learning: dependence, independence, and interdependence. These passages of learning ability from childhood to adulthood, labeled by Covey (1990) as the "maturity continuum," are identified as follows:

- Dependence is characteristic of the infant and young child, who are totally dependent on others for direction, support, and nurturance from a physical, emotional, and intellectual stand-

Table 5–1 Stage-Appropriate Teaching Strategies

Learner	General Characteristics	Teaching Strategies	Nursing Interventions
INFANCY–TODDLERHOOD			
Approximate age: Birth–2 years Cognitive stage: Sensorimotor Psychosocial stage: Trust vs. mistrust (Birth–12 mo) Autonomy vs. shame and doubt (1–2 yr)	Dependent on environment Needs security Explores self and environment Natural curiosity	Orient teaching to caregiver Use repetition and imitation of information Stimulate all senses Provide physical safety and emotional security Allow play and manipulation of objects	Welcome active involvement Forge alliances Encourage physical closeness Provide detailed information Answer questions and concerns Ask for information on child's strengths/limitations and likes/dislikes
EARLY CHILDHOOD			
Approximate age: 3–5 years Cognitive stage: Preoperational Psychosocial stage: Initiative vs. guilt	Egocentric Thinking precausal, concrete, literal Believes illness self-caused and punitive Limited sense of time Fears bodily injury Cannot generalize Animistic thinking (objects possess life or human characteristics) Centration (focus is on one characteristic of an object) Separation anxiety Motivated by curiosity Active imagination, prone to fears Play is his/her work	Use warm, calm approach Build trust Use repetition of information Allow manipulation of objects and equipment Give care with explanation Reassure not to blame self Explain procedures simply and briefly Provide safe, secure environment Use positive reinforcement Encourage questions to reveal perceptions/feelings Use simple drawings and stories Use play therapy, with dolls and puppets Stimulate senses: visual, auditory, tactile, motor	Welcome active involvement Forge alliances Encourage physical closeness Provide detailed information Answer questions and concerns Ask for information on child's strengths/limitations and likes/dislikes

154

MIDDLE AND LATE CHILDHOOD

Approximate age:	6–11 years	More realistic and objective	Encourage independence and active participation	Welcome active involvement
Cognitive stage:	Concrete operations	Understands cause and effect	Be honest, allay fears	Forge alliances
Psychosocial stage:	Industry vs. inferiority	Deductive/inductive reasoning	Use logical explanation	Encourage physical closeness
		Wants concrete information	Allow time to ask questions	Provide detailed information
		Able to compare objects and events	Use analogies to make invisible processes real	Answer questions and concerns
		Variable rates of physical growth	Establish role models	Ask for information on child's strengths/limitations and likes/dislikes
		Reasons syllogistically	Relate care to other children's experiences; compare procedures	
		Understands seriousness and consequences of actions	Use subject-centered focus	
		Subject-centered focus	Use play therapy	
		Immediate orientation	Provide group activities	
			Use drawings, models, dolls, painting, audio- and videotapes	

ADOLESCENCE

Approximate age:	12–19 years	Abstract, hypothetical thinking	Establish trust, authenticity	Explore emotional and financial support
Cognitive stage:	Formal operations	Can build on past learning	Know their agenda	Determine goals and expectations
Psychosocial stage:	Identity vs. role confusion	Reasons by logic and understands scientific principles	Address fears/concerns about outcomes of illness	Assess stress levels
		Future orientation	Identify control focus	Respect values and norms
		Motivated by desire for social acceptance	Include in plan of care	Determine role responsibilities and relationships
		Peer group important	Use peers for support and influence	Engage in 1:1 teaching without parents present, but with adolescent's permission inform family of content covered
		Intense personal preoccupation, appearance extremely important (imaginary audience)	Negotiate changes	
		Feels invulnerable, invincible/immune to natural laws (personal fable)	Focus on details	
			Make information meaningful to life	
			Ensure confidentiality and privacy	

Table 5–1 Stage-Appropriate Teaching Strategies *(Continued)*

Learner	General Characteristics	Teaching Strategies	Nursing Interventions
YOUNG ADULTHOOD			
Approximate age: 20–40 years Cognitive stage: Formal operations Psychosocial stage: Intimacy vs. isolation	Autonomous Self-directed Uses personal experiences to enhance or interfere with learning Intrinsic motivation Able to analyze critically Makes decisions about personal, occupational, and social roles Competency-based learner	Use problem-centered focus Draw on meaningful experiences Focus on immediacy of application Encourage active participation Allow to set own pace, be self-directed Organize material Recognize social role Apply new knowledge through role-playing and hands-on practice	Explore emotional, financial, and physical support system Assess motivational level for involvement Identify potential obstacles and stressors
MIDDLE-AGED ADULTHOOD			
Approximate age: 41–64 years Cognitive stage: Formal operations Psychosocial stage: Generativity vs. self-absorption and stagnation	Sense of self well-developed Concerned with physical changes At peak in career Explores alternative lifestyles Reflects on contributions to family and society Reexamines goals and values Questions achievements and successes Has confidence in abilities Desires to modify unsatisfactory aspects of life	Focus on maintaining independence and reestablishing normal life patterns Assess positive and negative past experiences with learning Assess potential sources of stress due to midlife crisis issues Provide information to coincide with life concerns and problems	Explore emotional, financial, and physical support system Assess motivational level for involvement Identify potential obstacles and stressors
OLDER ADULTHOOD			
Approximate age: 65 years and older Cognitive stage: Formal operations	**Cognitive changes** Decreased ability to think abstractly, process information	Use concrete examples Build on past life experiences Make information relevant and meaningful Present one concept at a time	Involve principal caregivers Encourage participation

Psychosocial stage:	Ego integrity vs. despair		
	Decreased short-term memory	Allow time for processing/response (slow pace)	Provide resources for support (respite care)
	Increased reaction time	Use repetition and reinforcement of information	Assess coping mechanisms
	Increased test anxiety	Avoid written exams	Provide written instructions for reinforcement
	Stimulus persistence (afterimage)	Use verbal exchange and coaching	Provide anticipatory problem solving (what happens if …)
	Focuses on past life experiences	Establish retrieval plan (use one or several clues)	
	Sensory/motor changes	Encourage active involvement	
	Auditory changes	Keep explanations brief	
	Hearing loss, especially high-pitched tones, consonants (*S, Z, T, F,* and *G*), and rapid speech	Use analogies to illustrate abstract information	
	Visual changes	Speak slowly, distinctly	
	Farsighted (needs glasses to read)	Use low-pitched tones	
	Lenses become opaque (glare problem)	Face client when speaking	
	Smaller pupil size (decreased visual adaptation to darkness)	Minimize distractions	
	Decreased peripheral perception	Avoid shouting	
	Yellowing of lenses (distorts low-tone colors: blue, green, violet)	Use visual aids to supplement verbal instruction	
	Distorted depth perception	Avoid glares, use soft white light	
	Fatigue/decreased energy levels	Provide sufficient light	
	Pathophysiology (chronic illness)	Use white backgrounds and black print	
	Psychosocial changes	Use large letters and well-spaced print	
	Decreased risk taking	Avoid color coding with pastel blues, greens, purples, and yellows	
	Selective learning	Increase safety precautions/provide safe environment	
	Intimidated by formal learning	Ensure accessibility and fit of prostheses (i.e., glasses, hearing aid)	
		Keep sessions short	
		Provide for frequent rest periods	
		Allow for extra time to perform	
		Establish realistic short-term goals	
		Give time to reminisce	
		Identify and present pertinent material	
		Use informal teaching sessions	
		Demonstrate relevance of information to daily life	
		Assess resources	
		Make learning positive	
		Identify past positive experiences	
		Integrate new behaviors with formerly established ones	

point (unfortunately, some adults are considered to be stuck in this stage if they demonstrate manipulative behavior, do not listen, are insecure, or do not accept responsibility for their own actions).

- Independence occurs when a child develops the ability to physically, intellectually, and emotionally care for himself or herself and make his or her own choices, including taking responsibility for learning.

- Interdependence occurs when an individual has advanced in maturity to achieve self-reliance, a sense of self-esteem, the ability to give and receive, and when that individual demonstrates a level of respect for others. Full physical maturity does not guarantee simultaneous emotional and intellectual maturity.

If the health professional educator is to encourage learners to take responsibility for their own health, then learners must be recognized as an important source of data regarding their health status. Before any learning can occur, the educator must assess how much knowledge the learner already possesses with respect to the topic to be taught. With the child as client, for example, new content should be introduced at appropriate stages of development and should build on the child's previous knowledge base and experiences.

The major question underlying the planning for educational experiences is: When is the most appropriate or best time to teach the learner? The answer is when the learner is ready—the teachable moment as defined by Havighurst (1976), that point in time when the learner is most receptive to a teaching situation. It is important to remember that the health professional does not always have to wait for teachable moments to occur; the teacher can create these opportunities by taking an interest in and attending to the needs of the learner. When assessing readiness to learn, the health professional must determine not only whether an interpersonal relationship has been established, prerequisite

knowledge and skills have been mastered, and the learner exhibits motivation, but also whether the plan for teaching matches the developmental level of the learner (Leifer & Hartston, 2004; Polan & Taylor, 2003; Santrock, 2006; Vander Zanden et al., 2007).

The Developmental Stages of Childhood

Pedagogy is the art and science of helping children to learn (Knowles, 1990). The different stages of childhood are divided according to what developmental theorists and educational psychologists define as specific patterns of behavior seen in particular phases of growth and development. One common attribute throughout all phases of childhood is that learning is subject centered. The following is a review of the developmental characteristics in the four stages of childhood and the teaching strategies to be used in relation to the physical, cognitive, and psychosocial maturational levels indicative of learner readiness (see **Table 5–1**).

Infancy (First 12 Months of Life) and Toddlerhood (1–2 Years of Age)

The field of growth and development is highly complex, and at no other time is physical, cognitive, and psychosocial maturation so changeable as during the very early years of childhood. Because of the dependency of this age group, the main focus of instruction for health maintenance of children is geared toward the parents, who are considered to be the primary learners rather than the very young child (Palfrey et al., 2005; Richmond & Kotelchuck, 1984; Santrock, 2006; Vander Zanden et al., 2007). However, the older toddler should not be excluded from healthcare teaching and can participate to some extent in the education process.

PHYSICAL, COGNITIVE, AND PSYCHOSOCIAL DEVELOPMENT

At no other time in life is physical maturation so rapid as during the period of development from infancy to toddlerhood (London, Ladewig, Ball, & Bindler, 2003). Exploration of self and the environment becomes paramount and a stimulant for further physical development (Vander Zanden et al., 2007). Patient education must focus on teaching the parents of very young children the importance of stimulation, nutrition, the practice of safety measures to prevent illness and injury, and health promotion (Polan & Taylor, 2003; Richmond & Kotelchuck, 1984).

Piaget (1951, 1952, 1976), the noted expert in defining the key milestones in the cognitive development of children, labels the stage of infancy to toddlerhood as the *sensorimotor period*. This period refers to the coordination and integration of motor activities with sensory perceptions. As children mature from infancy to toddlerhood, learning is enhanced through sensory experiences and through movement and manipulation of objects in the environment. Toward the end of the second year of life, the very young child begins to develop **object permanence**, that is, realizing that objects and events exist even when they cannot be seen, heard, or touched (Santrock, 2006). Motor activities promote their understanding of the world and an awareness of themselves as well as others' reactions in response to their own actions. Encouraging parents to create a safe environment can allow their child to develop with a decreased risk for injury.

The toddler has the rudimentary capacity for basic reasoning, understands object permanence, has the beginnings of memory, and begins to develop an elementary concept of **causality**, which refers to the ability to grasp a cause-and-effect relationship between two paired, successive events (Vander Zanden et al., 2007). With limited ability to recall past happenings or anticipate future events, the toddler is oriented primarily to the here and now and has little tolerance for delayed gratification. The child who has lived with strict routines and plenty of structure has more of a grasp of time than the child who lives in an unstructured environment.

Children at this stage have short attention spans, are easily distracted, are egocentric in their thinking, and are not amenable to correction of their own ideas. Unquestionably, they believe their own perceptions to be reality. Asking questions is the hallmark of this age group, and curiosity abounds as they explore places and things. They can respond to simple, step-by-step commands and obey such directives as "give Grandpa a kiss" or "go get your teddy bear" (Santrock, 2006).

Language skills are acquired rapidly during this period, and parents should be encouraged to foster this aspect of development by talking with and listening to their child. As they progress through this phase, children begin to engage in fantasizing and make-believe play. Because they are unable to distinguish fact from fiction and have limited cognitive capacity for understanding cause and effect, children may feel that illness and hospitalization are a punishment for something they did wrong (London et al., 2003). Children attributing the cause of illness to the consequences of their own transgressions is known as egocentric causation (Richmond & Kotelchuck, 1984).

According to Erikson (1963), the noted authority on psychosocial development, the period of infancy is one of *trust versus mistrust*. During this time, children must work through their first major dilemma of developing a sense of trust with their primary caretaker. As the infant matures into toddlerhood, autonomy versus shame and doubt emerges as the central issue. During this period of psychosocial growth, toddlers must learn to balance feelings of love and hate and learn to cooperate and control willful desires (see **Table 5–2**).

Children progress sequentially through accomplishing the tasks of developing basic trust in their environment to reaching increasing levels of independence and self-assertion. Their newly discovered sense of independence often is expressed by demonstrations of negativism. Children may have difficulty in making up their minds, and, aggravated by personal and external limits, they may express their level of frustration and feelings of ambivalence in words and behaviors, such as in exhibiting temper tantrums to release tensions (Falvo, 1994). With peers, play is a parallel activity, and it is not unusual for them to end up in tears because they have not yet learned about tact, fairness, or rules of sharing (Babcock & Miller, 1994; Polan & Taylor, 2003).

Toddlers like routines because they give these children a sense of security, and they gravitate toward ritualistic ceremonial-like exercises when carrying out activities of daily living. Separation anxiety is also characteristic of this stage of development and is particularly apparent when children are hospitalized and feel insecure in an unfamiliar environment. This anxiety is often compounded when they are subjected to medical procedures and other healthcare interventions performed by people who are strangers to them (London et al., 2003).

TEACHING STRATEGIES

Patient education for infancy through toddlerhood need not be illness related. Usually less time is devoted to teaching parents about illness care, and considerably more time is spent teaching aspects of normal development, safety, health promotion, and disease prevention. When the child is ill or injured, the first priority for teaching interventions would be to assess the parents' and child's anxiety levels and to help them cope with their feelings of stress related to uncertainty and guilt about the cause of the illness or injury. Anxiety on the part of the child and parents can adversely affect their readiness to learn.

Although teaching activities primarily are directed to the main caregiver(s), children at this developmental stage in life have a great capacity for learning. Toddlers are capable of some degree of understanding procedures and interventions that they may experience. Because of the young child's natural tendency to be intimidated by unfamiliar people, it is imperative that the health professional

---

Table 5–2 ERIKSON'S EIGHT STAGES OF PSYCHOSOCIAL DEVELOPMENT

Developmental Stages	Psychosocial Crises	Strengths
Infancy	Trust vs. mistrust	Hope
Toddlerhood	Autonomy vs. shame and doubt	Will
Early childhood	Initiative vs. guilt	Purpose
Middle and late childhood	Industry vs. inferiority	Competence
Adolescence	Identity vs. role confusion	Fidelity
Young adulthood	Intimacy vs. isolation	Love
Middle-aged adulthood	Generativity vs. self-absorption and stagnation	Care
Older adulthood	Ego integrity vs. despair	Wisdom

Source: Adapted from Ahroni, J. H. (1996). Strategies for teaching elders from a human development perspective. *Diabetes Educator, 22*(1), 48.

takes the time to establish a relationship with the child and parents. This approach not only provides consistency in the teaching–learning process but also helps to reduce the child's fear of strangers. Parents should be present whenever possible during formal and informal teaching and learning activities to allay stress, which could be compounded by separation anxiety (London et al., 2003).

Ideally, health teaching should take place in an environment familiar to the child, such as the home or day-care center. When the child is hospitalized, the environment selected for teaching and learning sessions should be as safe and secure as possible, such as the child's bed or the playroom, to increase the child's sense of feeling protected.

Movement is an important mechanism by which toddlers communicate. Immobility resulting from illness, hospital confinement, or disability tends to increase children's anxiety by restricting activity. Interventions that promote children's use of gross motor abilities and that stimulate their visual, auditory, and tactile senses should be chosen whenever possible.

Developing rapport with children through simple teaching helps to elicit their cooperation and active involvement. The approach to children should be warm, honest, calm, accepting, and matter-of-fact. A smile, a warm tone of voice, a gesture of encouragement, or a word of praise goes a long way in attracting children's attention and helping them adjust to new circumstances. Fundamental to the child's response is how the parents respond to healthcare personnel and medical interventions.

The following teaching strategies are suggested to convey information to members of this age group. These strategies feed into children's natural tendency for play and their need for active participation and sensory experiences.

For Short-Term Learning

- Read simple stories from books with lots of pictures.
- Use dolls and puppets to act out feelings and behaviors.
- Use simple audiotapes with music and videotapes with cartoon characters.
- Role-play to bring the child's imagination closer to reality.
- Give simple, concrete, nonthreatening explanations to accompany visual and tactile experiences.
- Perform procedures on a teddy bear or doll first to help the child anticipate what an experience will be like.
- Allow the child something to do—squeeze your hand, hold a Band-Aid, cry if it hurts—to channel their responses to an unpleasant experience.
- Keep teaching sessions brief (no longer than about 5 minutes each) because of the child's short attention span.
- Cluster teaching sessions close together so that children can remember what they learned from one instructional encounter to another.
- Avoid analogies and explain things in straightforward and simple terms because children take their world literally and concretely.
- Individualize the pace of teaching according to the child's responses and level of attention.

For Long-Term Learning

- Focus on rituals, imitation, and repetition of information in the form of words and actions to hold the child's attention. For example, practice washing hands before and after eating and toileting.
- Use reinforcement as an opportunity for children to achieve permanence of learning through practice.
- Employ the teaching methods of gaming and modeling as a means by which children can learn about the world and test their ideas over time.
- Encourage parents to act as role models because their values and beliefs serve to reinforce healthy

behaviors and significantly influence the child's development of attitudes and behaviors.

Early Childhood (3–5 Years of Age)

Children in the preschool years continue with development of skills learned in the earlier years of growth. Their sense of identity becomes clearer, and their world expands to encompass involvement with others external to the family unit. Children in this developmental category acquire new behaviors that give them more independence from their parents and allow them to care for themselves more autonomously. Learning during this time period occurs through interactions with others and through mimicking or modeling the behaviors of playmates and adults (Richmond & Kotelchuck, 1984; Whitener et al., 1998).

Physical, Cognitive, and Psychosocial Development

The physical maturation during early childhood is an extension of the child's prior growth. Fine and gross motor skills become increasingly more refined and coordinated so that children are able to carry out activities of daily living with greater independence (Santrock, 2006; Vander Zanden et al., 2007). Although their efforts are more coordinated, supervision of activities is still required because they lack judgment in carrying out the skills they have developed.

The early childhood stage of cognitive development is labeled by Piaget (1951, 1952, 1976) as the *preoperational period*. This stage emphasizes the child's inability to think things through logically without acting it out and it is the transitional period when the child starts to use symbols (letters and numbers) to represent something (Santrock, 2006; Snowman & Biehler, 2006; Vander Zanden et al., 2007).

Children in the preschool years begin to develop the capacity to recall past experiences and anticipate future events. They can classify objects into groups and categories, but have only a vague understanding of their relationships. The young child continues to be egocentric and is essentially unaware of others' thoughts or the existence of others' points of view. Thinking remains literal and concrete—they believe what is seen and heard. Precausal thinking allows young children to understand that people can make things happen, but they are unaware of causation as the result of invisible physical and mechanical forces. They often believe that they can influence natural phenomena, and their beliefs reflect **animistic thinking**—the tendency to endow inanimate objects with life and consciousness (Pidgeon, 1977; Santrock, 2006).

Preschool children are very curious, can think intuitively, and pose questions about almost anything. They want to know the reasons, cause, and purpose for everything (the why) but are unconcerned at this point with the process (the how). Fantasy and reality are not well differentiated. Children in this cognitive stage mix fact and fiction, tend to generalize, think magically, develop imaginary playmates, and believe they can control events with their thoughts. At the same time, they do possess self-awareness and realize that they are vulnerable to outside influences (Santrock, 2006; Vander Zanden et al., 2007).

The young child also continues to have a limited sense of time. For children of this age, being made to wait 15 minutes before they can do something can feel like an eternity. They do, however, understand the timing of familiar events in their daily lives, such as when breakfast or dinner is eaten and when they can play or watch their favorite television program. Their attention span (ability to focus) begins to lengthen such that they can usually remain quiet long enough to listen to a song or hear a short story read (Santrock, 2006).

In the preschool stage, children begin to develop sexual identity and curiosity, an interest that may cause considerable discomfort for their parents. Cognitive understanding of their bodies related to structure, function, health, and illness becomes more specific and differentiated. They can name external body parts but have only an ill-defined concept of the size and shape of internal organs and the function of body parts (Kotchab-hakdi, 1985).

Explanations of the purpose and reasons for a procedure remain beyond the young child's level of reasoning, so explanations have to be kept very simple and matter-of-fact (Pidgeon, 1985). Children at this stage have a fear of body mutilation and pain, which not only stems from their lack of understanding of the body but also is compounded by their active imagination. Their ideas regarding illness also are primitive with respect to cause and effect; illness is seen as a punishment for something they did wrong, either through omission or commission (Richmond & Kotelchuck, 1984). Health, on the other hand, may be identified with doing things right. Health allows them to play with friends and participate in desired activities; illness prevents them from doing so (Hussey & Hirsh, 1983).

Erikson (1963) has labeled the psychosocial maturation level in early childhood as the period of *initiative versus guilt*. Children take on tasks for the sake of being involved and on the move (see Table 5–2). Excess energy and a desire to dominate may lead to frustration and anger on their part. They show evidence of expanding imagination and creativity, are impulsive in their actions, and are curious about almost everything they see and do. Their growing imagination can lead to many fears—of separation, disapproval, pain, punishment, and aggression from others. Loss of body integrity is the preschool child's greatest threat, which significantly affects his or her willingness to interact with healthcare personnel (Poster, 1983; Vulcan, 1984).

In this phase of development, children begin interacting with playmates rather than just playing alongside one another. Appropriate social behaviors demand that they learn to wait for others, give

others a turn, and recognize the needs of others. Play in the mind of a child is equivalent to the work performed by adults. Play can be as equally productive as adult work and is a means for self-education of the physical and social world (Whitener et al., 1998). It helps the child act out feelings and experiences to master fears, develop role skills, and express joys, sorrows, and hostilities. Through play, children in the preschool years also begin to share ideas and imitate parents of the same sex. Role-playing is typical of this age as the child attempts to learn the responsibilities of family members and others in society (Santrock, 2006).

TEACHING STRATEGIES

During interactions with the child, the health professional should take every opportunity to teach parents about health promotion and disease prevention measures, to provide guidance regarding normal growth and development, and to offer instruction about medical recommendations related to illness or disability. Parents can be a great asset to the health professional in working with children in this developmental phase, and they should be included in all aspects of the educational plan and the actual teaching experience. Parents can serve as the primary resource to answer questions about children's disabilities, their idiosyncrasies, and their favorite toys—all of which may affect their ability to learn (Hussey & Hirsh, 1983; Ryberg & Merrifield, 1984; Woodring, 2000).

Children's fear of pain and bodily harm is uppermost in their minds, whether they are well or ill. Because young children have fantasies and active imaginations, it is most important for the health professional to reassure them and allow them to express themselves openly about their fears (Heiney, 1991). Health professionals should choose their words carefully when describing procedures and interventions. Preschool children are familiar with many words, but using terms like *cut* or *knife* is frightening to them. Instead, educators should use less threatening words such as *fix*, *sew*, and *cover up the hole*. *Band-Aids* rather than *dressings* is a much more understandable term, and bandages are often thought by children to have magical healing powers (Babcock & Miller, 1994).

Although still dependent on family, the young child has begun to have increasing contact with the outside world and is usually able to interact more comfortably with others. Nevertheless, significant adults in a child's life should be included as participants during teaching sessions. They can provide support to the child, substitute as the teacher if their child is reluctant to interact with the health professional, and reinforce teaching at a later point in time. The primary caretakers, usually the mother and father, are the recipients of the majority of the health professional's teaching efforts. They are the learners to assist the child in achieving desired health outcomes (Hussey & Hirsh, 1983; Kennedy & Riddle, 1989; Whitener et al., 1998).

The following specific teaching strategies are recommended:

FOR SHORT-TERM LEARNING

- Provide physical and visual stimuli because language ability is still limited, both for expressing ideas and for comprehending verbal instructions.
- Keep teaching sessions short (no more than 15 minutes) and scheduled sequentially at close intervals so that information is not forgotten.
- Relate information needs to activities and experiences familiar to the child. For example, ask the child to pretend to blow out candles on a birthday cake to practice deep breathing.
- Encourage the child to participate in selecting between a limited number of teaching–learning options, such as playing with dolls or reading a story, which promotes active involvement and helps to establish health professional–client rapport.

- Arrange small group sessions with peers as a way to make teaching less threatening and more fun.
- Give praise and approval, through both verbal expressions and nonverbal gestures, which are real motivators for learning.
- Give tangible rewards, such as badges or small toys, immediately following a successful learning experience as reinforcers in the mastery of cognitive and psychomotor skills.
- Allow the child to manipulate equipment and play with replicas or dolls to learn about body parts. Special kidney dolls, ostomy dolls with stomas, or orthopedic dolls with splints and tractions provide opportunity for hands-on experience.
- Use storybooks to emphasize the humanity of healthcare personnel; to depict relationships between the child, parents, and others; and to assist with helping the child identify with particular situations.

FOR LONG-TERM LEARNING

- Enlist the help of parents, who can play a vital role in modeling a variety of healthy habits, such as practicing safety measures and eating a balanced diet.
- Reinforce positive health behaviors and the acquisition of specific skills.

Middle and Late Childhood (6–11 Years of Age)

In middle and late childhood, children have progressed in their physical, cognitive, and psychosocial skills to the point where most begin formal training in structured school systems. They approach learning with enthusiastic anticipation, and their minds are open to new and varied ideas.

Children at this developmental level are motivated to learn because of their natural curiosity and their desire to understand more about themselves, their bodies, their world, and the influence that different things in the world have on them (Whitener et al., 1998). This stage is a period of great change for them, when attitudes, values, and perceptions of themselves, their society, and the world are shaped and expanded. Visions of their own environment and the cultures of others take on more depth and breadth (Santrock, 2006).

PHYSICAL, COGNITIVE, AND PSYCHOSOCIAL DEVELOPMENT

The gross- and fine-motor abilities of school-aged children are increasingly more coordinated so that they are able to control their movements with much greater dexterity than ever before. Involvement in all kinds of curricular and extracurricular activities helps them to fine-tune their psychomotor skills. Physical growth during this phase is highly variable, with the rate of development differing from child to child. Toward the end of this developmental period, girls more so than boys on the average begin to experience prepubescent bodily changes and tend to exceed the boys in physical maturation. Growth charts, which monitor the rate of growth, are a more sensitive indicator of health or disability than actual size (Burkett, 1989; Santrock, 2006; Vander Zanden et al., 2007).

Piaget (1951, 1952, 1976) labeled the cognitive development in middle and late childhood as the period of *concrete operations*. During this time, logical, rational thought processes and the ability to reason inductively and deductively develop. Children in this stage are able to think more objectively, are willing to listen to others, and selectively use questioning to find answers to the unknown. At this stage, they begin to use **syllogistic reasoning**—that is, they can consider two premises and draw a logical conclusion from them (Elkind, 1984). For example, they comprehend that mammals are warm-blooded, whales are mammals, and so whales must be warm-blooded.

Also, they are intellectually able to understand cause and effect in a concrete way. Concepts such as **conservation**, which is the ability to recognize that the properties of an object stay the same even though its appearance and position may change, are beginning to be mastered. For example, they realize that a certain quantity of liquid is the same amount whether it is poured into a tall, thin glass or into a short, squat one (Snowman & Biehler, 2006). Fiction and fantasy are separate from fact and reality. The skills of memory, decision making, insight, and problem solving are all more fully developed (Protheroe, 2007).

Children in this developmental phase are capable of engaging in systematic thought through inductive reasoning. They are able to classify objects and systems, express concrete ideas about relationships and people, and carry out mathematical operations. Also, they begin to understand and use sarcasm as well as to employ well-developed language skills for telling jokes, conveying complex stories, and communicating increasingly more sophisticated thoughts (Snowman & Biehler, 2006).

Nevertheless, thinking remains quite literal, with only a vague understanding of abstractions. Early on in this phase, children are reluctant to do away with magical thinking in exchange for reality thinking. They cling to cherished beliefs, such as the existence of Santa Claus or the tooth fairy, for the fun and excitement that the fantasy provides them, even when they have information that proves contrary to their beliefs.

Children passing through elementary and middle schools have developed the ability to concentrate for extended periods, can tolerate delayed gratification, are responsible for independently carrying out activities of daily living, have a good understanding of the environment as a whole, and can generalize from experience (Vander Zanden et al., 2007). They understand time, can predict time intervals, are oriented to the past and present, have some grasp and interest in the future, and have a vague appreciation for how immediate actions can have implications over the course of time. Special interests in topics of their choice begin to emerge, and they can pursue subjects and activities with devotion to increase their talents in particular areas.

Children at this cognitive stage can make decisions and act in accordance with how events are interpreted, but they understand only to a limited extent the seriousness or consequences of their choices. Children in the early period of this developmental phase know the functions and names of many common body parts, whereas older children have a more specific knowledge of anatomy and can differentiate between external and internal organs with a beginning understanding of their complex functions (Kotchabhakdi, 1985).

In the shift from precausal to causal thinking, the child begins to incorporate the idea that illness is related to cause and effect and can recognize that germs create disease. Illness is thought of in terms of social consequences and role alterations, such as the realization that they will miss school and outside activities, people will feel sorry for them, and they will be unable to maintain their usual routines (Banks, 1990).

Research indicates, however, that systematic differences exist in children's reasoning skills with respect to understanding body functioning and the cause of illness as a result of their experiences with illness. Children suffering from chronic diseases have been found to have more sophisticated conceptualization of illness causality and body functioning than do their healthy peers. Piaget (1976) postulated that experience with a phenomenon catalyzes a better understanding of it.

On the other hand, the stress and anxiety resulting from having to live with a chronic illness or disability can interfere with a child's general cognitive performance. Chronically ill children have a less refined understanding of the physical world than healthy children do, and the former often are unable to generalize what they learned about a specific illness to a broader understanding of illness causality (Perrin, Sayer, & Willett, 1991). Thus, illness may act as an intrusive factor in overall cognitive development (Palfrey et al., 2005).

Erikson (1963) characterized school-aged children's psychosocial stage of life as *industry versus inferiority*. During this period, children begin to gain an awareness of their unique talents and special qualities that distinguish them from one another (see Table 5–2). They begin to establish their self-concept as members of a social group larger than their own nuclear family and start to compare family values with those of the outside world.

The school environment, in particular, facilitates their gaining a sense of responsibility and reliability. With less dependency on family, they extend their intimacy to include special friends and social groups (Santrock, 2006). Relationships with peers and adults external to the home environment become important influences in their development of self-esteem and their susceptibility to social forces outside the family unit. School-aged children fear failure and being left out of groups. They worry about their inabilities and become self-critical as they compare their own accomplishments to those of their peers. They also fear illness and disability that could significantly disrupt their academic progress, interfere with social contacts, decrease their independence, and result in loss of control over body functioning.

TEACHING STRATEGIES

Woodring (2000) emphasizes the importance of following sound educational principles with the child and family, such as identifying individual learning styles, determining readiness to learn, and accommodating particular learning needs and abilities to achieve positive health outcomes. With their increased ability to comprehend information and their desire for active involvement and control of their lives, it is very important to include school-aged children in patient education efforts. The health professional should explain illness, treatment plans, and procedures in simple, logical terms in accordance with the child's level of understanding and reasoning. Although children at this stage of development are able to think logically, their ability for abstract thought remains limited. Therefore, teaching should be presented in concrete terms with step-by-step instructions (Pidgeon, 1985; Whitener et al., 1998). It is imperative that the health professional observe children's reactions and listen to their verbal feedback to confirm that information shared has not been misinterpreted or confused.

To the extent feasible, parents should be informed of what their child is being taught. Teaching parents directly is encouraged so that they may be involved in fostering their child's independence, providing emotional support and physical assistance, and giving guidance regarding the correct techniques or regimens in self-care management. Siblings and peers should also be considered as sources of support. In attempting to master self-care skills, children thrive on praise from others who are important in their lives as rewards for their accomplishments and successes (Hussey & Hirsh, 1983; Santrock, 2006).

According to *Healthy People 2010* (U.S. Department of Health and Human Services, 2000), health promotion regarding healthy eating, exercise, and prevention of injuries, as well as avoidance of tobacco, alcohol, and drug use, are just a few examples of goals set forth to improve the health of American children. The school nurse can play a vital role in providing education to the school-aged child to meet these goals (Leifer & Hartson, 2004). The school nurse has the opportunity to educate children in a group when teaching a class and on a one-to-one basis when encountering an individual child in the nurse's office for a particular problem or need. All health professionals should make an effort to routinely include health promo-

tion information during their regular encounters with children.

The specific conditions that may come to the attention of the health professional in caring for children at this phase of development include problems such as behavioral disorders, hyperactivity, learning disorders, obesity, diabetes, asthma, and enuresis. Extensive teaching may be needed to help children and parents understand a particular condition and learn how to overcome or deal with it.

The need to sustain or bolster their self-image, self-concept, and self-esteem requires that children be invited to participate, to the extent possible, in planning for and carrying out learning activities (Snowman & Biehler, 2006). For young children receiving an X-ray or other imaging procedure, for example, it would be beneficial to have them initially simulate the experience by positioning a doll or stuffed animal under the machine as the technician explains the procedure. This strategy allows them to participate and can decrease their fear. Because of children's fears of falling behind in school, being separated from peer groups, and being left out of social activities, teaching must be geared toward fostering normal development despite any limitations that may be imposed by illness or disability (Falvo, 1994; Leifer & Hartston, 2004).

Because children in middle and late childhood are used to the structured, direct, and formal learning in the school environment, they are receptive to a similar teaching–learning approach when hospitalized or confined at home. The following teaching strategies are suggested when caring for children in this developmental stage of life:

FOR SHORT-TERM LEARNING

- Allow school-aged children to take responsibility for their own health care because they are not only willing but also capable of manipulating equipment with accuracy. Because of their adeptness in relation to manual dexterity, mathematical operations, and logical thought processes, they can be taught, for example, to apply their own splint or use an asthma inhaler as prescribed.

- Teaching sessions can be extended to last as long as 30 minutes each because the increased cognitive abilities of school-aged children aids in the retention of information. However, lessons should be spread apart to allow for comprehension of large amounts of content and to provide opportunity for the practice of newly acquired skills between sessions.

- Use diagrams, models, pictures, videotapes, printed materials, and computers as adjuncts to various teaching methods because an increased facility with language (both spoken and written) as well as with mathematical concepts allows for these children to work with more complex instructional tools.

- Choose audiovisual and printed materials that show peers undergoing similar procedures or facing similar situations.

- Clarify any scientific terminology and medical jargon used.

- Use analogies as an effective means of providing information in meaningful terms, such as "Having a chest X-ray is like having your picture taken" or "White blood cells are like police cells that can attack and destroy infection."

- Use one-to-one teaching sessions as a method to individualize learning relevant to the child's own experiences and as a means to interpret the results of interventions particular to the child's own condition.

- Provide time for clarification, validation, and reinforcement of what is being learned.

- Select individual instructional techniques that provide opportunity for privacy, an increasingly important concern for this group of learners, who often feel quite self-conscious and modest when learning about bodily functions.

- Employ group teaching sessions with others of similar age and with similar problems or needs

to help children avoid feelings of isolation and to assist them in identifying with their own peers.

- Prepare children for procedures and interventions well in advance to allow them time to cope with their feelings and fears, to anticipate events, and to understand what the purpose of each procedure is, how it relates to their condition, and how much time it will take.

- Encourage participation in planning for procedures and events because active involvement helps the child to assimilate information more readily.

- Provide much-needed nurturance and support, always keeping in mind that young children are not just small adults. Praise and rewards help motivate and reinforce learning.

For Long-Term Learning

- Help school-aged children acquire skills that they can use to assume self-care responsibility for carrying out therapeutic treatment regimens on an ongoing basis with minimal assistance.

- Assist them in learning to maintain their own well-being and prevent illnesses from occurring.

Research suggests that lifelong health attitudes and behaviors begin in the early childhood phase of development and remain intrapersonally consistent throughout the stage of middle to late childhood. The development of cognitive understanding of health and illness has been shown to follow a systematic progression parallel to the stage of general cognitive development (Santrock, 2006). As the child matures, beliefs about health and illness become less concrete and more abstract, less egocentric, and increasingly differentiated and consistent.

Motivation, self-esteem, and positive self-perception are personal characteristics that influence health behavior. Research has shown that the higher the grade level of the child, the greater the understanding of illness and an awareness of body cues. Thus, children become more actively involved in their own health care as they progress developmentally (Farrand & Cox, 1993; Whitener et al., 1998). Teaching should be directed at assisting them to incorporate positive health actions into their daily lives. Because of the importance of peer influence, group activities are an effective method of teaching health behaviors, attitudes, and values.

Adolescence (12–19 Years of Age)

The stage of adolescence marks the transition from childhood to adulthood. During this prolonged and very change-filled period of time, many adolescents and their families experience much turmoil. How adolescents think about themselves and the world significantly influences many healthcare issues facing them, from anorexia to diabetes. Teenage thought and behavior give insight into the etiology of some of the major health problems of this group of learners (Elkind, 1984). Adolescents are known to be among the nation's most at-risk populations (American Association of Colleges of Nursing, 1994). For patient education to be effective, an understanding of the characteristics of the adolescent phase of development is crucial (Ackard & Neumark-Sztainer, 2001; Girod, Pardales, Cavanaugh, & Wadsworth, 2005; Michaud, Stronski, Fonseca, & MacFarlane, 2004).

PHYSICAL, COGNITIVE, AND PSYCHOSOCIAL DEVELOPMENT

Adolescents vary greatly in their biological, psychological, social, and cognitive development. From a physical maturation standpoint, they must adapt to rapid, dramatic, and significant bodily changes, which can temporarily result in clumsiness and poorly coordinated movement. Alterations in physical size, shape, and function of their bodies, along with the appearance and development of secondary sex characteristics, bring about a significant preoccupation with their appearance and a strong desire to express sexual urges (Santrock, 2006; Vander Zanden et al., 2007).

Piaget (1951, 1952, 1976) termed this stage of cognitive development as the period of *formal operations*. Adolescents have attained a new, higher-order level of reasoning superior to earlier childhood thoughts. They are capable of abstract thought and complex logical reasoning described as propositional as opposed to syllogistic. Their reasoning is both inductive and deductive, and they are able to hypothesize and apply the principles of logic to situations never encountered before. Adolescents can conceptualize and internalize ideas, debate various points of view, understand cause and effect, comprehend complex explanations, imagine possibilities, make sense out of new data, discern relationships among objects and events, and respond appropriately to multiple-step directions (Aronowitz, 2006; Vander Zanden et al., 2007).

Formal operational thought enables adolescents to conceptualize invisible processes and make determinations about what others say and how they behave. With this capacity, teenagers can become obsessed with what they think as well as what others are thinking, a characteristic known as adolescent egocentrism. They begin to believe that everyone is focusing on the same things they are—namely, themselves and their activities. Elkind (1984) labels this belief as the **imaginary audience**, a type of social thinking that has considerable influence over an adolescent's behavior. The imaginary audience explains the pervasive self-consciousness of adolescents, who, on the one hand, may feel embarrassed because they believe everyone is looking at them and, on the other hand, desire to be looked at and thought about because this attention confirms their sense of being special and unique (Santrock, 2006; Snowman & Biehler, 2006; Vander Zanden et al., 2007).

Adolescents are able to understand the concept of health and illness, the multiple causes of diseases, the influence of variables on health status, and the ideas associated with health promotion and disease prevention. Parents, healthcare providers, and the Internet are all potential sources of health-related information for adolescents. At this developmental stage, adolescents recognize that illness and disability are processes resulting from a dysfunction or nonfunction of a part or parts of the body and can comprehend the outcomes or prognosis of an illness. They can also identify health behaviors but may reject practicing them or begin to engage in risk-taking behaviors because of the social pressures they receive from peers as well as their feelings of invincibility (Girod et al., 2005). Elkind (1984) labels this second type of social thinking as the **personal fable**. The personal fable leads adolescents to believe that they are invulnerable—other people grow old and die, but not them; other people may not realize their personal ambitions, but they will.

This personal fable has value in that it allows individuals to carry on with their lives even in the face of all kinds of dangers. Unfortunately, it also leads teenagers to believe they are cloaked in an invisible shield that will protect them from bodily harm despite any risks to which they may subject themselves. They can understand implications of future outcomes, but their immediate concern is with the present.

Recent research, however, reveals that adolescents 15 years of age and older are not as susceptible to the personal fable as once thought (Cauffman & Steinberg, 2000). Although children in the mid- to late-adolescent period appear to be aware of the risks they take, it is important, nevertheless, to recognize that this population continues to need support and guidance (Brown, Teufel, & Birch, 2007).

Erikson (1968) has identified the psychosocial dilemma adolescents face as one of *identity versus role confusion*. These children indulge in comparing their self-image with an ideal image (see Table 5–2). Adolescents find themselves in a struggle to establish their own identity, match their skills with career choices, and determine their self. They work to emancipate themselves from their parents, seeking independence and autonomy so that they can emerge as more distinct individual personalities.

Teenagers have a strong need for belonging to a group, friendship, peer acceptance, and peer support. They tend to rebel against any actions or recommendations by adults whom they consider authoritarian. Their concern over personal appearance and their need to look and act like their peers drive them to conform to the dress and behavior of this age group, which is usually contradictory, nonconformist, and in opposition to the models, codes, and values of their parents' generation. Conflict, toleration, stereotyping, or alienation characterizes the relationship between adolescents and their parents and other authority figures (Hines & Paulson, 2006). Adolescents seek to develop new and trusting relationships outside the home but remain vulnerable to the opinions of those they emulate (Santrock, 2006).

Adolescents demand personal space, control, privacy, and confidentiality. To them, illness, injury, disability, and hospitalization mean dependency, loss of identity, a change in body image and functioning, bodily embarrassment, confinement, separation from peers, and possible death. The provision of knowledge alone is, therefore, not sufficient for this population. Because of the many issues apparent during the adolescent period, the need for coping skills is profound and can influence the successful completion of this stage of development (Grey, Kanner, & Lacey, 1999).

TEACHING STRATEGIES

Although the majority of individuals at this phase of development remain relatively healthy, an estimated 20% of U.S. teenagers have at least one serious health problem, such as asthma, learning disabilities, eating disorders (e.g., obesity, anorexia, or bulimia), diabetes, a range of disabilities as a result of injury, or psychological problems as a result of depression or physical and/or emotional maltreatment. In addition, adolescents are considered at high risk for teen pregnancy, the effects of poverty, drug or alcohol abuse, and sexually transmitted diseases such as venereal disease and AIDS. The three leading causes of death in this age group are accidents, homicide, and suicide (London et al., 2003). More than 50% of all adolescent deaths are a result of accidents and most involve motor vehicles (Santrock, 2006).

Despite all of these potential threats to their well-being, adolescents use medical services the least frequently of all age groups. Compounding this problem is the realization that adolescent health has not been a national priority and their health issues have been largely ignored by the healthcare system (American Association of Colleges of Nursing, 1994; Michaud et al., 2004). Thus, the educational needs of adolescents are broad and varied. The potential topics for teaching are numerous, ranging from sexual adjustment, contraception, and venereal disease to accident prevention, nutrition, and substance abuse.

Healthy teens have difficulty imagining themselves as sick or injured. Those with an illness or disability often comply poorly with medical regimens and continue to indulge in risk-taking behaviors. Because of their preoccupation with body image and functioning and the perceived importance of peer acceptance and support, they view health recommendations as a threat to their autonomy and sense of control.

Probably the greatest challenge to the health professional responsible for teaching the adolescent, whether healthy or ill, is to be able to develop a mutually respectful, trusting relationship (Brown et al., 2007). Adolescents, because of their well-developed cognitive and language abilities, are able to participate fully in all aspects of learning, but

they need privacy, understanding, an honest and straightforward approach, and unqualified acceptance in the face of their fears of embarrassment, losing independence, identity, and self-control (Ackard & Neumark-Sztainer, 2001). The Society of Adolescent Medicine cites availability, visibility, quality, confidentiality, affordability, flexibility, and coordination to be important factors in providing education effectively to the adolescent population (Girod et al., 2005; Leifer & Hartston, 2004).

The existence of an imaginary audience and personal fable can contribute to the exacerbation of existing problems or cause new ones. Adolescents with disfiguring disabilities, who as young children exhibited a great deal of spirit and strength, may now show signs of depression and lack of will. For the first time, they look at themselves from the standpoint of others and reinterpret behavior once seen as friendly as actually condescending. Teenagers may fail to use contraceptives because the personal fable tells them that other people will get pregnant or get venereal disease, but not them. Teenagers with chronic illnesses may stop taking prescribed medications because they feel they can manage without them to prove to others that they are well and free of medical constraints; other people with similar diseases need to follow therapeutic regimens, but not them.

Adolescents' language skills and ability to conceptualize and think abstractly give the health professional a wide range of teaching methods and instructional tools from which to choose (Brown et al., 2007). The following teaching strategies are suggested when caring for adolescents:

For Short-Term Learning

- Use one-to-one instruction to ensure confidentiality of sensitive information.
- Choose peer group discussion sessions as an effective approach to deal with health topics such as smoking, alcohol and drug use, safety measures, obesity, and teenage sexuality. Ado-

lescents benefit from being exposed to others who have the same concerns or who have successfully dealt with problems similar to theirs.

- Use face-to-face or computer group discussion, role-playing, and gaming as methods to clarify values and problem solve, which feed into the teenager's need to belong and to be actively involved. Getting groups of peers together in person or via technology can be very effective in helping teens confront health challenges and learn how to significantly change behavior (Snowman & Biehler, 2006).
- Employ adjunct instructional tools, such as complex models, diagrams, and specific, detailed written materials, which can be used competently by many adolescents. Using technology is a comfortable approach to learning for adolescents, who generally have facility with technological equipment after years of academic and personal experience with telecommunications in the home and at school.
- Clarify any scientific terminology and medical jargon used.
- Share decision making whenever possible because control is an important issue for adolescents.
- Include them in formulating teaching plans related to teaching strategies, expected outcomes, and determining what needs to be learned and how it can best be achieved to meet their needs for autonomy.
- Suggest options so that they feel they have a choice about courses of action.
- Give a rationale for all that is said and done to help adolescents feel a sense of control.
- Approach them with respect, tact, openness, and flexibility to elicit their attention and encourage their responsiveness to teaching–learning situations.
- Expect negative responses, which are common when their self-image and self-integrity are threatened.

- Avoid confrontation and acting like an authority figure. Instead of directly contradicting their opinions and beliefs, acknowledge their thoughts, and then casually suggest an alternative viewpoint or choices, such as "Yes, I can see your point, but what about the possibility of . . . ?"

For Long-Term Learning

- Accept adolescents' personal fable and imaginary audience as valid, rather than challenging their feelings of uniqueness and invincibility.
- Acknowledge that their feelings are very real because denying them their opinions simply will not work.
- Allow them the opportunity to test their own convictions. Let them know, for example, that although some other special people may get away without taking medication, others cannot. Suggest, if medically feasible, setting up a trial period with medications scheduled farther apart or in lowered dosages to determine how they can manage.

Although much of patient education should be done directly with adolescents to respect their right to individuality, privacy, and confidentiality, teaching effectiveness may be enhanced by including their families to some extent (Brown et al., 2007). The health professional can give guidance and support to families, helping them to better understand adolescent behavior (Hines & Paulson, 2006). Parents should be taught how to set realistic limits and at the same time foster the adolescent's sense of independence. Through prior assessment of potential sources of stress, teaching both the parents and the adolescent (as well as siblings) can be enhanced. Because of the ambivalence the adolescent feels while in this transition stage from childhood to adulthood, healthcare teaching, to be effective, must consider the learning needs of the adolescent as well as the parents (Ackard & Neumark-Sztainer, 2001; Falvo, 1994).

The Developmental Stages of Adulthood

Andragogy, the term coined by Knowles (1990) to describe his theory of adult learning, is the art and science of teaching adults. Education within this framework is more learner centered and less teacher centered; that is, instead of one party imparting knowledge to another, the power relationship between the educator and the adult learner is much more horizontal (Milligan, 1997). The concept of andragogy has served for years as a useful framework in guiding instruction for patient teaching and for continuing education of staff. Recently, based on emerging research and theory from a variety of disciplines, Knowles, Holton, and Swanson (1998) discussed new perspectives on andragogy that have refined and strengthened the core adult learning principles that Knowles originally proposed.

The following basic assumptions about Knowles's framework have major implications for planning, implementing, and evaluating teaching programs for adults as the individual matures:

1. His or her self-concept moves from one of being a dependent personality to being an independent, self-directed human being.
2. He or she accumulates a growing reservoir of previous experience that serves as a rich resource for learning.
3. Readiness to learn becomes increasingly oriented to the developmental tasks of social roles.
4. The perspective of time changes from one of postponed application of knowledge to one of immediate application; there is a shift in orientation of learning to being problem centered rather than subject centered.

A limitation of Knowles's assumptions about child versus adult learners is that they are derived from studies conducted on healthy people. It is important to keep in mind, however, that illness and injury have the potential for significantly changing cognitive and psychological processes used for learning (Best, 2001).

The period of adulthood constitutes three major developmental stages—the young adult stage, the middle-aged adult stage, and the older adult stage (see Table 5–1). Although adulthood, like childhood, can be divided into various developmental phases, the focus for learning is quite different. Whereas a child's readiness to learn depends on physical, cognitive, and psychosocial development, adults have essentially reached the peak of their physical and cognitive capacities.

The emphasis for adult learning revolves around differentiation of life tasks and social roles with respect to employment, family, and other activities beyond the responsibilities of home and career (Boyd, Gleit, Graham, & Whitman, 1998). In contrast to childhood learning, which is subject centered, adult learning is problem centered. The prime motivator to learn in adulthood is to be able to apply knowledge and skills for the solution of immediate problems. Unlike children, who enjoy learning for the sake of gaining an understanding of themselves and the world, adults must clearly perceive the relevancy in acquiring new behaviors or changing old ones for them to be willing and eager to learn. In the beginning of any teaching–learning encounter, therefore, adults want to know the benefit they will derive from their efforts at learning (Knowles et al., 1998).

In contrast to the child learner, who is dependent on authority figures for learning, the adult is much more self-directed and independent in seeking information. For adults, past experiences are internalized and form the basis for further learning. Adults already have a rich resource of stored information on which to build a further understanding of relationships between ideas and concepts. They are quicker than children at grasping relationships, and they do not tolerate learning isolated facts as well as children do (see **Table 5–3**).

Because adults already have established ideas, values, and attitudes, they also tend to be more resistant to change. In addition, adults must overcome obstacles to learning to a greater extent than children. For example, they have the burden of family, work, and social responsibilities, which can diminish their time, energy, and concentration for learning. Also, their need for self-direction may present problems because various stages of illness, as well as the healthcare setting in which they may find themselves, can force dependency. Anxiety, too, may negatively affect their motivation and ability to learn (Kessels, 2003). Furthermore, they may feel too old or too out of touch with the formal learning of the school years, and if past experiences with learning were not positive, they may shy away from assuming the role of learner for fear of the risk of failure (Boyd et al., 1998).

Although health professional educators can consider adult learners as autonomous, self-directed, and independent, these individuals often want and need structure, clear and concise specifics, and direct guidance. As such, Taylor, Marienau, and Fiddler (2000) label adults as "paradoxical" learners.

Only recently has it been recognized that learning is a lifelong process that begins at birth and does not cease until the end of life. Growth and development are a process of becoming, and learning is inextricably a part of that process. As a person matures, learning is a significant and continuous task to maintain and enhance oneself (Knowles, 1990; Knowles et al., 1998). Social scientists now recognize that adulthood "is not a single monolithic stage, not an undifferentiated phase of life

Table 5–3 SUMMARY OF ADULT LEARNING PRINCIPLES

Adults learn best when:

Principle No. 1	Learning is related to an immediate need, problem, or deficit.
Principle No. 2	Learning is voluntary and self-initiated.
Principle No. 3	Learning is person centered and problem centered.
Principle No. 4	Learning is self-controlled and self-directed.
Principle No. 5	The role of the teacher is one of facilitator.
Principle No. 6	Information and assignments are pertinent.
Principle No. 7	New material draws on past experiences and is related to something the learner already knows.
Principle No. 8	The threat to self is reduced to a minimum in the educational situation.
Principle No. 9	The learner is able to participate actively in the learning process.
Principle No. 10	The learner is able to learn in a group.
Principle No. 11	The nature of the learning activity changes frequently.
Principle No. 12	Learning is reinforced by application and prompt feedback.

Source: Adapted from Burgireno, J. (1985). Maximizing learning in the adult with SCI. *Rehabilitation Nursing, 10*(5), 20–21.

between adolescence and old age" (Vander Zanden et al., 2007, p. 443).

A variety of reasons explains why adults pursue learning throughout their lives. Basically, three categories describe the general orientation of adults toward continuing education (Babcock & Miller, 1994):

1. Goal-oriented learners engage in educational endeavors to accomplish clear and identifiable objectives. Continuing education for them is episodic and occurs as a recurring pattern throughout their lives as they realize the need for or an interest in expanding their knowledge and skills. Adults who attend night courses or professional workshops do so to build their expertise in a particular subject or for advancement in their professional or personal lives.
2. Activity-oriented learners select educational activities primarily to meet social needs. The learning of content is secondary to their need for human contact. Although they may choose to participate in support groups, special-interest groups, or self-help groups, or attend academic classes because of an interest in a particular topic being offered, they join essentially out of their desire to be around others and converse with people in similar circumstances—retirement, parenting, divorce, or widowhood. Their drive is to alleviate social isolation or loneliness.
3. Learning-oriented learners view themselves as perpetual students who seek knowledge for knowledge's sake. They are active learners all of their lives and tend to join groups, classes, or organizations with the anticipation that the experience will be educational and personally rewarding.

In most cases, all three types of learners initiate the learning experience for themselves. In planning educational activities for adults, it is important to determine their motives for wanting to be involved. That is, it is advantageous for the health professional educator to understand the purpose and expectations of the individuals who participate in continuing education programs. In that way, the health professional can best serve learners in the role as facilitator for referral or resource information, thus embracing the adults' state of independence and interdependence (Musinski, 1999).

Obviously, there are many differences between child and adult learners (see Table 5–1). As the following discussion clearly reveals, there also are differences in the characteristics of adult learners within the three developmental stages of adulthood.

Young Adulthood (20–40 Years of Age)

The transition from adolescence to becoming a young adult has recently been termed emerging adulthood. Early adulthood comprises the cohort currently between 20 and 24 years of age who belong to the millennial or Net generation (Prensky, 2001) and the cohort currently aged 25–40, who are known as Generation X. Both generations exhibit their own characteristic traits and present different challenges to the educator (Billings & Kowalski, 2004). These two age ranges of people constitute about 80 million Americans (Vander Zanden et al., 2007).

Young adulthood is a time for establishing long-term, intimate relationships with other people, choosing a lifestyle and adjusting to it, deciding on an occupation, and managing a home and family. All of these decisions lead to changes in the lives of young adults that can be a potential source of stress for them. It is a time when intimacy and courtship are pursued and spousal and/or parental roles are developed (Santrock, 2006).

PHYSICAL, COGNITIVE, AND PSYCHOSOCIAL DEVELOPMENT

During this period, physical abilities for most young adults are at their peak, and the body is at its optimal functioning capacity (Vander Zanden et al., 2007). The vast majority of individuals at this stage can master, if they so desire, almost any psychomotor skill they undertake to accomplish (Santrock, 2006).

The cognitive capacity of young adults is fully developed, but with maturation, they continue to accumulate new knowledge and skills from an expanding reservoir of formal and informal experiences. Young adults continue in the *formal operations* stage of cognitive development (Piaget, 1951, 1952, 1976). These experiences add to their perceptions, allow them to generalize to new situations, and improve their abilities to critically analyze, problem solve, and make decisions about their personal, occupational, and social roles. Their interests for learning are oriented toward those experiences that are relevant for immediate application to problems and tasks in their daily lives. Young adults are motivated to learn about the possible implications of various lifestyle choices (Vander Zanden et al., 2007).

Erikson (1963) describes the young adult's stage of psychosocial development as the period of *intimacy versus isolation*. During this time, individuals work to establish a trusting, satisfying, and permanent relationship with others (see Table 5–2). They strive to establish commitment to others in their personal, occupational, and social lives. They are now working to maintain the independence and self-sufficiency they worked to obtain in adolescence.

Young adults face many challenges as they take steps to control their lives. Many of the events they experience are happy and growth promoting from an emotional and social perspective, but they also can prove disappointing and psychologically draining. The new experiences and multiple decisions they must make regarding choices for a career, marriage, parenthood, and higher education can be quite stressful. Young adults realize that the avenues they pursue will affect their lives for years to come (Santrock, 2006).

Teaching Strategies

Based on the paucity of literature on health teaching of individuals who belong specifically to this age cohort, young adulthood is considered to be the life-span period that has received the least attention by health professional educators. At this developmental stage, prior to the emergence of the chronic diseases that characterize the middle-age and older years, young adults are generally very healthy and tend to have limited exposure to health professionals. Their contact with the healthcare system is usually for preemployment, college, or presport physicals; for a minor episodic complaint; or for pregnancy and contraceptive care (Orshan, 2008). At the same time, young adulthood is a crucial period for the establishment of behaviors that help individuals to lead healthy lives, both physically and emotionally. Many of the choices young adults make, if not positive ones, will be difficult to modify later. As Havighurst (1976) points out, this stage is full of teachable moment opportunities, but it is the most devoid of efforts by health providers to teach (Johnson-Saylor, 1980).

Health promotion is the most neglected aspect of healthcare teaching at this stage of life. Adults aged 20–24 are the most likely group to lack health insurance coverage (Vander Zanden et al., 2007). Yet, many of the health issues related to risk factors and stress management are important to deal with to help young adults establish positive health practices for preventing problems with illness in the future. The major factors associated with increased risk of death in later life, such as high blood pressure, elevated cholesterol, obesity, smoking, overuse of alcohol and drugs, and pertinent family history of major illnesses such as cancer and heart disease all need to be addressed (Santrock, 2006).

The health professional must find a way of reaching and communicating with this audience about health promotion and disease prevention measures. Readiness to learn does not always require the educator to wait for it to develop. Rather, such readiness can be fostered through experiences the health professional creates. Knowledge of the individual's lifestyle can provide cues to concentrate on when determining specific aspects of education for the young adult. For example, if the individual is planning marriage, then family planning, contraception, and parenthood are potential topics to address (Orshan, 2008). The motivation for adults to learn comes in response to internal drives, such as need for self-esteem, a better quality of life, or job satisfaction, and in response to external motivators, such as job promotion, more money, or more time to pursue outside activities (Babcock & Miller, 1994; Vander Zanden et al., 2007).

When young adults are faced with acute or chronic illnesses, or disabilities, many of which may significantly alter their lifestyles, they are stimulated to learn so as to maintain their independence and return to normal life patterns. It is likely they will view an illness or disability as a serious setback to achieving their immediate or future life goals.

Because adults typically desire active participation in the educational process, whenever possible, it is important for the health professional to allow them the opportunity for mutual collaboration in health education decision making. They should be encouraged to select what to learn (objectives), how they want material to be presented (instructional methods and tools), and which indicators will be used to determine the achievement of learning goals (evaluation) (Knowles, 1990). Also, it must be remembered that adults bring to the teaching–learning situation a variety of experiences that can serve as a foundation on which to build new learning. Consequently, it is important to draw on their experiences to make learning relevant, useful, and motivating. Young adults tend to be reluctant to expend the resources of time, money, and energy to learn new information, skills, and attitudes if they do not see the content of instruction as relevant to their current lives or anticipated problems (Collins, 2004).

Teaching strategies must be directed at encouraging young adults to seek information that expands their knowledge base, helps them control their lives, and bolsters their self-esteem. Whether they are well or ill, young adults need to know about the opportunities available for learning. Making them aware of health issues and learning opportunities can occur in a variety of settings, such as physicians' offices, community clinics, outpatient clinics, or hospitals. In all cases, these educational opportunities must be convenient and accessible to them in terms of their lifestyle with respect to work and family responsibilities. Relevant, applicable, and practical information is what adults desire and value—they want to know "what's in it for me" (WIIFM), according to Collins (2004).

Because they tend to be very self-directed in their approach to learning, young adults do well with written patient education materials and audiovisual tools, including computer-assisted instruction, that allow them to self-pace their learning independently. Group discussion is an attractive method for teaching and learning because it provides young adults with the opportunity to interact with others of similar age and situation, such as parenting groups, prenatal classes, exercise classes, or marital adjustment sessions. Although assessment prior to teaching helps to determine the level at which to begin teaching, no matter what the content, the enduring axiom is to make learning easy and relevant. To facilitate learning, present concepts logically from simple to complex and establish conceptual relationships through specific application of information (Collins, 2004; Musinski, 1999).

Middle-Aged Adulthood (41–64 Years of Age)

Just as adolescence is the link between childhood and adulthood, midlife is the transition period between young adulthood and older adulthood. Middle-aged Americans make up about one fifth of the population, and this current cohort has typically been labeled the baby-boom generation. Although this was once one of the most neglected age periods, baby boomers, who now make up this cohort, are receiving increasingly more attention by developmental psychologists and healthcare providers. This is because not only do they constitute the largest cohort of any current generation, but because current middle-aged adults are the best educated, most affluent in history, and they have the potential for a healthier life than ever before as a result of medical discoveries that can stave off the aging process. In just one century, the average life expectancy has increased by 30 years (Vander Zanden et al., 2007).

Thus, the concept of what has been thought of as middle age is being nudged upward. As more people live longer, middle age is now coming later in life than ever before. Adults are no longer considered to be over the hill when they celebrate their 40th birthday. Middle age for many healthy adults is starting later and lasting longer. Remember, chronological age is one factor, but biological, psychological, and social age also must be taken into account (Santrock, 2006).

During middle age, many individuals are highly accomplished in their careers, their sense of who they are is well developed, their children are grown, and they have time to share their talents, serve as mentors for others, and pursue new or latent interests. It is a time for them to reflect on the contributions they have made to family and society, relish in their achievements, and reexamine their goals and values.

PHYSICAL, COGNITIVE, AND PSYCHOSOCIAL DEVELOPMENT

During this stage of maturation, a number of physiological changes begin to take place. Skin and muscle tone decreases, metabolism slows down, body weight tends to increase, endurance and energy levels lessen, hormonal changes bring about a variety of symptoms, and hearing and visual acuity start to diminish. All these physical changes and others affect middle-aged adults' self-image, ability to learn, and motivation for learning about health promotion, disease prevention, and maintenance of health (Vander Zanden et al., 2007).

The ability to learn from a cognitive standpoint remains at a steady state for middle-aged adults as they continue in what Piaget (1951, 1952, 1976) labeled the *formal operations* stage of cognitive development. He maintained that cognitive development stopped with this stage (the ability to perform abstract thinking) that was achieved during adolescence. However, over the years critics of Piaget's theory have begun to assert the existence of *postformal operations*. That is, adult thought processes go beyond logical problem solving to include what is known as **dialectical thinking**. This is defined as the ability to search for complex and changing understandings to find a variety of solutions to any given situation or problem. In other words, adults are able to see the bigger picture (Vander Zanden et al., 2007).

For many adults, the accumulation of life experiences and their proven record of accomplishments often allow them to come to the teaching–learning situation with confidence in their abilities as learners. However, if their past experiences with learning were minimal or not positive, their motivation likely will not be at a high enough level to easily facilitate learning. Physical changes, especially with respect to hearing and vision, may impede learning as well (Santrock, 2006).

Erikson (1963) labels this psychosocial stage of adulthood as *generativity versus self-absorption and stagnation*. Midlife marks a point at which adults realize that half of their potential life has been spent. This realization may cause them to question their level of achievement and success. Middle-aged adults, in fact, may choose to modify aspects of their lives that they perceive as unsatisfactory or adopt a new lifestyle as a solution to dissatisfaction.

Developing concern for the lives of their grown children, recognizing the physical changes in themselves, dealing with the new role of being a grandparent, and taking responsibility for their own parents whose health may be failing—all are factors that may cause them to become aware of their own mortality (see Table 5–2). At this time, middle-aged adults may either feel greater motivation to follow health recommendations more closely or, just the opposite, may deny illnesses or abandon healthy practices altogether (Falvo, 1994).

The later years of middle adulthood are the phase in which productivity and contributions to society are valued. They offer an opportunity to feel a real sense of accomplishment from having cared for others—children, spouse, friends, parents, and colleagues for whom they have served as mentor. During this time, individuals often become oriented away from self and family to the larger community. New social interests and leisure activities are pursued as they find more free time from family responsibilities and career demands. As they move toward their retirement years, individuals begin to plan for what they want to do after culminating their career. This transition sparks their interest in learning about financial planning, alternative lifestyles, and ways to remain healthy as they approach the later years (Vander Zanden et al., 2007).

TEACHING STRATEGIES

Depending on individual situations, middle-aged adults may be facing either a more relaxed lifestyle or an increase in stress level because of midlife crisis issues such as menopause, obvious physical changes in their bodies, responsibility for their own parents' declining health status, or concern about how finite their life really is. They may have regrets and feel they did not achieve the goals or

live up to the values they had set for themselves in young adulthood or the expectations others had of them as young adults. Santrock (2006) cites research that indicates that this stage in life is not so much seen as a crisis, but as a period of midlife consciousness.

When teaching members of this age group, the health professional must be aware of their potential sources of stress, the health risk factors associated with this stage of life, and the concerns typical of midlife. Misconceptions regarding physical changes such as menopause are common. Stress may interfere with their ability to learn or may be a motivational force for learning (Leifer & Hartston, 2004). Those who have lived healthy and productive lives are often motivated to make contact with health professionals to ensure maintenance of their healthy status. It is an opportune time for the health professional to reach out to assist these middle-aged adults in coping with stress and maintaining optimal health status. Many need and want information related to chronic illnesses that can arise at this phase of life (Orshan, 2008).

Adult learners need to be reassured or complimented on their learning competencies. Reinforcement for learning is internalized and serves to reward them for their efforts. Teaching strategies for learning are similar to those instructional methods and tools used for the young adult learner, but the content is different to coincide with the concerns and problems specific to this group of learners.

Older Adulthood (65 Years of Age and Older)

The percentage of middle-aged adults in the United States has tripled since 1900, and in 2011, the first wave of baby boomers turns 65 years of age. Older persons constitute approximately 12% of the U.S. population, but in the next 30 years, the number of those older than age 65 will increase to one out of five (20%), or 70 million Americans. Those aged 85 and older make up the fastest-growing segment of the population in the country today, and that segment is expected to double by 2030. Some developmentalists, as Santrock (2006) points out, distinguish three categories of older adults: the young-old (65–74 years of age), the old-old (75–84 years of age), and the oldest-old (85 years and older). With more than 40% of the 2006 federal budget allocated for Medicare, Medicaid, and Social Security, a considerable portion of this country's fiscal resources is used for programs that support those 65 years and older (Vander Zanden et al., 2007).

Most older people suffer from at least one chronic condition, and many have multiple conditions. On the average, they are hospitalized longer than persons in other age categories and require more teaching overall to broaden their knowledge of self-care. In addition, it is approximated that as of 2001, 46% of Black Americans, 63% of those of Asian descent, and 74% of Caucasians older than 65 years of age have a high school education. However, only 16% have a college degree at the bachelor's level or higher (Leifer & Hartston, 2004). Low educational levels, sensory impairments, the disuse of literacy skills once learned, and cognitive changes in the older adult population may contribute to these individuals' decreased ability to read and comprehend written materials (Best, 2001).

For these reasons, their patient education needs are generally greater and more complex than those for persons in any of the other developmental stages. Numerous studies have documented that older adults can benefit from health education programs. Their compliance, if they are given specific health directions, can be quite high. In light of considerable healthcare expenditures for older people, education programs to improve their health status would be a cost-effective measure (Best, 2001; Jackson, Davis, Murphy, Bairnsfather, & George, 1994; Pearson & Wessman, 1996).

Ageism describes prejudice against the older adult. This discrimination based on age, which exists in most segments of American society, perpetuates the negative stereotype of aging as a period of decline (Gavan, 2003). Ageism, in many respects, is similar to the discriminatory attitudes of racism and sexism (Vander Zanden et al., 2007).

Because American society values physical strength, beauty, social networking, productivity, and integrity of body and mind, people fear the natural losses that accompany the aging process. Growing older is a normal event, yet the inevitable continuation of human development that results in biological, psychological, and social changes with the passage of time is a reminder of mortality. Health professional educators must recognize that many older persons respond to these changes as challenges rather than defeats. Many aspects of older adulthood can be pleasurable, such as becoming a grandparent and experiencing retirement that gives one time to pursue lifelong interests, as well as freedom to explore new avenues of endeavor (Santrock, 2006).

Ageism, which interferes with interactions between the older adult and younger age groups, must be counteracted because it "prevents older people from living lives as actively and happily as they might" (Ahroni, 1996, p. 48). Given that the aging process is universal, eventually everyone is potentially subjected to this type of prejudice. New research that focuses on healthy development and positive lifestyle adaptations, rather than on illnesses and impairments in the older adult, can serve to reverse the stereotypical images of aging. Education to inform people of the significant variations that occur in the way that individuals age and education to help the older adult learn to cope with irreversible losses can combat the prejudice of ageism as well (Vander Zanden et al., 2007).

The teaching of older persons, known as **gerogogy**, is different from teaching younger adults (andragogy) and children (pedagogy). For teaching to be effective, gerogogy must accommodate the normal physical, cognitive, and psychosocial changes that occur at this phase of growth and development (Best, 2001). Until recently, little has been written about the special learning needs of older adults that acknowledge the physiological and psychological aging changes that affect their ability to learn.

Age changes, which begin in young and middle adulthood, progress significantly at this older adult stage of life. These changes often create obstacles to learning unless health professionals understand them and can adapt appropriate teaching interventions to meet the older person's needs. The following discussion of physical, cognitive, and psychosocial maturation is based on findings reported by numerous authors (Ahroni, 1996; Best, 2001; Gavan, 2003; Matsuda & Saito, 1998; Pearson & Wessman, 1996; Santrock, 2006; Theis & Merritt, 1994; Vander Zanden et al., 2007; Weinrich & Boyd, 1992).

Physical, Cognitive, and Psychosocial Development

With advancing age, so many physical changes occur that it becomes difficult to establish normal boundaries. As a person grows older, natural physiological changes in all systems of the body are universal, progressive, decremental, and intrinsic. Alterations in physiological functioning can lead secondarily to changes in learning ability. The senses of sight, hearing, touch, taste, and smell are usually the first areas of decreased functioning noticed by adults.

The sensory perceptive abilities that relate most closely to learning capacity are visual and auditory changes. Hearing loss, which is very common beginning in the late 40s and 50s, includes diminished ability to discriminate high-pitched, high-frequency sounds. Visual changes such as cataracts, macular degeneration, reduced pupil size, decline in depth perception, and presbyopia prevent older persons from being able to see small print, read words printed on glossy paper, or drive a car. Yellowing of the ocular lens produces color distortions and diminished color perceptions.

Other physiological changes affect organ functioning and result in decreased cardiac output, lung performance, and metabolic rate; these changes reduce energy levels and lessen the ability to cope with stress. Nerve conduction velocity also is thought to decline by as much as 15%, influencing reflex times and muscle response rates. The interrelatedness of each body system has a total negative cumulative effect on individuals as they grow older.

Aging affects the mind as well as the body. Cognitive ability changes with age as permanent cellular alterations invariably occur in the brain itself, resulting in an actual loss of neurons, which have no regenerative powers. Physiological research has demonstrated that people have two kinds of intellectual ability—crystallized and fluid intelligence. **Crystallized intelligence** is the intelligence absorbed over a lifetime, such as vocabulary, general information, understanding social interactions, arithmetic reasoning, and ability to evaluate experiences. This kind of intelligence actually increases with experience as people age. However, it is important to understand that crystallized intelligence can be impaired by disease states, such as the dementia seen in Alzheimer's disease. **Fluid intelligence** is the capacity to perceive relationships, to reason, and to perform abstract thinking. This kind of intelligence declines as degenerative changes occur.

The decline in fluid intelligence results in the following specific changes:

1. *Slower processing and reaction time:* Older persons need more time to process and react to information, especially as measured in terms of relationships between actions and results.

However, if the factor of speed is removed from IQ tests, for example, older people can perform as well as younger people. In performance of activities of daily living when speed is not a factor, older adults can demonstrate their true abilities to function well and independently (Kray & Lindenberger, 2000).

2. *Persistence of stimulus (afterimage):* Older adults can confuse a previous symbol or word with a new word or symbol just introduced.

3. *Decreased short-term memory:* Older adults sometimes have difficulty remembering events or conversations that occurred just hours or days before. However, long-term memory often remains strong, such as the ability to clearly and accurately remember something from their youth.

4. *Increased test anxiety:* People in the older adult years are especially anxious about making mistakes when performing; when they do make an error, they become easily frustrated. Because of their anxiety, they may take an inordinate amount of time to respond to questions, particularly on tests that are written rather than verbal.

5. *Altered time perception:* For older persons, life becomes more finite and compressed. Issues of the here and now tend to be more important, and some adhere to the philosophy, "I'll worry about that tomorrow." This way of thinking can be detrimental when applied to health issues because it serves as a vehicle for denial or delay in taking action.

Despite the changes in cognition as a result of aging, most research supports the premise that the ability of older adults to learn and remember is virtually as good as ever if special care is taken to slow the pace of presenting information, to ensure relevance of material, and to give appropriate feedback when teaching (see **Figure 5–1**).

Erikson (1963) labels the major psychosocial developmental task at this stage in life as *ego integ-*

rity versus despair. This phase of older adulthood includes dealing with the reality of aging, the acceptance of the inevitability that all persons die, the reconciling of past failures with present and future concerns, and developing a sense of growth and purpose for those years remaining (see Table 5–2). The most common psychosocial tasks of aging involve changes in lifestyle and social status as a result of the following:

- Retirement
- Illness or death of spouse, relatives, and friends
- The moving away of children, grandchildren, and friends
- Relocation to an unfamiliar environment such as an extended care facility or senior residential living center

Depression, grief, loneliness, and isolation, once thought to be common traits among older adults, have now been found by researchers to vary from less frequent to no more frequent than the incidence rate found in middle adulthood. This is because older adults overall have fewer economic hardships and increased religiosity. However, depressive symptoms do increase in the oldest-old and are thought to be associated with more physical disability, more cognitive impairment, and lower socioeconomic status.

For those who experience major depression (the "common cold" of mental disorders), the most likely predictors are multiple losses over a short period of time with respect to a previous support network of home, friends, family, and job (Santrock, 2006). These losses, which signify a threat to one's own autonomy, independence, and decision making, result in isolation, financial insecurity, diminished coping mechanisms, and a decreased sense of identity, personal value, and societal worth. With aging, some individuals, particularly the oldest-old, begin to question their perception of a meaningful life—that is, the potential for further enjoyment, pleasure, and satisfaction.

Figure 5–1 (a) Elderly Client Variables Influencing Learning; (b) Gerontological Teaching Strategies to Optimize Learning

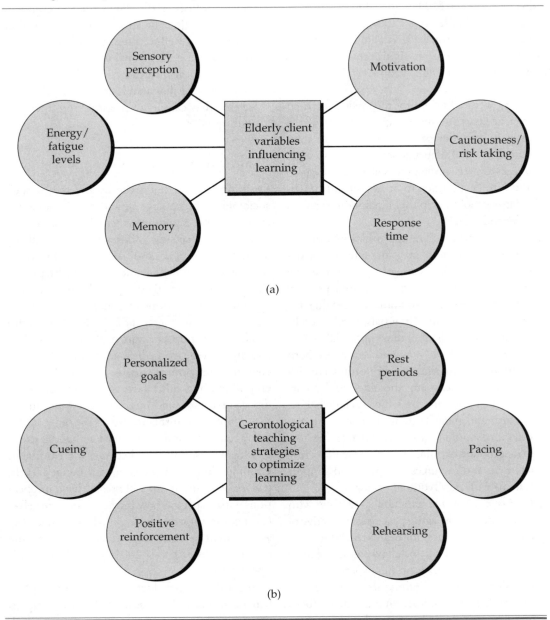

(a)

(b)

Source: Reprinted with permission from Rendon, D. C., David, D. K., Gioiella, E. C., & Tranzillo, M. J. (1986). The right to know, the right to be taught. *Journal of Gerontological Nursing, 12*(12), 34.

Separate from biological aging but closely related are the many sociocultural factors that affect how older adults see themselves as competent individuals (Leifer & Hartston, 2004; Santrock, 2006; Vander Zanden et al., 2007). The following traits regarding personal goals in life and the values associated with them are significantly related to motivation and learning:

1. *Independence:* The ability to provide for their own needs is the most important aim of the majority of older persons, regardless of their state of health. Independence gives them a sense of self-respect, pride, and self-functioning so as not to be a burden to others. Health teaching is the tool to help them maintain or regain independence.

2. *Social acceptability:* The approval from others is a common goal of many older adults. It is derived from health, a sense of vigor, and feeling and thinking young. Despite declining physical attributes, the older adult often has residual fitness and functioning potentials. Health teaching can help to channel these potentials.

3. *Adequacy of personal resources:* Resources, both external and internal, are important considerations when assessing the older adult's current status. Life patterns, which include habits, physical and mental strengths, and economic situation, should be assessed to determine how to incorporate teaching to complement existing regimens and resources (financial and support system) with new required behaviors.

4. *Coping mechanisms:* The ability to cope with change during the aging process is indicative of the person's readiness for health teaching. Positive coping mechanisms allow for self-change as older persons draw on life experiences and knowledge gained over the years. Negative coping mechanisms indicate an individual's focus on losses and show that his or her thinking is immersed in the past. The emphasis in teaching is on exploring alternatives, determining

realistic goals, and supporting large and small accomplishments.

5. *Meaning of life:* For well-adapted older persons, having realistic goals allows them the opportunity to enjoy the smaller pleasures in life, whereas less well-adapted individuals may be frustrated and dissatisfied with personal inadequacies. Health teaching must be directed at ways older adults can maintain optimal health so that they can derive pleasure from their leisure years.

Teaching Strategies

Learning in older adults can be affected by such sociological, psychological, and cognitive factors as retirement, economics, mental status, and information processing abilities (Santrock, 2006; Vander Zanden et al., 2007). Understanding older persons' developmental tasks allows health professionals to alter how they approach both well and ill individuals in terms of counseling, teaching, and establishing a therapeutic relationship. Health professionals must be aware of the fact that older patients may delay medical attention. Decreased cognitive functioning, sensory deficits, lower energy levels, and other factors may prevent early disease detection and intervention. A decline in psychomotor performance affects the older adults' reflex responses and their ability to handle stress. Coping with simple tasks becomes more difficult. Chronic illnesses, depression, and literacy levels, particularly among the oldest-old, have implications with respect to how they care for themselves (eating, dressing, and taking medications) as well as the extent to which they understand the nature of their illnesses (Best, 2001; Katz, 1997; Phillips, 1999).

In working with older adults, reminiscing is a beneficial approach to use to establish a therapeutic relationship. Memories can be quite powerful. Talking with older persons about their experiences—marriage, children, grandchildren, jobs, community involvement, and the like—can be very stimulating. Furthermore, their answers will give the health professional insight into their humanness, their abilities, and their concerns.

Too many times health professionals believe the adage, "You can't teach an old dog new tricks." Gavan (2003) warns that it is easy to fall into the habit of believing the myths associated with the intelligence, personality traits, motivation, and social relations of older adults. She outlined the following prevalent false stereotypes that must be dispelled to prevent harmful outcomes in the older adult when these myths are assumed to be true:

MYTH NO. 1: SENILITY Intelligence test scores indicate that many older adults maintain their cognitive functioning well into their 80s and 90s and mental decline is not always caused by the aging process itself but by disease processes, medication interactions, sensory deficits, dehydration, and malnutrition.

MYTH NO. 2: RIGID PERSONALITIES Personality traits, such as agreeableness, satisfaction, and extraversion, remain stable throughout the older adult years. Although diversity in personality traits among individuals in the older population exists as it does in all other stages of life, labeling older adults as cranky, stubborn, and inflexible does a disservice to them.

MYTH NO. 3: LONELINESS As mentioned earlier, the belief that older adults are more frequently vulnerable to depression, isolation, and feelings of being lonely has not been upheld by research, which indicates that their satisfaction with life continues at a steady level throughout the period of adulthood.

MYTH NO. 4: ABANDONMENT It is untrue that older adults are abandoned by their children, siblings, or good friends. The amount of contact older adults have with significant others remains con-

stant over time. Successful aging depends on an extended family support network.

Also, Vander Zanden et al. (2007) point out that American culture is preoccupied with youthfulness and has distorted notions about late adulthood that perpetuate negative views of this generation. There is no typical older adult—not all of them are unhealthy, unhappy, fearful, institutionalized, disengaged, dwell on their own mortality, or find themselves in financial straits.

Health professionals may not even be aware of their stereotypical attitudes toward older adults. Furthermore, healthcare providers make assumptions about older clients that can cause them to overlook problems that could be treatable (Gavan, 2003). To check their assumptions, health professional educators can think about the last time they gave instruction to an older patient and ask themselves the following questions:

- Did I talk to the family and ignore the patient when I described some aspect of care or discharge planning?
- Did I tell the older person not to worry when he or she asked a question? Did I say, "Just leave everything up to us"?
- Did I eliminate information that I normally would have given a younger patient?
- Did I attribute a decline in cognitive functioning to the aging process without considering common underlying causes in mental deterioration, such as effects of medication interactions, fluid imbalances, poor nutrition, or sensory impairments?

Health professionals must remember that older people can learn, but their abilities and needs differ from those of younger persons. The process of teaching and learning is much more rewarding and successful for both the health professional and the patient if it is tailored to fit the older adult's physical, cognitive, motivational, and social differences.

Because changes as a result of aging vary considerably from one individual to another, it is essential to assess each learner's physical, cognitive, and psychosocial functioning levels before developing and implementing any teaching plan. It is important to keep in mind that older adults have an overall lower educational level of formal schooling than does the population as a whole. Also, they were raised in an era when consumerism and health education were practically nonexistent. As a result, older people may feel uncomfortable in the teaching–learning situation and may be reluctant to ask questions. In the future, as the older population becomes more educated and in tune with consumer activism in the health field, these individuals will likely have an increased desire to participate more in decision making and demand more detailed and sophisticated information. The proliferation of self-help literature and today's expectations for patients and families to take responsibility for self-care result in the present-day need for health professionals to involve clients more fully in decisions affecting their health (Morra, 1991).

Health education for older persons should be directed at promoting their involvement and changing their attitudes toward learning (Ahroni, 1996; Weinrich & Boyd, 1992). A climate of mutual respect in which they are made to feel important for what they once were as well as for what they are today should be cultivated. Interaction needs to be supportive, not judgmental.

Interventions work best when they take place in a casual, informal atmosphere. In the primary care setting, where time is often limited, it may be beneficial to schedule additional time, if possible, to allow for a more relaxed environment. Individual and situational variables such as motivation, life experiences, educational background, socioeconomic status, health or illness status, and motor, cognitive, and language skills may all influence the ability of the older adult to learn.

Some of the more common aging changes that affect learning and the teaching strategies specific to meeting the needs of the older adult are summarized in Table 5–1. When teaching older persons, abiding by the following specific tips can create an environment for learning that takes into account major changes in their physical, cognitive, and psychosocial functioning (Best, 2001; Doak, Doak, & Root, 1996; Fisher, 1999; Katz, 1997; Kessels, 2003; Phillips, 1999; Santrock, 2006; Vander Zanden et al., 2007; Weinrich & Boyd, 1992):

Physical Needs

1. To compensate for visual changes, teaching should be done in an environment that is brightly lit but without glare. Visual aids should include large print, well-spaced letters, and the use of primary colors. The educator should wear bright colors and a visible name tag. Use white or off-white, flat matte paper and black print for posters, diagrams, and other written materials.

   Because of older persons' difficulty in discriminating certain shades of color, avoid blue, blue-green, and violet hues. Keep in mind that tasks that require recognizing different shades of color, such as test strips measuring the presence of sugar in the urine, may present learning difficulties for older patients. Color distortions can have an especially devastating effect on learning if, for example, the type of pills are referred to by color in guiding patients to take medications as prescribed. Green, blue, and yellow pills may all appear gray to older persons. Additional accommodations should be made to meet physical needs, such as arranging seats so that the learner is reasonably close to the instructor and to any visual aids that may be used. For patients who wear glasses, be sure they are readily accessible, lenses are clean, and frames are properly fitted.

2. To compensate for hearing losses, eliminate extraneous noise, avoid covering your mouth when speaking, directly face the learner, and speak slowly. Female instructors should wear

bright lipstick. These techniques assist the learner who may be seeking visual confirmation of what is being said.

Low-pitched voices are heard best, but be careful not to drop your voice at the end of words or phrases. Do not shout, because it distorts sounds and the decibel level is usually not a problem for individuals with hearing impairments. The intensity of sound seems to be less important than the pitch and rate of auditory stimuli.

Word speed should not exceed 140 words spoken per minute. If the learner uses hearing aids, be sure they have working batteries. Ask for feedback from the learner to determine whether you are speaking too softly, too fast, or not distinctly enough. When addressing a group, microphones are useful aids. Be alert to nonverbal cues from the audience. Participants who are having difficulty with hearing your message may try to compensate by leaning forward, turning the good ear to the speaker, or cupping their hands to their ears. Ask older persons to repeat verbal instructions to be sure they heard and interpreted correctly the entire message.

3. To compensate for musculoskeletal problems, decreased efficiency of the cardiovascular system, and reduced kidney function, keep sessions short, schedule frequent breaks to allow for use of bathroom facilities, and allow time for stretching to relieve painful, stiff joints and to stimulate circulation. Provide pain medication and encourage the learner to follow his or her usual pain management routine. Also, provide comfortable seating.

4. To compensate for any decline in central nervous system functioning and decreased metabolic rates, set aside more time for the giving and receiving of information and for the practice of psychomotor skills. Also, do not assume that older persons have the psychomotor skills necessary to handle technological equipment

for self-paced learning, such as computers, Mp3 players, and DVD players. In addition, they may have difficulty with independently applying prostheses or changing dressings because of decreased strength and coordination. Be careful not to misinterpret the loss of energy and motor skills as a lack of motivation.

COGNITIVE NEEDS

1. To compensate for a decrease in fluid intelligence, provide older persons with more opportunities to process and react to information and to see relationships between concepts. Research has shown that older adults can learn anything if new information is tied to familiar concepts drawn from relevant past experiences.

When teaching, health professional educators should avoid presenting long lists by dividing a series of directions for action into short, discrete, step-by-step messages and then waiting for a response after each one. For instance, to give directions about following different menus depending on exercise levels, they can use an active voice to personalize the message. For example, instead of saying, "Use menu A if not active; use menu B if fairly active; use menu C if very active," they should say, "You should use menu A if you are not active." Then wait for the learner's response, which might be, "That's what I should eat if I'm not very active?" The educator can follow up with the response, "That's right. And if you are fairly active, you should …"

Older persons also tend to confuse previous words and symbols with a new word or symbol being introduced. Again, educators can wait for a response before introducing a new concept or word definition. For decreased short-term memory, coaching and repetition are very useful strategies that assist with recall. Memory can also be enhanced by involving the learner in devising ways to remember how or when to perform a procedure. Because many older adults experience test anxiety, try to explain procedures simply and thoroughly, reassure them, and, if possible, give verbal rather than written tests.

2. Be aware of the effects of medications and energy levels on concentration, alertness, and coordination. Try to schedule teaching sessions before or well after medications are taken and when the person is rested. For example, the patient who has just returned from physical therapy or a diagnostic procedure will likely be too fatigued to attend to learning.

3. Be certain to ask what an individual already knows about a healthcare issue or technique before explaining it. Repetition for reinforcement of learning is one thing; repeating information already known may seem patronizing. Educators should never assume that because someone has been exposed to information before that they, in fact, learned it. Confirm their level of knowledge before beginning to teach. Basic information should be understood before progressing to more complex information.

4. Convincing older persons of the usefulness of what the educator is teaching is only half the battle in getting them motivated. Educators may also have to convince them that the information or technique they are teaching is correct. Anything that is entirely strange or that upsets established habits is likely to be far more difficult for older adults to learn. Information that confirms existing beliefs (cognitive schema) is better remembered than that which contradicts these beliefs. Patients with chronic illnesses frequently have established schemas about their medical conditions that they have embraced for years.

   As perception slows, the older person's mind has more trouble accommodating to new ways than does the mind of a younger person. Find out about older persons' health habits and beliefs before trying to change their ways or teach something new. For example, many older adults

were taught as children that pain is a sign that something is wrong and they should always stop whatever they are doing if it causes pain. Educators need to identify this belief before trying to teach them that they sometimes need to move through their pain to avoid stiffness and joint contractures.

5. Arrange for brief teaching sessions because a shortened attention span (attentional narrowing) requires scheduling a series of sessions to provide for sufficient time for learning. In addition, if the material is relevant and focused on the here and now, older persons are more likely to be attentive to the information being presented. If procedures or treatments are perceived as stressful or emotionally threatening, attentional narrowing occurs.

6. Take into account that the process of conceptualizing and the ability to think abstractly become more difficult with aging. Conclude each teaching session with a summary of the information presented and allow for a question and answer period to correct any misconceptions (see **Figure 5–2** for strategies to meet cognitive needs of older adults).

PSYCHOSOCIAL NEEDS

1. Assess family relationships to determine how dependent the older person is on other members for financial and emotional support. In turn, educators can explore the level of involvement by family members in reinforcing the lessons they are teaching and in giving assistance with self-care measures. Do family members help the older person to function independently, or do they foster dependency? With permission of the patient, include family members in teaching sessions and enlist their support.

2. Determine availability of resources. A lack of resources can sabotage any teaching plan, especially if the recommendations include expecting older adults to carry out something they cannot afford or lack the means to do, such as buying

Figure 5–2 A Basic Gerontological Teaching–Learning Model

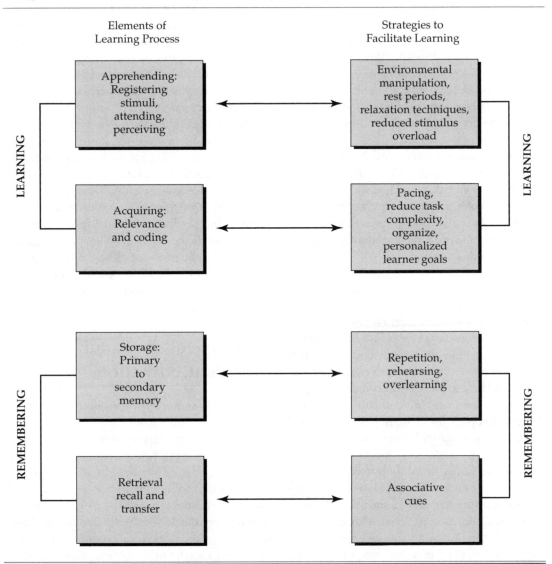

Source: Reprinted with permission from Rendon, D. C., Davis, D. K., Gioiella, E. C., & Tranzillo, M. J. (1986). The right to know, the right to be taught. *Journal of Gerontological Nursing, 12*(12), 36.

or renting equipment, having transportation to get to therapy or teaching sessions, purchasing medications, and the like.

3. Encourage active involvement of older adults to improve their self-esteem and to stimulate them both mentally and socially. Teaching must be directed at helping them find meaningful ways to use talents acquired over their lifetime. Establishing a rapport based on trust can provide them contact with others as a means to bolster their sense of self-worth.

4. Identify coping mechanisms. No other time in the life cycle carries with it the number of developmental tasks associated with adaptation to loss of roles, social and family contacts, and physical and cognitive capacities that this time does. Teaching must include offering constructive methods of coping.

The older person's ability to learn may be affected by the methods and materials chosen for teaching. One-to-one instruction provides a nonthreatening environment for older adults in which to meet their individual needs and goals. This teaching approach helps them to compensate for their special deficits and promotes their active participation in learning. Group teaching also can be a beneficial approach for fostering social skills and maintaining contact with others through shared experiences.

Self-paced instructional tools may be very appropriate, but it is important to know the client's previous learning techniques, mental and physical abilities, and comfort levels with certain approaches before assigning any such tools. Many older adults grew up in a time when technology did not exist to the extent that it does today, and those who have always learned by reading and discussion may not like mediated devices. Introducing new teaching methods and tools, such as the use of computer and interactive video formats without adequate instructions on how to operate these technical devices, may inhibit learning by

increasing anxiety and frustration levels and may adversely affect self-esteem.

Games, role-playing, demonstration, and return demonstration can be used to rehearse problem-solving and psychomotor skills as long as these methods, and the tools used to complement them, are designed appropriately to accommodate the various developmental characteristics of this age group. For example, speed or competition should not be factors in the games chosen and plenty of time should be reserved for return demonstrations. These teaching methods stimulate learning and can offer active learning opportunities to put knowledge into practice. Written materials, with attention being paid to appropriateness in terms of literacy level and visual impairments in the older adult, are excellent adjuncts to augment, supplement, and reinforce verbal instructions (see Chapters 7, 11, and 12 for specific information on literacy and the design and use of instructional methods and materials).

The Role of the Family in Patient Education

The role of the family is considered one of the key variables influencing positive patient care outcomes. The primary motives in patient education for involving family members in the care delivery and decision-making process are to decrease the stress of hospitalization, reduce costs of care, and effectively prepare the client for self-care management outside the healthcare setting. Family caregivers provide critical emotional, physical, and social support to the patient (Gavan, 2003; Reeber, 1992).

Under the most recent Joint Commission accreditation standards, new demands have been placed on healthcare organizations to show evidence that the family is included in patient education efforts. The standards mandate that the instruction of patients and significant others be considered an essential part in the healthcare team approach to providing care. Providers are responsible for assisting both patients and their family members to gain the knowledge and skills necessary to meet ongoing healthcare goals, particularly the first of the *Healthy People 2010* initiatives to increase the quality and years of a healthy life (U.S. Department of Health and Human Services, 2000). Interdisciplinary collaboration is a major resource for ensuring continuity of client teaching about healthy lifestyles in and across healthcare settings.

Including the family members in the teaching–learning process helps to ensure that the situation is win-win for both the client and the health professional. Family role enhancement and increased knowledge on the part of the family have positive benefits for the learner as well as the teacher. Clients derive increased satisfaction and greater independence in self-care, and health professionals experience increased job satisfaction and personal gratification in helping clients to reach their potentials and achieve successful outcomes (Barnes, 1995; Gavan, 2003).

Numerous nursing, life-span development, and educational psychology theories provide the conceptual frameworks for understanding the dynamics and importance of family relationships as influential in achieving teaching–learning outcomes. Although a great deal of attention has been given to the ways in which young and adolescent families function, unfortunately minimal attention has been paid to the dynamics of the complex interactions that characterize the aging family (Gavan, 2003).

In patient education, the health professional may be tempted to teach as many family members as possible. In reality, it is difficult to coordinate the instruction of so many different people. The more individuals involved, the greater the potential for misunderstanding of instruction. The family must make the deliberate decision as to who is the most appropriate person to take the primary responsibility as the caregiver.

Health professional educators must determine how caregivers feel about the role of providing supportive care and about learning the necessary information. They must also explore caregiver learning style preferences, cognitive abilities, fears and concerns, and current knowledge of the situation. Perceptions of the problem by both the family and the healthcare team must be determined to identify similarities and differences so that effective teaching can be provided (Leifer & Hartston, 2004). The caregiver needs information similar to what the patient is given to provide support, feedback, and reinforcement of self-care consistent with prescribed regimens of care.

Sometimes the family members need more information than the patient to compensate for any sensory deficits or cognitive limitations the patient may have. Anticipatory teaching with family caregivers can reduce their anxiety, uncertainty, and lack of confidence. What the family is to do is important, but what the family is to expect also is essential information to be shared during the teaching–learning process (Haggard, 1989). The greatest challenge for caregivers is to develop confidence in their ability to do what is right for the patient. Education is the means to help them confront this challenge.

The family can be the educator's greatest ally in preparing the patient for discharge and in helping the patient to become independent in self-care. The patient's family is perhaps the single most significant determinant of the success or failure of the education plan and achievement of successful aging (Gavan, 2003; Haggard, 1989). Rankin and Stallings's 2001 model for patient and family education serves as a foundation for assessing the family profile to determine the family members' understanding of the actual or potential health problem(s), the resources available to them, their ways of functioning, and their educational backgrounds, lifestyles, and beliefs.

Education is truly the most powerful tool health professionals have to ensure optimal care and the transfer of power to the patient–family dyad. It is imperative that attention be focused on both the assumed and the expected responsibilities of family caregivers. The role of the family has been stressed in each developmental section in this chapter. Table 5–1 outlines appropriate interventions for the family at different stages in the life cycle.

State of the Evidence

In an extensive review of the literature, a number of studies from primary and secondary sources by nurses and other healthcare professionals were found to support the application of teaching and learning principles to the education of middle-aged and older adult clients in various healthcare settings. However, current healthcare research focusing specifically on patient education approaches to the age cohorts of children, adolescents, and the young adult population, as well as instructional needs of family members as caregivers was lacking. For example, the article by Richmond and Kotelchuck (1984) was an excellent and thorough examination of health maintenance in children, including children's cognitive understanding of health and disease, their psychological control over health, parental and media influences on health behaviors, the impact of school health education, and the role of health professionals in the management of childhood illness and health services for children, but it was written more than 2 decades ago. Present knowledge of new approaches to foster child health is sorely needed.

To bolster general understanding of the physical, cognitive, and psychosocial (emotional) traits of human development across the life span, plenty of excellent resources, well-grounded by research evidence, exist in the fields of psychology in general and educational psychology in particular. However, much of the educational psychology literature focuses extensively on the application of teaching and learning principles only to preschool and K–12 classrooms. Understandably so, life-span developmental scientists do not give specific consideration to health education of well individuals with respect to disease prevention, risk reduction, and health promotion efforts or the health promotion, maintenance, and rehabilitation measures for those who are acutely and chronically ill. The application and translation of developmental characteristics to the teaching and learning aspects of healthcare delivery is the responsibility of healthcare providers. Much more investigation needs to be done to demonstrate how to effectively teach clients of different developmental stages based on their learning needs, learning styles, and readiness to learn for the achievement of the most positive client-centered outcomes possible.

Malcolm Knowles's original 1973 theory about adult learning and his subsequent modifications and clarifications of his theory (Knowles, 1990; Knowles et al., 1998) seem to be well accepted and have stood the test of time. Piaget's theory on cognitive development also has been accepted and extensively applied over the years, but recent critics of Piaget have challenged the assumptions underlying his theory with respect to the last stage of development (formal operations). Now a number of psychologists speculate that a fifth and qualitatively higher level of thinking follows adolescence and is postulated as the postformal operations period of adulthood. Vygotsky's sociocultural theory adds another dimension to understanding cognitive development (Santrock, 2006; Vander Zanden et al., 2007) that was not addressed by Piaget.

Erickson's theory of eight stages of psychosocial development, whereby individuals are faced with unique stage-related tasks (crises that must be resolved to reduce one's vulnerability and enhance one's potentials) are still recognized as the unique turning points in life that require successful completion for healthy, normal development to occur. Erickson's theory continues to be widely applied to the field of life-span development.

Recently, increased attention has been paid to the appropriateness of instructional methods and materials (especially as they relate to multimedia technology) for college-aged students and adult learners to meet their expectations for lifelong learning. Given the fact that the population is steadily aging, health professionals are caring for an increasingly older audience of learners. Many of the current health professional students are somewhat older than the traditional college-aged students, and staff are adult continuing education learners. It is gratifying to witness the acknowledgment of these population changes with an emphasis on studying generational differences on learner preferences, modes of information processing, and on memory and recall with respect to the impact of standard versus newer technological methods and tools for the effective delivery of instruction. Articles, such as those written by Billings and Kowalski (2004), Lewis (2003), Oblinger (2003), and Prensky (2001), are beginning to highlight the different experiences, values, beliefs, and needs of learners from varied generational backgrounds.

Although there has been an upsurge of interest in educational strategies and techniques for teaching and learning as it applies to certain population groups in the broad healthcare arena, much more research needs to be done as it relates to the creative leadership role of the health professional functioning as facilitator rather than teacher of patients and family members (at all stages of development) and of students and staff (Donner, Levonian, & Slutsky, 2005). Research has only begun to scratch the surface on how teaching and learning are affected by situational variables, such as chronic illness, acute illness, disability, or wellness; by personality traits, such as motivation and learning styles; by temperament responses, such as anxiety and attention span; and by sociocultural influences, such as gender, economic status, and educational background.

Another area requiring further exploration is the importance of the role of family and other support systems on the success of educational endeavors to help Americans of all ages maintain and improve their health status. There is a paucity of research evidence on family structure and the many changing relationships in society that promote or hinder teaching and learning of clients in various healthcare settings.

The national initiatives of *Healthy People 2010* and *Healthy People 2020*, as well as pending policy goals at local and state levels, will not be realized unless a better understanding is gained of the impact of physical, cognitive, psychological/emotional, and sociocultural changes that occur across the life course that can serve as a guideline for teaching and learning in healthcare practice.

Summary

It is important to understand the specific and varied tasks associated with each developmental stage to individualize the approach to education in meeting the needs and desires of clients and their families. Assessment of physical, cognitive, and psychosocial maturation within each developmental period is crucial in determining the strategies to be used to facilitate the teaching–learning process. The younger learner is, in many ways, very different from the adult learner. Issues of dependency, extent of participation, rate of and capacity for learning, and situational and emotional obstacles to learning vary significantly across the various phases of development.

Readiness to learn in children is very subject centered and highly influenced by their physical, cognitive, and psychosocial maturation. Motivation to learn in the adult is very problem centered and more oriented to psychosocial tasks related to roles and expectations of work, family, and community activities.

For client education to be effective, the health professional must create an environment conducive to learning by presenting information at the learner's level, inviting participation and feedback, and identifying whether parental, family, and/or peer involvement is appropriate or necessary. Health professionals are an important source of health information. In concert with the client, they must facilitate the teaching–learning process by determining what needs to be taught, when to teach, how to teach, and who should be the focus of teaching in light of the developmental stage of the learner.

When health professional students and staff are the audience of learners, the educator also is responsible for assuming the leadership role as facilitator of the learning process. In conjunction with these adult learners, educators can establish objectives and learner-centered approaches that challenge the educator's creativity to foster self-direction, motivation, interest, and active participation for independence and interdependence in learning.

REVIEW QUESTIONS

1. What are the seven stages of development?
2. What are the definitions of pedagogy, andragogy, and gerogogy?
3. Who is the expert in cognitive development? What are the terms or labels used by this expert to identify the key cognitive milestones?
4. Who is the expert in psychosocial development? What are the terms or labels used by this expert to identify the key psychosocial milestones?
5. What are the salient characteristics at each stage of development that influence the ability to learn?
6. What are three main teaching strategies for each stage of development?
7. How do people you know in each stage of development compare with what you have learned about physical, cognitive, and psychosocial characteristics at the various developmental stages?
8. What is the role of the family in the teaching and learning process in each stage of development?
9. How does the role of the health professional vary when teaching individuals at different stages of development?

CASE STUDY

Potomac University's Lillian Case Asthma Center is developing a new program that focuses on a family-centered approach to asthma management. Expected client outcomes of the program are to reduce hospitalizations and days off from work or school. Your role as a consultant to this program is to help the team develop a comprehensive, family-oriented educational program that covers important asthma topics such as pathophysiology, peak flow meter (PFM) use, and exercise. Mauricio, a member of the team, suggests, "Let's do our teaching with all the family members together in a group," while Liza, another team member, states, "We should separate the family members into similar age groups for the teaching—that way, we can better keep their interest." You suggest that the team integrate Mauricio's and Liza's suggestions and plan a total of five teaching sessions with four of the sessions grouping participants according to developmental stages and the final session grouping families together. Participants range from 6 to 50 years of age.

1. Describe how you will determine the different age range groupings of the participants for the first four sessions. Explain the different age ranges, cognitive and psychosocial stages, and general characteristics of each group.
2. Choose two different developmental stage groupings and give examples of teaching strategies you will use with each group for the specific teaching sessions. Explain why you chose these strategies for the individuals with asthma and their families.
3. What are some advantages to grouping participants by developmental stages? What are some disadvantages?

References

Ackard, D. M., & Neumark-Sztainer, D. (2001). Health care information sources for adolescents: Age and gender differences on use, concerns, and needs. *Journal of Adolescent Health, 29*(3), 170–176.

Ahroni, J. H. (1996). Strategies for teaching elders from a human development perspective. *Diabetes Educator, 22*(1), 47–52.

American Association of Colleges of Nursing. (1994). *AACN issue bulletin.* Washington, DC: Author.

Aronowitz, T. (2006). Teaching adolescents about adolescence: Experiences from an interdisciplinary adolescent health course. *Nurse Educator, 31*(2), 84–87.

Babcock, D. E., & Miller, M. A. (1994). *Client education: Theory & practice.* St. Louis, MO: Mosby–Year Book.

Banks, E. (1990). Concepts of health and sickness of preschool- and school-aged children. *Children's Health, 19*(1), 43–48.

Barnes, L. P. (1995). Finding the "win/win" in patient/family teaching. *MCN: American Journal of Maternal Child Nursing, 20*(4), 229.

Best, J. T. (2001). Effective teaching for the elderly: Back to basics. *Orthopedic Nursing, 20*(3), 46–52.

Billings, D., & Kowalski, K. (2004). Teaching learners from varied generations. *Journal of Continuing Education, 35*(3), 104–105.

Boyd, M. D., Gleit, C. J., Graham, B. A., & Whitman, N. I. (1998). *Health teaching in nursing practice: A professional model* (3rd ed.). Norwalk, CT: Appleton & Lange.

Brown, S. L., Teufel, J. A., & Birch, D. A. (2007). Early adolescents' perceptions of health and health literacy. *Journal of School Health, 77*(1), 7–15.

Burkett, K. W. (1989). Trends in pediatric rehabilitation. *Nursing Clinics of North America, 24*(1), 239–255.

Cauffman, E., & Steinberg, L. (2000). (Im)maturity of judgment in adolescence: Why adolescents may be less culpable than adults. *Behavioral Science Law, 18,* 741–760.

Collins, J. (2004). Education techniques for lifelong learners. *RadioGraphics, 24*(5), 1483–1489.

Covey, S. (1990). *The seven habits of highly effective people.* New York: Simon & Schuster.

Doak, C. C., Doak, L. G., & Root, J. H. (1996). *Teaching patients with low literacy skills* (2nd ed.). Philadelphia: Lippincott.

Donner, C. L., Levonian, C., & Slutsky, P. (2005). Move to the head of the class: Developing staff nurses as teachers. *Journal for Nurses in Staff Development, 21*(6), 277–283.

Elkind, D. (1984). Teenage thinking: Implications for health care. *Pediatric Nursing, 10*(6), 383–385.

Erikson, E. H. (1963). *Childhood and society* (2nd ed.). New York: Norton.

Erikson, E. H. (1968). *Identity: Youth and crisis.* New York: Norton.

Falvo, D. R. (1994). *Effective patient education: A guide to increased compliance* (2nd ed.). Gaithersburg, MD: Aspen.

Farrand, L. L., & Cox, C. L. (1993). Determinants of positive health behavior in middle childhood. *Nursing Research, 42*(4), 208–213.

Fisher, E. (1999). Low literacy levels in adults: Implications for patient education. *Journal of Continuing Education in Nursing, 30*(2), 56–61.

Gavan, C. S. (2003). Successful aging families: A challenge for nurses. *Holistic Nursing Practice, 17*(1), 11–18.

Girod, M., Pardales, M., Cavanaugh, S., & Wadsworth, P. (2005). By teens, for teachers: A descriptive study of adolescence. *American Secondary Education, 33*(2), 4–19.

Grey, M., Kanner, S., & Lacey, K. O. (1999). Characteristics of the learner: Children and adolescents. *Diabetes Educator, 25*(6), 25–33.

Haggard, A. (1989). *Handbook of patient education.* Rockville, MD: Aspen.

Havighurst, R. (1976). Human characteristics and school learning: Essay review. *Elementary School Journal, 77,* 101–109.

Heiney, S. P. (1991). Helping children through painful procedures. *American Journal of Nursing, 91*(11), 20–24.

Hines, A. R., & Paulson, S. E. (2006). Parents' and teachers' perceptions of adolescent storm and stress: Relations with parenting and teaching styles. *Adolescence, 41*(164), 597–614.

Hussey, C. G., & Hirsh, A. M. (1983). Health education for children. *Topics in Clinical Nursing, 5*(1), 22–28.

Jackson, R. H., Davis, T. C., Murphy, P., Bairnsfather, L. E., & George, R. B. (1994). Reading deficiencies in older patients. *American Journal of the Medical Sciences, 308*(2), 79–82.

Johnson-Saylor, M. T. (1980). Seize the moment: Health promotion for the young adult. *Topics in Clinical Nursing, 2*(2), 9–19.

Katz, J. R. (1997). Back to basics: Providing effective patient education. *American Journal of Nursing, 97*(5), 33–36.

Kennedy, C. M., & Riddle, I. I. (1989). The influence of the timing of preparation on the anxiety of preschool children experiencing surgery. *Maternal-Child Nursing Journal, 18*(2), 117–132.

Kessels, R. P. C. (2003). Patients' memory for medical information. *Journal of the Royal Society of Medicine, 96,* 219–222.

Knowles, M. (1990). *The adult learner: A neglected species* (4th ed.). Houston: Gulf.

Knowles, M. S., Holton, E. F., & Swanson, R. A. (1998). *The adult learner: The definitive classic in adult education and human resource development* (5th ed.). Houston: Gulf.

Kotchabhakdi, P. (1985). School-age children's conceptions of the heart and its function. Monograph 15. *Maternal-Child Nursing Journal, 14*(4), 203–261.

Kray, J., & Lindenberger, U. (2000). Adult age differences in task switching. *Psychology and Aging, 15*(1), 126–147.

Leifer, G., & Hartston, H. (2004). *Growth and development across the lifespan: A health promotion focus.* St. Louis, MO: Saunders.

Lewis, D. (2003). Computers in patient education. *Computer Informatics in Nursing, 21*(2), 88–96.

London, M. C., Ladewig, P. W., Ball, J. W., & Bindler, R. C. (2003). *Maternal-newborn & child nursing: Family-centered care.* Upper Saddle River, NJ: Prentice Hall.

Matsuda, O., & Saito, M. (1998). Crystallized and fluid intelligence in elderly patients with mild dementia of the Alzheimer type. *International Psychogeriatrics, 10*(2), 147–154.

Michaud, P.-A., Stronski, S., Fonseca, H., & MacFarlane, A. (2004). The development and pilot-testing of a training curriculum in adolescent medicine and health. *Journal of Adolescent Health, 35*(1), 51–57.

Milligan, F. (1997). In defense of andragogy. Part 2: An educational process consistent with modern nursing's aims. *Nurse Education Today, 17,* 487–493.

Morra, M. E. (1991). Future trends in patient education. *Seminars in Oncology Nursing, 7*(2), 143–145.

Musinski, B. (1999). The educator as facilitator: A new kind of leadership. *Nursing Forum, 34*(1), 23–29.

Oblinger, D. (2003, July/August). Boomers, Gen-Xers & millennials: Understanding the new students. *Educause,* 37–45.

Orshan, S. A. (2008). *Maternity, newborn, and woman's health nursing: Comprehensive care across the lifespan.* Philadelphia: Lippincott Williams & Wilkins.

Palfrey, J. S., Hauser-Cram, P., Bronson, M. B., Warfield, M. E., Sirin, S., & Chan, E. (2005). The Brookline early education project: A 25-year follow-up study of family-centered early health and development intervention. *Pediatrics, 116*(1), 144–152.

Pearson, M., & Wessman, J. (1996). Gerogogy. *Home Healthcare Nurse, 14*(8), 631–636.

Perrin, E. C., Sayer, A. G., & Willett, J. B. (1991). Sticks and stones may break my bones … Reasoning about illness causality and body functioning in children who have a chronic illness. *Pediatrics, 88*(3), 608–619.

Phillips, L. D. (1999). Patient education: Understanding the process to maximize time and outcomes. *Journal of Intravenous Nursing, 22*(1), 19–35.

Piaget, J. (1951). *Judgement and reasoning in the child.* London: Routledge and Kegan Paul.

Piaget, J. (1952). *The origins of intelligence in children.* New York: International Universities Press.

Piaget, J. (1976). *The grasp of consciousness: Action and concept in the young child.* (S. Wedgwood, Trans.). Cambridge, MA: Harvard University Press.

Pidgeon, V. A. (1977). Characteristics of children's thinking and implications for health teaching. *Maternal-Child Nursing Journal, 6*(1), 1–8.

Pidgeon, V. (1985). Children's concepts of illness: Implications for health teaching. *Maternal-Child Nursing Journal, 14*(1), 23–35.

Polan, E., & Taylor, D. (2003). *Journey across the lifespan: Human development and health promotion* (2nd ed.). Philadelphia: F. A. Davis.

Poster, E. C. (1983). Stress immunization: Techniques to help children cope with hospitalization. *Maternal-Child Nursing Journal, 12*(2), 119–134.

Prensky, M. (2001). Digital natives, digital immigrants. *On the Horizon, 9*(5), 1–6.

Protheroe, N. (2007). How children learn. *Principal, 86*(5), 40–44.

Rankin, S. H., & Stallings, K. D. (2001). *Patient education: Principles and practices* (4th ed.). Philadelphia: Lippincott.

Reeber, B. J. (1992). Evaluating the effects of a family education intervention. *Rehabilitation Nursing, 17*(6), 332–336.

Richmond, J. B., & Kotelchuck, M. (1984). Personal health maintenance for children. *Western Journal of Medicine, 141*(6), 816–823.

Ryberg, J. W., & Merrifield, E. B. (1984). What parents want to know. *Nurse Practitioner, 9*(6), 24–32.

Santrock, J. W. (2006). *Life-span development* (10th ed.). Boston: McGraw-Hill.

Snowman, J., & Biehler, R. (2006). *Psychology applied to teaching.* Boston: Houghton Mifflin.

Taylor, K., Marienau, C., & Fiddler, M. (2000). *Developing adult learners: Strategies for teachers and trainers.* San Francisco: Jossey-Bass.

Theis, S. L., & Merritt, S. L. (1994). A learning model to guide research and practice for teaching of elder clients. *Nursing and Health Care, 15*(9), 464–468.

U.S. Department of Health and Human Services. (2000). *Healthy People 2010.* McClean, VA: International Publishing.

Vander Zanden, J. W., Crandell, T. L., & Crandell, C. H. (2007). *Human development* (8th ed.). Boston: McGraw-Hill.

Vulcan, B. (1984). Major coping behaviors of a hospitalized 3-year-old boy. *Maternal-Child Nursing Journal, 13*(2), 113–123.

Weinrich, S. P., & Boyd, M. (1992). Education in the elderly. *Journal of Gerontological Nursing, 18*(1), 15–20.

Whitener, L. M., Cox, K. R., & Maglich, S. A. (1998). Use of theory to guide nurses in the design of health messages for children. *Advances in Nursing Science, 20*(3), 21–35.

Woodring, B. C. (2000). If you have taught—have the child and family learned? *Pediatric Nursing, 26*(5), 505–509.

Chapter 6

Compliance, Motivation, and Health Behaviors of the Learner

Eleanor Richards
Kirsty Digger

KEY TERMS

- compliance
- motivation
- adherence
- noncompliance
- locus of control
- hierarchy of needs
- motivational incentives

- motivational axioms
- concept mapping
- motivational interviewing
- health belief model
- self-efficacy theory
- protection motivation theory
- stages of change model

❏ theory of reasoned action
❏ therapeutic alliance model

❏ concordance
❏ educational contracting

OBJECTIVES

After completing this chapter, the reader will be able to

1. Define the terms *compliance*, *adherence*, and *motivation* relevant to behaviors of the learner.
2. Discuss compliance and motivation concepts and theories.
3. Identify incentives and obstacles that affect motivation to learn.
4. State axioms of motivation relevant to learning.
5. Assess levels of learner motivation.
6. Outline strategies that facilitate motivation and improve compliance.
7. Compare and contrast selected health behavior frameworks and their influence on learning.
8. Recognize the role of the health professional as educator in health promotion.

The concepts of compliance and motivation are used implicitly or explicitly in many health behavior models. This chapter discusses these concepts as they relate to health behaviors of the learner and presents an overview of selected theories and models for consideration in the teaching–learning process. When in the role of educator, the health professional needs to understand which factors promote or hinder the acquisition and application of knowledge and what drives the learner to learn.

Factors that determine health behaviors and outcomes are complex. Knowledge alone does not guarantee that the learner will engage in health-promoting behaviors or that the desired outcomes will be achieved. The most well-thought-out educational program or plan of care cannot achieve the prescribed goals if the learner is not understood in the context of complex factors associated with compliance and motivation.

Compliance

The literature reveals continuing controversy about the use of the term **compliance** to describe client behavior. By definition, *compliance* is a term that means submission or yielding to the recommendations or will of others. Defined as such, it has an authoritative undertone. Specifically, when applied to health care, it implies that the healthcare provider or educator is viewed as the authority, and the consumer or learner is in a submissive role. Many health professionals object to this hierarchical stance because they believe that clients have the right to make their own healthcare decisions and not necessarily follow predetermined courses of action set by healthcare professionals.

Healthcare literature suggests that compliance is a statement of outcome and indicates achievement of a goal identified in a health-related regimen. Compliance, as an end result, is different from **motivation**, which is viewed as means to an end. For example, a teenager with an eating disorder may not be compliant with the prescribed daily caloric requirement because she may not have the desire or motivation to gain weight. Compliance to a health regimen is an observable behavior and as such can be directly measured. Motivation, by comparison, is a precursor to action that can be indirectly measured through behavioral consequences or results. Commitment or attachment to a regimen is known as **adherence**, which may be long-lasting. Both compliance and adherence refer to health-promoting regimens, which are determined largely by the healthcare provider. A subtle difference separates the terms *compliance* and *adherence*.

The term *compliance* implies obedience or passive acceptance of the healthcare regimen. In comparison, the term *adherence* implies support of or commitment to a plan of care. It is possible for an individual to comply with a regimen and not necessarily be committed to it. For example, a patient who is experiencing sleep disturbances may comply with medication as directed for a period of 1 week. The same patient may not continue to adhere to the regimen for an extended period of time, even though the sleep disturbances continue. In this situation, there is no support of the plan or commitment to follow through.

Nonadherence can be intentional or unintentional and can be affected by such variables as cognitive function, social support, and financial constraints. Erlen (2006) and colleagues continue to investigate "maintenance strategies, booster programs, and specific factors that can impede or enhance adherence" (p. 17). Both *compliance* and *adherence* are terms used in the measurement of health outcomes. Therefore, for the purpose of this chapter, these terms are used interchangeably.

Research, as evidenced by the multidisciplinary healthcare literature, has focused on the compliance or adherence of healthcare consumers to their healthcare plans. The number of studies on compliance reflects the importance of the concept to practice. **Noncompliance** places a client under unnecessary health risk and can result in increased medical expenditures (Heiby, Lukens, & Frank, 2005). This phenomenon may also be the result of an emphasis on cost-effective health care, as seen, for example, in shorter lengths of hospital stays. The successes of educational programs in a fiscally responsible system ultimately are linked to measurement of patient compliance relative to outcomes.

Perspectives on Compliance

Theories and models of compliance, as described by Eraker, Kirscht, and Becker (1984) and Levanthal and Cameron (1987), can be viewed from various perspectives and are useful in explaining or describing compliance from a multidisciplinary approach including psychology and education. These theories and models are as follows:

1. Biomedical theory, which links compliance with patient characteristics such as demographics, severity of disease, and complexity of treatment regimen.
2. Behavioral/social learning theory, which focuses on external factors that influence the client's adherence such as rewards, cues, contracts, and social supports.
3. Communication models, which attempt to explain compliance on the basis of the communication between the client and the healthcare professional. These models address aspects such as the feedback loop of sending, receiving, comprehending, retaining, and accepting information.
4. Rational belief theory, which suggests that clients make a decision to comply or not comply by weighing the benefits of treatment and the risks of disease through the use of cost-benefit logic.
5. Self-regulatory systems, in which patients are seen as problem solvers whose regulation of behavior is based on perception of illness, cognitive skills, and past experiences that affect their ability to plan and cope with illness.

Although these theories and models shed some light on the very complex issue of compliance, most agree that each of them has limitations and no one theory or model alone has proven to be superior to the others (Heiby et al., 2005; Munro,

Lewin, Swart, & Volmink, 2007). In recent years, researchers have attempted to use a multivariate approach to explaining compliance. For example, Heiby et al. (2005) has proposed the Health Compliance-II Model, which incorporates variables from several theories and models. Further research is needed to identify a model that incorporates some of the multiple variables described subsequently.

Locus of Control

The authoritative aspect of compliance infers that the educator makes an attempt to control, in part, decision making on the part of the learner. Some models of compliance have attempted to balance the issue of control by using terms such as *mutual contracting* (Steckel, 1982) or *consensual regimen* (Fink, 1976).

One way to view the issue of control in the learning situation is through the concept of locus of control (Rotter, 1954) or health locus of control (Wallston, Wallston, & DeVellis, 1978). This term **locus of control** refers to an individual's sense of responsibility for his or her own behavior and the extent to which motivation to take action originates from within the self (internal) or is influenced by others (external). Through objective measurement, individuals can be categorized as internals, whose health behavior is self-directed, or externals, whereby others are viewed as more powerful in influencing health outcomes. Externals believe that fate is a powerful external force that determines life's course, whereas internals believe that they control their own destiny. For instance, an external might say, "Osteoporosis runs in my family, and it will catch up with me." An internal might say, "Although there is a history of osteoporosis in my family, I will have necessary screenings, eat an appropriate diet, and do weight-bearing exercise to prevent or control this problem."

Researchers in the health professions have attempted to link locus of control with compliance.

Study results have been mixed. Locus of control has been linked to compliance in some therapeutic regimens and has shown no relationship in others (Rosno, Steele, Johnston, & Aylward, 2008; Sin-Jae, Sug-Joon, & Tae-Woo, 2008). Shillinger (1983) suggests that different teaching strategies are indicated for internals and externals. The literature, however, remains inconclusive as to the nature of the relationship between compliance and internals versus externals.

Noncompliance

Noncompliance describes resistance of the individual to follow a predetermined regimen. Noncompliance often results in blaming behavior when patient goals are not achieved (Yach, 2003). Ward-Collins (1998) notes that *noncompliance* can be a highly subjective judgmental term sometimes used synonymously with the term *noncooperative* or *disobedient*. Helme and Harrington (2004) studied patients who were noncompliant with their diabetes regimen and found that although the largest number of people admitted their failure to comply with their healthcare plan, many offered excuses or justifications and some denied that noncompliance had occurred. Even though in this study participants had nothing to lose by admitting their noncompliance, many felt the need to explain or deny their failure to follow orders.

The literature is replete with studies on patient noncompliance. Nevertheless, the question of why clients are noncompliant remains largely unanswered. This is largely because of the complexity of the issue. Noncompliance can be related to patient issues such as knowledge or motivation, treatment factors such as side effects, disease issues such as prognosis, lifestyle issues such as transportation, sociodemographic factors such as social and economic status, and psychosocial variables such as depression and fear (Rosner, 2006). The expectation of total compliance in all spheres of behavior and at all times is unrealistic. At times, noncompliant behavior may be desirable and could be viewed as a necessary defensive response to stressful situations. The learner may use time-outs as the intensity of the learning situation is maintained or escalates. This mechanism of temporary withdrawal from the learning situation may actually prove beneficial. Following withdrawal, the learner could reengage, feeling renewed and ready to continue with an educational program or regimen. Viewed in this way, noncompliance is not an obstacle to learning and does not carry a negative connotation.

Motivation

Motivation, from the Latin word *movere*, means to set into motion. Motivation has been defined as a psychological force that moves a person toward some kind of action (Haggard, 1989). It has also been described as a willingness of the learner to embrace learning, with readiness as evidence of motivation (Redman, 2007). According to Kort (1987), motivation is the result of both internal and external factors and not the result of external manipulation alone. Implicit in motivation is movement in the direction of meeting a need or toward reaching a goal.

Lewin (1935), an early field theorist, conceptualized motivation in terms of positive or negative movement toward goals. Once an individual's equilibrium is disturbed, such as in the case of illness, forces of approach and avoidance may come into play. He noted that if avoidance endured in an approach–avoidance conflict, there would be negative movement away from a goal. His theory implies the existence of a critical time factor relative to motivation. This time factor, however, is generally not a serious consideration in motivational models of health behavior or motivational research.

Ideally, the health educator's role is to facilitate the learner's approach toward a desired goal and to prevent untimely delays. For example, staff may request an in-service program about evidence-based practice. The in-service educator may delay this request to the extent that the staff loses interest in the topic. Although untimely delays may be beyond the control of the educator, every effort should be made to capitalize on the staff's desire and readiness to learn.

Maslow (1943), another well-known early theorist, developed a theory of human motivation that is still widely used in the social sciences. The major premises of Maslow's motivation theory are integrated wholeness of the individual and a hierarchy of goals. Acknowledging the complexity of the concept of motivation, he noted that not all behavior is motivated and that behavior theories are not synonymous with motivation. Many determinants of behavior other than motives exist, and many motives can be involved in one behavior. Using the principles of **hierarchy of needs**—physiological, safety, love/belonging, self-esteem, and self-actualization—Maslow noted the relatedness of needs, which are organized by their level of potency. Some individuals are highly motivated, whereas others are weakly motivated. When a need is fairly well satisfied, then the next potent need emerges. An example of the hierarchy of basic needs is the potent need to satisfy hunger. This need may be met by the caregiver who assists the poststroke patient with feeding. The health professional–patient interaction may also satisfy the next most potent needs, those of love/belonging and self-esteem.

Relationships exist between motivation and learning; between motivation and behavior; and among motivation, learning, and behavior. Motivation may be viewed in relation to learning in many ways. Redman (2007) categorizes theories of motivation that direct learning as behavioral reinforcers, need satisfaction, reduction of discomforting inconsistencies as a result of cognitive dissonance, allocating causal factors known as attributions, personality in which motivation is acknowledged to be a stable characteristic, expectancy theory encompassing value and perceived chance of success, and humanistic interpretations of motivation that emphasize personal choice. Each theory attempts to address the complex and somewhat elusive quality of motivation.

Motivational Factors

Factors that influence motivation can serve as incentives or obstacles to achieve desired behaviors. Both creating incentives and decreasing obstacles to motivation pose a challenge for the health professional as educator. The cognitive (thinking processes), affective (emotions and feelings), social, and psychomotor (behavioral) domains of the learner can be influenced by the educator, who can act as a motivational facilitator or blocker.

Motivational incentives need to be considered in the context of the individual. What may be a motivational incentive for one learner may be a motivational obstacle to another. For example, a student who is assigned to work with an elderly woman may be motivated when the student holds older persons in high regard. Another student may be motivationally blocked by the same emotional domain because previous experiences with older women, such as a grandmother, were unrewarding.

Facilitating or blocking factors that shape motivation to learn can be classified into the following three major categories, which are not mutually exclusive:

1. Personal attributes, which consist of physical, developmental, and psychological components of the individual learner
2. Environmental influences, which include the physical and attitudinal climate
3. Learner relationship systems, such as those of significant other, family, community, and teacher–learner interaction

PERSONAL ATTRIBUTES

Personal attributes of the learner, such as developmental stage, age, gender, emotional readiness, values and beliefs, sensory functioning, cognitive ability, educational level, actual or perceived state of health, and severity or chronicity of illness, can shape an individual's motivation to learn. Functional ability to achieve behavioral outcomes is determined by physical, emotional, and cognitive dimensions. One's perception of disparity between current and expected states of health can be a motivating factor in health behavior and can drive readiness to learn.

The learner's views about the complexity or extent of changes that are needed can shape motivation. Values, beliefs, and natural curiosity can be firmly entrenched and enduring factors that can also shape desire to learn new behaviors. Other factors, such as sensory input and processing of information and short-term and long-term memory, can affect motivation to learn as well. Emerging interest about male–female behavioral and learning differences indicates the need for in-depth research on gender-related characteristics affecting motivation to learn (see Chapter 8).

ENVIRONMENTAL INFLUENCES

Physical characteristics of the learning environment, accessibility and availability of human and material resources, and different types of behavioral rewards influence the motivational level of the individual. The environment can create, promote, or detract from a state of learning receptivity. Pleasant, comfortable, and adaptable individualized surroundings can promote a state of readiness to learn. Conversely, noise, confusion, interruptions, and lack of privacy can interfere with the capacity to concentrate and to learn.

The factors of accessibility and availability of resources include physical and psychological aspects. Can the client physically access a health facility, and once there, will the healthcare personnel be psychologically available to the client? Psychological availability refers to whether the healthcare system is flexible and sensitive to patients' needs. It includes factors such as promptness of services, sociocultural competence, emotional support, and communication skills. Attitude influences the client's engagement with the healthcare system.

The manner in which the healthcare system is perceived by the client affects the client's willingness to participate in health-promoting behaviors. Behavioral rewards permeate the foundations of the learner's motivation. Rewards can be extrinsic, such as praise or acknowledgment from the educator or caretaker. Alternatively, they can be intrinsically based, such as feelings of a personal sense of fulfillment, gratification, or self-satisfaction.

RELATIONSHIP SYSTEMS

Family or significant others in the support system; cultural identity; work, school, and community roles; and teacher–learner interaction all influence an individual's motivation. The interactional aspects of motivation are perhaps the most salient because the learner exists in the context of interlocking relationship systems. Individuals are viewed in the context of family/community/cultural systems that have lifelong effects on the choices that individuals make, including healthcare seeking and healthcare decision making. These significant other systems may have even more of an influence on health outcomes than commonly acknowledged, and the health professional when in the role of educator needs to take into account the health-promoting use of these systems. All of these factors interact to address the motivation of the learner. They are not meant to be construed as comprehensive theory constructs, but rather as forces that act on motivation, serving to facilitate or block the desire to learn.

Motivational Axioms

Axioms are premises on which an understanding of a phenomenon is based. The health professional

as educator needs to understand the premises involved in promoting motivation of the learner. **Motivational axioms** are rules that set the stage for motivation. They include (1) the state of optimum anxiety, (2) learner readiness, (3) realistic goal setting, (4) learner satisfaction/success, and (5) uncertainty-reducing or uncertainty-maintaining dialogue.

STATE OF OPTIMUM ANXIETY

Learning occurs best when a state of moderate anxiety exists. In this optimum state for learning, the learner's ability to observe, focus attention, learn, and adapt is operative (Peplau, 1979). Perception, concentration, abstract thinking, and information processing are enhanced. Behavior is directed at a learning or challenging situation. Above this optimum level, at high or severe levels of anxiety, the ability to perceive the environment, concentrate, and learn is reduced. A moderate state of anxiety can be comfortably managed and is known to promote learning (Kessels, 2003; Ley, 1979; Stephenson, 2006). As anxiety escalates, however, attention to external stimuli is reduced, the learner becomes increasingly self-absorbed, and behavior becomes defensively reactionary rather than being cognitively generated (Shapiro, Boggs, Melamed, & Graham-Pole, 1992).

For example, a patient who has been recently diagnosed with a serious health problem and who has a high level of anxiety will not respond at an optimum level of retention of information when instructed about treatment options. When the health professional is able to aid the client in reducing anxiety, through techniques such as guided imagery, use of humor, or relaxation tapes, the patient will respond with a higher level of information retention.

LEARNER READINESS

Desire to move toward a goal and readiness to learn are factors that influence motivation. Desire cannot be imposed on the learner. It can, however, be critically influenced by external forces and be promoted by the health professional in the role of educator. Incentives are specific to the individual learner. An incentive for one individual can be a deterrent to another. For example, suggesting a method of weight reduction that includes physical exercise may be an incentive for one client, while totally unappealing for another. Incentives in the form of reinforcers and rewards can be tangible or intangible, external or internal.

As a facilitator to the learner, the health educator offers positive perspectives and encouragement, which shape the desired behavior toward goal attainment. By ensuring that learning is stimulating, making information relevant and accessible, and creating an environment conducive to learning, educators can facilitate motivation to learn (see Chapter 4 on readiness to learn).

REALISTIC GOALS

Goals that are within a person's grasp and possible to achieve are goals toward which an individual will work. Goals that are beyond the person's reach are frustrating and counterproductive. Unrealistic goals with loss of valuable time can set the stage for the learner to give up.

Setting realistic goals is a motivating factor. The belief that one can achieve the task set before him or her facilitates behavior geared toward achieving that goal. Goals should parallel the extent to which behavioral changes are needed. Determining what the learner wants to change is a critical factor in setting realistic goals. Mutual goal setting between learner and educator reduces the negative effects of hidden agendas or the sabotaging of educational plans.

LEARNER SATISFACTION/SUCCESS

The learner is motivated by success. Success is self-satisfying and feeds the learner's self-esteem. In a cyclical process, success and self-esteem escalate,

moving the learner toward accomplishment of goals. When a learner feels good about step-by-step accomplishments, motivation is enhanced. For example, in the instructor–student relationship, evaluations can be a valuable method of promoting learner success. Clinical evaluations, when focused on demonstration of positive behaviors, can encourage movement toward performance goals. Focusing on successes as a means of positive reinforcement promotes learner satisfaction and instills a sense of accomplishment. On the other hand, focusing on weak clinical performance can reduce students' self-esteem.

UNCERTAINTY REDUCTION OR MAINTENANCE

Uncertainty is a common experience in the healthcare arena. Healthcare consumers and health professionals alike are often asked to make decisions about treatment and care with outcomes that are unclear. An individual's response to this type of uncertainty may vary and is dependent upon the individual's characteristics (Politi, Han, & Col, 2007). Uncertainty (as well as certainty) can be a motivating factor in the learning situation. Individuals may have ongoing internal dialogues that can either reduce or maintain uncertainty. Individuals carry on "self-talk"; they think things through. When a person wants to change a state of health, behaviors often follow a dialogue that examines uncertainty, such as, "If I stop smoking, then my chances of getting lung cancer will be reduced." On the other hand, when the probable outcome of health behaviors is more uncertain, behaviors may maintain uncertainty. The person might say, "I am not sure that I need this surgery because the survival rates are no different for those who had this surgery and those who did not." Some learners may maintain current behaviors, given probabilities of treatment outcomes, thus maintaining uncertainty.

Mishel (1990) reconceptualizes the concept of uncertainty in illness. She views uncertainty as a necessary and natural rhythm of life, rather than an adverse experience. Uncertainty in sufficient concentration influences choices and decision making, and it can capitalize on receptivity or readiness for change. Premature uncertainty reduction can be counterproductive to the learner who has not sufficiently explored alternatives. For example, when a staff member is uncertain about how to position a patient for a particular treatment and is presented with alternatives, then a thinking dialogue is carried out. If the decision to use a particular position is not premature, then uncertainty will promote exploration of alternative positions.

Assessment of Motivation

How does the health professional know when the learner is motivated? As a generic concept, assessment of motivation to learn has not been adequately addressed in the literature. The lack of adequate conceptually based measurement tools could be a factor in this neglect.

Redman (2001) views motivational assessment as a part of general health assessment and states that it includes such areas as level of knowledge, client skills, decision-making capacity of the individual, and screening of target populations for educational programs. The educator can pose several questions in terms of the learner, such as those focusing on previous attempts, curiosity, goal setting, self-care ability, stress factors, survival issues, and life situations. Motivational assessment of the learner needs to be comprehensive, systematic, and conceptually based. Cognitive, affective, physiological, experiential, environmental, and learning relationship variables need to be considered. **Table 6–1** shows parameters for a comprehensive motivational assessment of the learner.

These multitheory-based parameters incorporate several perspectives, including Bandura's (1986) construction of incentive motivators; Ajzen and Fishbein's (1980) intent and attitude; Becker, Drachman, and Kirscht's (1974) notion of likeli-

Table 6–1 COMPREHENSIVE PARAMETERS FOR MOTIVATIONAL ASSESSMENT OF THE LEARNER

Cognitive Variables
- Capacity to learn
- Readiness to learn
  - Expressed self-determination
  - Constructive attitude
  - Expressed desire and curiosity
  - Willingness to contract for behavioral outcomes
- Facilitating beliefs

Affective Variables
- Expressions of constructive emotional state
- Moderate level of anxiety

Physiological Variables
- Capacity to perform required behavior

Experiential Variables
- Previous successful experiences

Environmental Variables
- Appropriateness of physical environment
- Social support systems
  - Family
  - Group
  - Work
  - Community resources

Educator–Learner Relationship System
- Prediction of positive relationship

hood of engaging in action; Pender's (1996) commitment to a plan of action; and Barofsky's (1978) focus on alliance in the learning situation. Additionally, the presence of cognitions in the form of facilitative beliefs proposed by Wright, Watson, and Bell (1996) provides a comprehensive and multidimensional assessment. This multidimensional guide allows for assessment of the level of learner motivation. If responses to dimensions are positive, the learner is likely to be motivated.

Assessment of learner motivation involves the judgment of the educator because teaching–learning is a two-way process. In particular, motivation can be assessed through both subjective and objective means. A subjective means of assessing level of motivation is through dialogue. By being present and using therapeutic communication skills, the health professional can obtain verbal information from the client, such as, "I really want to maintain my weight" or "I want to be able to take care of myself." Both of these statements indicate an energized desire with direction of movement toward an expected health outcome. Nonverbal cues can also indicate motivation, such as browsing through lay literature about diet strategies. Likewise, a staff member or student may express a verbal desire to know more about a specific advanced procedure. A nonverbal motivational cue might be expressed by the staff member or student carefully observing a clinician performing an advanced technique, for example.

Measurement of motivation is another aspect to be considered. Subjective self-reports indicate the level of motivation from the learner's perspective. If desired, self-report measurements could be developed for educational programs. Objective measurement of motivation—an indirect measurement—can be quantified through observation of expected behaviors, the consequence of motivation. These behaviors can be observed in increments as the learner moves toward preset realistic health or practice goals.

Motivational Strategies

Finding the spark that motivates the learner to learn is challenging to the educator. The question remains, how does an educator motivate a seemingly unmotivated individual or help a motivated person to remain motivated? As noted earlier, incentives viewed as appeals or inducements to motivation can be either intrinsically or extrinsically generated. Incentives and motivation are both stimuli to action. Bandura (1986) associates motivation with incentives. He notes, however, that intrinsic motivation, although highly appealing, is elusive. Only rarely does motivation occur without extrinsic influence. Green and Kreuter (1999) note that "strictly speaking we can appeal to people's motives, but we cannot motivate them" (p. 30). Extrinsic incentives are used for motivational strategizing in the educational situation.

Cognitive evaluation theory (Ryan & Deci, 2000) posits that knowing how to foster motivation becomes essential because educators cannot rely on intrinsic motivation to promote learning. They note, however, that autonomy and competence are intrinsic motivators that can be fostered by selected teaching strategies. One contemporary educational strategy used in a variety of health disciplines that can be used to promote motivation is **concept mapping**, which enables the learner to integrate previous learning with newly acquired knowledge through diagrammatic "mapping." As a motivational technique, concept mapping facilitates the acquisition of complex new knowledge through visual links that acknowledge previous learning. Learner interest is sustained by perceived competence and autonomy. Concept mapping as a less instructor-regulated learning activity promotes interest and value. A review of the health professions' literature indicates that students and faculty find concept mapping to be a valuable learning exercise (Torre et al., 2007; Wilkes, Cooper, Lewin, & Batts, 1999).

Motivational strategies for the health professional in the role of educator are extrinsically generated through the use of specific incentives. The critical question for the health educator to ask is, "What specific behavior, under what circumstances, in what time frame, is desired by this learner?" Strategizing begins with a systematic assessment of learner motivation, like that outlined in Table 6–1. When an applicable dimension is absent or reduced, incentive strategizing is likely to move the individual away from the desired outcome. When considering strategies to improve learner motivation, Maslow's (1943) hierarchy of needs can also be taken into consideration. An appeal can be made to the innate need for the learner to succeed, known as achievement motivation (Atkinson, 1964).

In the educational situation, clear communication, including clarification of directions and expectations, is critical. Organization of material in a way that makes information meaningful to the learner, environmental manipulation, positive verbal feedback, and providing opportunities for success are motivational strategies proposed by Haggard (1989). Reducing or eliminating barriers to achieve goals is an important aspect of maintaining motivation.

One particular model developed by Keller (1987), the Attention, Relevance, Confidence, and Satisfaction (ARCS) model, focuses on creating and maintaining motivational strategies used for instructional design. This model emphasizes strategies that the educator can use to effect changes in the learner by creating a motivating learning environment:

- **A**ttention introduces opposing positions, case studies, and variable instructional presentations.
- **R**elevance capitalizes on the learners' experiences, usefulness, needs, and personal choices.
- **C**onfidence deals with learning requirements, level of difficulty, expectations, attributions, and sense of accomplishment.
- **S**atisfaction pertains to timely use of a new skill, use of rewards, praise, and self-evaluation.

In motivational strategizing, it would also be beneficial to consider Damrosch's (1991) proposal that client health beliefs, personal vulnerability, efficacy of proposed change, and ability to effect the change are important in patient education efforts.

Beliefs are a major construct proposed by Wright, Watson, and Bell (1996) as the heart of healing in families. Facilitating beliefs can promote a desired change, whereas constraining beliefs can restrict options. Challenging constraining beliefs and promoting facilitating beliefs are, therefore, offered as motivational strategies.

An understanding of the individual's mental representations or beliefs is also foundational to the commonsense model in the representational approach to patient education (Levanthal & Diefenbach, 1991). Beliefs constitute an underacknowledged and understudied phenomenon that needs to be further developed in the education literature in terms of motivational strategizing.

Motivational interviewing is a method of staging readiness to change for the purpose of promoting desired health behaviors. It is an individualized, flexible, patient-centered approach that is supportive, empathetic, and goal directed. It takes into consideration problem solving, confidence in change, and resistance to change. The interviewer seeks to gain knowledge about health beliefs (Rollnick, Mason, & Butler, 1999). This method has been used as a strategy to explore client motivation for adherence to health regimens (Gance-Cleveland, 2005). Zimmerman, Olsen, and Bosworth (2000) developed a readiness to change ruler for motivational interviewing in which the client self-reports preparedness to change. This could be a useful tool for the health professional when in the role of educator in motivational strategizing.

Selected Models and Theories

Compliance and motivation are concepts germane to health behaviors of the learner. The health professional in the role of educator focuses on health education as well as the expected health behaviors.

Health behavior frameworks are blueprints and, as such, serve as tools for the health professional that can be used to maintain desired patient behaviors or promote changes (Syx, 2008). As a consequence, a familiarity with models and theories that describe, explain, or predict health behaviors can increase the range of health-promoting strategies for the health professional educator. When the educator understands these frameworks, the principles inherent in each can be used either to promote compliance to a health regimen or facilitate motivation. This chapter presents an overview of the following selected models and theories: health belief model, self-efficacy theory, protection motivation theory, stages of change model, theory of reasoned action, and the therapeutic alliance model.

Health Belief Model

The original **health belief model** was developed in the 1950s from a social psychology perspective to examine why people did not participate in health screening programs (Rosenstock, 1974). This model was modified by Becker et al. (1974) to address compliance to therapeutic regimens.

The two major premises on which the model is built are the eventual success of disease prevention and curing regimens that involve the clients' willingness to participate and the belief that health is highly valued (Becker, 1990). Both of these premises need to be present for the model to be relevant in explaining health behavior. The model is grounded on the supposition that it is possible to predict health behavior given these three major interacting components: individual perceptions, modifying factors, and likelihood of action (**Figure 6–1**).

Figure 6–1 shows the direction and flow of these interacting components, each of which is further divided into subcomponents:

1. *Individual perceptions:* Subcomponents of perceived susceptibility or perceived severity of a specific disease.

2. *Modifying factors:* Demographic variables (age, sex, race, ethnicity), sociopsychological variables (personality, locus of control, social class, peer and reference group pressure), and structural variables (knowledge about and prior contact with disease). These variables, in conjunction with cues to action (mass media, advice, reminders, illness, reading material), influence the subcomponent of perceived threat of the specific disease.

3. *Likelihood of action:* Subcomponents of perceived benefits of preventive action minus perceived barriers to preventive action.

All of the components are directed toward the likelihood of taking recommended preventive health action as the final phase of the model. In sum, individual perceptions and modifying factors interact. An individual appraisal of the preventive action occurs, which is followed by a prediction of the likelihood of action.

The health belief model has been the predominant explanatory model since the 1970s for uncovering differences in preventive health behaviors as well as differences in preventive use of health services (Langlie, 1977). Used to predict preventive health behavior and to explain sick-role behavior, it has been used widely in health behavior research across disciplines such as medicine, psychology, social behavior, and gerontology. The model has also been broadly used to study patient behaviors in relation to preventive behaviors and acute and chronic illnesses.

Over time, studies have supported the validity of this model. For instance, Turner, Kiviahan, Sloan, and Haselkorn (2007) found that the health belief model was effective in predicting adherence to a medication regimen among patients with multiple sclerosis. Charron-Prachnowik et al. (2001) studied reproductive health behaviors in adolescents with Type 1 diabetes and found that preconception counseling is a motivational cue that triggers positive health actions.

Figure 6–1 The Health Belief Model Used as a Predictor of Preventive Health Behavior

Source: From Becker, M., Drachman, R., & Kirscht, J. (1974). A new approach to explaining sick-role behavior in low-income populations. *American Journal of Public Health, 64*(3), 206. Copyright by American Public Health Association. Reprinted with permission.

Findings from studies such as these can be operationalized through educational programs specific to high-risk populations. In an historical 10-year review of the health belief model literature, Janz and Becker (1984) found that the model was robust in predicting health behaviors, with perceived barriers being the most influential factor. As it applies today, the health professional in the role of educator needs to take into consideration the availability of barrier-free educational resources.

Dutta-Bergman (2004) suggests a relationship between health beliefs, information seeking, and active versus passive learners with implications for type of health education delivery. They indicate that health educators need to be concerned with consumer health-seeking behaviors in the technology age.

Self-Efficacy Theory

Developed from a social-cognitive perspective, the **self-efficacy theory** is based on a person's expectations relative to a specific course of action (Bandura, 1977a, 1977b, 1986, 1997). It is a predictive theory in the sense that it deals with the belief that one can accomplish a specific behavior. The belief of competency and capability relative to certain behaviors is a precursor to expected outcomes. **Figure 6–2** shows an adaptation of Bandura's efficacy expectations model extended to include expected outcomes. In this adapted model, self-efficacy is used as an outcome determinant.

According to Bandura (1986, 1997), self-efficacy is cognitively appraised and processed through the following four principal sources of information:

1. Performance accomplishments evidenced in self-mastery of similarly expected behaviors
2. Vicarious experiences, such as observing successful expected behavior through the modeling of others

3. Verbal persuasion by others who present realistic beliefs that the individual is capable of the expected behavior
4. Emotional arousal through self-judgment of physiological states of distress

Bandura (1986, 1997) notes that the most influential source of efficacy information is that of previous performance accomplishments. Efficacy expectations (expectations relative to a specific course of action) are induced through certain modes. Modes of induction include, but are not limited to, desensitization, self-instruction, exposure, suggestion, and relaxation.

Self-efficacy has proved useful in predicting the course of health behavior. For example, Strachan and Brawley (2009) studied the eating habits of university students and staff. They found that self-efficacy was a strong predictor of healthy eating among this population. In a study designed to measure the effectiveness of a training program for older adults designed to improve memory and self-efficacy West, Bagwell, and Dark-Freudeman (2008) found that memory improvement could be predicted based on self-efficacy scores. The use of the self-efficacy theory for health professionals is particularly relevant in developing educational programs. The behavior-specific predictions of the theory can be used for understanding the likelihood of individuals to participate in existing or projected educational programs. Educational strategies such as modeling, demonstration, and verbal reinforcement parallel modes of self-efficacy induction.

Protection Motivation Theory

Protection motivation theory (Prentice-Dunn & Rogers, 1986) explains behavioral change in terms of threat and coping appraisal. A threat to health is considered a stimulus to protection motivation. This linear theory includes sources of informa-

Figure 6–2 Determinants of Expected Outcomes Using Self-Efficacy Perceptions

Source: Bandura, A. (1977, p. 80). "Determinants of expected outcomes using self-efficacy perceptions," *Social learning theory.* © 1977 Prentice-Hall. Reproduced by permission of Pearson Education, Inc.

tion (environmental and intrapersonal) that are cognitively processed by appraisal of threat and coping to form protective motivation, which leads to intent and ultimately to action.

Influenced by crisis and self-efficacy theories, protection motivation theory has tested antecedents to health behaviors such as drug abuse, AIDS, smoking, sun protection, and drinking behaviors.

Wu, Stanton, Li, Galbraith, and Cole (2005) found that adolescent drug trafficking can be predicted by an overall level of health protection motivation. They suggest that the theory be considered in the design of drug-trafficking prevention programs. Prentice-Dunn, McMath, and Cramer (2009) found that protection motivation theory was useful in creating a "readiness to change" sun-protective intentions among young women.

Evidence-based research can uncover motivational information that can be used to inform health educators in the design of educational programs that specifically target high-risk individuals or groups for selected risk behaviors. The protection motivation theory goes beyond the likelihood of action in the health belief model and self-efficacy intent to health behavior action.

Stages of Change Model

Another model that informs about the phenomenon of health behaviors of the learner is the **stages of change model**, also known as the transtheoretical model (Prochaska & Di Clemente, 1982). Originating from the field of psychology, this model (see **Table 6–2**) was developed around addictive and problem behaviors. Prochaska (1996) notes six distinct time-related stages of change:

1. *Precontemplation:* Individuals have no current intention of changing. Strategies involve simple observations, confrontation, or consciousness raising.
2. *Contemplation:* Individuals accept or realize that they have a problem and begin to think seriously about changing it. Strategies involve increased consciousness raising.
3. *Preparation:* Individuals are planning to take action within the time frame of 1 month. Strategies include a firm and detailed plan for action.
4. *Action:* There is overt/visible modification of behavior. This is the busiest stage, and strategies include commitment to the change, self-

***Table 6–2* Six Stages of Change**

- Precontemplation
- Contemplation
- Preparation
- Action
- Maintenance
- Termination

reward, countering (substitute behaviors), creating a friendly environment, and supportive relationships.

5. *Maintenance:* Maintenance is a difficult stage to achieve and may last 6 months to a lifetime. There are common challenges to this stage, including overconfidence, daily temptation, and relapse self-blame. The strategies in this stage are the same for the action stage.
6. *Termination:* This stage occurs when the problem no longer presents any temptation. However, some experts note that termination does not occur, only that maintenance becomes less vigilant.

The extent to which people are motivated and ready to change is seen as an important construct. It is useful in health care to stage the client's intentions and behaviors for change as well as strategies that will enable completion of the specific stage. More recent use of the model in health research has focused on its value in health promotion and the processes by which people decide to change (or not to change) behaviors.

The stages of change model has been used to investigate health behaviors such as sun protection (Prentice-Dunn et al., 2009) and exercise (Lowther, Mutrie, & Scott, 2007). Paul and Sneed (2004) examined readiness for behavior change in patients with heart failure and noted that it is "not realistic to expect patients to make changes that they are not prepared to make" (p. 313). This popular model can be used with children and adults, which has implications for a variety of educational settings. Recently, Kelly (2005) developed the commitment to health scale that shows potential as a research instrument for measuring the final stage of change. This stage could be viewed as an educational outcome in terms of health behaviors of the learner.

Theory of Reasoned Action

The **theory of reasoned action** emerged from a research program that began in the 1950s and is concerned with prediction and understanding of any form of human behavior within a social context (Ajzen & Fishbein, 1980). It is based on the premise that humans behave in a way that is consistent with their beliefs (Fishbein, 2008). This theory suggests that a person's behavior can be predicted by examining the individual's attitudes about the behavior as well as the individual's beliefs about how others might respond to the behavior. For example, if using this theory to predict how a client might respond to a weight reduction plan, it would not only be vital to consider the client's beliefs about food and exercise but also to examine what the client thinks about how the people around him would view his attempts to lose weight. It is important to note that "reasoned action" in this theory is not emotion free but rather based on beliefs that are influenced by emotion and mood (Fishbein, 2008) This theory is shown as a sequential model in **Figure 6–3**.

In a two-pronged linear approach, specific behavior is determined by (1) beliefs, attitude toward the behavior, and intention; and (2) motivation to comply with influential persons known as referents, subjective norms, and intention. The person's intention to perform can be measured by relative weights of attitude and subjective norms.

McGahee, Kemp, and Tingen (2000) suggest the use of the theory as a framework for conducting empirical studies for smoking prevention in preteens, which has implications for educational program development. Hanson (2005) investigated ethnic differences in cigarette smoking intention among female teenagers and found attitude to be the greatest predictor of intention to smoke in Hispanic as well as non-Hispanic White teenagers.

The theory of reasoned action is useful in predicting health behaviors, particularly for educators who want to understand the attitudinal context within which behaviors are likely to change. Health professionals need to take beliefs, attitudinal factors, and subjective norms into consideration when designing educational programs relating to intent to change a specific health behavior.

Therapeutic Alliance Model

Barofsky's (1978) **therapeutic alliance model** addresses a shift in power from the provider to a learning partnership in which collaboration and negotiation with the consumer are key. A therapeutic alliance is formed between the caregiver and receiver in which each participant in this affiliation is viewed as having equal power. The client is viewed as active and responsible, with an outcome expectation of self-care. The shift toward self-determination and control over one's own life is fundamental to this model (**Figure 6–4**).

The therapeutic alliance model compares the components of compliance, adherence, and alliance. According to Barofsky (1978), change is needed in treatment determinants—change from coercion in compliance and from conforming in adherence to collaboration in alliance. The power in the relationship between the participants is equalized by alliance. The role of the patient is neither passive nor rebellious, but rather active and responsible. The expected outcomes are not compliant dependence or counterdependence, but responsible self-care.

Figure 6–3 Factors Determining a Person's Behavior

Note: Arrows indicate the direction of influence.

Source: From Ajzen, I., & Fishbein, M. (1980, p. 8). "Factors Determining a Person's Behavior" figure from *Understanding attitudes and predicting social behavior.* © 1980 Prentice-Hall, Inc. Reproduced by permission of Pearson Education, Inc.

Although not originally developed as an educational model, the usefulness of this model to the health professional educator is nevertheless acknowledged in the partnership of learning. This interpersonal model is appropriate in the educational process when shifting the focus from the patient as a passive-dependent learner to one of an active learner. It serves as a guide to refocus education efforts on collaboration rather than on compliance. The health professional as educator and the patient as learner form an alliance with the goal of self-care.

Hobden (2006), in a recent exploration of the concepts of compliance and adherence, notes that these terms have a negative connotation. Instead, this author suggests emphasizing the consultative process known as **concordance**, which is "consultation that allows mutual respect for the patient's and professional's beliefs, and allows negotiation to take place about the best course of action for the patient" (p. 258). She notes there is a shift in the balance of power from the professional to the patient. Although concordance should lead to improved health outcomes, the focus is on the process.

Motivational interviewing also interfaces with the therapeutic alliance model. Duran (2003) notes that successful motivational interviewing

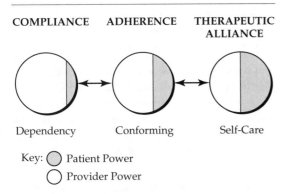

Figure 6–4 Continuum of the Therapeutic Alliance Model

COMPLIANCE   ADHERENCE   THERAPEUTIC
ALLIANCE

Dependency   Conforming   Self-Care

Key: ● Patient Power
○ Provider Power

takes place in an atmosphere of the client being understood and respected and is collaborative in nature with the highest priority placed on the client's autonomy and freedom of choice.

Models for Health Education

Selection of models for educational use can be made with respect to (1) similarities and dissimilarities, (2) the health professional's agreement with model conceptualizations, and (3) functional utility.

Similarities and Dissimilarities of Models

Models may be seen as so similar that there would be a negligible difference in choosing one over the other, or they may be seen as so dissimilar that one would be inappropriate for a specific educational purpose. A cursory comparative analysis of the different frameworks reveals that the self-efficacy theory and the theory of reasoned action are similar in that they focus on the predictions or expectations of specific behaviors. The theories lend themselves more easily to less complex model testing than the

health belief model because the former are more linear in conceptualization. Specificity of behaviors may aid in targeting outcomes of educational programs. The stages of change model is similar to the self-efficacy theory and the theory of reasoned action in the sense that these models focus on intent. The stages of change model appears to be less complicated and does not take into account personal characteristics or experiences. It differs from the self-efficacy theory, the protection motivation theory, and the theory of reasoned action in that change is time relevant with implications for educational interventions.

Protection motivation theory is similar to the theory of reasoned action in the sense that information is cognitively processed, followed by intent or commitment to action and the health behavior.

The health belief model, self-efficacy theory, protection motivation theory, and theory of reasoned action are similar in that they acknowledge factors such as experiences, perceptions, or beliefs relative to the individual and factors external to the individual that can modify health behaviors. These frameworks also recognize the multidimensional nature, complexity, and probability of health behaviors. One major difference between the health belief model and the protection motivation theory is that the latter has a component of fear appraisal and focuses on a specific vulnerability rather than general susceptibility to illness (Prentice-Dunn & Rogers, 1986).

All of the models acknowledge the importance of the client in decision making with respect to health behaviors. The differences relate to client focus, the relative importance of modifying factors, specificity of behavior, and outcomes.

The most dissimilar model is the therapeutic alliance model. Although it is relatively narrow in scope, its simplicity and parsimony are strengths. When applied to the educational arena, the educator–learner relationship is the critical factor. Addressing potentially frustrating patient education situations such as noncompliance, Hochbaum (1980) noted that patient educators, when frustrated, "are unable to understand the apparently irrational and self-destructive action of their patients, and sometimes throw their hands up in despair, bedeviled by the seeming irrationality of the patient's behavior. ... But this behavior may be altogether rational from the patient's perspective" (p. 7). Understanding of the client as learner can be uncovered in the therapeutic alliance model.

Educator Agreement With Model Conceptualizations

Health professionals as educators have belief systems, which may or may not agree with some of the tenets of each of the models presented. The choice of a model, therefore, can be based on the educator's level of agreement with salient factors in each framework.

Likelihood of action is best addressed by the health belief model, while attaining positive health outcomes is the focus of the protection motivation theory. Attitude and intention are best viewed through the theory of reasoned action. Belief in one's capabilities is best addressed by self-efficacy theory, and the therapeutic alliance model is best used for reduction of noncompliance through an educator–learner collaboration. Staging the individual's readiness for change and developing strategies for interventions are helpful in designing educational programs with the stages of change model.

Through in-depth analysis of each model, the attention of the educator may be drawn to other factors as well. Ultimately, the model or models that fit best with the educator's own beliefs are more likely to be chosen.

Functional Utility of Models

Model selection for educational purposes can also be based on functional utility. Questions to

be asked to determine functional utility are as follows:

- Who is the target learner?
- What is the focus of the learning?
- When is the optimal time?
- Where is the process to be carried out?

The question of *who* the learner is deals with whether the target learner is the individual, family, or group. The health belief model, self-efficacy theory, protection motivation theory, stages of change model, and theory of reasoned action can be used across the range of these target learners. The important notion for the health professional as educator to remember is the probability of individual variation. Another consideration in terms of the target learner is categorical groups, such as those considered at high risk and those diagnosed with acute or chronic illnesses.

The functional use of the models can also be determined by the content needed, the timing of the educational experience, and the setting in which the learning is to take place. *What* is needed relates to the focus of the learning and addresses the content to be taught, such as disease processes, specific disease, treatment, adaptation techniques, promotion of wellness, expectations of specific health practices, or focus on self-care.

The question of *when* is one of optimal timing and refers to the readiness of the learner, a mutually convenient time, and prevention of untimely delays in moving toward a desired goal. Although considered important in the context of health education, this critical factor has received little specific reference in terms of health promotion models. Except for the stages of change model, timing is an often neglected factor in the models discussed. It is apparent that determining optimal time can be a motivational incentive in terms of meeting the health needs of the learner.

Addressing the question of *where* the educational process is to be carried out is another aspect of functional utility. The settings of home, workplace, school, institution, or specific community locations are all options. All of the models discussed in this chapter lend themselves to these diverse settings.

Integration of Models for Use in Education

Theories provide blueprints for interventions. From the previous discussion, it is clear that the integration of various components of health behavior models is advantageous in the educational process. When salient factors are taken into consideration in light of developmental stages of the learner, an integrated motivational model of learning in health promotion could emerge.

Recent literature proposes model integration. For example, Gebhardt and Maes (2001) advocate for a multitheory approach to promote health behaviors. Cautioning against the use of unidirectional and nondynamic views of behavioral change, they propose an integrative approach using goal theories and stages of change. Poss (2001) developed a new model synthesizing the health belief model and the theory of reasoned action, noting that a synthesized model is appropriate for the study of persons from varying cultural backgrounds. The development of new models and/ or the revision of older models is a necessary step in the evolution and delivery of health care, and it necessarily affects the educator concerned with motivational behaviors of the learner.

Salient health promotion factors that health professional educators can use in a multitheory approach to health education include, but are not limited to, level of knowledge, attitudes, values, beliefs, perceptions, level of anxiety, self-confidence, skills mastery, past experiences, intention, physiological capacity, sociocultural enablers, environment, educator–learner alliance, resources and reinforcements, mutual and realistic goal setting, hierarchy of needs, quality of life, and voluntary participation in learning.

Developmental stages of the learner incorporate principles of pedagogy (teaching children), andragogy (teaching adults), and gerogogy (teaching older adults) to meet the needs of the learner. A more comprehensive and holistic model for the health professional as educator could emerge when learning is viewed along a unidirectional developmental continuum, in combination with salient health promotion factors. (For a discussion on educational approaches with learners at different stages of development, see Chapter 5.)

The Role of Health Professional as Educator in Health Promotion

Health professionals are in a position to promote healthy lifestyles. Combining content specific to their area of practice and knowledge from educational theories and health behavior models allows for an integrated approach to shaping the health behaviors of individuals through education. The roles of the health professional as educator include facilitator of change, contractor, organizer, and evaluator.

Facilitator of Change

The goal of the health professional as educator is, of course, to promote health. Health education and health promotion are integral to this effort. At the same time, the health professional as educator is an important facilitator of change. When learning is viewed as an intervention, it needs to be considered in the context of other interventions that will effect change. As far back as 1987, deTornay and Thompson proposed that explaining, analyzing, dividing complex skills, demonstrating, practicing, asking questions, and providing closure are effective in facilitating change in the learning situation.

Contractor

Contracting has been a popular means of facilitating learning. Informal or formal contracts can delineate and promote learning objectives. **Educational contracting** involves stating mutual goals to be accomplished, devising an agreed-upon plan of action, evaluating the plan, and deriving alternatives. (See the discussion of learning contracts in Chapter 10.) The plan of action needs to be as specific as possible and include the who, what, when, where, and how of the learning process. Responsibilities that are clearly stated aid in evaluating the plan and directing plan revisions.

In light of the changing healthcare system, there needs to be an emphasis on client–health professional partnerships because clients are expected to take increasingly more responsibility and control in the decisions that affect their own health. Educational contracting is the key to informed decision making.

When education is viewed in the context of the client, rather than the client in the context of education, learning is individualized. The fit between the client as learner and the health professional as educator has the capacity to facilitate learning. Indeed, the goodness of fit between these two educational participants can be a motivating factor. Do the client and educator share an understanding of backgrounds or language? Is there a mutual understanding of goal setting? Are health beliefs respected?

A contract involves a trusting relationship. In a mutually satisfying teacher–learner relationship system, trust is a key ingredient. The learner trusts that the health professional possesses a respectable, current body of theoretically based and clinically applicable knowledge. The health professional needs to be approachable, trustworthy, and culturally sensitive because the learner's own health status is often valued as a private matter. In turn, the health professional trusts that when the client enters into an agreement, the learner will demonstrate behaviors that will be health promoting. Newman and Brown (1986) list the following elements as part of the ideal relationship: Both parties have trust and respect; the teacher assumes the student can learn and is sensitive to individual needs; and both feel free to learn and make mistakes.

Organizer

Organization of the learning situation, including manipulation of materials and space, sequential organization of content from simple to complex, and determining priority of subject matter, is a task taken on by the health professional when in the role of educator. Organization of learning material decreases obstacles to learning. Attendance at educational programs or individual sessions can be organized around the target learner as well as significant others to facilitate the learning process and promote motivation to learn.

Evaluator

Educational programs, like other healthcare projects, need to be accountable to the learner or consumer of the health service. This accountability is ensured by evaluation in the form of outcomes. Self-evaluation, learner evaluation, organization evaluation, and peer evaluation are not new concepts. Evaluative processes are an integral part of all learning. Application of knowledge that improves the health of individuals, families, and groups is the evaluative measure of learning.

State of the Evidence

The evidence is less than adequate for implementing healthcare interventions that specifically address the variables of compliance and motivation as related to health behaviors of the learner. With the explosion of interest in evidence-based practice, further conceptually based research that identifies, describes, explains, and predicts health behaviors of the learner needs to be conducted.

Healthy People 2010 (U.S. Department of Health and Human Services, 2000) has established two major goals: (1) to increase the quality and years of healthy life, and (2) to eliminate health disparities among different segments of the population. This document sets the stage for the health professional educator to use theoretically based strategies to promote desirable health behaviors of the learner.

Carter and Kulbok (2002), in an integrative review of motivational research, conclude that no clear definition of motivation exists, certain populations have been underrepresented in motivational research, and that motivation may not be able to be effectively measured. They challenge researchers and practitioners to carefully examine the role of motivation in influencing health behaviors. Zinn (2005) argues that there is insufficient data to explain why people take health risks and that more research concerning how an individual's knowledge is shaped and how it affects health behaviors is needed. A clarion call is needed for both qualitative and quantitative conceptually grounded research to be infused into the teaching–learning process. Forums for evidence-based learning ought to be widely established and should include discussion relative to compliance, motivation, and health behaviors of the learner.

Summary

Critical components of this chapter include a discussion of concepts of compliance and motivation, assessment of level of learner motivation, identification of incentives and obstacles that affect motivation and compliance, and discussion of axioms of motivation relevant to learning. An overview of selected health behavior frameworks and their influence on learning have been compared and contrasted. In light of the role of health professional educators, strategies that facilitate health behaviors of the learner have been outlined and the need for continued evidence-based practice has been proposed.

When information is imparted, accepted, and applied, the foundation is set for change in health behaviors. When people are motivated and know that they can make a difference in their own lives, a barrier to health has been lifted.

REVIEW QUESTIONS

1. How are the terms *compliance*, *adherence*, and *motivation* defined?
2. How do the terms defined in question 1 relate to one another?
3. What are the three major motivational factors?
4. Which axioms (premises) are involved in promoting motivation of the learner?
5. What are the six parameters for a comprehensive motivational assessment of the learner?
6. What are six major models or theories used to describe, explain, or predict health behaviors?
7. Which models/theories are used to facilitate motivation, and which ones are used to promote compliance to a therapeutic healthcare regimen?
8. What are the basic concepts particular to each model or theory?
9. What are the similarities and differences among the models with respect to who is the target audience, what is the focus of the learning, and what are the implications for education?
10. What is the role of the health professional in shaping health behaviors of the learner?

CASE STUDY

"Keeping our employees healthy is not only the right thing to do, it is good for the bottom line." With this directive from the chief executive officer, Marie DeSantis, the staff in the Office of Human Resources at Jefferson Pharmaceuticals developed a "Let's Get Healthy" initiative for its 500 employees. Weight Watchers, a smoking cessation program, and yoga classes were brought on site and offered free of charge to all employees. Nicotine patches were offered at 50% of cost and gym memberships were provided at a significant reduction in price. The cafeteria began offering healthy, low-calorie meals and a walking club was started to support staff who chose to exercise before and after work or during lunch hours. Staff who were willing to submit an individual health plan and agreed to participate in one or more of the company's available health programs were offered a 10% discount in their health premiums.

One year after the start of Let's Get Healthy, the initiative is in trouble. Although initially met with a great deal of enthusiasm, staff compliance has declined. Attendance at Weight Watchers and smoking cessation classes is episodic and yoga classes were canceled because of lack of interest. Anecdotal information suggests that although the company has renewed gym memberships for about 20% of the staff, few are actually using them on a regular basis. Convinced that Let's Get Healthy is a good idea, the company has hired a health educator to evaluate the program and make recommendations for improvement.

1. Using one of the identified models and theories of compliance (health belief model, self-efficacy theory, protection motivation theory, stages of change model, theory of reasoned action, or therapeutic alliance model), provide a possible explanation for why the staff members at Jefferson Pharmaceuticals are not participating in the Let's Get Healthy campaign.
2. What motivational strategies did the human resources staff use in Let's Get Healthy? Why do you think these strategies did not work?
3. Do you think that if a health education campaign was offered in conjunction with the Let's Get Healthy program, the results would have been different?

References

Ajzen, I., & Fishbein, M. (1980). *Understanding attitudes and predicting social behavior*. Englewood Cliffs, NJ: Prentice Hall.

Atkinson, J. W. (1964). *An introduction to motivation*. Princeton, NJ: Van Nostrand.

Bandura, A. (1977a). Self-efficacy: Toward a unifying theory of behavioral change. *Psychological Review, 84*(2), 191–215.

Bandura, A. (1977b). *Social learning theory*. Englewood Cliffs, NJ: Prentice Hall.

Bandura, A. (1986). *Social foundations of thought and action: A social cognitive theory*. Englewood Cliffs, NJ: Prentice Hall.

Bandura, A. (1997). *Self-efficacy: The exercise of control*. New York: Freeman.

Barofsky, I. (1978). Compliance, adherence and the therapeutic alliance: Steps in the development of self-care. *Social Science and Medicine, 12*, 369–376.

Becker, M. (1990). Theoretical models of adherence and strategies for improving adherence. In S. A. Shumaker,

E. B. Schron, & J. K. Ockene (Eds.), *The handbook of human health behavior* (pp. 5–43). New York: Springer.

Becker, M. W., Drachman, R. H., & Kirscht, J. P. (1974). A new approach to explaining sick-role behavior in low-income populations. *American Journal of Public Health, 64*(3), 205–216.

Carter, K. F., & Kulbok, P. A. (2002). Motivation for health behaviours: A systematic review of the nursing literature. *Journal of Advanced Nursing, 40*(3), 316–330.

Charron-Prachnowik, D., Sereika, S., Becker, D., Jacober, S., Mansfield, J., White, N., et al. (2001). Reproductive health beliefs and behaviors in teens with diabetes: Application of the expanded health belief model. *Pediatric Diabetes, 2*, 30–39.

Damrosch, S. (1991). General strategies for motivating people to change their behavior. *Nursing Clinics of North America, 26*(4), 833–843.

deTornay, R., & Thompson, M. A. (1987). *Strategies for teaching nursing* (3rd ed.). New York: Wiley.

Duran, L. S. (2003). Motivating health: Strategies for the nurse practitioner. *Journal of the American Academy of Nurse Practitioners, 15*(5), 200–203.

Dutta-Bergman, M. J. (2004). Primary sources of health information: Comparisons in the domain of health attitudes, health cognitions, and health behaviors. *Health Communication, 16*(3), 273–288.

Eraker, S. A., Kirscht, J. P., & Becker, M. H. (1984). Understanding and improving patient compliance. *Annals of Internal Medicine, 100*, 258–268.

Erlen, J. (2006, Winter). Adherence is a concept. *Pitt Nurse*, 15–17.

Fink, D. L. (1976). Tailoring in the consensual regimen. In D. L. Sackett & R. B. Haynes (Eds.), *Compliance with therapeutic regimens*. Baltimore: Johns Hopkins University Press.

Fishbein, M. (2008). A reasoned action approach to health promotion. *Medical Decision Making, 28*, 834–844.

Gance-Cleveland, B. (2005). Motivational interviewing as a strategy to increase families' adherence to treatment regimens. *Journal of Specialists in Pediatric Nursing, 10*(3), 151–155.

Gebhardt, W. A., & Maes, S. (2001). Integrating social-psychological frameworks for health behavior research. *American Journal of Health Behavior, 25*(6), 528–536.

Green, L. W., & Kreuter, M. W. (1999). *Health promotion planning: An educational and ecological approach* (3rd ed.). Mountain View, CA: Mayfield.

Haggard, A. (1989). *Handbook of patient education*. Rockville, MD: Aspen.

Hanson, M. S. (2005). An examination of ethnic differences in cigarette smoking intention among female teenagers. *Journal of the American Academy of Nurse Practitioners, 17*(4), 149–155.

Heiby, E. M., Lukens, C. L., & Frank, M. R. (2005). The health compliance model. *Behavior Analyst Today, 6*(1), 27–36.

Helm, D. W., & Harrington, N. G. (2004). Patient accounts for non-compliance with diabetes self-care regimens and physician compliance-gaining response. *Patient Education and Counseling, 55*, 281–292.

Hobden, A. (2006). Concordance: A widely used term, but what does it mean? *British Journal of Community Nursing, 11*(6), 257–260.

Hochbaum, G. M. (1980). *Patient counseling vs. patient teaching: Education for self-care*. Rockville, MD: Aspen.

Janz, N. K., & Becker, M. H. (1984). The health belief model: A decade later. *Health Education Quarterly, 11*(1), 1–47.

Keller, J. M. (1987). Development and use of the ARCS model of instructional design. *Journal of Instructional Development, 10*(3), 2–10.

Kelly, C. W. (2005). Commitment to health scale. *Journal of Nursing Measurement, 13*(3), 219–229.

Kessels, R. P. C. (2003). Patients' memory for medical information. *Journal of the Royal Society of Medicine, 96*, 219–222.

Kort, M. (1987). Motivation: The challenge for today's health promoter. *Canadian Nurse, 83*(9), 16–18.

Langlie, J. K. (1977). Social networks, health beliefs, and preventive health behavior. *Journal of Health and Social Behavior, 18*, 244–260.

Levanthal, H. C., & Cameron, L. (1987). Behavior theories and the problem of compliance. *Patient Education and Counseling, 10*, 117–138.

Levanthal, H. C., & Diefenbach, M. (1991). The active side of illness cognition. In J. A. Skelton & R. T. Croyle (Eds.), *Mental representation in health and illness* (pp. 245–271). New York: Springer-Verlag.

Lewin, K. (1935). *A dynamic theory of personality*. New York: McGraw-Hill.

Ley, P. (1979). Memory for medical information. *British Journal of Social and Clinical Psychology, 18*, 245–255.

Lowther, M., Mutrie, N., & Scott, E. M. (2007). Identifying key processes of exercise behavior change associated with movement through the stages of exercise behaviour change. *Journal of Health Psychology, 12*, 261–271.

Maslow, A. H. (1943). A theory of human motivation. *Psychological Review, 50*(4), 371–396.

McGahee, T. W., Kemp, V., & Tingen, M. (2000). A theoretical model for smoking prevention studies in preteen children. *Pediatric Nursing, 26*(2), 135–138, 141.

Mishel, M. H. (1990). Reconceptualization of the uncertainty in illness theory. *Image: Journal of Nursing Scholarship, 22*(4), 256–262.

Munro, S., Lewin, S., Swart, T., & Volmink, J. (2007). A review of health behavior theories: How useful are these for developing interventions to promote long-term medication adherence for TB and HIV/AIDS. *BMC Public Health, 7*, 104. Retrieved August 3, 2009, from http://www.biomedcentral.com/1471-2458/7/104

Newman, F., & Brown, R. (1986). Creating optimal conditions for learning. *Educational Horizons, 64*(4), 188–189.

Paul, S., & Sneed, N. V. (2004). Strategies for behavior change in patients with heart failure. *American Journal of Critical Care, 13*(4), 305–313.

Pender, N. (1996). *Health promotion in nursing practice* (3rd ed.). Upper Saddle River, NJ: Pearson Education.

Peplau, H. E. (1979). *The psychotherapy of Hildegard E. Peplau*. Madison, WI: Atwood.

Politi, M. C., Han, K. J., & Col, N. F. (2007). Communicating the uncertainty of harms and benefits of medical interventions. *Medical Decision Making, 27*, 681–695.

Poss, J. E. (2001). Developing a new model for cross-cultural research: Synthesizing the health belief model and the theory of reasoned action. *Advances in Nursing Science, 23*(4), 1–15.

Prentice-Dunn, S., McMath, B. F., & Cramer, R. J. (2009). Protection motivation theory and change in sun protective behavior. *Journal of Health Behavior, 14*, 297–305.

Prentice-Dunn, S., & Rogers, W. R. (1986). Protection motivation theory and preventive health: Beyond the health belief model. *Health Education Research, 3*, 153–161.

Prochaska, J. O. (1996, September). Just do it isn't enough: Change comes in stages. *Tufts University Special Report Diet and Nutrition Letter*.

Prochaska, J. O., & Di Clemente, C. C. (1982). Trans-theoretical therapy: Towards a more integrative model of change. *Psychotherapy, Theory, and Practice, 19*(3), 276–288.

Redman, B. K. (2001). *The practice of patient education* (9th ed.). St. Louis, MO: Mosby.

Redman, B. K. (2007). *The practice of patient education: A case study approach* (10th ed.). St. Louis, MO: Mosby.

Rollnick, S., Mason, P., & Butler, C. (1999). *Health behavior change: A guide for practitioners*. London: Churchill Livingstone.

Rosenstock, I. M. (1974). Historical origins of the health belief model. In M. H. Becker (Ed.), *The health belief model and personal health behavior*. Thorofare, NJ: Slack.

Rosner, F. (2006). Patient noncompliance: Causes and symptoms. *Mount Sinai Journal of Medicine, 73*, 553–559.

Rosno, E. A., Steele, R. G., Johnston, C. A., & Aylward, B. S. (2008). Parental locus of control: Associations to adherence and outcomes in the treatment of pediatric overweight. *Children's Health Care, 37*(2), 126–144.

Rotter, J. B. (1954). *Social learning theory and clinical psychology*. Englewood Cliffs, NJ: Prentice Hall.

Ryan, R. M., & Deci, E. L. (2000). Intrinsic and extrinsic motivations: Classic definitions and new directions. *Contemporary Educational Psychology, 25*, 54–67.

Shapiro, D. E., Boggs, S. R., Melamed, B. G., & Graham-Pole, J. (1992). The effect of varied physician affect on recall, anxiety, and perceptions in women at risk for breast cancer: An analogue study. *Health Psychology, 11*(1), 61–66.

Shillinger, F. (1983). Locus of control: Implications for nursing practice. *Image: Journal of Nursing Scholarship, 15*(2), 58–63.

Sin-Jae, L., Sug-Joon, A., & Tae-Woo, K. (2008). Patient compliance and locus of control in orthodontic treatment: A prospective study. *American Journal of Orthodontics and Dentofacial Orthopedics, 133*(3), 354–358.

Steckel, S. B. (1982). Predicting, measuring, implementing and following up on patient compliance. *Nursing Clinics of North America, 17*(3), 491–497.

Stephenson, P. L. (2006). Before the teaching begins: Managing patient anxiety prior to providing education. *Clinical Journal of Oncology Nursing, 10*(2), 241–245.

Strachan, S. M., & Brawley, L. R. (2009). Healthy-eater identity and self efficacy predict healthy eating: A prospective view. *Journal of Health Psychology, 14*, 684–695.

Syx, R. (2008). The practice of patient education: The theoretical perspective. *Orthopaedic Nursing, 27*(1), 50–56.

Torre, D. M., Daley, B., Stark-Schweitzer, T., Siddartha, S., Petkova, J., & Seibert, M. (2007). A qualitative evaluation of medical student learning using concept maps. *Medical Teacher, 29*, 949–955.

Turner, A. P., Kiviahan, T. R., Sloan, A. P., & Haselkorn, J. K. (2007). Predicting ongoing adherence to disease modifying therapies in multiple sclerosis: Utility of the health beliefs model. *Multiple Sclerosis, 13*, 1146–1152.

U.S. Department of Health and Human Services. (2000). *Healthy People 2010* (Conference edition). Washington, DC: U.S. Government Printing Office.

Wallston, K. A., Wallston, B. S., & DeVellis, R. (1978, Spring). Development of the multidimensional health locus of control (MHLC) scales. *Health Education Monographs*, 160–170.

Ward-Collins, D. (1998). Noncompliant: Isn't there a better way to say it? *American Journal of Nursing, 98*(5), 17–31.

West, R. L., Bagwell, D. K., & Dark-Freudeman, A. (2008). Self efficacy and memory aging: The impact of memory intervention based on self efficacy. *Aging, Neuropsychology and Cognition, 15*, 302–329.

Wilkes, L., Cooper, K., Lewin, J., & Batts, J. (1999). Concepts mapping: Promoting science learning in BN learners in Australia. *Journal of Continuing Education in Nursing, 30*(1), 37–44.

Wright, L. M., Watson, W. L., & Bell, J. M. (1996). *Beliefs: The heart of healing in families and illness*. New York: Basic Books.

Wu, Y., Stanton, B. F., Li, X., Galbraith, J., & Cole, M. L. (2005). Protection motivation theory and adolescent drug trafficking: Relationship between health motivation and longitudinal risk involvement. *Journal of Pediatric Psychology, 30*(2), 127–137.

Yach, D. S. (2003). *Adherence to long term therapies: Evidence for action*. Geneva: World Health Organization.

Zimmerman, G. L., Olsen, C. G., & Bosworth, M. F. (2000). A stages of change approach to helping patients change behavior. *American Family Physician, 61*(5), 1409–1416.

Zinn, J. O. (2005). The biographical approach: A better way to understand behaviour in health and illness. *Health, Risk, and Society, 7*(1), 1–9.

Chapter 7

Literacy in the Adult Client Population

Susan B. Bastable

KEY TERMS

❑ literacy
❑ literate
❑ illiterate

❑ low literacy
❑ functional illiteracy
❑ health literacy

❑ reading   ❑ comprehension
❑ readability   ❑ numeracy

OBJECTIVES

After completing this chapter, the reader will be able to

1. Define the terms *literacy, illiteracy, health literacy, low literacy, functional illiteracy, reading, readability, comprehension,* and *numeracy.*
2. Identify the magnitude of the literacy problem in the United States.
3. Describe the characteristics of those individuals at risk for having difficulty with reading and comprehension of written and oral language.
4. Discuss common myths and assumptions about people with illiteracy.
5. Identify clues that are indicators of reading and writing deficiencies.
6. Assess the impact of illiteracy and low literacy on client motivation and compliance with healthcare regimens.
7. Recognize the role of the health professional as educator in the assessment of clients' literacy skills.
8. Use specific formulas and tests to critically analyze the readability and comprehension levels of printed materials and the reading skills of clients.
9. Describe specific guidelines for writing effective education materials.
10. Outline various teaching strategies useful in educating clients with low literacy skills.
11. Recognize the research and policy-making issues that must be addressed to solve the health literacy problem.

Over the past two decades, educators as well as government officials, employers, and media experts have focused interest on and expressed concern about literacy in the U.S. population. Adult illiteracy continues to be a major problem in this country despite public and private efforts at all levels to address the issue through testing of literacy skills and development of literacy training programs.

Today, the fact remains that many individuals do not possess the basic literacy abilities to function effectively in a technologically complex society. Many adult citizens have difficulty reading and comprehending information well enough to be

able to perform such common tasks as filling out job and insurance applications, interpreting bus schedules and road signs, completing tax forms, applying for a driver's license, registering to vote, and ordering from a restaurant menu (Weiss, 2003).

In the early 1980s, President Reagan launched the National Adult Literacy Initiative, which was followed by the United Nations' declaration of 1990 as International Literacy Year (Belton, 1991; Wallerstein, 1992). In 1992, the U.S. Department of Education conducted the National Adult Literacy Survey (NALS). The results of this survey revealed a shockingly high prevalence of illiteracy in this country (Weiss, 2003; Weiss et al., 2005; Zarcadoolas, Pleasant, & Greer, 2006). Since then, awareness about illiteracy, thought previously to be a problem mainly confined to developing countries, has taken on new meaning (Lasater & Mehler, 1998; Schwartzberg, VanGeest, & Wang, 2004).

However, in light of the relatively recent attention given to this problem in the last 20 years, it must be acknowledged that Literacy Volunteers of America and Lauback Literacy International have for many decades served as advocates for the most marginalized adult population in this country and around the globe. Today, ProLiteracy Worldwide, recently formed from the merger of these two entities, is the world's largest organization for adult literacy. It operates 1,200 literacy programs across the United States and partners with 120 other organizations in 62 countries worldwide. Syracuse, New York, has been the birthplace of all three of these organizations, and central New York is now recognized as the capital of the literacy movement. America's literacy problem has become a national crisis because for too long this country has ignored those who are unseen and unheard (Wedgeworth, 2007).

Particularly in the past 10 years as a result of the NALS report, the health professions literature has focused significant attention on the effects of patient illiteracy on healthcare delivery and health outcomes. Today, the emphasis is on health literacy—that is, the extent to which Americans can read and comprehend health information well enough to function successfully in a healthcare environment and make appropriate decisions for themselves. Although a great deal more research needs to be done on the causes and effects associated with poor health literacy as well as the methods available to screen and teach patients, much has been learned about the magnitude and consequences of the health literacy problem (Friedman & Hoffman-Goetz, 2008; Gazmararian, Curran, Parker, Bernhardt, & DeBuono, 2005; Paasche-

Orlow & Wolf, 2007a; Pignone, DeWalt, Sheridan, Berkman, & Lohr, 2005).

With respect to the subject of literacy, the health professional's attention specifically focuses on adult client populations. Literacy levels are not an issue in teaching staff or students because of their level of formal education. However, literacy levels remain a concern if the audience for in-service programs includes less educated, more culturally and socioeconomically diverse support staff (Hess, 1998), or if a member of the audience has been diagnosed with a learning disability, such as dyslexia.

What must be of particular concern to the healthcare industry are the numbers of consumers who are illiterate, functionally illiterate, or marginally literate. Researchers have discovered that people with poor reading and comprehension skills have disproportionately higher medical costs, increased number of hospitalizations and readmissions, and more perceived physical and psychosocial problems than do literate persons (Baker, Parker, Williams, & Clark, 1998; Baker, Williams, Parker, Gazmararian, & Nurss, 1999; DeWalt, Berkman, Sheridan, Lohr, & Pignone, 2004; Sudore & Yoffe, et al., 2006; Weiss, 2003; Weiss et al., 2005).

In today's world of managed care, the literacy problem is perceived to have grave consequences. Clients are expected to assume greater responsibility for self-care and health promotion, yet this expanded role depends on increased knowledge and skills. If people with low literacy abilities cannot fully benefit from the type and amount of information they are typically given, they cannot be expected to maintain health and manage independently. The result is a significant negative impact on the cost of health care and the quality of life (Kogut, 2004; Levy & Royne, 2009; Pignone et al., 2005; Williams, Davis, Parker, & Weiss, 2002; Wood, Kettinger, & Lessick, 2007).

Traditionally, healthcare professionals have relied heavily on printed education materials as a cost-effective and time-efficient means to communicate health messages. An assumption was made that the written materials commonly distributed to clients were sufficient to ensure informed consent for tests and procedures, to promote compliance with treatment regimens, and to guarantee adherence to discharge instructions.

Only recently have healthcare providers begun to recognize that the scientific and technical terminology inherent in the ubiquitous printed teaching aids is a bewildering set of written instructions little understood by the majority of people (Ache, 2009; Adkins, Elkins, & Singh, 2001; Morrow, Weiner, Steinley, Young, & Murray, 2007). Kessels (2003) points out that 40–80% of medical information provided by health professionals is forgotten immediately, not only because medical terminology is too difficult to understand, but too much information leads to poor recall. He also notes that half of the information remembered is incorrect. Unless education materials are written at a level and style appropriate for their intended audiences, clients cannot be expected to be able or willing to accept responsibility for self-care.

An essential prerequisite for implementing health education programs is to know the literacy skills of audiences for whom these programs are intended (Quirk, 2000). Yet calls for assessment of literacy and recommendations for appropriate interventions for clients with poor literacy skills have largely been ignored. Health professionals are sometimes reluctant to conduct a clinical assessment of literacy skill or place this information in the health record for fear of embarrassing or stigmatizing the client (Paasche-Orlow & Wolf, 2007b). Therefore, even though illiteracy and low literacy are quite prevalent in the U.S. population, problems with literacy frequently continue to go undiagnosed (Doak, Doak, & Root, 1996; Zarcadoolas et al., 2006).

This chapter examines the magnitude of the literacy problem, the myths associated with it, and the factors that influence literacy levels. Also, this chapter emphasizes the important role health professionals play in assessing clients' literacy skills and the effects of illiteracy on the health and well-being of the public. In addition, the formulas and tests used to evaluate readability of printed tools and to assess clients' comprehension and reading skills are reviewed, specific guidelines are put forth for writing effective health education materials, and teaching strategies are recommended as a means for breaking down the barriers of illiteracy.

Definition of Terms

For many years, there was no clear agreement of what it has meant to be literate in U.S. society. A literate person was loosely described as someone who possessed socially required and expected reading and writing abilities, such as being able to sign his or her name and read and write a simple sentence. Over time, performance on reading tests in school became the conventional method to measure grade-level achievement.

However, because it is difficult, if not impossible, to measure reading abilities on a population-wide basis, the U.S. Bureau of the Census still continues to this day to use the number of years of schooling attended to define literacy levels (Giorgianni, 1998). This remains, though, an imprecise estimation of someone's true reading skills. Many researchers have found that the reported grade level achieved in school is an inadequate predictor of reading ability (Chew, Bradley, & Boyko, 2004; Doak et al., 1996; Weiss, 2003; Winslow, 2001).

In the United States, the term **literacy** is generally defined as the ability to read and speak English (Andrus & Roth, 2002). In the 1992 National Adult Literacy Survey (NALS), the U.S. Department of Education defined literacy as "the ability to use printed and written information to function in society, to achieve one's goals, and to develop one's knowledge and potential" (National Center for Education Statistics, 1993, p. 6).

NALS categorized literacy into three general kinds of tasks (National Center for Education Statistics, 1993):

- Prose tasks, which measure reading comprehension and the ability to extract themes from newspapers, magazines, poems, and books
- Document tasks, which assess the ability of readers to interpret documents such as insurance reports, consent forms, and transportation schedules
- Quantitative tasks, which assess the ability to work with numerical information embedded in written material such as computing restaurant menu bills, figuring out taxes, interpreting paycheck stubs, or calculating calories on a nutrition checklist

Although no precise cut-off point defines the difference between literacy and illiteracy, the commonly accepted working definition of what is meant to be **literate** is the ability to write and to read, understand, and interpret information written at the eighth-grade level or above. On the other end of the continuum, **illiterate** is defined as someone who is unable to read or write at all or whose reading and writing skills are at the fourth-grade level or below.

Low literacy, also termed marginally literate or marginally illiterate, refers to the ability of adults to read, write, and comprehend information between the fifth- and eighth-grade levels of difficulty. Persons with low literacy have trouble using commonly printed and written information to meet their everyday needs such as reading a TV schedule, taking a telephone message, or filling out a relatively simple application form (Doak et al., 1996).

Functional illiteracy means that adults lack the fundamental reading, writing, and comprehension skills that are needed to operate effectively in today's society. Functional illiteracy is a relatively new term. People who are functionally illiterate have very limited competency to perform the tasks of everyday life (Giorgianni, 1998). They do not read well enough to understand and interpret what they have read or use the information as it was intended (Doak et al., 1996). For example, someone who is functionally illiterate may be able to read the simple words on a label of a can of soup that directs them to "Pour soup into pan. Add one can water. Heat until hot." However, they cannot comprehend the meaning and sequence of the words to carry through with these directions.

These operational definitions are, at best, approximations. Conventional grade-level definitions of literacy are considered conservative because even an adult with the ability to read at the eighth-grade level will encounter difficulties in functioning in this advanced society. However, although an individual may have poor reading skills, this does not necessarily imply a lack of intelligence. Low literacy or illiteracy cannot be equated with IQ level. A person can be illiterate or low literate, yet intellectually be within at least normal IQ range (Doak et al., 1996).

Health literacy refers to how well an individual can read, interpret, and comprehend health information for maintaining an optimal level of wellness. The Ad Hoc Committee on Health Literacy for the Council on Scientific Affairs of the American Medical Association (1999) defines health literacy as "a constellation of skills, including the ability to perform basic reading and numerical tasks required to function in the health care environment" (p. 553). This committee identified the scope and consequences of poor health literacy in the United States. They conclude that an individual's functional health literacy is likely to be significantly worse than his or her general literacy skills because of the complicated language (medicalese) used in the healthcare field.

The U.S. Department of Health and Human Services (2000) more explicitly defines health literacy as "the degree to which individuals have the capacity to obtain, process, and understand basic health information and services needed to make appropriate health decisions." Health literacy potentially enables individuals to make informed choices, reduce their health risks, and increase their quality of life (Wood et al., 2007). The 2003 National Assessment of Adult Literacy (NAAL), which was a 10-year follow-up to the original NALS study, was the first national assessment designed specifically to measure the literacy skills of adults in understanding health-related information (National Center for Education Statistics, 2006).

Health literacy is a complex issue and many variables have the potential to influence an individual's capacity to obtain, process, and understand information. Some have suggested that "if health literacy is the ability to function in the health care environment, it must be dependent upon the characteristics of both the individual and the health care system" (Baker, 2006, p. 878). Health literacy should be considered to be context specific and, as such, influenced by the client, the complexity of the condition and treatment, and the environment in which the treatment is taking place (Volandes, 2007).

With managed care requiring individuals to take more responsibility for self-care and symptom management, health literacy is becoming an important determinant of health status. Poor health literacy may lead to serious negative consequences, such as increased morbidity and mortality, when a person is unable to read and comprehend instructions for medications, follow-up appointments, diet, procedures, and other regimens. Patients cannot be expected to be compliant, autonomous, and self-directed in navigating the healthcare system if they do not have the ability to follow basic instructions (Bennett, Chen, Soroui, & White, 2009; Davis et al., 2006). *Reading, readability,* and *comprehension* also are terms frequently used when determining levels of literacy. Fisher (1999) defines **reading** or word recognition as "the process of transforming letters into words and being

able to pronounce them correctly" (p. 57). Word recognition test scores, which can be misleading because they indicate only a person's ability to identify words, not understand them, are usually three grade levels higher than comprehension scores (Fisher, 1999). Hirsch (2001) addresses the public's confusion between reading in the sense of being able to decode words fluently and reading in the sense of being able to comprehend the meaning of words.

Readability is defined as the ease with which written or printed information can be read. It is based on a measure of a number of different elements within a given text of printed material such as level of language being used and layout and design of the page (Hasselkus, 2009). These variables influence with what degree of success a group of readers will be able to read the style of writing of a selected printed passage.

Comprehension, on the other hand, is the degree to which individuals understand what they have read (Fisher, 1999; Koo, Krass, & Aslani, 2005). It is the ability to grasp the meaning of a message—to get the gist of it. A healthcare professional can determine whether comprehension of health instruction has occurred by noting whether clients are able to demonstrate correctly or recall in their own words the message that was received.

The ability to read does not alone guarantee reading comprehension. Comprehension is affected by the amount, clarity, and complexity of the information presented. If the elements of logic, language, and experience in health instruction are compatible with and culturally appropriate to the clients' background, the message likely will be clear and relevant to them (Doak et al., 1996). A mismatch will likely make the message confusing, incomprehensible, and useless to the individual.

Also, illness, medication, treatment, or disruptive life situations, which cause stress and anxiety, have been found to interfere significantly with comprehension. The ability to take in medical information, store it in memory, and recall it when necessary is affected by many other factors as well, such as the length of time between information disclosure and the need to remember the information, the nature of the information (how threatening), and the method of presentation (Doak et al., 1996; Doak, Doak, Friedell, & Meade, 1998; Kessels, 2003; Ley, 1979).

Readability and comprehension, therefore, are particularly complex activities involving many variables with respect to both the reader and the actual written material (Doak et al., 1996; Fisher, 1999). Both are commonly determined by using one or more measurement formulas (see the later discussions of measurement tools in this chapter). **Table 7–1** shows examples of elements that affect readability and comprehension.

Another term used when discussing literacy is **numeracy**, which is the ability to read and interpret numbers. Overwhelmingly, those with limited literacy also have limited skills in numeracy (Andrus & Roth, 2002; Doak et al., 1996; Fisher, 1999; Williams et al., 1995).

Literacy Relative to Oral Instruction

To date, very little attention has been paid to the role of oral communication in the assessment of illiteracy. Certainly, inability to comprehend the spoken word or oral instruction above the level of understanding simple words, phrases, and slang words should be considered an important element in the definition or assessment of literacy. Most health information can be provided verbally, and many clients prefer to learn in a face-to-face encounter (Morrow et al., 2007). However, oral instruction alone is not a very successful method of teaching. "Written information is better remembered and leads to better treatment adherence" (Kessels, 2003, p. 221).

Doak, Doak, and Root (1985) address the fact that there is no universally accepted way to test the degree of difficulty with oral language. However, as these authors observe, "It is believed that some of the same characteristics that are critical for written materials will also affect the comprehensibility of spoken language" (p. 40). Much more research

---

Table 7–1 EXAMPLES OF ELEMENTS THAT AFFECT READABILITY AND COMPREHENSION

Material Variables	Reader Variables
Legibility (e.g., print size, spacing)	Health status
Organization and flow of content	Perceived threat of illness
Concept level	Effects of illness/stress
Length of text	Physical and mental energy
Sentence structure	Level of motivation
Level of vocabulary	Visual and auditory acuity
Relevance to the reader	Educational attainment
Jargon (medical terminology)	Background knowledge
Number of polysyllabic words	Ability to decipher language of message

needs to be done on "iloralacy," or the inability to understand simple oral language, as a generic concept of illiteracy (Hirsch, 2001; Zarcadoolas et al., 2006).

Literacy Relative to Computer Instruction

The literacy issue has always been examined from the standpoint of readability and comprehension of printed materials. However, computer literacy is an increasingly popular concern as an important dimension of the literacy issue. More and more, educators and consumers are relying on computers as educational tools, and the potential of this technology is transforming the way healthcare information is accessed and shared. Clients who are well educated and career oriented are already likely to own a computer and be computer literate, but those with limited resources, literacy skills, and technological know-how are being left behind (Kerka, 2003; Zarcadoolas et al., 2006).

As healthcare organizations and agencies continue to invest more resources in computer technology and software programs for educational purposes, computer literacy in the overall client population must be addressed. Computers not only are used to convey instructional messages, but also serve as a valuable tool for access to a wide array of additional sources of information (see Chapters 12 and 13).

The opportunity to expand clients' knowledge base through telecommunications requires health professionals to attend to computer literacy levels of their audiences. In the same way that they now recognize the negative effects that illiteracy and low literacy have had in restricting the information base of consumers of health care when printed materials are relied upon, health professionals must begin to advocate for computer literacy in the public they serve (Doak et al., 1996; Moore, Bias, Prentice, Fletcher, & Vaughn, 2009). Computer software programs can be made suitable for use by low-literate learners as long as these individu-

als have the basic capacity to access and operate computers and the information is simplified for readability and comprehension.

Scope and Incidence of the Problem

Literacy has been termed the "silent epidemic," the "silent barrier," the "silent disability," and "the dirty little secret" (Conlin & Schumann, 2002; Doak & Doak, 1987; Kefalides, 1999; Wedgeworth, 2007). Based on available statistics over the past 20 years, it is evident that the United States has significant literacy problems. In fact, this country only ranked among the middle of industrialized nations on most measures of adult literacy, and yet many of its educators, elected representatives, and social advocates have remained blind to this significant problem (Kogut, 2004).

In 1985, the U.S. Department of Education undertook the first national assessment of adult literacy, known as the Young Adult Literacy Survey. Since then, the federal government has conducted two subsequent large-scale assessments (U.S. Department of Health and Human Services, 2003).

The 1992 National Adult Literacy Survey (NALS), considered to be a highly accurate and detailed profile on the condition of English language literacy in the United States, revealed surprising statistics. NALS interviewed and collected data from a representative sample of 26,000 individuals, age 16 years and older. Based on the findings from an assessment of literacy skills in three areas (prose, document, and quantitative), literacy abilities were categorized into five levels, with Level 1 being the lowest and Level 5 being the highest.

About 21–23%, or approximately 40–44 million of the 191 million adults in the country at that time, scored in the lowest level of the three skill areas. They were considered to be functionally illiterate. Another 25–28%, or approximately 50 million adults, scored in the Level 2 category.

That is, they were considered to have low literacy skills. Thus, the number of illiterate and low-literate adults in the United States conservatively was estimated to be approximately 90–94 million in total (**Figure 7–1**).

This figure represents about one half of the adult population in this country who had deficiencies in reading, writing, and math skills (Fisher, 1999; Weiss, 2003). The researchers found that those individuals with poor literacy skills (Levels 1 and 2) were disproportionately more often from minority populations, from lower socioeconomic groups, and had poorer health status (Andrus & Roth, 2002; Fisher, 1999; Weiss, 2003).

In 2003, building on the NALS of 10 years earlier, the National Assessment of Adult Literacy (NAAL) was the first study to identify the literacy of America's adults in the 21st century.

New, more sensitive instruments were designed to enhance measurement of the literacy abilities of the least-literate adults. Most important, this evaluation included a health literacy component to assess adults' understanding of health-related materials and forms (National Center for Education Statistics, 2006).

The NAAL categorized literacy skills into four levels, and the findings revealed the following percentages and total numbers: below basic, 14%, or 30 million; basic, 29%, or 63 million; intermediate, 44%, or 95 million; and proficient, 13%, or 28 million. Of the overall 216 million adults in the U.S. population in 2003, 43% (93 million) fell into the lowest two categories (National Center for Education Statistics, 2006).

The average score results indicated no significant change in prose and document literacy and

Figure 7–1 Literacy Levels in U.S. Adults

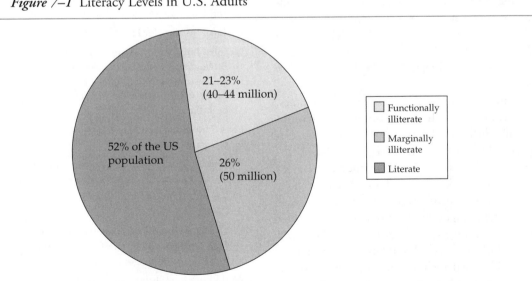

Source: Bastable, L. C., Chojnowski, D., Goldberg, L., McGurl, P., & Riegel, B. (2005). *Comparing heart failure patient literacy levels with available educational materials.* Poster presented at the Heart Failure Society of America, 9th Annual Scientific Conference, September 18–21, 2005, Boca Raton, FL.

only a slight increase in quantitative literacy between 1992 and 2003. However, a higher proportionate percentage of several population groups, such as those who did not graduate from high school, Hispanics, and those older than 65 years of age, fell into the below basic level of prose literacy (Kutner, Greenberg, Jin, & Paulsen, 2006). The NAAL's Health Literacy Report specifically found that 36% (47 million) of adults had basic or below basic health literacy and older adults (65 years and older) had the lowest health literacy levels (National Center for Education Statistics, 2006). For more detailed information on the NAAL survey, visit the National Center for Education Statistics at http://www.nces.ed.gov/NAAL.

In addition to the NAAL survey, in 2004, the Institute of Medicine (IOM), the Agency for Healthcare Research and Quality (AHRQ), and the American Medical Association (AMA) issued their own reports on the status of health literacy in this country. All three reports revealed that as many as 50% of all American adults lack the basic reading and numerical skills essential to function adequately in the healthcare environment (Aldridge, 2004; Institute of Medicine, 2004; Schwartzberg et al., 2004; Weiss et al., 2005). For more information on health literacy, see **Table 7–2** for Web sites.

Limited literacy leads to poor health outcomes. In fact, literacy skills are "a stronger predictor of an individual's health status than age, income, employment status, education level, and racial or ethnic group" (Weiss, 2003, p. 11). Individuals with limited literacy skills are less knowledgeable about their health problems and have higher hospitalization rates, higher healthcare costs, and poorer health status (Weiss et al., 2005). The American College of Physicians Foundation has created a short video that includes interviews with actual patients to illustrate the consequences of limited literacy. To view this video go to http://www.foundation.acponline.org/hl/hlvideo.htm. Also

Table 7–2 Health Literacy Web Sites

American Medical Association, Health Literacy: http://www.ama-assn.org/ama/no-index/physician-resources/8115.shtml

America's Literacy Directory: http://www.literacydirectory.org

Center for Health Care Strategies, Inc.: http://www.chcs.org

Harvard School of Public Health, Health Literacy Studies: http://www.hsph.harvard.edu/healthliteracy

Health Literacy Consulting: http://www.healthliteracy.com

Healthy People 2010: http://www.health.gov/healthypeople

National Center for Education Statistics: http://nces.ed.gov/naal

National Center for Family Literacy: http://www.famlit.org

National Center for the Study of Adult Learning and Literacy (NCSALL): http://www.ncsall.net

National Institute for Literacy: http://www.nifl.gov

National Library of Medicine, Current Bibliographies in Medicine 2004-1, Understanding Health Literacy and Its Barriers: http://www.nlm.nih.gov/pubs/cbm/healthliteracybarriers.html

Pfizer Health Literacy: http://www.pfizerhealthliteracy.com

ProLiteracy Worldwide: http://www.proliteracy.org/NetCommunity/Page.aspx?pid=191&srcid=-2

System for Adult Basic Education Support (SABES): http://www.sabes.org

U.S. Department of Health and Human Services/Office of Minority Health Resource Center: http://www.omhrc.gov

World Education: http://www.worlded.org

see **Table 7–3** for a list of additional audiovisuals on health literacy.

Thus, according to the findings of NALS and NAAL reports, about 4 to 5 out of every 10 Americans lack the basic reading and comprehension skills to perform simple, everyday literacy tasks (National Center for Education Statistics, 2006). Because the mean reading level of the U.S. population is at or below the eighth grade and many people read two to four grades below their reported level of formal education achieved, millions are challenged by the demands of common, day-to-day activities (Winslow, 2001). For example, one needs to be able to read at the 6th-grade level to understand a driver's license manual, at the 8th-

grade level to follow directions on a frozen dinner package, and at the 10th-grade level to read instructions on a bottle of aspirin (Doak et al., 1985). The literacy problem is so widespread that the government, in an effort to reduce traffic accidents, has replaced some conventional printed road signs with road signs using symbols (Loughrey, 1983).

Because of the difficulty inherent in defining and testing literacy, the lack of inclusion of unidentified illegal immigrants in the sample populations studied, and the fact that few people with limited reading skills admit to having any difficulty, the scope of the literacy problem is thought to be much greater than the estimates found in for-

Table 7–3 HEALTH LITERACY AUDIOVISUALS

Health Literacy: Help Your Patients Understand. (2003). VHS tape. American Medical Association. Chicago (20 minutes in length).

Health Literacy: A Prescription to End Confusion. (2004). CD-ROM. Institute of Medicine (IOM) of The National Academies. Includes an executive summary of the report *Health Literacy* and video clips of patients discussing their health literacy experiences. Requires Windows Media Player, Adobe Acrobat Reader, and a Web browser. For more information, contact ORAC@NAS.edu.

In Plain Language. (2002). This 15-minute online video on adult literacy is available at the Harvard School of Public Health-Health Literacy Studies: http://www.hsph.harvard.edu/healthliteracy/overview.html#Two

Low Health Literacy: You Can't Tell by Looking. (2000). VHS tape. American Medical Association. Chicago. Case studies of four patients with low health literacy (20 minutes in length).

Overcoming Patient Language Barriers: Caring for Patients With Limited English Proficiency. (2001). VHS tape. Concept Media. ISBN 156437653-2 (25 minutes in length).

Patient Education Takes Center Stage. (1999). VHS tape. Creative Health Care Management. Underscores the value of helping patients and families learn. Expands perspectives on patient education as the central aspect of health care by providing a real-life example of a person with a kidney transplant (28 minutes in length).

Providing Patient Education to Meet JCAHO Standards. (2003). DVD. MedCom. Cypress, California (23 minutes in length).

Reading Between the Lines. (2003). VHS tape. Medical Library Association. Chicago. Concepts of health information literacy to enhance knowledge of information professionals in the provision of quality consumer health with patient education information services.

Teaching Patients With Low Literacy Skills. (2001). VHS tape. Concept Media, Inc. Irvine, California ISBN 1564376524 (26 minutes in length).

mal studies (Brownson, 1998; Doak et al., 1996; Weiss, 2003).

The rates of illiteracy and low literacy in general and health literacy in particular continue to pose a major threat to many segments of society. The problem is expected to grow worse in light of the many forces operating in this country and worldwide unless specific measures are taken to curb the tide. To be literate 100 years ago meant that people could read and write their own name. Today, being literate means that one is able to learn new skills, think critically, problem solve, and apply general knowledge to various situations (Weiss, 2003).

Trends Associated With Literacy Problems

The trend toward an increased proportion of Americans with literacy levels that are inadequate for active participation in this advanced society is to the result of such factors as the following (Gazmararian et al., 1999; Giorgianni, 1998; Hayes, 2000; Hirsch, 2001; Kogut, 2004; Weiss, 2003):

- A rise in the number of immigrants
- The aging of the population
- The increasing amount and complexity of information
- The increasing sophistication of technology
- More people living in poverty
- Changes in policies and funding for public education
- Disparities between minority versus nonminority populations

All of these factors correlate significantly with the level of formal schooling attained and the level of literacy ability. Although research indicates the number of years of schooling is not a good predictor of literacy level, there remains a correlation between someone's educational background and the ability to read. As society becomes more

and more high tech, with new products and more complicated functions to perform, the basic language requirements needed for survival continue to rise. Many more people are beginning to fall behind, unable to keep up with an increasingly sophisticated world.

In cases of both illiteracy and low literacy, the level of readability is measured in terms of performance, not years of school attendance. The mean literacy level of the U.S. population is at or below eighth grade. Medicaid enrollees, on average, read at the fifth-grade level (Andrus & Roth, 2002; Giorgianni, 1998; Winslow, 2001). Many people read at least two to four grade levels below their reported level of formal education. For those in poverty, the gap between grade level completed and actual reading level is even greater (Andrus & Roth, 2002). This deficiency persists because schools have a tendency to promote students for social and age-related reasons rather than for academic achievement alone (Feldman, 1997), because clients may report inaccurate histories of years of school attended, and because reading skills may be lost over time through lack of practice (Davidhizar & Brownson, 1999; Miller & Bodie, 1994; Weiss, 2003; Williams et al., 2002).

Levels of literacy are often seen as indicators of the well-being of individuals, and the literacy problem has greater implications for the social and economic status of the country as a whole (Kogut, 2004). Low levels of literacy have been associated with marginal productivity, high unemployment, minimum earnings, high costs of health care, and high rates of welfare dependency (Andrus & Roth, 2002; Giorgianni, 1998; Winslow, 2001; Ziegler, 1998).

Also, illiteracy is considered to be an element that is contributing to many of the grave social issues confronting the United States today, such as homelessness, teen pregnancy, unemployment, delinquency, crime, and drug abuse (Fleener & Scholl, 1992; Kogut, 2004). Deficiencies in basic literacy skills compound to create devastating cumulative effects on individuals, which creates a social burden that is extremely costly for the American people. Illiteracy and low literacy are not necessarily the reasons for these ills, but the high correlation between literacy levels and social problems is a marker for disconnectedness from society in general (Kogut, 2004; U.S. Department of Health and Human Services, 2003).

Those at Risk

Illiteracy has been portrayed "as an invisible handicap that affects all classes, ethnic groups, and ages" (Fleener & Scholl, 1992, p. 740). It is a silent disability. Illiteracy knows no boundaries and exists among persons of every race and ethnic background, socioeconomic class, and age category (Duffy & Snyder, 1999; Weiss, 2003). It is true, however, that illiteracy is rare in the higher socioeconomic classes, for example, and that certain segments of the U.S. population are more likely to be affected than others by lack of literacy skills.

According to recent research (Cole, 2000; Hayes, 2000; Kogut, 2004; Montalto & Spiegler, 2001; Nath, Sylvester, Yasek, & Gunel, 2001; Rothman et al., 2004; Schillinger et al., 2002; Schultz, 2002; Williams, Baker, Parker, & Nurss, 1998; Winslow, 2001; Wood, 2005), populations that have been identified as having poorer reading and comprehension skills than the average American include the following:

- Those who are economically disadvantaged
- Older adults
- Immigrants (particularly illegal ones)
- Racial minorities
- High school dropouts
- Those who are unemployed
- Prisoners
- Inner-city and rural residents
- Those with poor health status resulting from chronic mental and physical problems

With respect to demographics, statistics indicate that 34 million Americans are presently living in poverty and that nearly half (43%) of all adults with low literacy live in poverty (Darling, 2004). Although those who are disadvantaged represent many diverse cultural and ethnic groups, including millions of poor White people, one third of disadvantaged people in this country are minorities, and a larger percentage of minorities fall into the disadvantaged category (Giorgianni, 1998; Weiss et al., 2005).

In this 21st century, the major growth in the population will come from the ranks of minority groups. By 2050, 53% of the people in the United States are projected to belong to a racial or ethnic minority and one in five will be foreign born (Passel & Cohn, 2008). In 2000, the U.S. Bureau of the Census reported that approximately 31 million immigrants reside in this country, more than triple the number in 1970. One third of the foreign-born population has arrived since 1990, one in five children is from an immigrant family, and 30% of immigrants do not have a high school diploma (3.5 times the rate for native Americans). Of the 1,200 community-based adult literacy programs run by ProLiteracy of America, 90% are teaching English as a second language (ESL) (Kogut, 2004). Health professionals must recognize how these demographic changes will affect the way in which services need to be rendered, educational materials need to be developed, and information needs to be marketed (Andrus & Roth, 2002; Borrayo, 2004; Nurss et al., 1997; Robinson, 2000).

Many minority and economically disadvantaged people, as well as the prison population—which has the highest concentration of adult illiteracy (Duffy & Snyder, 1999)—are not benefactors of mainstream health education activities, which often fail to reach them. Overall, they are not active seekers of health information because they tend to have weaker communication skills and inadequate foundational knowledge on which to better understand their needs. Many lack enough fluency to make good use of written health education materials. Also, not only are the majority of printed education materials written in English, but fluency in verbal skills in another language does not guarantee functional literacy in that native language (Horner, Surratt, & Juliusson, 2000). Areas with the highest percentage of minorities and high rates of poverty and immigration also have the highest percentage of functionally illiterate people. When these people need medical care, they tend to require more resources, have longer hospital stays, and have a greater number of readmissions (Weiss, 2003). The challenge now and in the future will be to find improved ways of communicating with these population groups and to develop innovative strategies in the delivery of health care.

Of the Americans older than 65 years of age, two out of five adults (approximately 40%) are considered functionally illiterate (Davidhizar & Brownson, 1999; Gazmararian et al., 1999; Williams et al., 2002). In 2003, the population of older adults was approximately 36 million (more than 12% of the total population) and the individuals older than 85 years of age make up the fastest-growing age group in the country. At the turn of the century, they numbered 4.2 million people, but it is projected that by 2050 that number could reach 21 million. Children born today can expect to live to an average age of at least 80. Statistics indicate that the U.S. population is growing older as people live longer. By 2030, it is expected that the 65-and-older population will double from what it was at the beginning of the 21st century (Santrock, 2006; Vander Zanden, Crandell, & Crandell, 2007).

As time goes on, the older population will be more educated and demand more services. In 1960, only 20% of older people were high school graduates, whereas by the beginning of the 21st century, 64% were educated at the high school level. Although these statistical trends indicate there will be a more highly educated group of older adults in the future, the information explosion and rapid technological advances may cause them to fall behind relative to future standards of education. Today, the illiteracy problem in the aged is caused by the facts that not only did these individuals have less education in the past, but also their reading skills have declined over time because of disuse. If a person does not use a skill, he or she loses the skill. Reading ability can deteriorate over time if not exercised regularly (Brownson, 1998).

In addition, cognition and some types of intellectual functioning are affected by aging (Kessels, 2003; Santrock, 2006; Vander Zanden et al., 2007). The vast majority of older people have some degree of cognitive changes and sensory impairments, such as vision and hearing loss. About one fourth of people age 65 and one half older than 75 years of age have serious hearing impairment (Vander Zanden et al., 2007). Along with these normal physiological changes, many suffer from chronic diseases, and large numbers are taking prescribed medications. All of these conditions can interfere with the ability to learn or can negatively affect thought processes, which contributes to the high incidence of illiteracy in this population group.

Beyond the issue of prevalence, illiteracy also presents unique psychosocial problems for the older adult. Because older persons tend to process information more slowly than do young adults, they may become more easily frustrated in a learning situation (Kessels, 2003; Vander Zanden et al., 2007). Furthermore, many older individuals have developed ways to compensate for missing skills through their support network. Lifetime patterns of behavior have been set such that they may lack the motivation to improve their literacy skills. Today and in the years to come, those involved with providing health education will be challenged to overcome these obstacles to learning in the older adult.

Cultural diversity, although not considered to be directly related to illiteracy, may also serve as a barrier to effective client education. According to

Davidhizar and Brownson (1999) and backed up by the NAAL's 2003 statistics, most adults with illiteracy problems in this country are White, native-born, English-speaking Americans. However, when examining the proportion of the population that has poor literacy skills, minority ethnic groups are at a disproportionately higher risk (Andrus & Roth, 2002).

When healthcare providers communicate with clients from cultures different from their own, it is important for them to be aware that their clients may not be fluent in English. Furthermore, even if people speak the English language, the meanings of words and their understanding of facts may vary significantly based on life experiences, family background, and culture of origin, especially if English is the client's second language (Purnell & Paulanka, 2003). In conversation, an individual must be able to understand undertones, voice intonations, and in what context (slang, terminology, or customs) the message is being delivered.

Purnell and Paulanka (2003) stress the importance of assessing other elements of verbal and nonverbal communication, such as emotional tone of speech, gestures, eye contact, touch, voice volume, and stance, between persons of different cultures that may affect the interpretation of behavior and the validating of information received or sent (see Chapter 8). Educators must be aware of these potential barriers to communication when interacting with clients from other cultures whose literacy skills may be limited. Given the increasing diversity of the U.S. population, most currently available written materials are inadequate based on the literacy level of minority groups and the fact that the majority of printed education materials are available only in English.

Thus, individuals with less education, which often includes the groups of low-income persons, older adults, racial minorities, and people with ethnic origins for whom English is a second language, are likely to have more difficulty with reading and comprehending written materials as well as understanding oral instruction (Winslow, 2001). This profile is not intended to stereotype people who are illiterate but rather to give a broad picture of who most likely lacks literacy skills. When carrying out assessments on their patient populations it is essential that healthcare providers be aware of those susceptible to having literacy problems.

Myths, Stereotypes, and Assumptions

Rarely do people voluntarily admit that they are illiterate. Illiteracy is a stigma that creates feelings of shame, inadequacy, fear, and low self-esteem (Paasche-Orlow & Wolf, 2007b; Weiss, 2003; Williams et al., 2002; Wolf et al., 2007). Most individuals with poor literacy skills have learned that it is dangerous to reveal their illiteracy because of fear that others such as family, strangers, friends, or employers would consider them dumb or incapable of functioning responsibly. In fact, the majority of people with literacy problems have never told their spouse or children of their disability (Quirk, 2000; Williams et al., 2002).

People also tend to underreport their limited reading abilities because of embarrassment or lack of insight about the extent of their limitation. The NALS report reveals that the majority of adults performing at the two lowest levels of literacy skill describe themselves as proficient in being able to read and/or write English (Ad Hoc Committee on Health Literacy, 1999). Because self-reporting is so unreliable and because illiteracy and low literacy are so common, many experts suggest that screening of all patients should be done to identify clients who have reading difficulty to determine the extent of their impairment (Andrus & Roth, 2002; Weiss, 2003; Weiss et al., 2005). However, health professionals must recognize that many clients would approach testing reluctantly and be fearful of having their literacy report recorded in their health record (Paasche-Orlow & Wolf, 2007b; Wolf et al., 2007).

Most people with limited literacy abilities are masters at concealment. Typically, they are ashamed by their limitation and attempt to hide the problem in clever ways. Often, they are resourceful and intelligent about trying to conceal their illiteracy and have developed remarkable memories to help them cope with family and career situations (Doak et al., 1996; Kanonowicz, 1993). Many have discovered ways to function quite well in society without being able to read by memorizing signs and instructions, by making intelligent guesses, or by finding employment opportunities that are not heavily dependent on reading and writing skills.

An important thing to remember is that there are many myths about illiteracy. It is very easy for healthcare providers to fall into the trap of labeling someone as illiterate or, for that matter, assuming that they are literate based on stereotypical images. Some of the most common myths about people who struggle with literacy skills are outlined next (Andrus & Roth, 2002; Doak et al., 1996; Weiss, 2003; Williams et al., 2002; Winslow, 2001).

Myth No. 1: They are intellectually slow learners or incapable of learning at all. (In fact, many have average or above-average IQs.)

Myth No. 2: They can be recognized by their appearance. (In fact, appearance alone is an unreliable basis for judgment; some very articulate, well-dressed people have no visible signs of a literacy disability.)

Myth No. 3: The number of years of schooling completed correlates with literacy skills. (In fact, grade-level achievement does not correspond well to reading ability. The number of years of schooling completed overestimates reading levels by four to five grade levels.)

Myth No. 4: Most are foreign-born, poor, and of ethnic or racial minority. (In fact, they come from very diverse backgrounds and the majority are White, native-born Americans.)

Myth No. 5: Most will freely admit that they do not know how to read or do not understand. (In fact, most try to hide their reading deficiencies and will go to great lengths to avoid discovery, even when directly asked about their possible limitations.)

Assessment: Clues to Look For

So, the question remains: How does one recognize an illiterate person? Identifying illiteracy is not easy because there is no stereotypical pattern. It is an impairment easily overlooked because illiteracy has no particular face, age, socioeconomic status, or nationality (Cole, 2000; Hayes, 2000).

Health professionals, because of their role with healthcare consumers, are in an ideal position to determine the literacy levels of individuals (Cutilli, 2005; Monsivais & Reynolds, 2003). Because of the prevalence of illiteracy, health professionals must never assume that a client is literate. Knowing a person's ability to read and comprehend is critical in providing teaching–learning encounters that are beneficial, efficient, and cost effective.

Health professionals can watch out for a number of informal clues or red flags that indicate reading and writing deficiencies. The caveat is: Do not rely on the obvious, but look for the unexpected. In so many instances when someone does not fit the stereotypical image, health professionals have never even considered the possibility that an illiteracy problem exists.

Overlooking the problem has the potential for grave consequences in treatment outcomes and has resulted in frustration for both the client and the caregiver (Cole, 2000; Weiss, 2003). Unfortunately, healthcare providers are often hesitant to infer that a patient may have low literacy skills because there is an implication of personal inadequacy associated with the failure to have learned to read (Quirk, 2000).

Because people with illiteracy or marginal literacy skills often have had many years of practice at disguising the problem, they will go to elaborate lengths to hide the fact that they do not possess a skill already acquired by most elementary schoolchildren. The observant practitioner should always be on the lookout for possible signs of poor reading abilities. If healthcare providers become aware of a client's literacy problem, they must convey sensitivity and maintain confidentiality to prevent increased feelings of shame (Quirk, 2000).

During assessment, the health professional should take note of the following clues that clients with illiteracy or low literacy may demonstrate (Andrus & Roth, 2002; Carol, 2007; Davis, Michielutte, Askov, Williams, & Weiss, 1998; Weiss, 2003):

- Reacting to complex learning situations by withdrawal, complete avoidance, or being repeatedly noncompliant
- Using the excuse that they were too busy, too tired, too sick, or too sedated with medication to maintain their attention span when given a booklet or instruction sheet to read
- Claiming that they just did not feel like reading, that they gave the information to their spouse to take home, or that they lost, forgot, or broke their glasses
- Camouflaging their problem by surrounding themselves with books, magazines, and newspapers to give the impression they are able to read
- Circumventing their inability by insisting on taking the information home to read or having a family member or friend with them when written information is presented
- Asking you to read the information for them under the guise that their eyes are bothersome, they lack interest, or they do not have the energy to devote to the task of learning
- Showing nervousness as a result of feeling stressed by the threat of the possibility of getting caught or having to confess to illiteracy

- Acting confused, talking out of context, holding reading materials upside down, or expressing thoughts that may seem totally irrelevant to the topic of conversation
- Showing a great deal of frustration and restlessness when attempting to read, often mouthing words aloud (vocalization) or silently (subvocalization), substituting words they cannot decipher (decode) with meaningless words, pointing to words or phrases on a page, or exhibiting facial signs of bewilderment or defeat
- Standing in a location clearly designated for authorized personnel only
- Listening and watching very attentively to observe and memorize how things work
- Demonstrating difficulty with following instructions about relatively simple activities such as breathing exercises or with operating the TV, electric bed, call light, and other simple equipment, even when the operating instructions are clearly printed on them
- Failing to ask any questions about the information they received
- Turning in registration forms or health questionnaires that are incomplete, illegible, or not attempted
- Revealing a discrepancy between what is understood by listening and what is understood by reading

In summary, although it has been clearly pointed out that the level of completed formal education is an inaccurate presumption by which to predict reading level, it is certainly one estimate that health professionals should incorporate into their methods of assessment. Also, negative feedback and clues from the client in the form of puzzled looks, inappropriate behaviors, excuses, or irrelevant statements may give the health professional the intuitive feeling that the message being communicated has neither been received nor understood. Not only do illiterate people become confused and frustrated in their attempts to deal with the complex system of health care, which is so dependent on written and verbal information, but they also become stressed in their efforts to cover up their disability.

Healthcare providers, in turn, can feel frustrated when those who have undiagnosed literacy problems seem at face value to be unmotivated and noncompliant in following self-care instructions. Many times, health professionals wonder why clients make caregiving so difficult for themselves as well as for the provider. It is not unusual for them to conclude, "He's too proud to bend," "She's in denial," or "He's just being stubborn—it's a control issue."

Health professionals in their role as educators must go beyond their own assumptions, look beyond a client's appearance and behavior, and seek out the less than obvious by conducting a thorough initial assessment of variables to uncover the possibility that a literacy problem exists. An awareness of this possibility and good skills at observation are key to diagnosing illiteracy or low literacy in learners. Early diagnosis enables health professionals to intervene appropriately to avoid disservice to those who do not need condemnation but caregivers' support and encouragement.

Impact of Illiteracy on Motivation and Compliance

In addition to the fact that poor literacy skills affect the ability to read as well as to understand and interpret the meaning of written and verbal instructions, a person with illiteracy or semiliteracy struggles with other significant interrelated limitations with communication that negatively influence healthcare teaching (Doak et al., 1998; Kalichman, Ramachandran, & Catz, 1999). The person's organization of thought, perception, vocabulary and language/fluency development, and problem-solving skills are adversely affected, too (Giorgianni, 1998).

Fleener and Scholl (1992) investigated characteristics of those who had self-identified themselves as literacy disabled. For the functionally illiterate, the most common deficiencies found were in phonics, comprehension, and perception. Difficulties in perception were evident in the reversal of letters and words, miscalling letters, and adding and omitting letters. Also, a major problem was comprehension, identification of words without knowing their meaning. Some individuals needed to read aloud to understand, and others read so slowly that they lost the meaning of a paragraph before they had finished it. Still other subjects perceived difficulty in remembering as a factor in their lack of reading skill.

People with poor reading skills have difficulty analyzing instructions, assimilating and correlating new information, and formulating questions (Giorgianni, 1998). They may be reluctant to ask questions because of concerns that their inquiries will be regarded as incomprehensible or irrelevant. Often they do not even know what to ask, but they also fear if they try, others will think of them as ignorant or lacking in intelligence. These individuals have great difficulty navigating the healthcare delivery system that relies on written information and printed forms at every juncture. Studies have shown that Health Insurance Portability and Accountability Act (HIPAA) privacy notices, informed consent forms, drug warning labels, and insurance forms all present obstacles for individuals with poor reading skills (Davis et al., 2006; McCormack, Bann, Uhrig, Berkman, & Rudd, 2009; Sudore & Landefeld, et al., 2006; Walfish & Ducey, 2007).

Most professionals can recount a story of a situation where a client failed to follow advice because he or she did not understand the instructions that were given. Hussey and Guilliland (1989) provide a poignant example, which remains as relevant today as it was then, of a young pregnant girl prescribed antiemetic suppositories to control her nausea. When she had no relief of symptoms, questioning revealed that she was swallowing the medication. Obviously, not only did she not understand how to take the medicine, but she also likely had never seen a suppository and was not even able to read or understand the word. She did not ask what it was, probably because she did not know what to ask in the first place, and she may have been reluctant to question the treatment out of fear that she would be regarded as ignorant.

If their past experiences with learning have been less than positive, some people may prefer not knowing the answers to questions and may withdraw altogether to avoid awkward or embarrassing learning situations. Also, they may react to complicated, fast-paced instruction with discouragement, feelings of low self-esteem, and refusal to participate because their process of interpretation is so slow. Even when questioned about their understanding, persons with low literacy skills most likely claim that they understood the information even when they did not (Doak et al., 1996).

Another characteristic of illiterate individuals is that they have difficulty synthesizing information in a way that fits into their behavior patterns. If they are unable to comprehend a required behavior change or cannot understand why it is needed, they will disregard any health teaching (Vanderhoff, 2005; Weiss, 2003). For example, patients recovering from fractured hips who are taught via demonstration and written instructions how to climb stairs and how to do strengthening exercises may fail to comply with this regimen because of lack of understanding of the information and how to go about incorporating these changes into their lifestyle (Schultz, 2002).

Persons with poor literacy skills may also think in only concrete, specific, and literal terms. An example of this limitation is the diabetic patient whose glucose levels were out of control even when the patient insisted he was taking his insulin as instructed—injecting the orange and then eating the fruit (Hussey & Guilliland, 1989).

The person with limited literacy also may experience difficulty handling large amounts of information and classifying it into categories. Older adults, in particular, who need to take several different medications at various times and in different dosages may either become confused with the schedule or ignore the instruction. If asked to change their daily medication routine, a great deal of retraining may be needed to convince them of the benefits of the new regimen (Kessels, 2003).

Another major factor in noncompliance is the lack of adequate and specific instructions about prescribed treatment regimens. Unfortunately, poor literacy skills are seldom assessed by healthcare personnel when, for example, teaching a patient about medications. Literacy problems tend to limit the patient's ability to understand the array of instructions regarding medication labels, dosage scheduling, adverse reactions, drug interactions, and complications (Davis et al., 2006; Elliot, 2007; Williams et al., 2002). No wonder those who lack the required vocabulary, organized thinking skills, and the ability to formulate questions, coupled with inadequate instruction, become confused and easily frustrated to the point of taking medications incorrectly or refusing to take them at all.

Thus, illiteracy, functional illiteracy, and low literacy significantly affect both motivation and compliance levels (see Chapter 6). What is often mistaken for noncompliance is, instead, the simple inability to comply. Although almost one half of the adult population is functionally illiterate, this statistic is overlooked by many healthcare professionals as a major factor in noncompliance with prescribed regimens, follow-up appointments, and measures to prevent medical complications (Andrus & Roth, 2002; Doak et al., 1996; Weiss, 2003; Williams et al., 2002).

A number of studies have correlated literacy levels with noncompliance (Doak et al., 1998; Kalichman et al., 1999; Mayeaux, et al., 1996; Weiss, 2003). Individuals with poor literacy skills that coincide with inadequate language skills have difficulty following instructions and providing accurate and complete health histories, which are vital to the delivery of good health care. The burden of illiteracy leads patients into noncompliance not because they do not want to comply, but rather because they are unable to do so (Hayes, 2000; Williams, Counselman, & Caggiano, 1996).

Numerous research studies indicate that the impact of illiteracy is broader than just the inability to read; it alters the way a person organizes, interprets, analyzes, and summarizes information (Giorgianni, 1998). Caregivers often overestimate an individual's ability to understand instructions and are quick to label someone as uncooperative. In reality, the underlying problem may be limited cognitive processing that impedes comprehending and following written and oral communication.

Ethical, Financial, and Legal Concerns

Sources of printed education materials (PEMs) include healthcare facilities, commercial vendors, government services, voluntary health agencies, nonprofit charitable organizations, pharmaceutical firms, and medical equipment supply companies. These materials are distributed primarily by health professionals and are the major sources of information for clients participating in health programs in many settings.

Written health information materials are intended to reinforce learning about health promotion, disease prevention, illness management, diagnostic procedures, drug and treatment modalities, rehabilitative course, and self-care regimens. Unfortunately, many of these sources fail to take into account the educational level, preexisting knowledge base, cultural influences, language barriers, or socioeconomic backgrounds of persons with limited literacy skills.

As compared with people who have adequate health literacy, it is estimated that expenditures for health care for those with limited literacy cost the country between $32 billion and $58 billion in 2001 (Center for Health Care Strategies, 2003; Wood, 2005). Unless patients are competent in reading and comprehending the literature given to them, these tools are useless as adjuncts for health education. They are neither a cost-effective nor a time-efficient means for teaching and learning. Materials that are widely distributed, but little or not at all understood, pose not only a health hazard for clients but also an ethical, financial, and legal liability for healthcare providers (Ad Hoc Committee, 1999; French & Larrabee, 1999; Gazmararian et al., 2005; Giorgianni, 1998; Ryhanen et al., 2008; Schultz, 2002; Vallance, Taylor, & LaVallee, 2008).

Materials that are too difficult to read or comprehend serve little purpose. Health education cannot be considered to have taken place if the written information that has been distributed to clients does not enhance their knowledge and requisite skills necessary for self-care. Ultimately, indiscriminate or nonselective use of PEMs can result in complete or partial lack of communication between healthcare providers and consumers (Andrus & Roth, 2002; Fisher, 1999; Villaire & Mayer, 2007; Weiss, 2003; Winslow, 2001).

Initial standards for health education put forth in 1993 by the Joint Commission for Accreditation of Healthcare Organizations (JCAHO)—now known as the Joint Commission (JC)—still remain as a current standard requiring "the patient and/or, when appropriate, his/her significant other(s) [be] provided with education that can enhance their knowledge, skills, and those behaviors necessary to fully benefit from the health care interventions provided by the organization" (JCAHO, 1993, p. 1030).

In 1996, JCAHO identified additional standards necessary for client care to meet accreditation mandates. Not only is patient and family (or significant other) instruction required, but education must be provided by all relevant members of the interdisciplinary healthcare team, with special consideration being given to the client's literacy level, educational level, and language. All clients must have an assessment of their readiness to learn and an identification of any obstacles to learning (Weiss, 2003).

Emphasis on such standards has prompted healthcare agencies and providers to reexamine their teaching practices, educational materials, and systems of documenting evidence of teaching interventions to better match the reading levels and cultural diversity of the clients being served. These JC standards further specify that education relevant to a person's healthcare needs must be understandable and culturally appropriate to the patient and/or significant others. Therefore, PEMs must be written in ways that assist clients in comprehending their health needs and problems to undertake self-care regimens such as medications, diet, exercise therapies, and use of medical equipment (Fisher, 1999; Weiss, 2003).

Furthermore, the federally mandated Patient's Bill of Rights has established the rights of patients to receive complete and current information regarding their diagnoses, treatments, and prognoses in terms they can understand (Duffy & Snyder, 1999). It is imperative that the reading levels of PEMs match the patients' reading abilities and vice versa. Compounding the need for appropriately written materials is the fact that research reveals that people forget almost immediately about one half of any instruction they receive orally (Kessels, 2003). Failure to retain information combined with inappropriate reading levels of materials used to reinforce or supplement verbal teaching methods decreases compliance, increases morbidity, and results in misuse of healthcare facilities (Weiss et al., 2005).

Encouraging self-care through client education for purposes of health promotion, disease preven-

tion, health maintenance, and rehabilitation is not a new concept to either consumers or providers of health care. However, the trends in the current healthcare system in the United States have impinged on the professional ability of health professionals to provide needed information to ensure self-care that is both safe and effective. Patient education has assumed an even more vital role in assisting clients to independently manage their own healthcare needs given such factors as follows:

- Early discharge
- Decreased reimbursement for direct care
- Increased emphasis on delivery of care in the community and home setting
- Greater demands on health professionals in all settings
- Increased technological complexity of treatment
- Assumption by caregivers that printed information is an adequate substitute for direct instruction of patients

These constraints do not allow for sufficient opportunities for clients in the home or various healthcare settings to receive the necessary education they need for self-management. Most outpatient care, such as that given in clinics; doctors', physical therapists', and other health professional offices; and same-day surgery centers, requires patients and their families to understand both written and oral instruction (Wood, 2005). Consequently, health professionals are relying to a greater extent than ever before on PEMs to supplement their teaching (Horner et al., 2000; Vanderhoff, 2005).

Thus, the burden of becoming adequately educated falls on the shoulders of patients, their families, and significant others. Often unprepared because of shortened hospital stays or limited contact with healthcare providers, consumers have to assume a greater role in their own recovery and the maximization of their health potential (Weiss, 2003; Wood, 2005).

The burden also falls on healthcare providers to safeguard the lives of their clients by becoming better, more effective communicators of written health information. Since 1990, the Maine Area Health Education Center (AHEC) Literacy Center at the University of New England has been holding summer institutes for healthcare professionals to learn about literacy issues, to share resources with colleagues from around the world, and to acquire skills in writing and critiquing health information documents (Andrus & Roth, 2002; Osborne, 1999).

It is only recently that research in the area of written health education materials in relation to clients' literacy skills has examined and attempted to answer even the most basic questions, such as the following:

- Do consumers read the health education literature provided them?
- Are they capable of reading it?
- Can they comprehend what they read?
- Are written materials appropriate and sufficient for the intended target audience?

In this increasingly litigious and ethically conscious society, growing attention is being paid by health professionals to informed consent and teaching for self-care via both verbal and written healthcare instruction (Gazmararian et al., 2005). The potential for misinterpretation of instructions not only can adversely affect treatment but also raises serious concerns about the ethical and legal implications with respect to professional responsibility and liability when information is written at a level incomprehensible to many patients (French & Larrabee, 1999; Weiss, 2003). A properly informed consumer is not only a legal concern in health care today but an ethical one as well (see Chapter 2).

Readability of Printed Education Materials

Many studies on literacy have attempted to document the disparity between the reading levels of consumers and the estimated readability demand of printed health information. Given that the health of people depends in part on their ability to understand information contained in food labeling, over-the-counter and prescription medication instructions, environmental safety warnings, discharge instructions, health promotion and disease prevention flyers, and the like, the focus of attention on identifying this discrepancy is more than warranted.

A substantial body of evidence in the literature indicates that there is a significant gap between patients' reading and comprehension levels and the level of reading difficulty of printed education materials (PEMs) (Andrus & Roth, 2002; Vallance et al., 2008; Weiss, 2003; Wilson, 2009; Winslow, 2001). A variety of education materials available from sources such as the government, health agencies, professional associations, health insurance companies, and industries are written beyond the reading ability of the majority of clients.

Healthcare providers are beginning to recognize that the reams of written materials relied on by so many of them to convey health information to consumers are essentially closed to those with illiteracy and low literacy problems. For example, look at the following text on information about colonoscopy:

Your naicisyhp has dednemmocer that you have a ypocsonoloc. A ypocsonoloc is a test for noloc rec- nac. It sevlovni gnitresni a elbixelf gniweiv epocs into your mutcer. You must drink a laiceps diuqil the thgin erofeb the noitanimaxe to naelc out your noloc.

Does it make sense, or are you confused? If the words appear unreadable, that is exactly what written teaching instructions look like to someone who cannot read (Weiss, 2003).

Many researchers have assessed specific population groups in a variety of healthcare settings based on the ability of clients to meet the literacy demands of written materials related to their care. All of these investigators used commonly accepted readability formulas to test consumers' understanding of printed health information. Their findings revealed the following information:

- Emergency department instructional materials (average 10th-grade readability) are written at a level of difficulty out of the readable range for most patients (Duffy & Snyder, 1999; Lerner, Jehle, Janicke, & Moscati, 2000; Williams et al., 1996).
- A significant mismatch exists between the reading ability of older adults and the readability levels of documents essential to their gaining access to health-related services offered through local, state, and federal government programs (Kim, 2006; Winslow, 2001).
- A large discrepancy exists between clients' average reading comprehension levels and the readability demand of PEMs used in ambulatory care and home care settings (Ache, 2009; Lerner et al., 2000; Schillinger et al., 2002; Walfish & Ducey, 2007; Wood, 2005).
- Standard consent forms used in hospitals, private physician offices, and clinics, as well as by institutional review boards (IRBs) to protect potential research subjects, require high school– to college-level reading comprehension (Doak et al., 1998; Paasche-Orlow, Taylor, & Brancati, 2003; Sudore & Landefeld, et al., 2006).
- Physicians' letters to their patients required an average of 16th- to 17th-grade reading ability, and, likewise, health articles in newspapers ranged from 12th- to 14th-grade level (Conlin & Schumann, 2002).

- The reading grade levels of 15 psychotropic medication handouts for patient education ranged from 12th to 14th grade, well above the 5th-grade level recommended by the National Cancer Institute guidelines (Myers & Shephard-White, 2004).

Thus, numerous investigators have demonstrated that PEMs for the purpose of disseminating health information are written at grade levels that far exceed the reading ability of the majority of consumers. Results from these studies reveal that most health education literature is written above the 8th-grade level, with the average level falling between the 10th and 12th grades. Many PEMs exceed this upper range, even though the average reading level of adults falls at the 8th-grade level. Millions of people in the population read at considerably lower levels and need materials written at the 5th-grade level or lower (Bastable, Chojnowski, Goldberg, McGurl, & Riegel, 2005; Brownson, 1998; Davis, Williams, Marin, Parker, & Glass, 2002; Doak et al., 1998).

Furthermore, the health education literature indicates that people typically read at least two grade levels below their highest level of schooling and prefer materials that are written below their literacy abilities. In fact, contrary to popular belief, sophisticated readers also prefer simplified PEMs when ill because of low energy and concentration levels, and even when they are well because of the demands of their busy schedules and the fact that even highly educated people do not know the vocabulary of medicine, known as medicalese (Giorgianni, 1998; Lasater & Mehler, 1998; Winslow, 2001).

The conclusion to be drawn is that complex and lengthy PEMs serve no useful teaching purpose if healthcare consumers are unable to understand them or unwilling to read them. Literacy levels of clients compared with literacy demands of PEMs, whether in hospital or community-based settings, are an important factor in the rehabilitation and recidivism of those who are recipients of healthcare services.

The Internet is an excellent resource for health educators to locate easy-to-read PEMs. See **Table 7–4** for sources of low literacy education materials.

Measurement Tools to Test Literacy Levels

Healthcare professionals continually struggle with the task of effectively communicating highly complex and technical information to their consumers, who often lack sufficient background knowledge to understand the sophisticated content of instruc-

tion relevant to their care. Whether they author or merely distribute printed education information, healthcare practitioners are responsible for ensuring the appropriate literacy level of the materials given to their clients.

If the literacy of education materials matches the readers' literacy skills, consumers may be better able to understand and comply with healthcare regimens, thereby reducing the costs of care and improving their quality of life (Ad Hoc Committee, 1999). Because health professionals rely heavily on PEMs to convey necessary information to their clients, the usefulness and efficacy of these materials must be determined in relation to the readers' abilities to decipher information.

To objectively evaluate the difficulty of written materials, two basic measurement methods exist:

Table 7-4 Sources of Low-Literacy Education Materials

Agency for Healthcare Research and Quality (AHRQ). Web site: www.ahcpr.gov; phone: (315) 594-1364

National Institutes of Health (NIH). Web site: www.nih.gov

National Heart, Lung, and Blood Institute (NHLBI). Web site: www.nhlbi.nih.gov; phone: (301) 251-1222

United States Pharmacopeia (Library of Pictograms). Web site: www.usp.org; phone: (800) 227-8772

The Indian Health Service. Web site: www.ihs.gov

National Cancer Institute, Cancer Information Services. Web site: www.nci.nih.gov; phone: (800) 4-CANCER

American Cancer Society. Web site: www.cancer.org; phone: (800) ACS-2345

American Heart Association. Web site: www.americanheart.org; phone: (800) 242-1793

National Institute for Literacy. Web site: www.nifl.gov; phone: (202) 632-1500

American Dietetic Association. Web site: www.eatright.org; phone: (312) 899-0400

Office of Minority Health. Web site: www.omhrc.gov; phone: (800) 444-6472

Channing L. Bete Company, Inc. Web site: www.channing-bete.com; phone: (800) 477-4776

Krames Communication. Web site: www.krames.com; phone: (800) 333-3032

U.S. Elsevier Health Bookshop. Web site: www.elsevierhealth.com; phone: (800) 325-4177

Executive Secretariat: The Plain Language Initiative. Web site: execsec.od.nih.gov/plainlang/guidelines/index.html

National Cancer Institute. Web site: cancer.gov/cancerinformation/clearandsimple formulas and tests. Various formulas measure readability of PEMs and are based on ascertaining the average length of sentences and words (vocabulary difficulty) to determine the grade level at which they are written. Standardized tests, which measure actual comprehension and reading skills, involve readers' responses to instructional materials or the ability to decode and pronounce words to determine their grade level (see Appendix A).

Both methods, although not ideal, are considered to have a sufficient relationship to literacy ability to justify their use. The most widely used readability formulas and standardized tests for comprehension and reading skill rate high on reliability and predictive validity. They also do not require elaborate training to use, but they do vary in the amount of time required to administer. In addition, the advent of computerized readability analysis (nearly all word-processing programs, such as Microsoft Word, will produce readability statistics with just a click of the mouse) has made evaluating the reading grade level of written materials much easier and quicker. All of these methods are most useful to health educators for designing and evaluating PEMs.

Formulas to Measure Readability of PEMs

Readability is not a new concept and has been a concern of primary and secondary school educators and educational psychologists for years. In the 1940s, there was a great upswing in attempts by educators and reading specialists to develop systematic procedures by which to objectively evaluate reading materials. Readability is defined as "characteristics of reading materials that make material 'easy' or 'difficult' to read" (Aldridge, 2004). Today, more than 40 formulas are available to measure the readability levels of PEMs.

Readability indices have been devised to determine the grade level demand of specific written information. Although they can predict a level of reading difficulty of material based on an analysis of sentence structure and word length, they do not take into account the inherent individual variables that affect the reader, such as interest in or familiarity with the subject itself or the actual content of the materials (Doak et al., 1996).

Even though materials may have similar readability levels as measured by some formula, not all readers have equal competence in reading them. For example, a patient with a long-standing chronic illness may already be familiar with vocabulary related to the disease and, therefore, may be able to read similar grade-level materials much more easily than a newly diagnosed patient, even though both individuals may have equal literacy skill with other types of material (Doak et al., 1985).

As assessment tools, readability formulas are useful but must be employed with caution because the match between reader and material does not necessarily guarantee comprehension (Aldridge, 2004; Davis et al., 1998). Readability formulas originally were designed as predictive averages to rank the difficulty of books used in specific grades of school—not to determine exactly which factors contribute to the difficulty of a text. Educators should be careful in assuming that people can or cannot read instructional material simply because a formula-based readability score does or does not match their educational level.

Even though these simple instruments are practical for assessment of literacy, they are limited in that they cannot determine the cause or type of reading and learning problems (Davis et al., 1998). Therefore, while readability formulas are easily applied and have proved useful in determining the reading grade level of a text, when used alone they are not an adequate index of readability (Davis et al., 1998; Doak et al., 1996).

Readability formulas are merely one useful step in determining reading ease of a document. Many researchers suggest using a multimethod approach to ascertain readability—that is, they suggest applying a number of readability formulas to any given piece of written material as well as taking into consideration the reader and other material variables (Doak et al., 1996; Ley & Florio, 1996). Formula scores are simply rough approximations of text difficulty. Human judgment is always needed in conjunction with formula-based estimates to determine the quality of PEMs.

Readability formulas are mathematical equations derived from multiple regression analysis that describe the correlation between an author's style of writing and a reader's ability at identifying words as printed symbols within a context (Doak et al., 1996). Most of them provide fairly accurate grade-level estimates, give or take one grade level, with 68% confidence. In many respects, a readability formula is like a reading test, except that it does not test people but rather written material (Fry, 1977).

The first guideline to remember is that readability formulas should not be the only tool used for assessing PEMs. The second rule is to select readability formulas that have been validated on the reader population for whom the PEM is intended. Several formulas are geared to specific types of materials or population groups.

Ley and Florio (1996) and Meade and Smith (1991) conducted extensive studies of the most commonly used formulas and reported on their reliability and validity when used to measure health-related information. In particular, the Flesch, Fog, and Fry formulas showed strong correlations with health-based literature (Horner et al., 2000). Because so many readability formulas are available for assessment of reading levels of PEMs, only those that are relatively simple to work with, are accepted as reliable and valid, and are in widespread use have been chosen for review here.

Spache Grade-Level Score

What is unique about the Spache grade-level formula (Spache, 1953) is that, unlike the other lead-ing formulas that focus largely on the evaluation of materials written for adults, this score is specifically designed to judge materials written for children at grade levels below fourth grade (elementary grades 1 through 3). The Spache grade-level score should not be used to assess adult reading materials (Spache, 1953). The elements used to estimate reading difficulty using the Spache formula are sentence length and the number of words outside the Dale easy word list of 769 words required for formula calculation. See Appendix A for the method of formula analysis.

Flesch-Kincaid Scale

The Flesch-Kincaid formula was developed as an objective measurement of readability of materials between grade 5 and college level. Its use has been validated repeatedly over more than 50 years for assessing news reports, adult education materials, and government publications. The Flesch formula is based on a count of two basic language elements: average sentence length (in words) of selected samples and average word length measured as syllables per 100 words of sample. The reading ease (RE) score is calculated by combining these two variables (Flesch, 1948; Spadero, 1983; Spadero, Robinson, & Smith, 1980). See Appendix A for the method of formula analysis.

Fog Index

The Fog formula developed by Gunning (1968) is appropriate for use in determining readability of materials from fourth grade to college level. It is calculated based on average sentence length and the percentage of multisyllabic words in a 100-word passage. The Fog index is considered one of the simpler methods because it is based on a short sample of words (100), it does not require counting syllables of all words, and the rules are easy to follow (Spadero, 1983; Spadero et al., 1980). See Appendix A for the method of formula analysis.

Fry Readability Graph—Extended

The contribution of the Fry formula comes from the simplicity of its use without sacrificing accuracy, as well as its wide and continuous range of testing readability of materials (especially books, pamphlets, and brochures) at the level of grade 1 through college (grade 17). It is well accepted by literature and reading specialists and is not copyrighted (Doak et al., 1996). A series of simple rules can be applied to plot two language elements—the number of syllables and the number of sentences in three 100-word selections (Fry, 1968, 1977; Spadero et al., 1980). If a very long text is being analyzed, such as a 50-page or more book, one should use six 100-word samples rather than three (Doak et al., 1996). With some practice, this formula takes only about 10 minutes to determine the readability level of a document. See Appendix A for directions on how to use the Fry readability graph.

SMOG Formula

The SMOG (simplified measure of gobbledygook) formula by McLaughlin (1969) is recommended not only because it offers relatively easy computation (simple and fast) but also because it is one of the most valid tests of readability. The SMOG formula measures readability of PEMs from grade 4 to college level based on the number of polysyllabic words within a set number of sentences (Doak et al., 1996). It evaluates the readability grade level of PEMs to within 1.5 grades of accuracy (Myers & Shepard-White, 2004). Thus, when using the SMOG formula to calculate the grade level of material, the SMOG results are usually about two grades higher than the grade levels calculated by the other methods (Spadero, 1983).

The SMOG formula has been used extensively to judge grade-level readability of patient education materials. It is one of the most popular measurement tools because of its reputation for reading-level accuracy, its simple directions, and its speed of use, which is a particularly important factor if computerized resources for analysis of test samples are not available (Meade & Smith, 1991). See Appendix A for the method of formula analysis and for an example of how to apply the SMOG formula to a short passage.

In summary, Doak et al. (1996) state that it is critically important to determine the readability of all written materials at the time they are drafted or adopted by using one or more of the many available formulas. They contend that you cannot afford to fly blind by using health materials that are untested for readability difficulty. Pretesting PEMs before distribution is the way to be sure they fit the literacy level of the audience for which they are intended. It is imperative that the formulas used to measure grade-level readability of PEMs are appropriate for the type of material being tested (see **Table 7–5**).

Computerized Readability Software Programs

Computerized programs have helped tremendously in facilitating the use of readability formulas. Some software programs are capable of applying a number of formulas to analyze one text selection. In addition, some packages are able to identify difficult words in written passages that may not be understood by patients. Dozens of user-friendly, menu-driven commercial software packages can automatically calculate reading levels as well as provide advice on how to simplify text (Aldridge, 2004; Doak et al., 1996).

Computerized assessment of readability is fast and easy, and it provides a high degree of reliability, especially when several formulas are used. Determining readability by computer programs rather than doing so manually is also more accurate in calculating reading levels because it eliminates human error in scoring and because entire articles, pamphlets, or books can be scanned (Duffy & Sny-

Table 7–5 APPROPRIATE READABILITY FORMULA CHOICE

Formula	Selection Shorter Than 300 Words	Selection Longer Than 300 Words	Entire Piece	Grade Level
Spache score	Yes	Yes	Yes	1–3
Flesch formula	Yes	Yes	Yes	5 to college
Fog formula	Yes (minimum of 100 words)	Yes	Yes	4 to college
Fry graph	Not recommended	Yes	Yes	1 to college
SMOG formula	Yes	Yes	Yes	4 to college

Source: Adapted from Spadero, D. C., Robinson, L. A., & Smith, L. T. (1980), p. 216.

der, 1999). It is advisable to take an average across several pieces of literature, using several different formulas and software programs, when calculating estimates of readability.

Tests to Measure Comprehension of PEMs

A number of standardized tests have proved reliable and valid to measure comprehension of readers, a relatively new concept in health education (Doak et al., 1996). Usually pretests and posttests used in institutional settings measure recall of knowledge rather than comprehension. However, the determination of readers' abilities to comprehend information is essential. Health education materials must serve a useful purpose, both from the standpoint of assisting patients to assume self-care and for protecting the health professional from legal liability.

Comprehension implies that the reader has internalized the information found in PEMs (Aldridge, 2004). The two most popular standardized methods to measure comprehension of written materials are the cloze test and the listening test. These tests can be used to assess how much someone understands from reading or listening to a passage of text.

Cloze Procedure

The cloze test (derived from the term *closure*) has been specifically recommended for assessing understanding of health education literature. Although it takes more time and resources to compute than do readability formulas, the cloze procedure has been validated for its adequacy in ranking reading difficulty of medical literature, which typically has a high concept load. This procedure is not a formula that provides a school grade-type level of readability like the formulas already described, but rather takes into consideration the context of a written passage (Doak et al., 1996).

The cloze test can be administered to individual clients who demonstrate difficulty comprehending health materials used for instruction. Nevertheless, it is suggested that this test not be administered to every client in a particular health setting but rather to a representative sample of consumers. The cloze test should be used only with those individuals whose reading skills are at sixth grade or higher (approximately Level 1 on the NALS scale); otherwise, it is likely that the test will prove too difficult (Doak et al., 1996).

The cloze test is best used when reviewing the appropriateness of several texts of the same content for a particular audience. The reader may or may not be familiar with the material being tested. This procedure is designed so that every fifth word is systematically deleted from a portion of a text. The reader is asked to fill in the blanks with the exact word replacements. One point is scored for every missing word guessed correctly by the reader. The final cloze score is the total number of blanks filled in correctly by the reader.

To be successful, the reader must demonstrate sensitivity to clues related to grammar, syntax, and semantics. If the reader is able to fill in the blanks with appropriate words, this process is an indication of how well the material has been comprehended—that is, how much knowledge was obtained from the set surrounding the blank spaces and how well the information was used to supply the additional information (Dale & Chall, 1978; Doak et al., 1996). The underlying theory is that the more readable a passage is, the better it will be understood even when words are omitted. The resulting score can be converted to a percentage for ease in interpreting and analyzing the data (Pichert & Elam, 1985).

A score for the cloze test is obtained by dividing the number of exact word replacements by the total number of blanks. A score of 60% or better indicates that the passage was sufficiently understood by the patient. A score of 40–59% indicates a moderate level of difficulty, where supplemental teaching is required for the patient to understand the message. A score of less than 40% indicates the material is too difficult to be understood and is not suitable to be used for teaching (Doak et al., 1996).

Instead of using packaged cloze tests available from commercial sources, it is suggested that edu-

cators devise their own tests so that the resultant scores will indicate a client's comprehension of their own instructions. Then, problem words or sentences within these PEMs can be revised accordingly to make them more understandable. See Appendix A for an outline of the steps for constructing a cloze test, test scoring methodology, and a sample test.

Because the cloze procedure is a test of learners' ability to understand what they have read, health professional educators should be sure to be honest about the purpose of the test. For example, they might state that it is important for clients to understand what they are to do when on their own after discharge, so the educator wants to be sure they understand the written instructions they will need to follow. Doak et al. (1985) found that most people are willing to participate in the testing activity. They suggest that the following guidelines should be used before taking the cloze test:

1. Encourage participants to read through the entire test passage before attempting to fill in the blanks.
2. Tell them that only one word should be written in each blank.
3. Let them know that it is all right to guess, but that they should try to fill in every blank as accurately as possible.
4. Reassure them that spelling errors are all right just as long as the word they have put in the blank can be recognized.
5. Explain to them that this exercise is not a timed test. (If readers struggle to complete the test, tell them not to worry, that it is not necessary for them to fill in all the blanks, and set the test aside to go on to something else less frustrating or less threatening.)

Listening Test

Unlike the cloze test, which may be too difficult for clients who read below the sixth-grade level—

that is, those who likely lack fluency and read with hesitancy—the listening test is a good approach to determining what a low-literate person understands and remembers when listening to oral instruction (Doak et al., 1996). Although it may take a couple of hours to develop this test, it takes only about 10–20 minutes to administer.

The procedure for administering the listening test is to select a passage from instructional materials that takes about 3 minutes to read aloud and is written at approximately the fifth-grade level. Formulate 5–10 short questions relevant to the content of the passage by selecting key points of the text. Read the passage to the person at a normal rate. Ask the listener the questions orally and record the answers (Doak et al., 1996).

To determine the percentage score, divide the number of questions answered correctly by the total number of questions. The instructional material will be appropriate for the client's comprehension level if the score is approximately 75–89% (some additional assistance when teaching the material may be necessary for full comprehension). A score of 90% or higher indicates that the material is easy for the client and can be fully comprehended independently. A score of less than 75% means that the material is too difficult and simpler instructional material will need to be used when teaching the individual. Doak et al. (1996) provide an example of a sample passage and questions for a listening comprehension test.

Tests to Measure Reading Skills of Clients

The three most popular standardized methods to measure reading skill are the Wide Range Achievement Test (WRAT), the Rapid Estimate of Adult Literacy in Medicine (REALM), and the Test of Functional Health Literacy in Adults (TOFHLA). The Literacy Assessment for Diabetes (LAD) is a relatively new instrument specific to clients with diabetes.

WRAT (Wide Range Achievement Test)

The WRAT is a word recognition screening test. It is used to assess a learner's ability to recognize and pronounce a list of words out of context as a criterion for measuring reading skills. There are a number of word recognition tests available, but the WRAT requires the least time to administer (approximately 5 minutes as compared with 30 minutes or more for the other tests).

Although it is limited to measuring only word recognition and does not test other aspects of reading such as vocabulary and comprehension of text material, this test is nevertheless useful for determining an appropriate level of instruction and for establishing a client's level of literacy. It is based on the belief that reading skill is associated with the ability to look at written words and put them into oral language, a necessary first step in comprehension (Doak et al., 1996).

As designed, it should be used only to test people whose native language is English. The WRAT tests on two levels: Level I is designed for children 5 to 12 years of age, and Level II is intended for testing persons older than age 12. The WRAT scores are normed on age but can be converted to grade levels.

The WRAT consists of a graduated list of 42 words. Starting with the most easy and ending with the most difficult, the person taking the test is asked to pronounce the words from the list, starting from the top, where the easiest words are located. The individual administering the test listens carefully to the patient's responses and scores those responses on a master score sheet. Next to those words that are mispronounced, a checkmark should be placed. When five words are mispronounced, indicating that the patient has reached his or her limit, the test is stopped.

To score the test, the number of words missed or not tried is subtracted from the list of words on the master score sheet to get a raw score. Then a table of raw scores is used to find the equivalent grade rating (GR). For more information on this test, see Doak et al. (1996), Davis et al. (1998), and Quirk (2000).

REALM (Rapid Estimate of Adult Literacy in Medicine)

The REALM test has advantages over the WRAT and other word tests because it measures a patient's ability to read medical and health-related vocabulary, it takes less time to administer, the scoring is simpler, and is well received by most clients (Davis et al., 1998; Duffy & Snyder, 1999; Foltz & Sullivan, 1998). This instrument has been field tested on large populations in public health and primary care settings (Davis et al., 1993). Although it has established validity, this test offers less precision than other word tests (Hayes, 2000). The raw score is converted to a range of grade levels rather than an exact grade level, but this result correlates well with the WRAT reading scores.

The procedure for administering the test is to ask patients to read aloud words from three word lists. Sixty-six medical and health-related words are arranged in three columns of 22 words each, beginning with short, easy words such as *fat, flu, pill,* and *dose,* and ending with more difficult words such as *anemia, obesity, osteoporosis,* and *impetigo.* Clients are asked to begin at the top of the first column and read down, pronouncing all the words that they can from the three lists. If they come upon a word they cannot pronounce, they are told to skip it and proceed to the next word. There is no time limit. The examiner keeps score on a separate copy of the list and places a plus sign next to words correctly pronounced and a minus next to those mispronounced or skipped (Davis et al., 1993). The total number of words pronounced correctly

is the client's raw score, which is converted to a grade ranging from third grade and below (score of 0–18) to ninth grade and above (score of 61–66). Those whose scores fall at sixth grade or below have literacy skills equivalent to NALS Levels 1 and 2 (Schultz, 2002; Weiss, 2003).

TOFHLA (Test of Functional Health Literacy in Adults)

The TOFHLA is a relatively new instrument developed in the mid-1990s for measuring patients' literacy skills using actual hospital materials, such as prescription labels, appointment slips, and informed consent documents. The test consists of two parts: reading comprehension and numeracy. It has demonstrated reliability and validity, requires approximately 20 minutes to administer, and is available in a Spanish version (TOFHLA-S) as well as an English version (Parker, Baker, Williams, & Nurss, 1995; Quirk, 2000; Williams et al., 1995). A more recent abbreviated version, known as the S-TOFHLA, was developed in 1999; it takes only 12 minutes to administer. Not only has it been tested for reliability and validity, but it is a more practical measure of functional health literacy to determine who needs assistance with achieving learning goals (Baker et al., 1999). A copy of the TOFHLA instrument and directions can be accessed at http://www.peppercornbooks.com/catalog/information.php?info_id=5.

Readability formulas and standardized tests for comprehension and reading skills were never designed for the purpose of serving as writing guides. Patient educators may be tempted to write PEMs to fit the formulas and tests, but they should be aware that doing so places emphasis on structure, not content, and that comprehensibility of a written message may be greatly compromised. Pichert and Elam (1985) recommend that readability formulas should be used solely to judge material written without formulas in mind. Formulas are merely methods to check readability, and standardized tests are merely methods to check comprehension and word recognition. Neither method guarantees good style in the form of direct, conversational writing.

LAD (Literacy Assessment for Diabetes)

The LAD was specifically developed in 2001 to measure word recognition in adult patients with diabetes. This reading skills test, compared with WRAT3 (3rd version) and the REALM, was assessed to have strong reliability and validity. It consists of three word lists presented in ascending order of difficulty. The majority of terms are at the 4th-grade reading level, but the remaining words range from 6th- through 16th-grade levels. The LAD can be administered in 3 minutes or less. It was tested on a group of 200 people at a primary care clinic, a senior center, and three prisons. The subjects ranged in age from 20 to 85 years (mean age = 43.5). This standardized test was modeled after the REALM but emphasizes common words used when teaching self-care management of diabetes. The LAD instrument is copyrighted but is available with permission from Robert C. Byrd Health Sciences Center, Department of Family Medicine, PO Box 9152, Morgantown, WV 26505-9152, attn. Charlotte Nath, EdD (Nath et al., 2001) or via the Internet at http://tde.sage pub.com.

SAM (Instrument for Suitability Assessment of Materials)

In addition to using formulas and tests to measure readability, comprehension, and reading skills, Doak et al. (1996) designed a tool to rapidly and systematically assess the suitability of instructional materials for a given population of learners. Ideally, instructional tools should be evaluated with a sample of the intended audience, but limited time and resources may preclude such an approach. In response to this dilemma, these literacy experts developed the (suitability assessment of materials) SAM instrument. Not only can the SAM be used with print material and illustrations, but it has also been designed to be applied to video- and audiotaped instructions.

The SAM yields a numerical (percent) score, with materials tested falling into one of three categories: superior (70–100%), adequate (40–69%), or not suitable (0–39%). The application of the SAM can identify specific deficiencies in instructional materials that reduce their suitability. The SAM includes 22 factors to assess the content, literacy demand, graphics, layout and typography, learning stimulation and motivation, and cultural appropriateness of instructional materials being developed or already in use. The maximum score possible is 44 points (equals 100%). If one or more SAM factors do not apply to the material being tested, the test administrator should subtract two points each for every not applicable factor. For example, if the material tests at 36 but two factors did not apply, the maximum possible score would be 40. Thus, 36/40 = 90% (Doak et al., 1996). See Appendix A for the SAM instrument and directions for scoring.

Simplifying the Readability of PEMs

The suitability of written materials for different audiences depends not only on actual grade-level demand, which can be measured by readability formulas, but also on those elements within a text such as technical format, concept density, and accuracy and clarity of the message. It must never be forgotten that knowing the target audience in terms of the members' level of motivation, reading abilities, experiential factors, and cultural background is also of crucial importance in determining the appropriateness of printed health information as an effective communication tool (Meade & Smith,

1991; Weiss, 2003). Even good readers may fail to respond to important health education literature if they lack the motivation to do so or if the material is not appealing to them.

Despite the well-documented potential of written materials to increase knowledge, compliance, and satisfaction with care, PEMs are often too difficult for even motivated clients to read. Clearly, the technical nature of health education literature lends itself to high readability levels, often requiring college-level reading skills to fully comprehend (Winslow, 2001).

Even though printed materials are the most commonly used form of media, as currently written, they remain the least effective means for reaching a large proportion of the adult population who have marginal literacy skills (Monsivais & Reynolds, 2003). What the educator must strive to achieve when designing or selecting health-based literature is a good and proper fit between the material and the reader. Choosing and designing PEMs is a difficult, time-consuming, and challenging task that often becomes the responsibility of the health professional (Winslow, 2001).

Certainly the best solution for improving the overall comprehension and reading skills of clients would be to strengthen their basic general education, but this process would require decades to accomplish. What is needed now are ways in which to write or rewrite educational materials commensurate with the current comprehension and reading skills of learners. Nathaniel Hawthorne was once reported to have said, "Easy reading is damned hard writing" (Pichert & Elam, 1985, p. 181). He was correct in his perception that clear and concise writing is a task that takes effort and practice.

It is possible, though, to reduce the disparity between the literacy demand of written instructional materials and the actual reading level of clients by attending to some basic linguistic, motivational, organizational, and content principles. *Linguistics* refers to the type of language and grammatical style

used. Motivation principles focus on those elements that stimulate the reader, such as relevance and appeal of the material. Organizational factors deal with layout and clarity. Content principles relate to load and concept density of information (Bernier, 1993). Wood et al. (2007) describe the language, information, and design (LID) method to create easy-to-read materials. These elements are examined as they relate to designing or revising instructional materials for the marginally literate reader.

Prior to writing or rewriting a text for easier reading, however, some preliminary planning steps need to be taken to ensure that the final written material will be geared to the target audience (Davis et al., 1998; Doak et al., 1996; Kessels, 2003). The steps are as follows:

1. Decide what the client should do or know. In other words, what is the purpose of the instruction? What outcomes do you hope learners will achieve?

2. Choose information that is relevant and needed by the client to achieve the behavioral objectives. Limit or cut out altogether extraneous and nice-to-know information such as the history or detailed physiological processes of a disease. Include only survival skills and essential main ideas of who, what, where, and when, with new information related to what the reader already knows. Remember: A person does not have to know how an engine works to drive a car.

3. Select other media to supplement the written information, such as pictures, demonstrations, models, audiotapes, and videotapes. Even poor readers will benefit from written material if it is combined with other forms of delivering a message. Consider the field of advertising, for example. Advertisers get their message across with words but often in combination with strong, action-packed visuals.

4. Organize topics into chunks that follow a logical sequence. Prioritize to present the most im-

portant information first. If topics are of equal importance, proceed from the more general as a basis on which to build to the more specific. Begin with a statement of purpose. In a list of items, place key facts at the top and bottom because readers best remember information presented first and last in a series.

5. Determine the preferred reading level of the material. If the readers have been tested, preferably write two to four grades below the reading grade-level score. If the audience has not been tested, the group is likely to display a wide range of reading skills. When in doubt, write instructional materials at the 5th-grade level, which is the lowest common denominator, keeping in mind that the average reading level of the population is approximately 8th grade, that more than 20% read below the 5th-grade

level, and that fewer than 50% read above the 10th-grade level.

To cover a wide range of reading skills, it is also possible to develop two sets of instructions—one at a higher grade level and one at a lower grade level—and allow patients to select the one they prefer (**Table 7–6**). Once the reading grade level of a piece of written material is determined, it should be printed on the back of the document in coded form as, for example, RL = 7 (reading level = seventh grade), for easy reference.

The literature contains numerous references related to techniques for writing effective educational materials (Aldridge, 2004; Andrus & Roth, 2002; Buxton, 1999; Doak et al., 1996; Doak et al., 1998; Duffy & Snyder, 1999; Horner et al., 2000; Mayer & Rushton, 2002; Monsivais

---

Table 7–6 EXAMPLE OF LOWERED READABILITY LEVEL

NINTH-GRADE LEVEL

Smoking contributes to heart disease in the following ways:

1. When you smoke, you inhale carbon monoxide and nicotine, which causes your blood vessels to narrow, your heart rate to increase, and your blood pressure to go up. All of these factors increase the workload for your heart.

2. Carbon monoxide stimulates your body to produce more red blood cells. The presence of more red cells means that your blood will clot more readily, leading to increased risk of coronary artery disease and stroke.

3. Carbon monoxide and nicotine may also increase your risk of atherosclerotic buildup by causing damage to your artery walls.

4. Smoking raises blood cholesterol level and has been known to cause irregular heartbeats.

FOURTH-GRADE LEVEL

Smoking hurts your heart in many ways:

1. Smoking makes your heart beat faster, raises your blood pressure, and makes your blood vessels smaller. All these things cause your heart to work harder.

2. Smoking makes your blood clot easier. This increases your chance of having a heart attack or a stroke.

3. Smoking makes your cholesterol level go up. It may also damage your blood vessels.

4. Smoking may make your heartbeat less regular.

Source: From Wong, M. (1992, February). Self-care instructions: Do patients understand educational materials? *Focus on Critical Care, 19*(1), 47–49. Reprinted with permission of American Association of Critical-Care Nurses. © 1992 Elsevier.

& Reynolds, 2003; Pignone et al., 2005; Weiss, 2003). Recommendations have been put forth for developing written instructions that can be more easily understood by a wide audience.

The strategies described in this section are specific with regard to simplifying written health information for clients with low literacy skills. The key factor in accommodating low-literate readers is to write in plain, familiar language using an easy visual format. The following general guidelines are some basic linguistic, motivational, organizational, and content principles to adhere to when writing effective PEMs:

1. Write in a conversational style using the personal pronoun *you* and the possessive pronoun *your*. Use an active voice in the present tense rather than a passive voice in the past or future tense. The message is more personalized, more imperative, more interesting, and easier to understand if instruction is written as "Take your medicine …" instead of "Medicine should be taken …" This rule is considered to be the most important technique to reduce the level of reading difficulty and to improve comprehension of what is read. Directly addressing the reader through personal words and sentences engages the reader. For example:

   LESS EFFECTIVE

   People who sunburn easily and have fair skin with red or blond hair are most prone to develop skin cancer. The amount of time spent in the sun affects a person's risk of skin cancer.[1]

   MORE EFFECTIVE

   If you sunburn easily and have fair skin with red or blond hair, you are more likely to get skin cancer. How much time you spend in the sun affects your risk of skin cancer.

2. Use short words and common vocabulary with only one or two syllables as much as possible. Rely on sight words, known as high-frequency words, which are recognized by almost everyone. The key is to choose words that sound familiar and natural and are easy to read and understand, such as *shot* rather than *injection* and *use* instead of *utilize*. Avoid compound words, such as *lifesaver*, and words with prefixes or suffixes, such as *reoccur* or *emptying*, that create multisyllable words.

   Also, try to avoid technical words and medical terms (medicalese), and substitute common, nontechnical, lay terms such as *stroke* instead of *cardiovascular accident*. Be sure to select substitutions carefully because they may have a different meaning for some people than for others or in one context versus another. For example, if the word *medicine* is replaced with the word *drug*, the latter may be interpreted as the illegal variety. Using modest words is not considered talking down to readers; it is considered talking to them at a more comfortable level.

3. Spell out words rather than using abbreviations or acronyms. *That is* should be used instead of *i.e.* and *for example* instead of *e.g.* Abbreviations for the months of the year (such as *Sept.*) or the days of the week (*Wed.*, for example) are a real problem for clients with limited vocabulary. Also do not use acronyms, such as CVA or NPO, unless these medical abbreviations are clearly defined beforehand in the text.

4. Organize information into chunks, which improves recall. Also, use numbers sparingly and only when absolutely necessary. Statistics are usually meaningless and are another source of confusion for the low-literate reader. Limit the number of items in any list to no more than seven. People have a difficult time remembering more than seven consecutive items (Baddeley, 1994).

---

[1] *Fry Now, Pay Later*, American Cancer Society pamphlet, No. 2611, 1985.

5. Keep sentences short, preferably not longer than 20 words and fewer if possible, because they are easier to read and understand for clients with short-term memories or who struggle decoding words of a sentence. Avoid subordinate (dependent) clauses that make the reading more difficult. The use of commas, colons, or dashes results in long, complex sentences that turn off the reader. Titles also should be short and convey the purpose and meaning of the material that follows.

6. Clearly define any technical or unfamiliar words by using parentheses that include simple terms after difficult words—for example, "bacteria (germ)." A glossary that provides definitions of each difficult term is a helpful tool, but it is highly recommended to spell out terms phonetically immediately following the unfamiliar word within the text; for example, "Alzheimer's (pronounced Alts-hi-merz)." If a new technical vocabulary word needs to be introduced, such as *diabetes* or *hypertension*, it should be used and repeated frequently (Byrne & Edeani, 1984; Spees, 1991). Standal's (1981) method suggests identifying words whose meanings should be taught to the reader prior to introducing the instructional material to increase reader comprehension and to avoid having to make major revisions to a printed piece.

7. Use words consistently throughout the text and avoid interchanging words. For example, if discussing diet, adhere to the word *diet* rather than substituting other terms for it, such as *meal plan*, *menu*, *food schedule*, and *dietary prescription*, which merely confuse readers and can lead to misunderstanding of instruction.

8. Avoid value judgment words with many interpretations, such as *excessive*, *regularly*, and *frequently*. How much pain or bleeding is excessive? How often is regularly or frequently? Use exact terms to describe what you mean by

using, for example, a scale of 1–5 or explaining frequency in terms of minutes, hours, or days. Instead of saying, "drink milk frequently," you should be more specific by stating, "drink three full glasses of milk every day."

9. Put the most important information first by prioritizing the need to know. Place essential messages up front and get rid of extraneous details.

10. Use advance organizers (topic headings or headers) and subheadings. They clue in the reader to what is going to be presented and help focus the reader's attention on the message.

11. Limit the use of connectives such as *however*, *consequently*, *even though*, and *in spite of* that lengthen sentences and make them more complex. Also, avoid *and* if it connects two different ideas; instead break the ideas into two sentences.

12. Make the first sentence of a paragraph the topic sentence, and, if possible, make the first word the topic of the sentence. For example:
    LESS EFFECTIVE
    Even though overexposure to the sun is the leading cause, it isn't necessary to give up the outdoors in order to reduce your chances of developing skin cancer.[2]
    MORE EFFECTIVE
    Enjoying the outdoors is still possible if you take steps to reduce your risk of skin cancer when in the sun.
    OR
    You can reduce your chance of skin cancer even when enjoying the outdoors.

13. Reduce concept density by limiting each paragraph to a simple message or action and include only one idea per sentence. In the following example, the original paragraph con-

---

[2] *Fry Now, Pay Later*, American Cancer Society pamphlet, No. 2611, 1985.

tains at least six concepts. As rewritten, the revised paragraph has been reduced to four concepts (and is written using the second person pronoun, which is a much more personalized approach):

ORIGINAL PARAGRAPH

A person who has had a stroke may or may not be able to return to his or her former level of functioning, depending on the extent and location of brain damage. Mental attitude, efforts of the rehabilitation team, and the understanding of family and friends also affect the patient's progress. Recovery must be gradual, but it should begin the moment the patient is hospitalized. After the patient is tested to determine the extent of brain damage, rehabilitation such as physical, speech, and occupational therapy should begin. Family and friends should be told how to handle special problems the stroke victim may have, such as irrational behavior or difficulty communicating.[3]

REVISED PARAGRAPH

Getting back to your normal life after a stroke is an important part of your recovery. Each stroke patient is different. Your progress depends on where and how much your brain is damaged. Getting better will take time. The care you get will begin while you are in the hospital. How you think and feel about what happened to you will help you handle special problems. Also helpful to you is the care given by the nurses, doctors, and other health professionals. The support you get from your family and friends is important, too.

---

[3] Adapted from American Heart Association. (1983). *An Older Person's Guide to Cardiovascular Health*. National Center, 7320 Greenville Avenue, Dallas, TX 75321. The information from this book is not current and is used for illustration purposes only.

14. Keep density of words low by not exceeding 30–40 characters (letters) per line. The number of words in each line is influenced by the size of the font.

15. Allow for plenty of white space in margins, and use generous spacing between paragraphs and double spacing within paragraphs to reduce density. Pages that are not crowded seem less overwhelming to the reader with low-literacy skills.

16. Keep right margins unjustified because the jagged right margins help the reader distinguish one line from another. In this way, the eye does not have to adjust to different spacing between letters and words as it does with justified type.

17. Design layouts that encourage eye movement from left to right, as in normal reading. In simple drawings and diagrams, using arrows or circles that give direction is helpful, but do not add too many elements to a schematic.

18. Select a simple type style (serif, Times New Roman, or Courier) and a large font (14 or 16 point size) in the body of the text for ease of reading and to increase motivation to read. A sans serif font (without little hooks at the top and bottom of letters) or other type of clean style should be used only for titles to give style to the page. Avoid *italics*, *fancy lettering*, and ALL CAPITAL letters. Low-literate readers are not fluent with the alphabet and need to look at each letter to recognize a word. To facilitate their decoding of words in titles, headings, and subheadings, use uppercase and lowercase letters, which provide reading cues given by tall and short letters on the type line. Avoid using a large stylized letter to begin a new paragraph, such as:

This looks attractive, but it is confusing to a poor reader who cannot decode the word minus the first letter.

19. Highlight important ideas or key terms with bold type or underlining, but never use all capital letters or italics.

20. If using color, employ it consistently throughout the text to emphasize key points or to organize topics. Color, if applied appropriately, attracts the reader. Red, yellow, and orange are warm colors that are more eye-catching and easier to read than cold colors such as violet, blue, and green. Use bold, solid colors and avoid pastel colors that all look gray to older adults with vision problems, such as cataracts.

21. Create a simple cover page with a title (in uppercase and lowercase lettering) that clearly and succinctly states the topic to be addressed. The title should ideally be one to four words in length.

22. Limit the entire length of a document—the shorter, the better. It should be long enough just to cover the essential, need-to-know information. Too many pages with nice-to-know information will turn off even the most eager and capable reader.

23. Select paper that is attractive and on which the typeface is easy to read. Black print on white paper is most easily read and most economical. Dull finishes reduce the glare of light. Avoid high-gloss paper, which reflects light into the eyes of the reader and is usually too formal and not in harmony with the purpose and informal tone of your message.

24. Use bold line drawings and simple, realistic pictures and diagrams. Basic visuals aid the reader to better understand the text information. Use cartoons judiciously, however, because they can trivialize the message and make it less credible.

    Graphic designs that are strictly decorative should never be used because they are distracting and confusing. Also, never superimpose words on a background design because it makes reading the letters of the words very difficult. Only illustrations that enhance understanding of the text and that relate specifically to the message should be used.

    Be careful to use pictures that portray the messages intended. For example, avoid using a picture of a pregnant woman smoking or drinking alcohol because this negative message is dependent on careful reading of the text to correct a faulty impression. The visuals should clearly show only those actions that you want the reader to do and remember. Be sure that visuals do not communicate cultural bias.

    Use simple subtitles and captions for each picture. Also, be sure drawings are recognizable to the audience. For instance, if you draw a picture of the lungs, be certain they are within the outline of the person's body to accurately depict the location of the organs. The person with low literacy may not know what they are looking at if the lungs are not put in context with the body's torso. However, pictures do not necessarily make the text easier to read if the readability level remains high.

25. Include a summary section using bullet points or a numbered list to review what has already been presented. A question-and-answer format using the client's point of view is an effective way to summarize information in single units using a conversational style. The following example is adapted from an American Cancer Society pamphlet.[4]

    Q: Am I likely to get skin cancer?

    A: If you have spent a lot of time in the sun, you have a greater chance of getting skin cancer than people who have stayed out of the strong sunlight. If you sunburn easily, you are at more risk for skin cancer. If you have fair skin with red or blond hair, you are

---

[4] *Fry Now, Pay Later*, American Cancer Society pamphlet, No. 2611, 1985.

more likely to get skin cancer than people with dark skin.

Q: How can I tell if I have skin cancer?

A: The only way to know for certain is to see your doctor. Your doctor may want to take a sample of skin to test for cancer. If you have a red, scaly patch, a mole that has changed, or an area of the skin that does not heal, see your doctor right away.

Q: How can I prevent skin cancer?

A: Stay out of direct sunlight between 11:00 a.m. and 2:00 p.m. When outside in the sun, cover up with clothing, wear a wide-brimmed hat, and use sunscreens that block out the sun's harmful rays.

Ask for feedback after clients have read your instructions. Either have readers explain the information in their own words or have them demonstrate the desired behavior. If learners can do so correctly, it is a good indication that the information is understood. Do not ask questions such as "Do you understand?" because you are likely to get a "yes" or "no" answer, not a substantive response.

26. Put the reading level (RL) on the back of a PEM for future reference—for example, if the PEM is readable at the sixth-grade level, the designation would be RL6.

27. Determine readability by applying at least two formulas (SMOG, Fog, and Fry are suggested). Also, you can measure comprehension by applying the cloze or listening test and check reading skills by applying the WRAT, REALM, or TOFHLA.

It does not take a great deal of effort, just know-how and common sense, to improve the readability and comprehensibility of instructional materials (see **Table 7–7** for a summary of tips). The benefits are significant in terms of compliance and quality of care when marginally literate patients are given PEMs that effectively communicate messages they can read and understand.

Always remember to test any new materials before printing and distributing them. Not only will this effort save the cost of printing handouts that might not be useful, but patients will have the opportunity to participate in the evaluative process. Readily understandable materials also reduce time and frustration on the part of the health professional and avoid the possibility of litigation when better-quality and more appropriate healthcare instructions are used. The important role of printed media to communicate health information should compel all writers of PEMs to use the techniques recommended in this chapter. As Doak and Doak (1987) so aptly summarize, "With so much to be gained, the investments of a little time and thoughtful attention to the materials provided to patients can pay back dividends too important to ignore" (p. 8).

Teaching Strategies for Clients With Low Literacy

Working with clients who are illiterate and marginally literate requires more than designing simple-to-read instructional literature. It also calls for using alternative and innovative teaching strategies to break down the barriers of illiteracy. Using techniques to improve communication with clients has the potential to greatly enhance their understanding (Mayeaux et al., 1996; Weiss, 2003).

Teaching clients with poor reading skills does not have to be viewed as a problem, but rather can be seen as a challenge (Dunn, Buckwalter, Weinstein, & Palti, 1985). Existing teaching methods and tools can be adapted to meet the logic, language, and experience of the patient who has difficulty with reading and comprehension (Doak et al., 1998). Incidentally, many literate and highly motivated clients also can benefit from some of these same teaching strategies.

Many authors (Austin, Matlock, Dunn, Kesler, & Brown, 1995; Davis et al., 2002; Doak et al.,

1998; Houts et al., 1998; Kessels, 2003; Lerner et al., 2000; Mayeaux et al., 1996; Pignone et al., 2005; Rothman et al., 2004; Schultz, 2002; Webber, Higgins, & Baker, 2001; Weiss, 2003; Winslow, 2001) suggest the following tips as useful strategies for the health professional to employ when in the role of educator:

1. *Establish a trusting relationship before beginning the teaching–learning process.* Start by getting to know the clients to reduce their anxiety. Because many poor readers have a history of being defensive, the health professional must attempt to overcome their defense mechanisms by casting aside communication barriers such as any preconceived notions, including myths and stereotypes. Also, focus on clients' strengths. Demonstrate your belief in them as responsible individuals. Be open and honest about what specifically needs to be learned to build up their confidence in their ability to perform self-care activities. Encourage family and friends to help reinforce the clients' self-confidence. Remember, your role as educator is to facilitate learning by providing guidance and support.

2. *Use the smallest amount of information possible to accomplish the predetermined behavioral objectives.* Stick to the essentials, paring down the information you teach to what the client must learn. Prioritize behavioral objectives, and select only one or two concepts to present and discuss in any one session. Present the context of the message first before giving any new information. Remember, clients with poor comprehension and reading skills are easily overwhelmed. Information about the history of treatment, general principles, statistics, detailed physiology, and extraneous facts about a topic are not necessary for them to know. Keep teaching sessions short, limiting them to no more than 20–30 minutes, but 15–20 minutes is the ideal time limit.

3. *Make points of information as vivid and explicit as possible.* Explain information in simple, concrete terms using everyday, living-room language. Provide personal examples relevant to the client's background. Visual aids, such as signs and pictographs, should be large with readable print and contain only one or two messages. For example, a sign reading "NOTHING BY MOUTH" or, worse yet, "NPO" should be changed to "Do not eat or drink anything" (remember to avoid using all-capital letters and abbreviations).

   Underlining, highlighting, color coding, arrows, and common international symbols can be used effectively to give directions and draw attention to important information. For example, different-colored signs, pictorial cues, and other visual stimuli, such as strips on the floor tiles that lead to specific areas of the hospital, are valuable for increasing independence and safety.

4. *Teach one step at a time.* Teaching in increments and organizing information into segments of information (chunks) help to reduce anxiety and confusion and give enough time for clients to understand each item before proceeding to the next unit of information. Also, these techniques give clients a sense of order and a chance to ask questions after each block of information has been presented. In addition, you have the opportunity to assess their progress and reward them with words of encouragement, praise, and reinforcement every step of the way. Most important, the pacing of instruction allows for more adequate time between sessions for learners to assimilate information.

5. *Use multiple teaching methods and tools requiring fewer literacy skills.* Oral instruction contains cues such as tone, gestures, and expressions that are not found in written materials. However, the spoken word lacks other signals, such as punctuation and capital letters. Therefore, a

person with poor reading skills may likely have some trouble with understanding spoken language as well. The listening test, as previously described, can be used to measure comprehension of oral instruction. Another way to test the difficulty level of information presented verbally is to begin by taping a spoken message, converting it into a written form, and finally applying a readability formula to it.

Exposing clients to repetition and multiple forms of the same message is highly recommended. Audiotaped instruction, used in combination with other visual resources such as simple lists, pictorials, and videotapes, can help to improve comprehension and reduce learning time. These media forms, as more permanent sources of information, can also be sent home with the client for added reinforcement of health messages. Also, interactive computer programs, which allow clients to proceed at their own pace, can be programmed developmentally to match a user's literacy skill level.

6. *Allow patients the chance to restate information in their own words and to demonstrate any procedures being taught.* Use the "teach back" or "show me" method to verify that information shared with the learner was, in fact, understood. Encouraging them to explain something in their own words may take longer and requires patience on the part of the educator, but feedback in this manner can reveal gaps in knowledge or misconceptions of information. Return demonstration, hands-on practice, role-playing real-life situations, and sharing personal stories in dialogue form are communication modes that provide you with feedback as to the client's level of functioning.

Trying to elicit feedback by asking questions does not always work because people with low literacy skills often do not have the right vocabulary or fluency to explain what they do and do not understand. Remember, do not ask questions that will elicit only a yes or no response. This is because learners will likely respond in the affirmative, even when they have no clue as to what the health professional educator is talking about, just so they do not have to admit their ignorance.

Furthermore, they are unlikely to ask questions of the educator for fear of embarrassment at not understanding instructions. Use open-ended statements, such as "Tell me what you understand about … " to obtain feedback from them to verify their comprehension. Encouraging clients to repeat instructions in their own words or physically demonstrate an activity is an effective approach to verifying what they really understand.

Chew et al. (2004), based on their research, developed the following three questions as a practical and quick method for identifying literacy skills in patients: (1) "How often do you have someone help you read hospital materials?" (2) "How confident are you filling out medical forms by yourself?" and (3) "How often do you have problems learning about your medical condition because of difficulty understanding written information?" They found these three questions to be effective screening tests for inadequate health literacy in patients at the VA preop clinic, but not as effective for detecting patients with marginal health literacy.

7. *Keep motivation high.* It is important to recognize that people with limited literacy may feel like failures when they cannot work through a problem. Reassure them that it is normal to have trouble with new information and that they are doing well. Encouraging them to keep trying and recognizing any progress they make, even if in small increments, is motivating to the slow learner. Rewards—not punishments—are excellent motivators. Sticking to the basics and keeping the information relevant and succinct maintain a learner's interest and willingness to learn.

Table 7–7 SUMMARY OF TIPS FOR DESIGNING EFFECTIVE LOW-LITERACY PRINTED MATERIALS

CONTENT

Clearly define the purpose of the material.
Decide when and how the information will be used.
Use behavioral objectives that cover the main points.
Verify the accuracy of content with experts.
Give "how to" information for the learner to achieve objectives.
Present only the most essential information (three to four main ideas: who, what, where, and when).
Relate new information to what the audience already knows.
Present content relevant to the audience and avoid cultural bias in writing and graphics.

ORGANIZATION

Keep titles short, yet use words that clearly convey the meaning of the content.
Provide a table of contents for lengthy material and a summary to review content presented.
Present the most important information first.
Use topic headings (advance organizers).
Make the first sentence of each paragraph the topic sentence.
Include only a few concepts per paragraph.
Use short, simple sentences that convey only one idea at a time; limit the length of the entire text.
Limit lists to no more than seven items.
Present each idea in logical sequence.

LAYOUT/GRAPHICS

Select large, easily read print (minimum 12-point type) and use nonglossy paper.
Write headings and subheadings in both lowercase and uppercase letters; avoid fancy lettering.
Use bold type or underlining to emphasize important information.
Use lots of white space between segments of information.
Use generous margins and keep right-hand margins unjustified.
Provide a question-and-answer format for patient–nurse interaction.
Select double spacing (between lines of type), type style (serif), and font (print size) for ease of reading.
Design a colorful, eye-catching cover that suggests the message contained in the text.

LINGUISTICS

Keep sentences short (ideally 8–10 words, but no more than 20 words).
Write in the active voice, using the present tense and the pronouns *you* and *your* to engage the reader.
Use one- to two-syllable words as much as possible; avoid multisyllabic (polysyllabic) words.
Use words familiar and understandable to the target audience.
Avoid complex grammatical structures (i.e., multiple clauses).
Limit the number of concepts.
Focus content on what the audience should do as well as know.
Use positive statements; avoid negative messages.
Use questions throughout the text to encourage active learning.
Provide examples the audience can use to relate to personal experiences/circumstances.
Avoid using double negatives and value judgment words.
Clearly define terms likely to be unclear to audience.

Table 7–7 SUMMARY OF TIPS FOR DESIGNING EFFECTIVE LOW-LITERACY PRINTED MATERIALS *(Continued)*

VISUALS

Include simple, culturally sensitive illustrations and pictures.

Use simple drawings, but only if they improve the understanding of essential information.

Choose illustrations and photographs free of clutter and distractions.

Convey a single message or point of information in each visual.

Use visuals that are relevant to the text and meaningful to the audience.

Use drawings recognizable to the audience that reflect familiar images.

Use adult rather than childlike images (use cartoons sparingly).

Use captions to describe illustrations.

Use cues such as arrows, underlines, circles, and color to give direction to ideas and to highlight the most important information.

Use appealing and appropriate colors for the audience (for older adults, use black and white, and avoid pastel shades, especially blue, green, and violet hues).

READABILITY AND COMPREHENSION

Perform analysis with readability formulas and comprehension tests to determine reading level of material.

Write materials two to four grade levels below the determined literacy level of the audience.

Pilot test the material to determine readability, comprehensibility, and appeal before its widespread use.

Source: Adapted from Bernier, M. J. (1993). Developing and evaluating printed education materials: A prescriptive model for quality. *Orthopedic Nursing, 12*(6), 42, and from papers from the 16th Annual Conference on Patient Education, Nov. 17–20, 1994, Orlando, FL—sponsored by American Academy of Family Physicians and Society of Teachers of Family Medicine.

8. *Build in coordination of procedures.* A way to facilitate learning is to simplify information by using the principles of tailoring and cuing. *Tailoring* refers to coordinating recommended regimens into the daily schedules of clients rather than forcing them to adjust their lifestyles to these regimens. Otherwise, they may feel that changes are being imposed on them. Tailoring allows new tasks to be associated with old behaviors. It personalizes the message so that instruction is individualized to meet the client's learning needs. For example, coordinating a medication schedule to a patient's mealtimes does not drastically alter everyday lifestyle and tends to increase motivation and compliance. *Cuing* focuses on the appropriate combination of time and situation using prompts and reminders to get a person to perform a routine task. For example, placing medications where they best can be seen on a frequent basis or keeping a simple chart to check off each time a pill is taken serves as a reminder to comply with taking medications as prescribed.

Both of these principles are related to the behavior modification theory and are especially useful techniques to encourage compliance with medications. Because poor readers often cannot decipher schedules, tailoring and cuing can assist them to adhere to time frames.

9. *Use repetition to reinforce information.* Repetition, at appropriate intervals, is a key strategy to use with clients who have low literacy. Each major point made along the way should be reviewed. Therefore, time must be set aside to remind learners of what has come before and to prepare them for what is to follow. But this

is time well spent. Repetition, in the form of saying the same thing in different ways, is one of the most powerful tools to help clients understand their situations and learn important self-care measures.

All of these teaching strategies are especially well suited to the individual needs of people with low-literacy skills. As noted earlier, health professionals must empower consumers by providing health information that is culturally and linguistically appropriate. Creating an open, trusting, and accepting environment that makes it acceptable for the client to say "I don't understand" is the cornerstone of effective communication (Cole, 2000).

It is always a challenge to teach clients who, because of illness or a threat to their well-being, may be anxious, frightened, depressed, in denial, or in pain. Teaching patients, in particular, is even more of a special challenge in today's healthcare environment, when varying degrees of literacy compound the ability of a significant portion of the adult population to understand information vital to their health and welfare.

State of the Evidence

In 1999, the Ad Hoc Committee on Health Literacy for the Council on Scientific Affairs of the American Medical Association acknowledged that, although a great deal had been learned to that date about the magnitude and consequences of the problem of illiteracy and low literacy, further research efforts had to focus on four areas:

1. Literacy screening
2. Methods of health education
3. Medical outcomes and economic costs
4. Understanding the causal pathway of how health literacy influences health status

The committee also called for healthcare policies to address the issue of health literacy for the following reasons:

1. Low-literate patients cannot be empowered consumers in a market-driven healthcare system.
2. Patients who cannot understand healthcare instructions will not receive quality health care.
3. Healthcare professionals are subject to liability for adverse outcomes by patients who do not understand important health information.
4. Clinical management problems likely result in substantial but avoidable costs for the U.S. healthcare system.
5. Health literacy problems are more prevalent in certain populations (Medicare beneficiaries, Medicaid recipients, and uninsured individuals).

Indeed, as a result of the findings of the NALS and NAAL reports, a broad policy agenda on health literacy has been put forth in the 10-year goals and objectives of *Healthy People 2010* (U.S. Department of Health and Human Services, 2003). Specifically, objective 11-2 (Improvement of Health Literacy) addresses three major health literacy initiatives: prevention measures, interaction activities between healthcare providers and clients, and navigation of the healthcare system. Although the literacy and verbal skills of individuals are concerns of critical importance, so too are the demands made by PEMs, the need to improve communication skills of health professionals, and the need to make the healthcare system less complex.

The specific reports by the Institute of Medicine (IOM), the Agency for Healthcare Research and Quality (AHRQ), and the American Medical Association (AMA), all released in 2004, recognized that health literacy is a key priority in transforming the U.S. healthcare system (Aldridge, 2004; Weiss et al., 2005). In particular, AHRQ examined the relationship between literacy and adverse outcomes as well as interventions to improve outcomes for people who are low literate (Pignone et al., 2005).

The interest in the literacy problem has escalated tremendously in the past 5–10 years and numerous research studies have been conducted to examine many aspects of the problem. Pignone et al. (2005) conducted a systematic review of intervention studies designed to improve health outcomes of clients with low health literacy. These authors called for further research to understand the types of interventions that would be most effective and efficient. Also, Williams et al. (2002) examined patient–physician communication as a critical factor affecting health outcomes. These researchers, noted experts in the field of health literacy, have called for additional research on the optimal methods for interacting with people who have limited literacy skills. Healthcare research must specifically focus on client interaction techniques that improve understanding of health information, which would lead to a higher level of motivation and compliance.

Baker et al. (1998) studied health literacy and the risk of increased hospital admissions. They called for further research that would lead to a more accurate assessment of the impact of low literacy on healthcare costs. If the consequences of inadequate literacy result in poorer health outcomes and higher costs for health care, this would be an incentive for all types of payers to develop education programs to better reach patients with different levels of reading ability.

However, it is not yet well understood if health education materials for clients with low literacy do, in fact, improve health outcomes. In addition, more evidence is needed on the benefits of nonprint media, such as videos, audiotapes, and computers, in helping clients to overcome barriers of health illiteracy to improve their quality of life. In addition, much more attention must be paid to the ethical and legal implications of providing education materials to clients with limited literacy skills that are suitable to meet their health information needs. Health professionals, in the role of educators, must empirically explore teaching and learning approaches to find those most effective in working with clients who suffer the burden of illiteracy and low literacy.

Summary

The ability to learn from health instruction varies for clients, depending on such factors as educational background, motivational levels, reading and comprehension skills, and readability level of the materials used for instruction. The prevalence of functional illiteracy and low literacy is a major problem in the adult population of this country. Health professionals in the role of educators serve as communicators and interpreters of health information. They must always be alert to the potentially limited capacity of their clients to grasp the meaning of written and oral instruction. Health professionals need to know how to identify clients with literacy problems, assess their needs, and choose appropriate interventions that create a supportive environment directed toward helping those with poor reading and comprehension skills to better and more safely care for themselves. An awareness of the incidence of illiteracy, the populations most at risk, and the effects that literacy levels have on motivation and compliance with self-management regimens are key to understanding the barriers to communication between health professionals and clients.

The first half of this chapter focuses on the magnitude of the illiteracy problem, the myths and stereotypes associated with poor literacy skills, the assessment of variables affecting reading and comprehension of information, and the readability levels of patient education materials. The remainder of the chapter examines in detail the measurement tools available to test for readability, comprehension, and reading skills, guidelines for writing and evaluating education materials, and specific teaching strategies to be used to match the logic, language, and experience of clients with literacy problems.

Data suggest that written materials are an important source of health information to reinforce and complement other methods and tools of instruction. PEMs are the most cost-effective and time-efficient means to communicate health messages, but research suggests that there is a large discrepancy between the average comprehension and reading skills of clients and the readability level of current written instructional aids. Unless this gap is narrowed, printed sources of information can serve no useful purpose for adults who suffer with illiteracy and low literacy.

Removing the barriers to communication between clients and healthcare providers offers an ideal opportunity for health professionals to function as facilitators and work collaboratively with other health professionals to improve the quality of care delivered to consumers. It is their mandated responsibility to teach in understandable terms so that clients can fully benefit from interventions.

REVIEW QUESTIONS

1. What are the definitions of the terms *literacy, illiteracy, low literacy, functional illiteracy,* and *health literacy*?
2. Approximately how many millions of Americans are considered to be illiterate or functionally illiterate? This represents what percentage of the U.S. population?
3. Why are the rates of low literacy and illiteracy potentially on the rise in the United States?
4. Why is the number of years of schooling a poor indicator of someone's literacy level?
5. What segments of the U.S. population are more likely to be at risk for having poor reading and comprehension skills?
6. Why are problems with low literacy and functional illiteracy greater in older adults than in younger age groups?
7. What are three common myths about people who are illiterate?
8. What are seven clues that clients who are illiterate may demonstrate?
9. What impact does illiteracy or low literacy have on a person's level of motivation and compliance?
10. How does reliance on printed education materials to supplement teaching pose an ethical or legal liability for nurse educators?
11. Which measurement tools (formulas and standardized tests) are used specifically to test readability, comprehension, and reading skills?
12. What are 10 general guidelines to simplify written educational materials for clients with low literacy skills?
13. What five teaching strategies can be used by educators to make health information more understandable for clients with poor reading and comprehension skills?

CASE STUDY

As an institution committed to serving the community, Smithfield University Hospital has agreed to provide healthcare services to the women and children living in the Elias Domestic Violence Shelter (EDVS) located 5 miles from the hospital. These services include a special weekly clinic held at the shelter as well as in-hospital services as needed. It is anticipated that all units in the hospital will participate in the program.

EDVS is a 32-bed shelter for women and children seeking refuge from violence in their homes. The residents represent the most high risk segment of the domestic violence population. The violence they have experienced is severe and they have very limited social and material resources. They come to the shelter because they have nowhere else to go. Few of the women are employed and most have a high school diploma or less. Their healthcare needs range from emergency services to acute and preventive physical and mental health services. Several of the women and children have chronic conditions. The residents are a transient population and their contact with healthcare services is limited and infrequent. Health education is an important component of the care they receive from the hospital staff, who strive to teach them to care for themselves and their children.

1. What risk factors suggest that this population may have low literacy and inadequate health skills?
2. How would you assess the reading and comprehension levels of the residents? What clues will you look for?
3. Select a teaching strategy you would use with this population. Explain why this strategy would work when teaching groups with mixed literacy levels.
4. How will you evaluate the learning that has taken place as a result of your instruction?

References

Ache, K.A.(2009). Are end of life patient education materials readable? *Palliative Medicine*, *23*, 545–548.

Ad Hoc Committee on Health Literacy for the Council on Scientific Affairs, American Medical Association. (1999). Health literacy: Report of the Council on Scientific Affairs. *Journal of the American Medical Association*, *281*(6), 552–557.

Adkins, A. D., Elkins, E. N., & Singh, N. N. (2001). Readability of NIMH easy to read patient education materials. *Journal of Child and Family Studies*, *10*, 279–285.

Aldridge, M. D. (2004). Writing and designing readable patient education materials. *Nephrology Nursing Journal*, *31*(4), 373–377.

Andrus, M. R., & Roth, M. T. (2002). Health literacy: A review. *Pharmacotherapy*, *22*(3), 282–302.

Austin, P. E., Matlock, R., Dunn, K. A., Kesler, C., & Brown, C. K. (1995). Discharge instructions: Do il-lustrations help our patients understand them? *Annals of Emergency Medicine*, *25*(3), 317–320.

Baddeley, A. (1994). The magical number seven: Still magic after all these years? *Psychological Review*, *101*(2), 353–356.

Baer, J., Kunter, M., & Sabatini, J. (2009). *Basic reading skills and the literacy of America's least literate adults: Results from the 2003 National Assessment of Adult Literacy (NALS) Supplemental Studies* (NCES 2009-481). Washington, DC: National Center for Education Statistics, Institute of Education Sciences, U.S. Department of Education.

Baker, D.W. (2006). The meaning and measure of health literacy. *Journal of General and Internal Medicine*, *21*, 878–883.

Baker, D. W., Parker, R. M., Williams, M. V., & Clark, W. S. (1998). Health literacy and the risk of hospital admission. *Journal of General Internal Medicine, 13*, 791–798.

Baker, D. W., Williams, M. V., Parker, R. M., Gazmararian, J. A., & Nurss, J. (1999). Development of a brief test to measure functional health literacy. *Patient Education and Counseling, 38*, 33–42.

Bastable, L. C., Chojnowski, D., Goldberg, L., McGurl, P., & Riegel, B. (2005). *Comparing heart failure patient literacy levels with available educational materials.* Poster presentation at the Heart Failure Society of America, 9th Annual Scientific Conference, September 18–21, Boca Raton, FL.

Belton, A. B. (1991). Reading levels of patients in a general hospital. *Beta Release, 15*(1), 21–24.

Bennett, I. M., Chen, J., Soroui, J., & White, S. (2009). The contribution of health literacy to disparities in self-rated health status and preventative health behaviors in older adults. *Annals of Family Medicine, 7*, 204–211.

Bernier, M. J. (1993). Developing and evaluating printed education materials: A prescriptive model for quality. *Orthopedic Nursing, 12*(6), 39–46.

Borrayo, E. A. (2004). Where's Maria? A video to increase awareness about breast cancer and mammography screening among low-literacy Latinas. *Preventive Medicine, 39*, 99–110.

Brownson, K. (1998). Education handouts: Are we wasting our time? *Journal for Nurses in Staff Development, 14*(4), 176–182.

Buxton, T. (1999). Effective ways to improve health education materials. *Journal of Health Education, 30*(1), 47–50, 61.

Byrne, T., & Edeani, D. (1984). Knowledge of medical terminology among hospital patients. *Nursing Research, 33*(3), 178–181.

Carol, P. (2007). Health literacy: A critical patient safety tool. *RT: The Journal of Respiratory Care Practitioners, 20*(7), 36–39.

Center for Health Care Strategies. (2003). Impact of low health literacy skills on annual health care expenditures. Retrieved July 16, 2003, from http://www.chcs.org/usr_doc/health_literacy_fact_sheets.pdf

Chew, L. D., Bradley, K. A., & Boyko, E. J. (2004). Brief questions to identify patients with inadequate health literacy. *Family Medicine, 36*(8), 588–594.

Cole, M. R. (2000). The high risk of low literacy. *Nursing Spectrum, 13*(10), 16–17.

Conlin, K. K., & Schumann, L. (2002). Literacy in the health care system: A study on open heart surgery patients. *Journal of the American Academy of Nurse Practitioners, 14*(1), 38–42.

Cutilli, C. C. (2005). Do your patients understand? Determining your patient's health literacy skills. *Orthopaedic Nursing, 24*(5), 372–377.

Dale, E., & Chall, J. S. (1978). The cloze procedure: Measuring the readability of selected patient education materials. *Health Education, 9*, 8–10.

Darling, S. (2004, Spring). Family literacy: Meeting the needs of at-risk families. *Phi Kappa Phi Forum,* 18–21.

Davidhizar, R. E., & Brownson, K. (1999). Literacy, cultural diversity, and client education. *Health Care Manager, 18*(1), 39–47.

Davis, T. C., Long, S. W., Jackson, R. H., Mayeaux, E. J., George, R. B., Murphy, P. W., et al. (1993). Rapid estimate of adult literacy in medicine: A shortened screening instrument. *Family Medicine, 25*(6), 391–395.

Davis, T. C., Michielutte, R., Askov, E. N., Williams, M. V., & Weiss, B. D. (1998). Practical assessment of adult literacy in health care. *Health Education & Behavior, 25*(5), 613–624.

Davis, T. C., Williams, M. V., Marin, E., Parker, R. M., & Glass, J. (2002). Health literacy and cancer communication. *CA: A Cancer Journal for Clinicians, 52*(3), 134–151.

Davis, T. C., Wolf, M. S., Bass, P. F., Middlebrook, M., Kennen, E., Baker, D. W., Bennett, C. L., Durazo, R., Bocchioni, A., Savory, S., & Parker, R. (2006). Low literacy impairs comprehension of prescription drug warning labels. *Journal of General Internal Medicine, 21*, 847–851.

DeWalt, D. A., Berkman, N. D., Sheridan, S., Lohr, N., & Pignone, M. P. (2004). Literacy and health outcomes: A systematic review of the literature. *Journal of General Internal Medicine,* 19, 1228–1239.

Doak, C. C., Doak, L. G., Friedell, G. H., & Meade, C. D. (1998). Improving comprehension for cancer patients with low literacy skills: Strategies for clinicians. *CA: A Cancer Journal for Clinicians, 48*(3), 151–162.

Doak, C. C., Doak, L. G., & Root, J. H. (1985). *Teaching patients with low literacy skills.* Philadelphia: Lippincott.

Doak, C. C., Doak, L. G., & Root, J. H. (1996). *Teaching patients with low literacy skills* (2nd ed.). Philadelphia: Lippincott.

Doak, L. G., & Doak, C. C. (1987, July/August). Lowering the silent barriers to compliance for patients with low literacy skills. *Promoting Health,* 6–8.

Duffy, M. M., & Snyder, K. (1999). Can ED patients read your patient education materials? *Journal of Emergency Nursing, 25*(4), 294–297.

Dunn, M. M., Buckwalter, K. C., Weinstein, L. B., & Palti, H. (1985). Teaching the illiterate client does not have to be a problem. *Family & Community Health, 8*(3), 76–80.

Elliot, V. S. (2007). Literacy advocates call for drug label uniformity. Retrieved July 20, 2009, from http://

www.ama-assn.org/amednews/2007/11/19/hlsc1119.htm

Feldman, S. (1997). Passing on failure: Social promotion is not the way to help children who have fallen behind. *American Educator, 21*(3), 4–10.

Fisher, E. (1999). Low literacy levels in adults: Implications for patient education. *Journal of Continuing Education in Nursing, 30*(2), 56–61.

Fleener, F. T., & Scholl, J. F. (1992). Academic characteristics of self-identified illiterates. *Perceptual and Motor Skills, 74*(3), 739–744.

Flesch, R. (1948). A new readability yardstick. *Journal of Applied Psychology, 32*(3), 221–233.

Foltz, A., & Sullivan, J. (1998). Get real: Clinical testing of patients' reading abilities. *Cancer Nursing, 21*(3), 162–166.

French, K. S., & Larrabee, J. H. (1999). Relationships among educational material readability, client literacy, perceived beneficence, and perceived quality. *Journal of Nursing Care Quality, 13*(6), 68–82.

Friedman, D. B., & Hoffman-Goetz, L. (2008). Literacy and health literacy as defined in cancer education research: A systematic review. *Health Education Journal, 67*, 285–304.

Fry, E. (1968). A readability formula that saves time. *Journal of Reading, 11*, 513–516, 575–579.

Fry, E. (1977). Fry's readability graph: Clarifications, validity, and extension to level 17. *Journal of Reading, 21*, 242–252.

Gazmararian, J. A., Baker, D. W., Williams, M. V., Parker, R. M., Scott, T. L., Green, D. C., et al. (1999). Health literacy among Medicare enrollees in a managed care organization. *Journal of the American Medical Association, 281*(6), 545–551.

Gazmararian, J. A., Curran, J. W., Parker, R. M., Bernhardt, J. M., & DeBuono, B. A. (2005). Public health literacy in America: An ethical perspective. *American Journal of Preventive Medicine, 28*(3), 317–322.

Giorgianni, S. J. (Ed.). (1998). Perspectives on health care and biomedical research: Responding to the challenge of health literacy. *Pfizer Journal, 2*(1), 1–37.

Gunning, R. (1968). The Fog index after 20 years. *Journal of Business Communications, 6*, 3–13.

Hasselkus, A. (2009). Health literacy in clinical practice. *ASHA Leader, 14*(1), 28–29.

Hayes, K. S. (2000). Literacy for health information of adult patients and caregivers in a rural emergency department. *Clinical Excellence for Nurse Practitioners, 4*(1), 35–40.

Hess, V. T. (1998). Literacy and learning for hospital employees. *Journal for Nurses in Staff Development, 14*(3), 143–146.

Hirsch, E. D. (2001). Overcoming the language gap. *American Educator, 4*, 6–7.

Horner, S. D., Surratt, D., & Juliusson, S. (2000). Improving readability of patient education materials. *Journal of Community Health Nursing, 17*(1), 15–23.

Houts, P. S., Bachrach, R., Witmer, J. T., Tringali, C. A., Bucher, J. A., & Localio, R. A. (1998). Using pictographs to enhance recall of spoken medical instructions. *Patient Education and Counseling, 35*, 83–88.

Hussey, L. C., & Guilliland, K. (1989). Compliance, low literacy, and locus of control. *Nursing Clinics of North America, 24*(3), 605–611.

Institute of Medicine. (2004). IOM report calls for national effort to improve health literacy. Retrieved July 1, 2007, from http://www8.nationalacademies.org/onpinews/newsitem.aspx?RecordID=10883

Joint Commission on Accreditation of Healthcare Organizations. (1993). *Accreditation manuals for hospitals—1993.* Chicago: Author.

Kalichman, S. C., Ramachandran, B., & Catz, S. (1999). Adherence to combination antiretroviral therapies in HIV patients of low health literacy. *Journal of General Internal Medicine, 14*, 267–273.

Kanonowicz, L. (1993). National project to publicize link between literacy, health. *Canadian Medical Association Journal, 148*(7), 1201–1202.

Kefalides, P. T. (1999). Illiteracy: The silent barrier to health care. *Annals of Internal Medicine, 130*(4), 333–336.

Kerka, S. (2003). Health literacy beyond basic skills. *Eric Digest,* ED478948.

Kessels, R. P. C. (2003). Patients' memory for medical information. *Journal of the Royal Society of Medicine, 96*, 219–222.

Kim, K. (2006). The Medicare maze: Why consumers don't know which way to turn. Consumer Health Information Corporation. Retrieved July 27, 2009, from http://www.consumer-health.com/services/the_medicare_maze.htm

Kogut, B. H. (2004, Spring). Why adult literacy matters. *Phi Kappa Phi Forum,* 26–28.

Koo, M. M., Krass, I., & Aslani, P. (2005). Patient characteristics influencing evaluation of written medicine information: Lessons for patient education. *Annals of Pharmacotherapy, 39*(9), 1434–1440.

Kutner, M., Greenberg, E., Jin, Y., & Paulsen, C. (2006, September). The health literacy of America's adults: Results from the 2003 National Assessment of Adult Literacy. Retrieved July 1, 2007, from http://nces.ed.gov/pubsearch/pubsinfo.asp?pubid=2006483

Lasater, L., & Mehler, P. S. (1998). The illiterate patient: Screening and management. *Hospital Practice, 33*(4), 163–165, 169–170.

Lerner, E. B., Jehle, D. V. K., Janicke, D. M., & Moscati, R. M. (2000). Medical communication: Do our patients understand? *American Journal of Emergency Medicine, 18*(7), 764–766.

Levy, M., & Royne, M. (2009). The impact of consumers' health literacy on public health. *Journal of Consumer Affairs, 43,* 367–372.

Ley, P. (1979). Memory for medical information. *British Journal of Social and Clinical Psychology, 18*(2), 245–255.

Ley, P., & Florio, T. (1996). The use of readability formulas in health care. *Psychology, Health & Medicine, 1*(1), 7–28.

Loughrey, L. (1983). Dealing with the illiterate patient … You can't read him like a book. *Nursing, 13*(1), 65–67.

Mayeaux, E. J., Murphy, P. W., Arnold, C., Davis, T. C., Jackson, R. H., & Sentell, T. (1996). Improving patient education for patients with low literacy skills. *American Family Physician, 53*(1), 205–211.

Mayer, G. G., & Rushton, N. (2002). Writing easy-to-read teaching aids. *Nursing 2002, 32*(3), 48–49.

McCormack, L., Bann, C., Uhrig, J., Berkman, N., & Rudd, R. (2009). Health insurance literacy of older adults. *Journal of Consumer Affairs, 43,* 223–247.

McLaughlin, G. H. (1969). SMOG—grading: A new readability formula. *Journal of Reading, 12,* 639–646.

Meade, C. D., & Smith, C. F. (1991). Readability formulas: Cautions and criteria. *Patient Education and Counseling, 17,* 153–158.

Miller, B., & Bodie, M. (1994). Determination of reading comprehension level for effective patient health-education materials. *Nursing Research, 43*(2), 118–119.

Monsivais, D., & Reynolds, A. (2003). Developing and evaluating patient education materials. *Journal of Continuing Education in Nursing, 34*(4), 172–176.

Montalto, N. J., & Spiegler, G. E. (2001). Functional health literacy in adults in a rural community health center. *West Virginia Medical Journal, 97*(2), 111–114.

Moore, M., Bias, R. G., Prentice, K., Fletcher, R., & Vaughn, T. (2009). Web usability testing with a Hispanic medically underserved population. *Journal of the Medical Library Association, 97*(2), 114–121.

Morrow, D. G., Weiner, M., Steinley, D., Young, J., & Murray, M. D. (2007). Patients' health literacy and experience with instructions: Influence preferences for heart failure medication instructions. *Journal of Aging and Health, 19,* 575–592.

Myers, R. E., & Shepard-White, F. (2004). Evaluation of adequacy of reading level and readability of psychotropic medication handouts. *Journal of the American Psychiatric Nurses Association, 10,* 55–59.

Nath, C. R., Sylvester, S. T., Yasek, V., & Gunel, E. (2001).

Development and validation of a literacy assessment tool for persons with diabetes. *Diabetes Educator, 27*(6), 857–864.

National Center for Education Statistics. (1993). *Adult Literacy in America: National Adult Literacy Survey.* Washington, DC: U.S. Department of Education.

National Center for Education Statistics. (2004). *Adult Literacy in America: A first look at the National Adult Literacy Survey* (3rd ed.). Washington, DC: U.S. Department of Education. Retrieved July 15, 2009, from http://nces.ed.gov/pubs93/93275.pdf

National Center for Education Statistics. (2006). National Assessment of Adult Literacy (NAAL): Health Literacy Component. Retrieved April 29, 2006, from http://nces.ed.gov/NAAL/index.asp? file=highlights/health literacyfactsheet.asp

Nurss, J. R., El-Kebbi, I. M., Gallina, D. L., Ziemer, D. C., Musey, V. C., Lewis, S., et al. (1997). Diabetes in urban African Americans: Functional health literacy of municipal hospital outpatients with diabetes. *Diabetes Educator, 23*(5), 563–568.

Osborne, H. (1999). In other words … Getting through … Lives can depend on simplifying the written word. *On-Call, 2*(9), 42–43.

Paasche-Orlow, M. K., Taylor, H. A., & Brancati, F. L. (2003). Readability standards for informed-consent forms as compared with actual readability. *New England Journal of Medicine, 348*(8), 721–726.

Paasche-Orlow, M. K., & Wolf, M. (2007a). The causal pathway linking health literacy to health outcomes. *American Journal of Health Behavior, 31,* S19–S26.

Paasche-Orlow, M. K., & Wolf, M. (2007b). Evidence does not support clinical screening of literacy. *Journal of General Internal Medicine, 23,* 100–102.

Parker, R., Baker, D., Williams, M., & Nurss, J. (1995). The test of functional health literacy in adults (TOFHLA): A new instrument for measuring patients' literacy skills. *Journal of General Internal Medicine, 10,* 537–545.

Passel, J. S., & Cohn, D. (2008). U.S. population projections 2005–2050. The Pew Research Center. Retrieved July 10, 2009, from http://pewhispanic.org/files/reports/85.pdf

Pichert, J. W., & Elam, P. (1985). Readability formulas may mislead you. *Patient Education and Counseling, 7,* 181–191.

Pignone, B. D., DeWalt, D. A., Sheridan, S., Berkman, N., & Lohr, K. W. (2005). Interventions to improve health outcomes for patients with low literacy. *Journal of Internal Medicine, 20,* 185–192.

Purnell, L. D., & Paulanka, B. J. (2003). *Transcultural health care: A culturally competent approach* (2nd ed.). Philadelphia: F. A. Davis.

Quirk, P. A. (2000). Screening for literacy and readability: Implications for the advanced practice nurse. *Clinical Nurse Specialist, 14*(1), 26–32.

Robinson, J. H. (2000). Increasing students' cultural sensitivity: A step towards greater diversity in nursing. *Nurse Educator, 25*(3), 131–135, 144.

Rothman, R. L., DeWalt, D. A., Malone, R., Bryant, B., Shantani, A., Crigler, B., et al. (2004). Influence of patient literacy on the effectiveness of a primary care-based diabetes disease management program. *Journal of the American Medical Association, 292*(14), 1711–1716.

Ryhanen, A. M., Johansson, V. H., Salo, S., Salantera, S., & Leino-Kilpi, H. (2008). Evaluation of written patient educational materials in the field of diagnostic imaging. *Radiography, 15,* e1–e5.

Santrock, J. W. (2006). *Life-span development* (10th ed.). Boston: McGraw-Hill.

Schillinger, D., Grumbach, K., Piette, J., Wang, F., Osmond, D., Daher, C., et al. (2002). Association of health literacy with diabetes outcomes. *Journal of the American Medical Association, 288*(4), 475–482.

Schultz, M. (2002). Low literacy skills needn't hinder care. *RN, 65*(4), 45–48.

Schwartzberg, J., VanGeest, J., & Wang, C. (Eds.). (2004). *Understanding health literacy: Inspirations for medicine and public health.* Chicago: American Medical Association Press.

Spache, G. (1953). A new readability formula for primary-grade reading materials. *Elementary School Journal, 53*(7), 410–413.

Spadero, D. C. (1983). Assessing readability of patient information materials. *Pediatric Nursing, 9*(4), 274–278.

Spadero, D. C., Robinson, L. A., & Smith, L. T. (1980). Assessing readability of patient information materials. *American Journal of Hospital Pharmacy, 37,* 215–221.

Spees, C. M. (1991). Knowledge of medical terminology among clients and families. *Image: Journal of Nursing Scholarship, 23*(4), 225–229.

Standal, T. C. (1981). How to use readability formulas more effectively. *Social Education, 45,* 183–186.

Sudore, R., Landefeld, S., Williams, B., Barnes, D., Lindquist, K., & Schillinger, D. (2006). Use of modified informed consent process among vulnerable patients: A descriptive study. *Journal of General Internal Medicine, 21,* 867–873.

Sudore, R. L., Yaffe, K., Satterfield, S., Harris, T. B., Mehta, K. M., Simonsick, E. M., Newman, A. B., Rosana, C., Rooks, R., Rubin, S. M., Ayonayon, H., & Schillinger, D. (2006). Limited literacy and mortality in the elderly. *Journal of General Internal Medicine, 21,* 806–812.

U.S. Department of Health and Human Services. (2000).

Healthy People 2010 (Vol. II). Washington, DC: U.S. Government Printing Office.

U.S. Department of Health and Human Services. (2003). *Community health: Priorities and strategies for success.* Washington, DC: Office of Disease Prevention and Health Promotion. Retrieved April 6, 2004, from http://odphp.osophs.dhhs.gov/projects/healthcomm/

Vallance, J. K., Taylor, L. M., & LaVallee, C. (2008). Suitability and readability assessment of educational print resources related to physical activity: Implications and recommendations for practice. *Patient Education and Counseling, 72,* 342–349.

Vander Zanden, J. W., Crandell, T. L., & Crandell, C. H. (2007). *Human development* (8th ed.). Boston: McGraw-Hill.

Vanderhoff, M. (2005). Patient education and health literacy. *PT: The Magazine of Physical Therapy, 13*(9) 42–46.

Villaire, M. & Mayer, G. (2007). Low health literacy: The impact on chronic illness management. *Professional Case Management, 12*(4), 213–216.

Volandes, A. (2007). Health literacy, health inequality and a just healthcare system. *American Journal of Ethics, 7*(11), 5–8.

Walfish, S., & Ducey, B. B. (2007). Readability levels of health insurance portability and accountability act notices of privacy practices used by psychologists in clinical practice. *Professional Psychology; Research and Practice, 38,* 203–207.

Wallerstein, N. (1992). Health and safety education for workers with low-literacy or limited-English skills. *American Journal of Industrial Medicine, 22*(5), 751–765.

Webber, D., Higgins, L., & Baker, V. (2001). Enhancing recall of information from a patient education booklet: A trial using cardiomyopathy patients. *Patient Education and Counseling, 44,* 263–270.

Wedgeworth, R. (2007). *Fundraising letter.* Syracuse, NY: ProLiteracy Worldwide.

Weiss, B. D. (2003). *Health literacy: A manual for clinicians.* Chicago: American Medical Association and American Medical Association Foundation.

Weiss, B. D., Mays, M. Z., Martz, W., Castro, K. M., DeWalt, D. A., Pignone, M. A., et al. (2005). Quick assessment of literacy in primary care. *Annals of Family Medicine, 3*(8), 514–522.

Williams, D. M., Counselman, F. L., & Caggiano, C. D. (1996). Emergency department discharge instructions and patient literacy: A problem of disparity. *American Journal of Emergency Medicine, 14*(1), 19–22.

Williams, M. V., Baker, D. W., Parker, R. M., & Nurss, J. R. (1998, January 26). Relationship of functional health literacy to patients' knowledge of their chronic disease. *Archives of Internal Medicine, 158,* 166–172.

Williams, M. V., Davis, T., Parker, R. M., & Weiss, B. D. (2002). The role of health literacy in patient–physician communication. *Family Medicine, 34*(5), 383–389.

Williams, M. V., Parker, R. M., Baker, D. W., Parikh, W. S., Pitkin, K., Coates, W. C., et al. (1995). Inadequate functional health literacy among patients at two public hospitals. *Journal of the American Medical Association, 274*(21), 1677–1682.

Wilson, M. (2009). Readability and patient education materials used for low-income populations. *Clinical Nurse Specialist, 23,* 33–40.

Winslow, E. H. (2001). Patient education materials: Can patients read them, or are they ending up in the trash? *American Journal of Nursing, 101*(10), 33–38.

Wolf, M. S., Williams, M. V., Parerk, R. M., Parikh, N. S., Nowlan, A. W., & Baker, D. W. (2007). Patients' shame and attitudes toward discussing the results of literacy screening. *Journal of Health Communication, 12,* 1–12.

Wood, F. G. (2005). Health literacy in a rural clinic. *Journal of Rural Nursing and Health Care, 5*(1). Retrieved July 27, 2006, from http://www.rno.org/journal/index.php/online-journal/article/viewFile/53/145

Wood, M. R., Kettinger, C. A., & Lessick, M. (2007). Knowledge is power: How nurses can promote health literacy. *Nursing for Women's Health, 11*(2), 180–188.

Zarcadoolas, C., Pleasant, A. F., & Greer, D. J. (2006). *Advancing health literacy: A framework for understanding and action.* San Francisco: Jossey-Bass.

Ziegler, J. (1998). How literacy drives up health care costs. *Business & Health, 16*(4), 53–54.

Chapter 8

Gender, Socioeconomic, and Cultural Attributes of the Learner

Susan B. Bastable

CHAPTER HIGHLIGHTS

Gender Characteristics
  Cognitive Abilities
  Personality Traits
  Sexual Orientation and Gender Identity
Socioeconomic Characteristics
  Teaching Strategies
Cultural Characteristics
  Definition of Terms
  The Delivery of Culturally Sensitive Care
  General Assessment and Teaching
    Interventions

  Use of Interpreters
The Four Major Ethnic Subcultural Groups
  Hispanic/Latino Culture
  Black/African American Culture
  Asian/Pacific Islander Culture
  American Indian/Alaska Native Culture
Preparing Health Professionals for Diversity
  Care
Stereotyping: Identifying the Meaning, the
  Risks, and the Solutions
State of the Evidence

KEY TERMS

❏ gender-related cognitive abilities
❏ gender-related personality behaviors
❏ gender gap
❏ gender bias
❏ socioeconomic status (SES)
❏ poverty circle (cycle of poverty)
❏ acculturation
❏ assimilation
❏ cultural awareness
❏ cultural competence

❏ cultural diversity
❏ cultural relativism
❏ culture
❏ ethnic group
❏ ethnocentrism
❏ ideology
❏ subculture
❏ transcultural
❏ worldview
❏ primary characteristics of culture

- ❏ secondary characteristics of culture
- ❏ cultural assessment
- ❏ spirituality
- ❏ religiosity
- ❏ stereotyping

OBJECTIVES

After completing this chapter, the reader will be able to

1. Identify gender-related characteristics in the learner based on social and hereditary influences on brain functioning, cognitive abilities, and personality traits.
2. Recognize the influence of socioeconomics in determining health status and health behaviors.
3. Define the various terms associated with diversity.
4. Examine cultural assessment from the perspective of different models of care.
5. Distinguish between the beliefs and customs of the four predominant ethnic subcultural groups in the United States.
6. Suggest teaching strategies specific to the needs of learners belonging to each of the four ethnic groups.
7. Examine ways in which transcultural approaches to health care can serve as a framework for meeting the learning needs of various ethnic populations.
8. Identify the meaning of stereotyping, the risks involved, and ways to avoid stereotypical behavior.

Gender, socioeconomic level, and cultural background have a significant influence on teaching and learning. Not only do these three factors have an effect on a learner's willingness and ability to respond to and make use of the teaching–learning situation, they also play a role in how clients experience health and illness and their expectations of the health professional (Core, 2008). Two of these factors—gender and socioeconomic status—have been given very little attention to date by health educators. The third factor, cultural and ethnic diversity, has been the focus of considerable study in recent years with respect to its effects on learning. Understanding diversity, particularly those variations among learners related to gender, socioeconomics, and culture, is of major importance when

designing and implementing education programs to meet the needs of an increasingly unique population of learners.

This chapter explores how individuals respond differently to healthcare interventions through examination of gender-related variations resulting from heredity or social conditioning that affects how the brain functions for learning. Second, the chapter examines the influence of environment on the learner from a socioeconomic viewpoint. Third, consideration is given to the significant effects cultural norms have on the behaviors of learners from the perspective of the four major ethnic subcultural groups in the United States. In addition, models for cultural assessment and the planning of care are highlighted. This chapter also includes ways to prepare health professionals for diversity care and to deal with the issue of stereotyping.

Gender Characteristics

Most of the information on gender variations with respect to learning can be found in the educational psychology and neuroscience literature. The health professions literature contains scant information about this subject from a teaching–learning perspective. There are, however, characteristics of male and female orientations that affect learning, which need to be addressed more closely. Two well-established facts exist. First, individual differences within a group of males or females are usually greater than differences between groups of males versus groups of females. Second, studies that compare the sexes seldom are able to separate genetic differences from environmental influences on behavior (Santrock, 2006; Vander Zanden, Crandell, & Crandell, 2007).

There remains a gap in knowledge of what the sexes would be like if humans were not subject to behavioral conditioning. No person can survive outside a social matrix, and, therefore, individuals begin to be shaped by their environment right from birth. For example, U.S. culture exposes girls and boys, respectively, to pink and blue blankets in the nursery, dolls and trucks in preschool, ballet and basketball in the elementary grades, and cheerleading and football in high school. These social influences continue to affect the sexes throughout the life span.

Of course, men and women are different. But the question is: Are they different or the same when it comes to learning, and to what can the differences and similarities be attributed? Biological and behavioral scientists have, to date, been unable to quantify the exact impact that genetics and environment have on the brain. Opinions are rampant, and research findings are inconclusive.

To date, there has been a great divide between neuroscience and education. What is needed is multidisciplinary research to bridge the gap in the discoveries being made in cognitive science laboratories and the application of this information to teaching in the real world. To address this need, the National Science Foundation in 2005 pledged $90 million in grants over 5 years to support four teams of cognitive neuroscientists, psychologists, computer scientists, and educationalists to "give the craft of teaching a solid scientific underpinning" (Gura, 2005, p. 1156). By discovering how the brain works in learning, teaching methods and tools can be designed "to complement the brain's natural development" (Gura, 2005, p. 1156). This is "a massive effort to put the way children are taught on a sounder scientific footing" (Gura, 2005, p. 1156).

The fact remains that there are gender differences as to how males and females act, react, and perform in situations affecting every aspect of life (Cahill, 2006). As Cahill contends, the issue of gender influences is much too important to be ignored or marginalized. The National Academy of Sciences reports, "Sex does matter in ways that we did not expect. Undoubtedly, it matters in ways that we have not yet begun to imagine" (Cahill, 2006, p. 7).

For example, when it comes to human relationships, intuitively women tend to pick up subtle tones of voice and facial expressions, whereas men tend to be less sensitive to these communication cues. In navigation, women tend to have difficulty finding their way, while men seem to have a better sense of direction. In cognition, females tend to excel in languages and verbalization, and men are likely to demonstrate stronger spatial abilities and interest in mathematical problem solving. Scientists are beginning to believe that gender differences have as much to do with the biology of the brain as with the way people are raised (Baron-Cohen, 2005; Gorman, 1992). Kimura (1999) reports on the many different patterns of behavior and cognition between men and women that are thought to be caused by varying hormonal influences on brain development.

Some would argue that these examples are representative of stereotyping. But as generalizations, these statements seem to hold some truth. Neuroscientists have begun to detect structural as well as functional differences in the brains of males and females. These early findings have led to an upsurge in neuroscience research into the mental lives of men and women (Baron-Cohen, 2005).

Neurobiologists are just at the dawn of understanding how the human brain works and exactly the types of sensory input that wire the brain and how that input affects it. Scientists suspect that cognitive abilities work much like sensory ones in that they are promoted by those activities and experiences to which a person is exposed right from birth. Circuits in different regions of the brain are thought to mature at different stages of development. These circuits are critical windows of opportunity at different ages for the learning of math, music, language, and emotion.

Brain development is much more sensitive to life experiences than once believed (Begley, 1996; Hancock, 1996). A baby's brain is like "a work in progress, trillions of neurons waiting to be wired . . . to be woven into the intricate tapestry of the mind" (Begley, 1996, pp. 55–56). Some of the neurons of the brain have been hard wired by genes, but trillions more have almost infinite potential and are waiting to be connected by the influence of environment. The first 3 years of life, it is being discovered, are crucial in the development of the mind. The wiring of the brain, a process both of nature and nurture, dubbed the "dual sculptors," forms the connections that determine the ability to learn and the interest for learning different types of skills (Harrigan, 2007; Nash, 1997).

Thanks to modern technology, imaging machines are revolutionizing the field of neuroscience. Functional magnetic resonance imaging (fMRI)

and positron emission tomography (PET) are being used to observe human brains in the very act of thinking, feeling, or remembering (Kawamura, Midorikawa, & Kezuka, 2000; McRae, Ochsner, Mauss, Gabrieli, & Gross, 2008; Monastersky, 2001; Speck et al., 2000; Yee et al., 2000). Amazing discoveries through brain scanning have been made, such as where the emotion of love resides in the brain. Although machines can measure the brain's blood flow that supports nerve activity, no machines have been developed to date that can read or interpret a person's thoughts. The field of brain scanning still has far to go, but experts consider its potential to be incredible.

The trend in current studies is to focus on how separate parts of the brain interact while performing different tasks rather than focusing on only isolated regions of the brain associated with certain tasks (Monastersky, 2001). Researchers have already reported that men and women use different clusters of neurons when they read than when their brains are idling. For example, Kawamura and colleagues (2000) focused on the cerebral localization of the center for reading and writing music of a male patient. They concluded that the left side of the brain is involved in this type of task, just as it is in an individual's ability to read and write language.

Also, gender differences in brain activity during working memory—an important component for performing many higher functions—have been examined with fMRI. For example, in a study of verbal working memory by Speck et al. (2000), the amount of brain activity increased with task difficulty. Interestingly, male subjects demonstrated more right-sided hemispheric dominance, whereas females showed more left-sided hemispheric dominance, with higher accuracy and slightly slower reaction times than their male counterparts. The results revealed significant gender differences in the functional brain organization for working memory.

In general, the brains of men and women seem to operate differently. Provocative new studies are revealing that women engage more of their brains when thinking sad thoughts. When men and women subjects were asked to conjure up sad memories, the front of the limbic system in the brain of women glowed with activity eight times more than in men. Although men and women were able to perform equally well in math problems, tests indicated that they seemed to use the temporal lobes of the brain differently to figure out problems. Also, it has been found that men and women employ different parts of their brains to figure out rhymes. These results are just a few examples of some of the tentative, yet tantalizing, findings from research that are beginning to show that male and female identity is a creation of both nature and nurture. Along with genetics, life experiences and the choices men and women make in the course of a lifetime help to mold personal characteristics and determine gender differences in the very way the sexes think, sense, and respond (Begley, Murr, & Rogers, 1995).

In comparing how men and women feel, act, process information, and perform on cognitive tests, scientists have been able to identify only a few gender differences in the actual brain structure of humans (**Table 8–1**). Most differences that have been uncovered are quite small, as measured statistically. Even the largest differences in **gender-related cognitive abilities** are not as significant as, for example, the disparity found between male and female height. There seems to be, in fact, a great deal of overlap in how the brains of the two sexes work. Otherwise, "women could never read maps and men would always be left-handed. That flexibility within the sexes reveals just how complex a puzzle gender actually is, requiring pieces from biology, sociology, and culture" (Gorman, 1992, p. 44).

With respect to brain functioning, there is likely a mix between the factors of heredity and environment that accounts for gender characteristics. The following is a comparison of cognitive abilities between the genders based on developmental and educational psychology findings in Vander Zanden et al. (2007), Santrock (2006), Snowman and Biehler (2006), and Baron-Cohen (2005).

Cognitive Abilities

General intelligence: Various studies have not yielded consistent findings on whether males and females differ in general intelligence. But if any gender differences exist, they seem to be attributed to patterns of ability rather than IQ (Kimura, 1999). When mean differences have occurred, they are small. However, what is well documented is the strong correlation between IQ and heredity (Santrock, 2006). On IQ tests during preschool years, girls score higher; in high school, boys score higher on these tests. Differences may be the result of greater dropout rates in high school for low-ability boys and gender identity formation in adolescence. Thus, overall no dramatic differences between the sexes have been found on measures of general intelligence (Vander Zanden et al., 2007).

However, a very interesting trend in IQ scores has been noted. IQs (as measured by the Stanford-Binet intelligence test) are increasing rapidly worldwide. In the United States, children seem to be getting smarter. As compared with IQs tested in 1932, if people took the same test today, a large percentage would score much higher. Because the increase has occurred over such a relatively short time, heredity is not the cause. It is thought that increasing levels of education and the information-age explosion are the reasons. This increase in IQ scores is known as the Flynn effect after the researcher who discovered it (Santrock, 2006).

Verbal ability: Girls learn to talk, form sentences, and use a variety of words earlier than boys do. In addition, girls speak more clearly, read earlier, and do consistently better on tests of spelling and grammar. Originally, researchers believed females performed better than males on measures of verbal fluency, but recent research has questioned this early superiority of females in the verbal domain.

Table 8–1 Gender Differences in Brain Structure

	Men	Women
TEMPORAL LOBE		
Regions of the cerebral cortex help to control hearing, memory, and a person's sense of self and time.	In cognitively normal men, a small region of the temporal lobe has about 10% fewer neurons than it does in women.	More neurons are located in the temporal region where language, melodies, and speech tones are understood.
CORPUS CALLOSUM		
The main bridge between the left and right brain contains a bundle of neurons that carry messages between the two brain hemispheres.	This part of the brain in men takes up less volume than a woman's does, which suggests less communication between the two brain hemispheres.	The back portion of the callosum in women is bigger than in men, which may explain why women use both sides of their brains for language.
ANTERIOR COMMISSURE		
This collection of nerve cells, smaller than the corpus callosum, also connects the brain's two hemispheres.	The commissure in men is smaller than in women, even though men's brains are, on average, larger in size than women's brains.	The commissure in women is larger than in men, which may be a reason why their cerebral hemispheres seem to work together on tasks from language to emotional responses.
BRAIN HEMISPHERES		
The left side of the brain controls language, and the right side of the brain is the seat of emotion.	The right hemisphere of men's brains tends to be dominant.	Women tend to use their brains more holistically, calling on both hemispheres simultaneously.
BRAIN SIZE		
Total brain size is approximately 3 pounds.	Men's brains, on average, are larger than women's.	Women have smaller brains, on average, than men because the anatomical structure of their entire bodies is smaller. However, they have more neurons than men (an overall 11%) crammed into the cerebral cortex.

Source: Adapted from Begley, S., Murr, A., & Rogers, A. (1995, March 27). Gray matters. *Newsweek*, 51.

On tests of verbal reasoning, verbal comprehension, and vocabulary, the findings are not consistent. The conclusion is that no significant gender differences in verbal ability exist.

Mathematical ability: During the preschool years, there appear to be no gender-related differences in ability to do mathematics. By the end of elementary school, however, boys show signs of excelling in mathematical reasoning, and the differences in math abilities of boys over girls become even greater in high school. Recent studies reveal that any male superiority likely is related to the way math is traditionally taught—as a competitive individual activity rather than as a cooperative group learning endeavor.

When the approach to teaching math is taken into consideration, only about a 1% variation in quantitative skills is seen in the general population. In American culture, math achievement differences may result from different role expectations. The findings on math ability and achievement can also be extended to science ability and achievement because these two subjects are related.

Spatial ability: The ability to recognize a figure when it is rotated, to detect a shape embedded in another figure, or to accurately replicate a three-dimensional object is consistently better for males than for females. Of all possible gender-related differences in cognitive activity, the spatial ability of males is consistently higher than that of females and probably has a genetic origin. Rubin Gur, a noted researcher on gender differences in the brain, concurs with other research findings that men do perform better on spatial tasks than women do (Gur et al., 2000). However, the magnitude of this sex difference accounts for only about 5% of the variation in spatial ability.

Interestingly, women surpass men in the ability to discern and later recall the location of objects in a complex, random pattern (Kimura, 1999). Scientists have reasoned that historically men may have developed strong spatial skills so as to be successful hunters, while women may have needed other types of visual skills so as to excel as gatherers and foragers of food (Gorman, 1992).

Problem solving: The complex concepts of problem solving, creativity, analytical skill, and cognitive styles, when examined, have led to mixed findings regarding gender differences. Men tend to try new approaches in problem solving and are more likely to be field independent. That is, they are less influenced by irrelevant cues and more focused on common features in certain learning tasks (see Chapter 4 on learning styles). Males also show more curiosity and significantly less conservatism

than women in risk-taking situations. In the area of human relations, however, women perform better at problem solving than do men.

School achievement: Without exception, girls get better grades on average than boys, particularly at the elementary school level. Scholastic performance of girls is more stable and less fluctuating than that of boys.

Although no compelling evidence proves significant gender-linked differences in the areas of cognitive functioning, except in spatial ability as mentioned earlier, some findings do reveal sex differences when it comes to personality characteristics. Evidence reported by Vander Zanden and others (2007), Santrock (2006), and Snowman and Biehler (2006) was used to substantiate the following summary findings unless otherwise noted.

Personality Traits

Most of the observed **gender-related personality behaviors** are thought to be largely determined by culture but are, to some extent, a result of mutual interaction between environment and heredity.

Aggression: Males of all ages and in most cultures are generally more aggressive than are females (Baron-Cohen, 2005). The role of the gender-specific hormone testosterone is linked as a possible cause of the more aggressive behavior demonstrated by males (Kimura, 1999). However, anthropologists, psychologists, sociologists, and scientists in other fields continue to disagree about whether aggression is biologically based or environmentally influenced. Nevertheless, male and female roles differ widely in most cultures, with males usually being more dominant, assertive, energetic, active, hostile, and destructive.

Conformity and dependence: Females have been found generally to be more conforming and more influenced by suggestion. The gender biases of some studies have made these findings open to suspicion, however.

Emotional adjustment: The emotional stability of the sexes is approximately the same in childhood, but differences do arise in how emotional problems are manifested. Some evidence indicates that adolescent girls and adult females have more neurotic symptoms than males do. However, this tendency may reflect how society defines mental health in ways that coincide with male roles. Also, it has been pointed out that tests to measure mental health usually have been designed by men and, therefore, may be biased against females.

Values and life goals: In the past, men have tended to show greater interest in scientific, mathematical, mechanical, and physically active occupations as well as to express stronger economic and political values. Women have tended to choose literary, social service, and clerical occupations and to express stronger aesthetic, social sense, and religious values. These differences have become smaller over time because women have begun to think differently about themselves, have more freely pursued career and interest pathways, and society has begun to take a more equal opportunity viewpoint for both sexes.

Achievement orientation: Females are more likely to express achievement motivation in social skills and social relations, whereas men are more likely to try to succeed in intellectual or competitive activities. This difference is thought to be the result of sex-role expectations that are strongly communicated at very early ages.

How do the preceding observations on gender characteristics in intellectual functioning and personality relate to how the health professional educator can teach clients? It is very difficult to differentiate between biological and environmental influences simply because these two factors are intertwined and influence each other. The cause, meaning, and outcome of these differences remain speculative at this time, and further research needs to be conducted.

The behavioral and biological differences between males and females, known as the **gender gap**, are well documented. Also well documented is **gender bias**, "a preconceived notion about the abilities of women and men that prevented individuals from pursuing their own interests and achieving their potentials" (Santrock, 2006, p. 66). Females have an accelerated biological timetable and, in general, are more prone to have early verbal ability. Conversely, males lag behind females in biological development and attention span but tend to excel in visual-spatial ability and mathematical pursuits (Vander Zanden et al., 2007). During adolescence, they also are likely to surpass females in physical strength.

With respect to gender differences and aging, as suggested by current life-span mortality rates, females have a life expectancy of approximately 80.2 years compared to approximately 75.1 years for males. Also, men have higher mortality rates for 12 of the 15 leading causes of death (U.S. Department of Health and Human Services [USDHHS], 2009). However, more needs to be understood about women's health because for years their health issues have been underrepresented in research studies. Fortunately, this trend has changed within the last 2 to 3 decades and significant evidence is beginning to surface about the physical and mental health status of females (Dignam, 2000; Kato & Mann, 1996; USDHHS, 2000).

However, what has been known is that women are likely to seek health care more often than men do (U.S. Census Bureau, 2006). It is suspected that one of the reasons women have more contact with the healthcare system is that they traditionally have tended to be the primary caretakers of their children, who need pediatric services. In addition, during childbearing years, women seek health services for care surrounding pregnancy and childbirth (Kato & Mann, 1996).

Perhaps the reason that men tend not to rely as much as do women on care from health providers is because of the sex-role expectation of society that men should be stronger. They also have a tendency to be risk takers and to think of themselves as more independent. Although men are less likely to pursue routine health care for purposes of health and safety promotion and disease and accident prevention, they typically face a greater number of health hazards, such as a higher incidence of automobile accidents, use of drugs and alcohol, suicide, heart disease, and engaging in dangerous occupations. Furthermore, men are less likely to notice symptoms or report them to physicians (Kato & Mann, 1996).

Sexual Orientation and Gender Identity

The exact number of lesbian, gay, bisexual, and transgender (LGBT) individuals in the United States and around the world is unknown; however, it is estimated to be more than 8 million people (Fenway Institute, 2010a; Romero, Baumle, Badgett, & Gates, 2007). This number is based on U.S. Census data and represents a very conservative estimate of the LGBT population. Although the U.S. Census does gather information on same-sex couples, it does not ask questions about sexual orientation or gender identity (Gates, 2010). Therefore, single gays and lesbians are not included in U.S. Census data and neither are members of the transgender community. Because of hesitancy on the part of many members of the LGBT population to disclose their sexual preference and/or gender identity, underrepresentation is always an issue.

Lack of representation of the LGBT community is not restricted to the U.S. Census. Because questions about sexual preference or gender identity are not included on many health surveys, the LGBT population is also underrepresented in health research (National Coalition for LGBT Health, 2009; Sexual Minority Assessment Research Team, 2009). In an effort to rectify some of these issues, the Institute of Medicine (IOM) convened a panel to write the federal government's first report about the health issues of the LGBT community. The IOM report will explore the state of the science on LGBT health and outline a research agenda that will assist the National Institutes of Health to direct research in this area (Institute of Medicine of the National Academies, 2010).

When considering gender and the social and other factors that influence the unique learning styles and educational needs of men and women, it is important to include the LGBT community. The LGBT population represents a distinct cultural group whose needs are often overlooked by health professionals. Although members of the LGBT population have many of the same health problems as do the general population, disparities do exist, and as a group, their health outcomes are worse than those of the heterosexual community (Centers for Disease Control and Prevention, 2010; Krehely, 2009).

Three main problems contribute to the health disparities experienced by the LGBT population:

1. The social stigma associated with being lesbian, gay, bisexual, or transgender creates undue stress and contributes to negative health behavior patterns. For example, research demonstrates increased tobacco, alcohol, and drug use among the LGBT population as well as a high incidence of depression, anxiety, and other mental health problems (Woodiel & Brindle, 2008).
2. Structural barriers decrease access to health care for people who are lesbian, gay, bisexual, or transgender (Mayer et al., 2008). For example, unemployment in the LGBT community resulting from job discrimination and lack of insurance benefits for same-sex domestic partners have led to a higher than average number of people without health coverage (Krehely, 2009).
3. Lack of culturally appropriate care for the LGBT community results in limited or ineffective use of healthcare services. For example, in an attempt to avoid negative interactions with healthcare providers, LGBT clients are often reluctant to disclose their sexual preference or gender identity. Without this vital piece of information, health professionals are unable to

provide comprehensive care. Other members of the LGBT community simply avoid seeking health care unless absolutely necessary. As a result, they may not take advantage of preventive services or receive early treatment for serious health problems (McRae et al., 2008).

Although bias and misunderstanding remain, in recent years there has been greater awareness and acceptance of the LGBT lifestyle in the United States. Thanks to the national efforts of organizations such as the National Coalition for LGBT Health, the Williams Institute of the UCLA School of Law, and the Fenway Institute, tremendous efforts have been made in health-related public policy, research, and public and professional education. Also, local groups have been active in advocating for the needs of the LGBT community. Particular emphasis has been placed both at the local and national levels on educating health professionals in an attempt to improve LGBT health services. For example, the Fenway Institute published the first medical textbook on LGBT health and offers learning modules for health professionals on its Web site (Fenway Institute, 2010a).

TEACHING STRATEGIES

Davidson, Trudeau, van Roosmalen, Stewart, and Kirkland (2006) describe gender as a "multifaceted construct" (p. 731) that includes a number of modifiable attributes that influence health outcomes and health education. These attributes include personality, social supports, coping skills, values, and health-related behaviors. When planning teaching strategies, health professionals must be aware of the extent to which attributes such as these as well as heredity-related characteristics of the genders affect health-seeking behaviors and influence individual health needs. As stated previously, in some areas males and females display different orientations and learning styles (Severiens & Ten Dam, 1994). The differences seem to depend on interests and past experiences in the

biological and social roles of men and women in American society.

Women and men are part of different social cultures, too. They use different symbols, belief systems, and ways to express themselves, much in the same manner that different ethnic groups have distinct cultures (Tear, 1995). In the future, these gender differences may become less pronounced as the sex roles become more blended. Symbols are also very important to the LGBT community, the most common being the pink triangle and the rainbow pride flag. These symbols are used by the LGBT community as a show of pride and unity. However, some health professionals display these symbols as a sign of welcome to LGBT clients (Woodiel & Brindle, 2008).

When in the role of educator, it is important for health professionals to create an environment that is welcoming to all men and women regardless of lifestyle. Clients, particularly those living alternative lifestyles, look for subtle clues to determine whether the health professional will accept them without judgment (Woodiel & Brindle, 2008). For example, a women's or children's health clinic that only displays photos of traditional families may give the message that nontraditional families are not welcome. Brochures on LGBT health issues and unisex bathrooms are all strategies that give a welcoming message to a diverse client base.

When working with men and women, it is important that the health professional as educator avoid making assumptions about family structure, sexual preference, or lifestyle. Many families in the 21st century are structured differently from how families were structured in years past. For example, more and more men are assuming primary responsibility for child care. The health professional should never assume that a client is heterosexual, even if that person is or has been married. Almost half of self-identified lesbians have been or are currently married (Fenway Institute, 2010b).

To complete an accurate assessment of each client, the health professional educator should take every opportunity to gather accurate information from the client. Admission or intake forms are often designed for the traditional family. Clients are often not given an opportunity to identify a same-sex domestic partner. Transgender clients are usually forced to select either male or female. By adjusting the forms to be more inclusive, the health professional is not only creating a welcoming environment, he or she is creating an opportunity for the client to share important information.

One of the two major goals of *Healthy People 2010* (goal No. 2) is to eliminate health disparities among segments of the population. This includes differences that occur by gender, such as men are two times more likely to die from injuries than are women, and women are at greater risk for Alzheimer's disease and two times as likely to be affected by depression as are men (USDHHS, 2000). When considering health disparities that occur by gender, it is important also to consider differences among the LGBT population, such as transgender adults being 10 times more likely to suffer suicidal ideation or LGBT youth being twice as likely to be overweight (Krehely, 2009).

Health professionals are encouraged to include information on general health disparities when educating clients and staff. They also are encouraged to use versatile teaching style strategies so as not to perpetuate stereotypical approaches to teaching and learning with the two genders. In addition, health professions have a responsibility to incorporate gender issues into professional education curricula.

Socioeconomic Characteristics

Socioeconomic status (SES), in addition to gender characteristics, influences the teaching–learning process. SES is considered to be the single most important determinant of health in American society (Crimmins & Saito, 2001; Singh-Manoux, Ferrie, Lynch, & Marmot, 2005). Socioeconomic

class is an aspect of diversity that must be addressed in the context of education and in the process of teaching and learning.

Class is the "unmentionable five-letter word" (Rhem, 1998, p. 1). Many people are hesitant to categorize themselves according to class. They also are reluctant to discuss the issue of class differences because of the widespread idea that the United States should be a classless society (Felski, 2002; Rhem, 1998). It is a myth, though, that America is a country without classes (McGoldrick, 1995). Class, as universal as race or gender, hides in the shadows. However, class consciousness seems to be a commonality shared by everyone. Those who are privileged often feel guilty about their advantages. Those who are poor feel ashamed or embarrassed about their disadvantages (Rhem, 1998).

Social and economic levels of individuals have been found to be significant variables affecting health status and literacy levels and in determining health behaviors (Crimmins & Saito, 2001; Monden, van Lenthe, & Mackenbach, 2006). Health status can also affect socioeconomic status. For example, research shows that people with disabilities "represent more than half of those experiencing long term poverty," with inability to work, difficulty in achieving higher levels of education, and cost of care as contributing factors (She & Livermore, 2008, p. 254). Approximately 39.8 million Americans live in poverty. The poverty threshold for a family of four is defined as an income of $21,910 per year (DeNavas-Walt, Proctor, Smith, & U.S. Census Bureau, 2009).

Disadvantaged people—those with low incomes, low educational levels, and/or social deprivation—come from many different ethnic groups, including millions of poor White people (USDHHS, 2000). SES takes into account the variables of educational level, family income, and family structure (Vander Zanden et al., 2007). See **Figure 8–1** for the relationship between educational level and household income. All of these variables influence health beliefs, health practices,

Figure 8–1 Relationship Between Education and Median Household Income Among Adults Aged 25 Years and Older, by Gender, United States, 1996

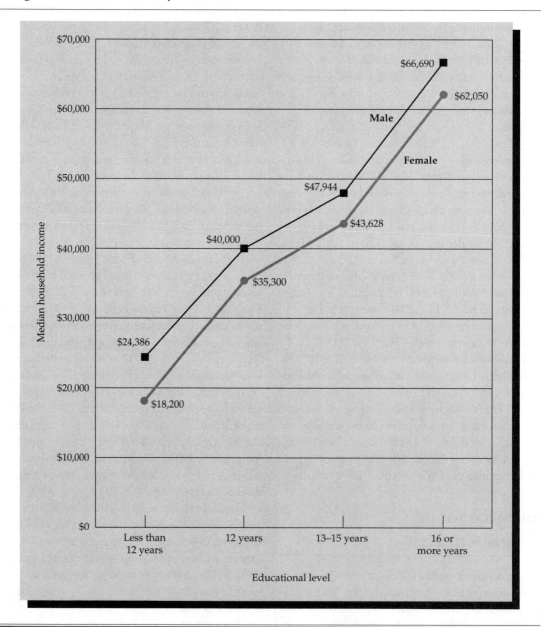

Source: U.S. Department of Commerce, Bureau of the Census. (1997, March). Current population survey. In *Healthy People 2010: Understanding and improving health* (p. 101). Rockville, MD: U.S. Department of Health and Human Services.

and readiness to learn (Darling, 2004; Mackenbach et al., 2003).

The relationships among socioeconomic position, cognitive ability, and health status have been explored, but the mechanics and processes involved are highly complex and remain poorly understood (Batty, Der, Macintyre, & Deary, 2006; Kroenke, 2007; Singh-Manoux et al., 2005). Heredity and environment usually vary together; that is, people who are genetically related (parents and their children) tend to have similar environments. Evidence suggests that variations in heredity are equally as powerful as variations in environmental conditions in producing individual differences in cognitive ability (Luciano et al., 2006; Santrock, 2006; Turkheimer, Haley, Waldron, D'Onofrio, & Gottesman, 2003; Vander Zanden et al., 2007). Krugman (2008) reports that children growing up in families with low SES have impaired language and memory development; in essence, high levels of stress hormones caused by poverty conditions in childhood "poison the brain" for a lifetime (p. 1). Also, low socioeconomic class is correlated with low educational levels and health inequalities (Mackenbach, Cavelaars, Kunst, Groenhof, and the EU Working Group on Socioeconomic Inequalities in Health, 2000). The significant correlation between literacy levels and SES is well documented in Chapter 7.

Although many educators, psychologists, and sociologists have recognized that a cause-and-effect relationship exists among low SES, low cognitive ability, and poor quality of health and life, they are hard pressed to know what to do about breaking the cycle (Batty, Deary, & Macintyre, 2006). So, too, are healthcare providers, who recognize that clients belonging to lower social classes have higher rates of illness, more severe illnesses, and reduced rates of life expectancy (Mackenbach et al., 2003). People with low SES, as measured by indicators such as income, education, and occupation, have increased rates of morbidity and mortality compared to those with higher SES (USDHHS, 2000, 2009).

An inverse relationship exists between SES and health status. Individuals who have higher incomes and are better educated live longer and healthier lives than those who are of low income and poorly educated (Crimmins & Saito, 2001; Rognerud & Zahl, 2005). Thus, the level of socioeconomic well-being is a strong indicator of health outcomes. See **Figure 8–2** for the relationship between SES and health status.

These findings raise serious questions about health differences among the nation's people as a result of unequal access to health care resulting from SES. These unfortunate health trends are costly to society in general and to the healthcare system in particular. Although adverse health-related behavior and less access to medical care have been found to contribute to higher morbidity and mortality rates, there is newer but still limited research on the effect socioeconomic status has on disability-free or active life expectancy (Crimmins & Saito, 2001; Mackenbach et al., 2003).

Social class is measured by one or more of the following types of indices:

- Occupation of parents
- Income of family
- Location of residence
- Educational level of parents

Vander Zanden et al. (2007) and Santrock (2006) explain that many factors, including poor health care, limited resources, family stress, discrimination, and low-paying jobs, maintain the cycle by which generation after generation is born into poverty. Elstad and Krokstad (2003) find that health inequalities as a result of socioeconomic factors are reproduced as people mature from young adulthood into middle age. That is, a social causation pattern exists whereby environments are the source of socioeconomic health inequalities. As such, people with good health tend to move up in the social hierarchy and those with poor health move downward.

Figure 8–2 Percentage of Persons with Perceived Fair or Poor Health Status by Household Income, United States, 1995

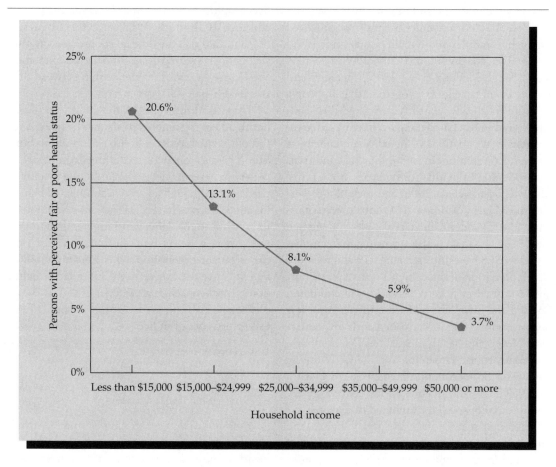

Source: Centers for Disease Control and Prevention, National Center for Health Statistics. (1995). National health interview survey. In *Healthy People 2010: Understanding and improving health* (p. 101). Rockville, MD: U.S. Department of Health and Human Services.

In addition, rates of illiteracy and low literacy have been linked to poorer health status, high unemployment, low earnings, and high rates of welfare dependency, all of which are common measures of a society's economic well-being (Giorgianni, 1998; Weiss, 2003). Whatever the factors that keep particular groups from achieving at higher levels, these groups are likely to remain on the lower end of the occupational structure. This cycle has been coined the **poverty circle** (Gage & Berliner, 1998) or the **cycle of poverty**. The poverty circle is described as follows:

Parents low in scholastic ability and consequently in educational level create an environment in their homes and neighborhoods that produce children who are also low in scholastic ability and academic attainment. These children grow up and become parents, repeating the cycle. Like them, their children are fit only for occupations at lower levels of pay, prestige, and intellectual demand (Gage & Berliner, 1998, p. 61).

Family structure and the home environment are not the only factors affecting proficiency in learning. Hirsch (2001) contends that the alarming verbal and reading gap between rich and poor students "represents the single greatest failure in American public schooling" (p. 5). Many low-income children entering kindergarten have heard only half the words and understand only half the meanings of language than the high-income child has heard and understands. This gap continues to widen along the same trajectory as students progress in each succeeding grade in school. Barriers to equal educational opportunity must be reduced by putting the responsibility on the educational system to become more intensive. That is, standards for each grade must be developed and the educational system must make sure each child meets these expectations before being allowed to progress to subsequent grades in school.

The lower socioeconomic class has been studied by social scientists more than other economic classes. This is probably because the health views of this group deviate the most from those viewpoints of health professionals who care for this group of individuals. People from the lower social stratum have been characterized as being indifferent to the symptoms of illness until poor health interferes with their lifestyle and independence. Their view of life is one of a sense of powerlessness, meaninglessness, and isolation from middle-class knowledge of health and the need for preventive measures, such as vaccination for their children (Lipman, Offord,

& Boyle, 1994; USDHHS, 2000; Winkleby, Jatulis, Frank, & Fortmann, 1992).

The high cost of health care may well be a major factor affecting health practices of people in the lower socioeconomic classes. Individuals with adequate financial and emotional resources are able to purchase services and usually have support systems on which to rely to sustain them during recovery or to augment their remaining functions after the course of an acute illness. Conversely, individuals deprived of monetary and psychosocial resources are at a much greater risk for failing to reach an optimal level of health and well-being. Unfortunately, the number of Americans at or below the national poverty level is at 12.6% and almost 47 million Americans lack health insurance, an increase of 1.3 million between 2004 and 2005 (U.S. Census Bureau, 2006).

Just as SES can have a negative effect on illness, so, too, can illness have devastating implications for a person's socioeconomic well-being (Elstad & Krokstad, 2003). A catastrophic or chronic illness can lead to unemployment, loss of health insurance coverage or ineligibility for health insurance benefits, enforced social isolation, and a strain on social support systems (Lindholm, Burstrom, & Diderichsen, 2001; Mulligan, 2004). Without the socioeconomic means to counteract these threats to their well-being, impoverished individuals may be powerless to improve their situation.

These multiple losses tax the individual, their families, and the healthcare system. Low-income groups are especially affected by changes in federal and state assistance in the form of Medicare and Medicaid. The spiraling costs associated with illness and consequent overuse of the healthcare system have resulted in increased interest on the part of the public and healthcare providers to control costs (Baker, Parker, Williams, & Clark, 1998). Today, more emphasis is being given to health promotion, health maintenance, and disease prevention.

Teaching Strategies

The current trends in health care, as a result of these economic concerns, are directed toward teaching individuals how to attain and maintain health. The health professional plays a key role in educating the consumer about avoiding health risks, reducing illness episodes, establishing healthful environmental conditions, and accessing healthcare services. Educational interventions by health professionals for those who are socially and economically deprived have the potential for yielding short-term benefits in meeting these individuals' immediate healthcare needs. However, more research must be done to determine whether teaching can ensure the long-term benefits of helping deprived people develop the skills needed to reach and sustain independence in self-care management.

Health professionals working in the role of educators must be aware of the probable effects of low SES on an individual's ability to learn as a result of suboptimal cognitive functioning, poor academic achievement, low literacy, high susceptibility to illness, and disintegration of social support systems. Low-income people are at greater risk for these factors that can interfere with learning. Stress hormones caused by poverty have been shown to "poison the brain for a lifetime" (Krugman, 2008). However, health professionals cannot assume that everyone at the poverty or near-poverty level is equally influenced by these threats to their well-being. To avoid stereotyping, it is essential that each individual or family be assessed to determine their particular strengths and weaknesses for learning. In this way, teaching strategies unique to particular circumstances can be designed to assist socioeconomically deprived individuals in meeting their needs for health care.

Nevertheless, it is well documented that individuals with literacy problems, poor educational backgrounds, and low academic achievement are likely to have low self-esteem, feelings of helplessness and hopelessness, and low expectations. They

also tend to think in concrete terms, are more focused on satisfying immediate needs, have a more external locus of control, and have decreased attention spans. They have difficulty in problem solving and in analyzing and synthesizing large amounts of information. With these individuals, the health educator will most likely have to rely on specific teaching methods and tools similar to those identified as appropriate for intervening with clients who have low literacy abilities (see Chapter 7).

Cultural Characteristics

At the beginning of the 21st century, the composition of the U.S. population was approximately 71.3% White, 12.2% Black/African American, 11.2% Hispanic/Latino, 3.8% Asian/Pacific Islander, 0.7% American Indian/Alaska Native, and 0.8% other. Thus, more than one quarter (28.7%) of the U.S. population consists of people from culturally diverse ethnic groups (U.S. Census Bureau, 2006). In addition, 7 million people indicated in their responses to the U.S. census survey taken in 2000 that they belonged to more than one race (Tashiro, 2002). The diversity of the U.S. population is anticipated to grow. By 2042, the non-Hispanic White population of the United States is expected to be in the minority and reach a level of about 46% by the year 2050 (U.S. Census Bureau, 2008). If predictions prove true, by the middle of this century, for the first time in U.S. history people from ethnic groups (subcultures) will constitute the majority of the total population.

To keep pace with a society that is increasingly more culturally diverse, health professionals need to have sound knowledge of the cultural values and beliefs of specific ethnic groups as well as be aware of individual practices and preferences (Price & Cortis, 2000; Purnell & Paulanka, 2003). Culture has been compared to an iceberg. The tip of the iceberg can be seen, but the very large area below the waterline is only visible with effort. So, too, with culture. When a person from a different culture is approached, the health provider is aware of the way the individual dresses and speaks but must seek to discover the values, beliefs, and practices that are part of the individual's cultural makeup (Core, 2008; National Mental Health Information Center, 2008; Phan et al., 2009). In the past, healthcare providers have experienced difficulties in caring for clients whose cultural beliefs differ from their own because beliefs about health and illness vary considerably among ethnic groups. Lack of cultural sensitivity by health professionals has resulted in millions of dollars wasted annually through misuse of healthcare services, the alienation of large numbers of people, and the misdiagnosis of health problems with often tragic and dangerous consequences.

In addition, underrepresented ethnic groups are beginning to demand culturally relevant health care that respects their cultural rights and incorporates their specific beliefs and practices into the care they receive. Although in recent years the curriculum in healthcare programs typically has been unicultural, an increasing awareness of this multicultural society has resulted in curriculum revision across many of the health professions. Education in the health professions is beginning to change as faculty are developing courses in culture and language and incorporating culture concepts into classroom and clinical experiences. A review of the literature reveals that much work still needs to be done but the important first steps have been taken to promote cultural competence in many of the health professions (Chun, Young, & Jackson 2009; Smith, Constantine, Dunn, Dinehart, & Montoya, 2009).

Definition of Terms

Before examining the major ethnic (subcultural) groups within the United States, it is imperative to define the following terms, as identified by Purnell and Paulanka (2003), which are commonly used in discussing the subject of culture:

Acculturation: A willingness to adapt or "to modify one's own culture as a result of contact with another culture" (p. 351).

Assimilation: The willingness of an individual or group "to gradually adopt and incorporate characteristics of the prevailing culture" (p. 351).

Cultural awareness: Recognizing and appreciating "the external signs of diversity" in other ethnic groups, such as their art, music, dress, and physical features (p. 352).

Cultural competence: A conscious process of recognizing one's own culture so as to avoid "undue influence on those from other cultural backgrounds" (p. 352).

Cultural diversity: A term meaning "representing a variety of different cultures" (p. 352).

Cultural relativism: "The belief that the behaviors and practices of people should be judged only from the context of their cultural system" (p. 352).

Culture: "The totality of socially transmitted behavioral patterns, arts, beliefs, values, customs, lifeways, and all other products of human work and thought characteristic of a population of people that guide their worldview and decision making. These patterns may be explicit or implicit, are primarily learned and transmitted within the family, and are shared by the majority of the cultures" (pp. 352–353).

Ethnic group: Also referred to as a subculture, a population of "people who have experiences different from those of the dominant culture" (p. 4).

Ethnocentrism: "The tendency of human beings to think that [their] own ways of thinking, acting, and believing are the only right, proper, and natural ones and to believe that those who differ greatly are strange, bizarre, or unenlightened" (p. 353).

Ideology: "Consists of the thoughts, attitudes, and beliefs that reflect the social needs and desires of an individual or ethnocultural group" (p. 3).

Subculture: A group of people "who have had different experiences from the dominant culture by status, ethnic background, residence, religion, education, or other factors that functionally unify the group and act collectively on each other" (p. 357).

Transcultural: "Making comparisons for similarities and differences between cultures" (p. 358).

Worldview: Refers to "the way individuals or groups of people look at the universe to form values about their lives and the world around them" (p. 4).

The Delivery of Culturally Sensitive Care

Given increases in immigration and birth rates in the United States as well as the significant increased geographical mobility of people around the globe, the U.S. system of health care and this country's educational institutions must respond by shifting from a dominant monocultural, ethnocentric focus to a more multicultural, transcultural focus (Narayan, 2003).

Tripp-Reimer and Afifi (1989) describe the interpretation of American cultural ideals from a historical perspective:

> In the United States, the myth of the melting pot emerged largely from a combination of a cultural ideal of equality and a European ethnocentric perspective. This myth promoted the notion that all Americans are alike—that is, like white, middle-class persons. For many years, the notion that ethnicity should be discounted or ignored was prominent in the delivery of health care, including health teaching programs. . . . (p. 613)

Madeline Leininger (1994), a noted nursing leader, asked, "How can nurses competently respond to and effectively care for people from diverse cultures who act, speak, and behave in ways different than their own?" Dr. Leininger's question is relevant to all health professions. How can health professionals respond to the needs of their clients when they see the world through a different cultural lens.

In her book *The Spirit Catches You and You Fall Down: A Hmong Child, Her American Doctors and the Collision of Two Cultures*, Anne Fadiman (1997) tells a story about what can happen when health professionals fail to recognize how differently diverse cultures may view health, illness, and treatment. In this true story, language issues and different interpretations of the child's health problem and the appropriate treatment resulted in noncompliance with a vitally important treatment regimen. All teaching efforts failed and despite the best intentions of all involved, the child is left with severe brain damage as a result of cultural miscommunication. The story highlights the importance of cultural competence in health care.

From a sociological perspective, the symbolic interaction theory provides a theoretical framework for interacting with ethnic groups. It emphasizes social and group identities rather than just individual identity. Tashiro (2002) points out that this framework is useful for understanding the situational nature of identity and the negotiation and renegotiation necessary when working with groups.

Purnell and Paulanka (2003) propose that there are a number of factors that influence an individual's identification with an ethnic group and that person's willingness to share his or her worldview of the ethnic group to which he or she belongs. They have labeled these factors as primary and secondary characteristics of culture. **Primary characteristics of culture** include nationality, race, color, gender, age, and religious affiliation. **Secondary characteristics of culture** include many of a person's attributes that are addressed in this chapter and this text, such as SES, physical characteristics, educational status, occupational status, and place of residence (urban versus rural). These two major characteristics affect one's worldview and belief system.

The Purnell model for cultural competence is presented as a popular organizing framework for understanding the complex phenomenon of culture and ethnicity. This framework "provides a comprehensive, systematic, and concise" approach that can assist healthcare providers in teaching students in educational settings and clients and staff in practice settings for the delivery of "holistic, culturally competent, therapeutic interventions" (Purnell & Paulanka, 2003, p. 8).

The Purnell model, depicted in a circle format, includes the macro layers of the following metaparadigm concepts:

1. Global society (outermost sphere)
2. Community (second sphere)
3. Family (third sphere)
4. Individual (innermost sphere)

The interior of the circle is cut into 12 equally sized, pie-shaped wedges that represent the following 12 cultural domains that should be assessed when planning for educational interventions for clients in any setting:

1. Communication (e.g., dominant language and nonverbal expressions and cues)
2. Family roles and organization (e.g., head of household, gender roles, developmental tasks, social status, alternative lifestyles, roles of older adults)
3. Workforce issues (e.g., language barriers, autonomy, acculturation)
4. Biocultural ecology (e.g., heredity, biological variations, genetics)
5. High-risk behaviors (e.g., smoking, alcoholism, physical activity, safety practices)
6. Nutrition (e.g., common foods, rituals, deficiencies, limitations)
7. Pregnancy (e.g., fertility, practices, views toward childbearing, beliefs about pregnancy, birthing practices)
8. Death rituals (e.g., views of death, bereavement, burial practices)

9. Spirituality (e.g., religious beliefs and practices, meaning of life, use of prayer)
10. Healthcare practices (e.g., traditions, responsibility for health, pain control, sick role, medication use)
11. Healthcare practitioners (e.g., folk practitioners, gender issues, perceptions of providers)
12. Overview/heritage (e.g., origins, economics, education, occupation)

These two authors also put forth 19 explicit assumptions upon which the model is based, some of which are most pertinent to this chapter, such as the following:

- One culture is not better than another—they are just different.
- The primary and secondary characteristics of culture determine the degree to which one varies from the dominant culture.
- Culture has a powerful influence on one's interpretation of and responses to health care.
- Each individual has the right to be respected for his or her uniqueness and cultural heritage.
- Prejudices and biases can be minimized with cultural understanding.
- Caregivers who intervene in a culturally competent manner improve the care of clients and their health outcomes.
- Cultural differences often require adaptations to standard professional practices.

Other models have been developed across the health professions to address the issue of cultural diversity and health care. The Multiple Dimensions of Cultural Competence model (MDCC) proposed by Sue (2001) originated within the field of psychology but defines cultural competence in a way that can be used to guide practice or education across many disciplines. This model identifies three primary dimensions of competence:

1. Race and culture-specific attributes that focus on knowledge of various racial and cultural groups

2. Components of cultural competence that stress the skills, values, beliefs, and knowledge of the professional
3. Foci of cultural competence that identifies the individual, the profession, the organization, and society as levels for analysis

Several important principles can be derived from the MDCC that are useful to the health professional when in the role of educator:

• Individuals are multidimensional, belonging to several cultural groups, all of which influence their worldview (Reynolds, 2001). This multidimensionality creates complexity in each person that must be assessed before teaching can begin.
• Cultural competence develops as a result of personal experiences with people from various cultural groups (Vaughn, 2008). The health professional as educator must continually strive to learn about culture from his or her clients.
• Self-awareness is critical. Health professionals must seek to develop an awareness of personal values, beliefs, and biases that may affect their relationships with clients (Vaughn, 2008).
• It is sometimes necessary to move beyond the individual client and address issues of culture within the profession and society (Reynolds, 2001). For health professional educators, this may involve advocating for change at the organizational level, sharing knowledge at the professional level, or supporting culture-related policy development at the national level.

Cultural brokering has also been suggested as a model for assisting health professionals to work with clients from diverse cultures. As a cultural broker, the healthcare provider uses knowledge of the client's culture and the culture of the healthcare system to mediate and achieve desired outcomes (Jezewski, 1993; National Center for Cultural Competence, 2004). Health educators who are knowledgeable about culture and competent in **cultural assessment** likely will be the most suc-

cessful at designing and implementing culturally effective teaching programs. When the values and beliefs of a client differ from those of the healthcare system, conflict can be created, and if not resolved, the client may be unfairly labeled. Health professionals with strong cultural assessment skills can assist their colleagues in working with clients who may be considered uncooperative, noncompliant, or difficult. In addition, they can help with identifying potential areas of cultural conflict and select teaching interventions that minimize conflict.

There is one very important caveat for the educator to remember when conducting a cultural assessment of any client:

> Health professionals must be especially careful not to over-generalize or stereotype clients on the basis of their ethnic heritage. Just because someone belongs to a particular subculture does not necessarily mean they adhere to all the beliefs, values, customs, and practices of that ethnic group. Health professionals should never assume a client's learning needs or preferences for treatment will be alike simply based on the individual's ethnicity.

As Andrews and Boyle (1995) so aptly explain, "Sometimes cultural stereotyping may be perpetuated when a recipe-like approach to clients from specific cultural groups is used" (p. 50). Each client is unique and health professionals must never allow their prior experiences or knowledge of a particular cultural group to lead them to make assumptions about the values and beliefs of an individual client. Knowledge of cultural variations should serve only as background cues for obtaining additional information through assessment.

General Assessment and Teaching Interventions

As a first step in the teaching process, assessment should determine health beliefs, values, and practices. In particular, the health professional must identify those aspects of culture that should be addressed in developing and implementing the teaching plan (Martinez-Cossio, 2008). The health professional in the role of educator must implement successful teaching interventions using the universal skills of establishing rapport, assessing readiness to learn, and using active listening to understand problems. Health professionals need to be aware of the established customs that influence the behavior they are attempting to change (Tripp-Reimer & Afifi, 1989). The health professional should, however, keep in mind that belonging to an ethnic group does not always mean a person follows or buys into all of the traditions or customs of the group to which they belong. Given that culture affects the way someone perceives a health problem and understands its course and possible treatment options, it is essential to carry out a thorough assessment prior to establishing a plan of action for long-term behavioral change.

Different cultural backgrounds not only create different attitudes and reactions to illness, but also can influence how people express themselves, both verbally and nonverbally, which may prove difficult to interpret. For example, asking patients to explain what they believe to be the cause of a problem can help to reveal whether they think it is caused by a spiritual intervention, a hex, an imbalance in nature, or other culturally based beliefs. The health professional should accept the client's explanation (most likely reflecting the beliefs of the support system as well) in a nonjudgmental manner.

Culture also guides the way a person who is ill is defined and treated. For example, some cultures believe that once the symptoms disappear, illness is no longer present. This belief can be problematic for individuals suffering from an acute illness, such as a streptococcal infection, when a 1- or 2-day course of antibiotic therapy relieves the soreness in the throat. This belief also can be a problem for the individual afflicted with a chronic disease that is manifested by periods of remission or exacerbation.

In addition, health professional educators must assess readiness to learn from the standpoint of a person's culture. Patients and their families, for instance, may believe that behavior change is context specific, such that they will adhere to a recommended medical regimen while in the hospital setting but fail to follow through with the guidelines once they return to the home setting. Also, healthcare providers must be cautious not to assume that the values adhered to by professionals are equally important or cherished by the patient and significant others. Consideration, too, must be given to barriers that might exist, such as time, financial, and environmental variables, which may hinder readiness to learn (see Chapter 4). Finally, the client needs to believe that new behaviors are not only possible, but also beneficial if the new information is to be remembered and interpreted correctly for behavioral change to be maintained over the long term (Kessels, 2003).

Health professional educators should use the following additional guidelines for assessment regardless of the particular cultural orientation of the client (Anderson, 1987; Martinez-Cossio, 2008; Uzundede, 2006):

1. Identify the client's primary language (which may be different from the health professional's) and assess his or her ability to understand, read, and speak the language of the health professional. Language should be one of the first considerations because it is of critical importance in establishing a relationship with the client and in determining the client's ability to participate in the education process.
2. Observe the interactions between the client and his or her family members as well as among family members. Determine who makes the decisions, how decisions are made, who is the primary caregiver, what type of care is given, and what foods and other objects are important to them.
3. Listen to the client. Find out what the person wants, how his or her wants differ from the

family's wants, and how they differ from what you think is appropriate.

4. Consider other communication abilities and patterns. For example, note manners of speaking (rate of speech, expressions used) and nonverbal cues that can enhance or hinder understanding. In addition, health professionals should be aware of their own nonverbal behaviors and etiquettes of interaction that may be acceptable or unacceptable to the client and family members.

5. Explore customs and taboos. Observe behaviors and clarify beliefs and practices that may interfere with care or treatment.

6. Determine the client's notion of time. Health professionals should become oriented to the individual's and family members' sense of time and importance of time frames.

7. Be aware of cues for interaction. Determine which communication approaches are appropriate with respect to what is the most comfortable way to address the person(s) with whom the health professional is interacting. Also, find out the symbolic objects or the activities that provide comfort and security.

8. Assess the client's religious practices and determine how their religious beliefs influence their perceptions of illness and treatment.

These guidelines can assist in the exchange of information between the educator and client. The health professional–client interaction is one in which the health professional is both learner and teacher and the client is also both learner and teacher. The goal of negotiation is to arrive at ways of working together to solve a problem or to determine a course of action (Anderson, 1987, 1990). The objective is not for the health professional to take a totally fact-centered approach or pretend he or she is completely color blind, but to recognize each person as an individual and to know that differences exist within ethnic and racial groups as well as between these groups.

Use of Interpreters

If the client speaks a foreign language, the health professional should use the client's primary language whenever possible. When the health professional does not fluently speak the same language, it is necessary to secure the assistance of an interpreter, who may be a family member, neighbor, friend, other healthcare staff, or professional healthcare interpreter.

For many reasons, the use of family or friends for interpretation of the spoken word (or translation of the written word) is not as desirable as using professionally trained individuals for provider–client interaction. First, family members and friends may not be sufficiently fluent to assume the role. Second, they may choose to omit portions of the content they believe to be unnecessary or unacceptable. Third, their presence may inhibit peer communication and violate the patient's right to privacy and confidentiality (Baker, Parker, Williams, Coates, & Pitkin, 1996; Poss & Rangel, 1995; Schenker, Lo, Ettinger, & Fernandez, 2008), especially in light of the recent Health Insurance Portability and Accountability Act (HIPAA) regulations.

Thus, it is optimal to use professionally trained interpreters for oral communication. They can convey instructional messages verbatim, they work under an established code of ethics and confidentiality, and they are available without fee for patients who require their services. When determining whether a healthcare interpreter is required, the educator should consider the criticality and complexity of the teaching situation, the degree to which the educator can be understood by the client, the client's preferences, and the availability of resources (Schenker et al., 2008). If there is no bilingual person available to facilitate communication, the AT&T Language Line provides 24-hour access to interpreters of 144 languages (Duffy & Snyder, 1999).

In teaching clients who are only partially fluent in the language being spoken, the following strategies are recommended (Poss & Rangel, 1995; Stanislav, 2006; Tripp-Reimer & Afifi, 1989) to help alter the style of interaction when no interpreter is used:

- Speak slowly and distinctly, allowing for twice as much time as a typical teaching session would take.
- Use simple sentences, relying on an active rather than a passive voice.
- Avoid technical terms (e.g., use *heart* rather than *cardiac*, or *stomach* rather than *gastric*). Also avoid medical jargon (e.g., use *blood pressure* rather than *BP*) and idioms (e.g., *it's just red tape you have to go through* or *I heard it straight from the horse's mouth*).
- Organize instructional material in the sequence in which the plan of action should be carried out.
- Make no assumptions that the information given has been understood. Ask for clients to explain in their own words what they heard, and, if appropriate, request a return demonstration of a skill that has been taught.

The Four Major Ethnic Subcultural Groups

The U.S. Census Bureau (2000) defines the major ethnic groups in this country as follows: Black/African American (of African, Haitian, and Dominican Republic descents), Hispanic/Latino (of Mexican, Cuban, Puerto Rican, and other Latin descents), Asian/Pacific Islander (of Japanese, Chinese, Filipino, Korean, Vietnamese, Hawaiian, Guamian, Samoan, and Asian Indian descents), and American Indian/Alaska Native (descendents of hundreds of tribes of Native Americans and of Inuit descent).

Given the fact that there are many ethnic groups (subcultures) in the United States, and hundreds worldwide, it is impossible to address the cultural

characteristics of each one. The following is a review of the beliefs and health practices of the four major ethnic groups in the United States identified as subcultures by the U.S. Census Bureau. These groups, who have been historically underrepresented, account for almost one third (28.7%) of the total U.S. population. These groups are recognized by the U.S. government as disadvantaged because of low income, low education, and/or sociocultural deprivation. The Hispanic/Latino and Asian/Pacific Islander groups are the fastest-growing ethnic subcultures in this country (U.S. Census Bureau, 2006).

Health professional educators must remember that one of their most important roles is to serve as an advocate for clients—as a representative of client interests. If health professionals are to assume this role, then their efforts should be directed at making the healthcare setting as similar to the client's natural environment as possible. To do so, they must be aware of clients' customs, beliefs, and lifestyles.

In addition to the following information on the four major ethnic groups, the following references are recommended as sources of additional information on particular tribes or subcultures not specifically addressed: Purnell and Paulanka (2003); Kelley and Fitzsimons (2000); Vivian and Dundes (2004); Chideya (1999); Chachkes and Christ (1996); Cantore (2001); Lowe and Struthers (2001); Parker and Kiatoukaysy (1999); Young, McCormick, and Vitaliano (2002); Cohen (1991); Kniep-Hardy and Burkhardt (1977); Pang (2007); Horton and Freire (1990); and Smolan, Moffitt, and Naythons (1990).

Hispanic/Latino Culture

According to the U.S. Census Bureau (2006), the Hispanic/Latino group is the largest and the fastest-growing subculture in the United States. As of the 2000 census survey, this group represents 11.9% of the total population of the United States. The number of Hispanic Americans has increased significantly since 1970 as a result of a higher birth rate in this group than the rest of the population, an increase in immigration, as well as improved census procedures.

Hispanic or Latino Americans derive from diverse origins. This heterogeneous group of Americans with varied backgrounds in culture and heritage are of Latin American or Spanish origin and use Spanish (or a related dialect) as their dominant language. Those of Mexican heritage comprise the largest number of people (approximately 60%) of this subculture, followed by Puerto Rican, Central and South American, and Cuban Americans. They are found in every state but are concentrated in just nine states. California and Texas together have one half of the Hispanic population, but other large concentrations are found in New York, New Jersey, Florida, Illinois, Arizona, New Mexico, and Colorado (U.S. Census Bureau, 2006). Health educators who practice in the southwestern states are most likely to encounter clients of Mexican heritage, those practicing in the northeast states most likely are caregivers of clients of Puerto Rican heritage, and health professionals in Florida deliver care to a large number of Cuban Americans. Also, Hispanic people are more likely to live in metropolitan or rural areas than are non-Hispanic Americans (Purnell & Paulanka, 2003). Although Hispanic Americans have many common characteristics, each subgroup has unique characteristics.

The people of Hispanic heritage have particular healthcare needs that must be addressed. They are disproportionately affected by certain cancers, alcoholism, drug abuse, obesity, hypertension, diabetes, adolescent pregnancy, dental disease, and HIV/AIDS. Unlike in non-Hispanic Whites, homicide, AIDS, and perinatal conditions rank as the top 10 causes of mortality. Hispanics are more prone to certain diseases, are less likely to receive preventive care, often lack health insurance, and

have less access to health care than do Whites living in the United States (Fernandez & Hebert, 2000; Hebert & Fernandez, 2000; Pacquiao, Archeval, & Shelley, 2000; Purnell & Paulanka, 2003; USDHHS, 2000).

Unfortunately, both the curricula in schools preparing health professionals nationwide and the literature with respect to patient education efforts geared toward Hispanic Americans pay little attention to the healthcare needs of this minority group. Although Hispanics are a culturally diverse group of people with varying health needs, avenues for including Hispanic healthcare issues in health professions curricula have been minimal and especially need to be developed in schools located in areas with high population concentrations of this ethnic group (Kelley & Fitzsimons, 2000; Sullivan & Bristow, 2007).

Fluency in Spanish as a foreign language is a necessity or at least is highly recommended when practitioners are responsible for delivering care to this growing, underserved, culturally diverse ethnic group. Spanish-speaking people represent 54% of all non–English-speaking persons in the United States (U.S. Census Bureau, 2006). However, the percentage of healthcare professionals of Hispanic heritage is very small across the health professions. For example, only 2% of the RN population and 4.9% of physicians are Hispanic (USDHHS, 2003a). The lack of representation of people from this subculture in the health professions is not thought to result from their low aspirations. Indeed, many Hispanic high school students rank health/medical services among their top 10 career choices. Unfortunately, the often poor academic achievement of Hispanic students in high schools and colleges is associated with a number of factors related to socioeconomic and educational disadvantages and prevents them from entering the health professions (Educating the Largest Minority Group, 2003).

Hispanics' access to health care is limited both by choice and availability of health services. Only one fifth of Puerto Rican, one fourth of Cuban, and one third of Mexican Americans see a physician during the course of a year. Even when Hispanic people have access to the healthcare system, they may not receive the care they need. Difficulty in obtaining services, dissatisfaction with the care provided, and inability to afford the rising costs of medical care are major factors that discourage them from using the healthcare system (Fernandez & Hebert, 2000; Purnell & Paulanka, 2003). The demographics of the community may play a role in access to health care. In their study of Mexican Americans, Gresenz, Rogowski, and Escarce (2009) found that access to health care was better when Mexican Americans lived among larger numbers of other Hispanic people. The researchers suggest that support systems such as Spanish-speaking healthcare providers and local groups that facilitate access may have an influence on the use of healthcare services.

Approximately 23% of Hispanic families live below the poverty line; members of this ethnic group are 2.5 times more likely to be below the poverty level than members of other subcultural groups in the United States. Economic disadvantage leaves little disposable income for paying out-of-pocket expenses for health care. When they do seek a regular source of care, many people of this minority group rely on public health facilities, hospital outpatient clinics, and emergency rooms (Fernandez & Hebert, 2000; Purnell & Paulanka, 2003). Also, they are very accepting of health care being delivered in their homes, where they feel a sense of control, stability, and security (Pacquiao et al., 2000).

The health beliefs of Hispanic people also affect their decisions to seek traditional care. Many studies dating back to the 1940s on Hispanic health beliefs and practices stress exotic folklore practices, such as their use of herbs, teas, home remedies, and over-the-counter drugs for treating symptoms of acute and chronic illnesses. In addition, they rely to a high degree on health healers, known as *curen-*

deros or *esperitistas*, for health advice and treatment (Fernandez & Hebert, 2000; Purnell & Paulanka, 2003). For example, illnesses of Mexican Americans as a Hispanic subgroup could be organized into the following categories (Caudle, 1993; Markides & Coreil, 1986; Purnell & Paulanka, 2003):

1. Diseases of hot and cold, believed to be caused by an imbalanced intake of foods or ingestion of foods at extreme opposites in temperature. In addition, cold air was thought to lead to joint pain, and a cold womb resulted in barrenness in women. Heating or chilling was the cure for parts of the body afflicted by disease.
2. Diseases of dislocation of internal organs, cured by massage or physical manipulation of body parts.
3. Diseases of magical origin, caused by *mal ojo*, or evil eye, a disorder of infants and children as a result of a woman's looking admiringly at someone else's child without touching the child, resulting in crying, fitful sleep, diarrhea, vomiting, and fever.
4. Diseases of emotional origin, attributed to sudden or prolonged terror called *susto*.
5. Folk-defined diseases, such as *latido*.
6. Standard scientific diseases.

Recent research reveals that overall health status of Hispanic Americans is determined by key health indicators on infant mortality, life expectancy, mortality from cardiovascular disease and cancer, and measures of functional health. This research concludes that the health of people of Hispanic heritage is much closer to that of White Americans than it is to African Americans, even though the Hispanic and Black populations share similar socioeconomic conditions. Concerning the incidence of diabetes and infectious and parasitic diseases, however, Hispanic people are clearly at a disadvantage in relation to White people.

Possible explanations for the relative advantages and disadvantages in health status of Hispanic

Americans involve such factors as the following, which were outlined by Purnell and Paulanka (2003):

- Cultural practices favoring reproductive success
- Early and high fertility contributing to low breast cancer but high cervical cancer rates
- Dietary habits linked to low cancer rates but high prevalence of obesity and diabetes
- Genetic heritage
- Extended family support reducing the need for psychiatric services
- Low socioeconomic status that contributes to increased infectious and parasitic diseases

Alcoholism also represents a serious health problem for many Hispanic Americans. Furthermore, as the Hispanic population becomes more acculturated, certain risk factors conducive to cardiovascular disease and certain cancers are expected to play larger roles in this group (Markides & Coreil, 1986; Purnell & Paulanka, 2003).

Today, the literature disagrees about the extent and frequency to which Hispanic people use home remedies and folk practices. In the southwestern United States, the Hispanic population has been found to use herbs and other home remedies to treat illness episodes—twice the proportion reported in the total U.S. population. Other studies claim that the use of folk practitioners has declined and practically disappeared in some Hispanic subgroups (Purnell & Paulanka, 2003).

Knowing where people get their health information can provide clues to practitioners as to how to reach particular population groups. For example, Mexican Americans receive almost as much information from mass media sources (TV, magazines, and newspapers) as they do from physicians and other healthcare providers. As a consequence, mass media could play an important role in disseminating information to a large portion of the Mexican American population (Purnell & Paulanka, 2003).

Because of the centrality of the family in Hispanic peoples' lives, the extended family serves as the single most important source of social support to people of Hispanic origin. This culture is characterized by a pattern of respect for and obedience to elders as well as a pattern of male dominance. Caregivers' focus, therefore, needs to be on the family rather than on the individual. It is likely, for example, that a woman would be reluctant to make a decision about her or her child's health care without consulting her husband first (Purnell & Paulanka, 2003).

Gender and family member roles are changing, however, as Hispanic women take jobs outside the home. Also, children are picking up the English language more quickly than their parents are and are ending up in the powerful position of acting as interpreters for their adult relatives. The heavy reliance on family has been linked to this minority group's low utilization of healthcare services. In addition, levels of education correlate highly with access to health care. That is, as clearly depicted in Figure 8–1, the less education members within a household have, the poorer the family's health status and access to health care (Purnell & Paulanka, 2003; USDHHS, 2000). Hispanic Americans are more likely than the general U.S. population to read English below the basic health literacy level (National Center for Education Statistics, 2006) and to have lower educational attainment than non-Hispanic Whites (Massett, 1996).

TEACHING STRATEGIES

Only about 40% of the Hispanic population has completed 4 years of high school or more, and only 10% have completed college, as compared with approximately 80% and 20%, respectively, of the rest of the non-Hispanic population (Educating the Largest Minority Group, 2003; Purnell & Paulanka, 2003). Both the educational level and the primary language of Hispanic clients need to be taken into consideration when selecting instructional materials

(Massett, 1996; National Center for Education Statistics, 2006). Sophisticated teaching methods and tools are inappropriate for those who have minimal levels of education.

The age of the population also can affect health and client education efforts. According to the U.S. Census Bureau (2006), the Hispanic population as a total group is young (30% are younger than 20 years of age). Thus, the school system is an important setting for educating members of the Hispanic community. In the school system, education programs for Hispanic students on alcohol and drug abuse and on cardiovascular disease risk reduction proved successful if the following factors were considered:

- Cultural beliefs were observed.
- The educator was first introduced by an individual accepted and respected by the learners.
- Family members were included.
- The community was encouraged to take responsibility for resolving the health problems discussed.

Morbidity, mortality, and risk factor data also provide clues to the areas in which patient education efforts should be directed. As mentioned earlier, Hispanic people have higher rates of diabetes, AIDS, obesity, alcohol-related illnesses, and mortality from homicide than does the general population. All of these topics should be targeted for educational efforts at disease prevention and health promotion (Caudle, 1993).

Until recently, few data existed regarding patient education for Hispanic Americans. Purnell and Paulanka (2003), Fernandez and Hebert (2000), Hebert and Fernandez (2000), Pacquiao and others (2000), and Caudle (1993) have contributed significantly to the understanding of the traditions and practices surrounding health and illness in the various Hispanic subgroups. The following general suggestions are useful when designing and implementing education programs for Hispanic Americans:

1. Identify the Hispanic American subgroups (e.g., Mexican, Cuban, and Puerto Rican) in the community whose needs differ in terms of health beliefs, language, and general health status. Design education programs that can be targeted to meet their distinct ethnic needs.

2. Be aware of individual differences within subgroups in regard to age, years of education, income levels, job status, and degree of acculturation.

3. Take into account the special health needs of Hispanic Americans with respect to incidences of diseases and risk factors to which they are vulnerable—breast cancer in women (Borrayo, 2004), diabetes, AIDS, obesity, alcohol-related illnesses, homicide, and accidental injuries.

4. Be aware of the importance of the family so as to direct education efforts to include all interested members. Remember that Hispanic families on the whole are very supportive of each other, and decision making rests with the male and elder authority figures in traditional families.

5. Provide adequate space for teaching to accommodate family members who typically accompany patients seeking health care.

6. Be cognizant of the importance of the Roman Catholic religion in the lives of the Hispanic people when dealing with such issues as contraception, abortion, and family planning.

7. Demonstrate cultural sensitivity to health beliefs by respecting ethnic values and taking time to learn about Hispanic beliefs.

8. Consider other sources of care that this ethnic group might be using, such as home remedies, before they enter or while they are within the healthcare system.

9. Be aware of the modesty felt by some Hispanic women and girls, who may be particularly uncomfortable in talking about sexual issues in mixed company.

10. Display warmth, friendliness, and tactfulness when developing a relationship with people of Hispanic heritage because they expect healthcare providers to be informal and interested in their lives.

11. Determine whether Spanish is the language with which the client best communicates. Many Hispanic Americans prefer to speak Spanish, but they are not always literate in reading their native language.

12. Speak slowly and distinctly, avoiding the use of technical words and slang if the client has limited proficiency in the language being spoken.

13. Do not assume that a nod of the head or a smile indicates understanding of what has been said. Even if Hispanic clients are not familiar with English, they respect authority, and, therefore, it is not uncommon for them to display nonverbal cues that may be misleading or misinterpreted by the healthcare provider. Ask clients to repeat in their own words what they have been told or use the teach back method to determine their level of understanding (Weiss, 2003).

14. If interpreters are used, be sure they speak the dialect of the learner. Be certain that the interpreter conveys instructions verbatim, rather than just summarizing the information, so that the real meaning gets conveyed. Also, be sure to talk to and with the client, not to the interpreter. If an interpreter is not available, use the AT&T hotline telephone number for a direct link to Spanish-speaking interpreters.

15. Provide written and audiovisual materials in Spanish that reflect linguistic appropriateness and cultural sensitivity. An increasing number of health education materials are available in Spanish (Borrayo, 2004).

Much more must be learned by health educators about the Hispanic American population with respect to their cultural beliefs and their health and education needs. It is evident that many members of this cultural group are not receiving the kind and amount of health services they desire and deserve. Health professionals need to extend themselves to Hispanics in a culturally sensitive manner to effectively and efficiently address the needs of this rapidly growing segment of the U.S. population (Borrayo, 2004).

Black/African American Culture

According to the 2000 U.S. Census, people of Black/African American descent make up the largest subcultural group in the United States. Currently, Black Americans constitute 12.2% of the U.S. population as compared with 11.9% for Hispanics. However, the most recent 2004 statistics indicate that the Hispanic population has surpassed this group in population growth (U.S. Census Bureau, 2006).

The cultural origins and heritage of Black Americans are quite diverse. Their roots are mainly from Africa and the Caribbean Islands. They speak a variety of languages, including French, Spanish, African dialects, and various forms of English. Depending on the age cohort group to which they belong, African Americans may prefer to identify themselves differently as a racial group. For example, the youngest generation often refers to themselves (and likes to be referred to by others) as *African American*. By contrast, middle-aged members of this ethnic group may prefer the term *Black* or *Black American*. Either designation is politically correct according to the U.S. Census Bureau's identification of this ethnic group as Black/African American. However, because the diversity of cultural heritage varies within the many Black subgroups, healthcare providers need to be aware of intraethnic differences in cultural beliefs, customs, and traditions (Purnell & Paulanka, 2003).

The one distinguishing factor of this ethnic group, in comparison to other subcultures, is that quite a few Black families have ancestry dating back to the early colonization of America in the 1600s when millions of Africans were brought forcibly to this country as slaves. The rich history of African heritage and American slavery has been passed on from generation to generation (Purnell & Paulanka, 2003).

The majority of this ethnic population resides in the South (54%). Approximately 19% live in the Midwest, 18% in the Northeast, and 9% in the West. The greatest concentration resides in large metropolitan areas, such as New York City; Chicago; Atlanta, Georgia; Washington, D.C.; Baltimore; Detroit, Michigan; and New Orleans, Louisiana (U.S. Census Bureau, 2006).

Unfortunately, African Americans have suffered a long history of inequality in educational opportunity. They were victims of school segregation and inferior facilities until the 1954 Supreme Court decision *Brown v. Board of Education of Topeka* outlawed the separation of Blacks and Whites in the public school systems. However, this educational deprivation has had long-term consequences, such as unequal access to higher paying and higher status job opportunities, which has led to low wages and a disproportionate number (approximately one third) of African Americans living at or below the poverty level (U.S. Census Bureau, 2006). In turn, poverty has resulted in low educational attainment, high rates of school dropout, drug and alcohol abuse, decreased health status, and a lower quality of life altogether (Forrester, 2000; Purnell & Paulanka, 2003). Nevertheless, many African Americans value education, which they see as the means to raise their standard of living by being able to secure better jobs and a higher social status.

Black Americans constitute a large segment of blue-collar workers and are not well represented in managerial and professional positions of employment. Discrimination in employment and job advancement is thought to be a major variable contributing to problems with career mobility. The government has taken major steps in the past 30 years to reverse discrimination in social and employment settings so as to give Black Americans more equal opportunities, but the majority of working-class Black people still do not typically advance to higher-level occupations.

Also, poverty and low educational attainment have had major consequences for the Black American community in terms of social and medical issues. Although Black families value education highly, there continues to be a greater than average high school dropout rate among Blacks, and many individuals remain poorly educated with concomitant literacy problems. Low educational levels and socioeconomic deprivation are strongly correlated with higher incidences of disease, poor nutrition, lower survival rates, and a decreased quality of life in general. Increased exposure to hazardous working conditions in low-paying, manual labor jobs has also resulted in a greater incidence of occupation-related diseases and illnesses among this population (Dignam, 2000; Mackenbach et al., 2000; Monden et al., 2006; Rognerud & Zahl, 2005). In addition, the majority of Blacks reside in inner-city areas where exposure to violence and pollution puts them at greater risk for disease, disability, and death. The average life span of Black Americans is shorter than that of White Americans as a result of high death rates from cancer, cardiovascular disease, cirrhosis, diabetes, accidents, homicides, and infant mortality (Anderson et al., 2000; Dignam, 2000; Forrester, 2000; Holt, Kyles, Wiehagen, & Casey, 2003; Keyserling et al., 2000; Samuel-Hodge et al., 2006; Yanek, Becker, Moy, Gettelsohn, & Koffman, 2001). Also, Blacks are at higher risk for drug addiction, teen-aged pregnancy, and sexually transmitted diseases (Purnell & Paulanka, 2003).

Purnell and Paulanka (2003) report findings that African Americans are pessimistic about human relationships and their belief system emphasizes three major themes:

1. The world is a hostile and dangerous place to live.
2. The individual is vulnerable to attack from external forces.

3. The individual is considered helpless with few internal resources to combat adversity.

Because many African Americans tend to be suspicious of Western ethnomedical practitioners, they often seek the assistance of physicians and other health professionals only when absolutely necessary (Purnell & Paulanka, 2003). Instead, folk practitioners are held in higher esteem than the Western biomedical healthcare team.

Common to the Black culture is the concept of extended family, consisting of several households, with the older adults often taking the leadership role within the family constellation. Respect for elders and ancestors is valued. They are held in high esteem because living a long life indicates that the individual had more opportunities to acquire much experience and knowledge. Decision making regarding healthcare issues is, therefore, often left to the elders. Family ties are especially strong between grandchildren and grandparents. It is not unusual for grandmothers to want to stay at the hospital bedside when their grandchildren are ill. This extended family network provides emotional, physical, and financial support to members during times of illness and other crises (Forrester, 2000; Purnell & Paulanka, 2003).

Single parenting within the African American culture is an accepted position without stigma attached to it. This cultural group does have a high tolerance for becoming a mother at a young age, although not highly desirable or condoned by Black women (Purnell & Paulanka, 2003). In fact, Black women do not perceive negative sanctions within their culture if they do not meet the ideal norm of getting an education or job prior to marriage and children. Relatives are supportive of each other if help is needed with childbearing and child rearing.

Spirituality and religiosity are very prominent cultural components of this ethnic group's community. They are at the center of and are a defining feature of African American life and serve as a source of hope, renewal, liberation, and unity among its members. **Spirituality** is defined as a belief in a higher power, a sacred force that exists in all things. **Religiosity** is defined as an individual's level of adherence to beliefs and ritualistic practices associated with religious institutions (Holt, Clark, & Kreuter, 2003; Mattis, 2000; Mattis & Jagers, 2001; Puchalski & Romer, 2000).

Both spirituality and religion play a role in the development and maintenance of social relationships throughout the developmental life span. Blacks, more so than Whites, turn to religion to cope with health challenges. Religious practices also have been found to influence health beliefs and positively influence health status and outcomes in the African American community (Newlin, Knafl, & Melkus, 2002). These strong religious values and beliefs may extend to their feelings about illness and health. A majority of Black Americans find inner strength from their trust in God. Some believe that whatever happens is God's will. This belief has led to the perception that Black Americans have a fatalistic view of life (Purnell & Paulanka, 2003) and are governed by a relatively strong external locus of control (Holt, Clark et al., 2003).

A traditional folk practice, known as voodoo, consists of beliefs about good or evil spirits inhabiting the world. Religious leaders or voodoo doctors have the power to appease or release hostile spirits. Illness, or disharmony, is thought to be caused by evil spirits because a person failed to follow religious rules or the dictates of ancestors. Curative measures involve finding the cause of an illness—a hex or a spell placed on a person by another or the breaking of a taboo—and then finding someone with magical healing powers or witchcraft to rid the afflicted individual of the evil spirit(s). Some Black American families also continue to practice home remedies such as the use of mustard plasters, herbal medicines and teas, and amulets to cure or ward off a variety of illnesses and afflictions (Purnell & Paulanka, 2003).

TEACHING STRATEGIES

In teaching Black Americans preventive and promotion measures, as well as caring for them during acute and chronic illnesses, the health professional must explore the client's value systems. Generally, any folk practices or traditional beliefs should be respected and allowed (if they are not harmful) and incorporated into the recommended treatment or healthcare interventions used by Western medicine. The following discussion offers more specific recommendations for rendering culturally appropriate care for Black Americans.

Black Americans tend to be very verbal, dynamic, animated, and interpersonal, whereby they express feelings openly to family and friends. However, they are much more private about family matters when in the company of strangers. Even though Black Americans are very informal when they interact among themselves, they prefer to be greeted in a more formal manner with the use of their surnames, which demonstrates the respect and pride they have in their family heritage.

Also, Black Americans tend to feel comfortable with less personal space than do some other ethnic groups. Humor, joking, and teasing one another are ways to reduce stress and tension, but these types of communications can be misinterpreted as aggressive behavior if not understood within the context of their culture (Purnell & Paulanka, 2003).

Generally, African Americans are also more present than past or future oriented. Thus, they tend to be more relaxed about specific time frames, evincing a more circular rather than linear sense of time, which is more characteristic of the dominant White culture. Health providers must be careful not to misinterpret nonverbal and verbal behaviors when delivering care and must be flexible in the timing of appointments because Blacks will usually keep their appointments but may not always be on schedule.

Traditionally, the family structure has been matriarchal; this pattern persists to the present day because of a high percentage of households run by a female single parent. It is imperative that healthcare providers acknowledge the dominant role that Black women play in decision making and the importance of sharing health information directly with them. Grandmothers continue to play a central role in the Black American family and are often involved in providing economic support and child care for their grandchildren (Forrester, 2000).

With respect to prevalent diseases and health issues within this population group, diabetes and hypertension continue to be the most serious health problems. The group as a whole suffers higher morbidity and mortality rates from these diseases than do other Americans (Samuel-Hodge et al., 2006; Yanek et al., 2001). Also, Blacks are at higher risk for being victims of violence, accidents, disabilities, and cancer (Forrester, 2000; Purnell & Paulanka, 2003). Obesity is another major problem among Black Americans. Food to them is a symbol of health and wealth, and a higher than ideal body weight is viewed as positive by this ethnic group.

Health educators must concentrate on disease prevention measures; institute early screening for high blood pressure, cancer, and diabetes, as well as for signs and symptoms of other diseases common in this population; and provide culturally congruent health education to improve the overall health status of Black Americans (Bailey, Erwin, & Belin, 2000; Powe, Daniels, Finnie, & Thompson, 2005). Strong family ties encourage individuals to be treated by the family before seeking care from health professionals. This cultural practice may be a factor contributing to the delay or failure of Blacks to seek treatment of diseases at the early stages of illness. An effective approach to providing care can be to conduct health screening programs in conjunction with community and church activities (Samuel-Hodge et al., 2006). "The church is a viable health education venue for this population" (Holt, Kyles et al., 2003).

Because of economic factors, Black Americans are likely to have less ready access to healthcare services. Identified barriers to Black Americans seeking the health care they need include lack of culturally relevant care, perceptions of racial discrimination, and a general distrust of both health professionals and the healthcare system. Establishing a trusting relationship, therefore, is an essential first step to be taken by health professionals if Blacks are to receive and accept the health services they require and deserve. Recognizing their unique responses to health and illness based on their spiritual and religious foundations, their strong family ties, and other traditional beliefs is essential if therapeutic interventions developed by the healthcare team are to be successful. Efforts to recruit more Blacks into the health professions would help most assuredly to reduce some of the barriers to caring for this population of Americans.

Asian/Pacific Islander Culture

People from Asian countries and the Pacific Islands constitute the third major ethnic subcultural group. Many Southeast Asian refugees have come to the United States mainly as a result of World War II, the Korean War in the 1950s, the fall of the South Vietnam government in 1975, and the successive disintegrations of the governments of Laos and Cambodia. Primarily, they have settled on the West Coast, particularly in the San Francisco Bay area of California and in Washington State (Villanueva & Lipat, 2000; Young et al., 2002). Also, the states of New York, New Jersey, and Texas have experienced a large influx of Asian peoples, particularly from China, the Philippines, and Japan. In the decades following political and social upheavals in Southeast Asia, almost three quarters of a million people of Asian/Pacific Islander origin immigrated into the United States. As of 2004, more than 12 million Asian/Pacific Islanders (3.8% of the total U.S. population) live in the country (U.S. Census Bureau, 2006).

Although Asian/Pacific Islander people have been classified as a single ethnic group by many researchers and census takers, this category represents different groups of people with distinct

health issues and unique cultures. Asian Americans, the largest group of people within this category, experience a number of extremes. Although some of the richest Americans are of Asian background, nearly 1 million Asian Americans live at or below the federal poverty level. Asian women have the highest life expectancy of any ethnic group. However, as a group, Asian Americans suffer from a higher than average incidence of many chronic illnesses such as tuberculosis, hepatitis B, and certain forms of cancer (Office of Minority Health and Health Disparities, 2010). Native Hawaiian and other Pacific Islanders represent less than 1% of the U.S. population. As a group, they experience poorer health outcomes than the general population, are more likely to die of cancer or heart disease, and have a high incidence of HIV/AIDS and hepatitis B (Office of Minority Health and Health Disparities, 2010).

A wide variety of cultural, religious, and language backgrounds is represented by the Asian/Pacific Islander people. Some similarities exist among members of this ethnic group, but there are also many differences (Purnell & Paulanka, 2003). By understanding the basic beliefs of the Asian/Pacific Islander people, healthcare practitioners can be better prepared to understand and accept their cultural differences and varied behavior patterns (Villanueva & Lipat, 2000; Young et al., 2002).

The major philosophical orientation of the Asian/Pacific Islander people is a blend of four philosophies—Buddhism, Confucianism, Taoism, and Phi. Four common values are strongly reflected in all of these philosophies:

1. Male authority and dominance
2. Saving face (behavior as a result of a sense of pride)
3. Strong family ties
4. Respect for parents, elders, teachers, and other authority figures

The following is a brief review of the beliefs and healthcare practices of the Asian/Pacific Islander people (Pang, 2007; Purnell & Paulanka, 2003).

BUDDHISM

The fundamental belief is that all existence is suffering. The continuation of life, and therefore suffering, arises from desires and passions. According to the Buddhist philosophy, no humans are limited to a single existence terminating in death. Instead, everyone is reincarnated. Cambodians, who are in particular strongly influenced by the Buddhist philosophy, strive to accumulate religious merits or good deeds to ensure a better life to come. They adhere to a deep belief in karma, whereby things done in this existence can help or hinder their ascension on the ladder to nirvana. Good deeds, sharing, donating, and being generous and kind are all ways to accumulate merits.

CONFUCIANISM

Moral values and beliefs are heavily influenced by this philosophy, which focuses on these aspects of one's personality. Two predominant moral qualities, developed through cultivation of the personality, include humaneness (the attitude shown toward others) and a sense of moral duty and obligation (attitudes persons display toward themselves). The principles that guide the social behavior of people who adhere to Confucianism are described as follows.

PATTERNS OF AUTHORITY   The following five relationships run from inferior to superior to form a pattern of obligation and authority in the family as well as in social and political realms:

1. Son (child) to father
2. Wife to husband
3. Younger brother to older brother
4. Friend to friend
5. Subject to ruler

These patterns of authority and obligation influence decision making and social interactions. For example, a friend is to regard a friend as a younger or older brother. Women's subservience to men is reflected in a woman's behavior to al-

ways seek the advice of her husband when making decisions. This authority needs to be respected by health professionals when, for instance, a woman refuses to choose a contraceptive method until she asks for her husband's advice and permission.

MAN IN HARMONY WITH THE UNIVERSE   In the Confucian system, people are seen as being between heaven and earth, and life has to be in harmony with the universe. An example of this principle in action is when an Asian responds passively to new information, quietly accepting it rather than actively seeking to clarify it. Given this perspective, it is important for the health professional when instructing the client to ask for an explanation of the information to ascertain whether it was understood.

ANCESTOR WORSHIP   Concern for the moral order of relationships is reflected in a deep reverence for tradition and prescribed rites. Great emphasis is placed on funerals, etiquette for mourning, and the sharing of a communal meal with the dead.

The Asian/Pacific Islander culture values harmony in life and a balance of nature. Shame is something to be avoided, families are the center of life, elders are respected, and ancestors are worshiped and remembered. Children are highly valued because they carry on the family name and are expected to care for aging parents. The woman's role is one of subservience throughout her entire life—she will follow the advice of parents while unmarried, the husband's advice while married, and the children's advice when widowed. This subservient role is in direct conflict with U.S. social and family values, which expect women to take a more independent, assertive, and self-determined role.

TAOISM

The Tao philosophy has its roots in the belief of two opposing magical forces in nature, the negative (yin) and the positive (yang), which affect the course of all material and spiritual life. The basic concepts of Chinese philosophy, the beliefs in tao (the way of nature), and yin and yang (the principle of balance) stress that human achievement in harmony with nature should be accomplished through nonaction.

Common also is the idea that good health depends on the balance between hot and cold. Equilibrium of hot and cold elements produces good health. Drugs, natural elements, and foods are classified as either hot or cold. It is believed that sickness can be caused by eating too much hot or cold food. Hot foods include meats, sweets, and spices. Cold foods include rice and vegetables.

The Chinese people believe in strong family ties, respect for elders, and the authority of men as the head of the household. As a consequence, sons are highly valued. Illness is believed to result from an imbalance in the forces of nature. Ill health is believed to be a curse from heaven, with mental illness being the worst possible curse, because the individual was irresponsible in not obtaining the right amount of rest, food, and work.

Phi

Phi worship is a belief in the spirits of dead relatives or the spirits of animals and nature. Phi ranges from bad to good. If a place has a strong phi, the individual must make an offering before doing anything in that place, such as building a house or tilling the land. If someone violates a rule of order, an atmosphere of bad phi can result in illness or death. Redemption can be sought from a phi priest as a hope of getting relief from suffering. Offerings are made and special rites are performed to rid the person of a bad phi.

Adherents to this philosophy respect elders and avoid conflict by doing things in a pleasant manner. Those who adhere to the phi philosophy are hospitable and generous. They show respect to others by the way a person is addressed and tend to prize hard work and ambition.

For people of the Asian/Pacific Islander ethnic group living in the United States, marked cultural differences confront them with respect to ways of life, ways of thinking, values orientation, social structure, and family interactions (Chao, 1994; Young et al., 2002). Children may adapt quickly, but the older generations tend to have difficulty acculturating.

Their medical practices, like their other unique cultural practices, differ significantly from Western ways. The health-seeking behaviors of immigrants tend to be crisis oriented, following the pattern in their homelands where medical care was not readily available. They are likely to seek health care only when seriously ill. Reinforcement is needed to encourage them to come for follow-up visits after an initial encounter with the healthcare system. Sometimes they are viewed by practitioners as noncompliant when they do not do exactly what is expected of them, when they withdraw from follow-up treatments, or when they do not keep prearranged appointments.

Asian people make great use of herbal remedies to treat various ills, such as fevers, diarrhea, and coughs. Dermabrasion, often misunderstood by U.S. practitioners, is a home remedy to cure a wide variety of problems such as headaches, cold symptoms, fever, and chills. In their traditional healthcare system, Asian individuals rely on folk medicines from healers, sorcerers, and monks.

Western medicine is thought to be "shots that cure," and Asian patients expect to get some form of medicine (injections or pills) whenever they seek medical help in the United States. If no medication is prescribed, the person, if not given an explanation, may feel that care is inadequate and fail to return for future care.

Common to many Southeast Asians is the idea that illnesses, just like foods, are classified as hot and cold. This belief coincides with the yin and yang philosophy of the principle of balance. If a disease is considered hot in origin, then giving cold foods is believed to be the proper treatment.

Conflict and fear are the most likely responses to laboratory tests and having blood drawn. It is the belief of this ethnic group that removing blood makes the body weak and that blood is not replenished. Fear of surgery may result from the conviction that souls inhabit the body and may be released. Another major fear is the loss of privacy leading to extreme embarrassment and humiliation.

TEACHING STRATEGIES

Respect is automatically endowed on most healthcare providers and teachers because they are seen as knowledgeable. Asians are sensitive and formal people, so making a friendly and nonthreatening approach to them is necessary before giving care. They must be given permission to ask a question but are not offended by questions from others.

One salient characteristic to be noted of the Japanese subculture is a childlike dependency known as *amae*, which continues through adulthood but is especially evident when people are ill or going through hardships. This behavior conflicts with the Western philosophy of many health professions of helping those they care for to become independent in self-care. Awareness of this characteristic dependent behavior allows American healthcare providers to approach clients of Japanese heritage in a culturally relevant and tolerant manner (Hisama, 2000).

Language barriers are usually the first and biggest obstacle to overcome in working with people of Asian/Pacific Islander descent. The learning style of Asians is essentially passive—no personal opinions, no confrontations, no challenges, and no outward disagreements. Healthcare practitioners should be aware that in the Asians' wish to save face for themselves and others, they avoid being disruptive and will agree to what is said so as not to be offensive.

The approach to learning is done primarily by repetition and rote memorization of information. It must be remembered that decision making is a family affair. Consequently, family members need to be included, especially the male authority figure,

in the process of deciding the best solution for a situation. They are easily shamed, so clients must be reassured and told what is considered acceptable behavior by Western moral and legal standards. Nods of the head do not necessarily mean agreement or understanding. Questions directed to them need to be asked in several ways to confirm that they understand any instructional messages given.

American Indian/Alaska Native Culture

The U.S. Census Bureau (2006) has identified more than 2.8 million people (approximately 1% of the U.S. population) who are of the American Indian/Alaska Native ethnic group living in the United States. There are more than 500 distinct tribes of American Indians and Native Alaskans, including Eskimo and Aleut tribes (Lowe & Struthers, 2001). The largest of these tribes is the Cherokee. Other tribes of significant size are the Navaho, Sioux, Chippewa, Choctaw, Pueblo, and the Latin American Indian. These tribes reside primarily in the northwestern, central, and southwestern regions of the United States (U.S. Census Bureau, 2006). The term *Native American* is used throughout this section of the chapter to include both the American Indian and Native Alaskan people.

Of these people, approximately one half are eligible for health services provided by the federal government. Medical care to American Indian people has a long history. As far back as 1832, the War Department undertook a smallpox vaccination campaign for tribes of American Indian people, largely to protect military troops from infection. In 1849, healthcare responsibility was transferred to the newly created Bureau of Indian Affairs. In 1954, the Department of Health, Education, and Welfare of the U.S. Public Health Service (USPHS) took over jurisdiction. Today, the Indian Health Service (IHS) of the USPHS maintains responsibility for providing health care to members of this ethnic group (Mail, McKay, & Katz, 1989).

The current challenge to healthcare practitioners is to integrate Western medicine with traditional non-Western tribal folk medicine to provide cross-cultural health education to Native Americans in reservation-based communities across the nation. To do so, health professionals must understand contemporary Native American cultural patterns, including theories of disease causality and associated therapies. It is also essential for health professionals to become focused on a more ethnomedical orientation. This means delineating the nature and consequences of illness problems and disease interventions from the ethnic group's perspective, rather than adhering to the biomedical orientation of defining diseases and illness interventions from only a Western perspective.

In the ethnomedical context, the concept of health and illness incorporates the relationship of humans with their universe—a concept that bridges culture with a sensitivity toward the daily practices inherent within specific ethnic groups. The challenge for the health educator is to understand the world perspective of contemporary American Indian and Native Alaskan people that sets them apart from non–Native Americans (Cantore, 2001; Lowe & Struthers, 2001; Mail et al., 1989).

As outlined by Purnell and Paulanka (2003), Lowe and Struthers (2001), Harding (1998), Scharnberg (2007), Joho and Ormsby (2000), and Cantore (2001), Native American culture has the following major characteristics:

1. A spiritual attachment to the land and harmony with nature
2. An intimacy of religion and medicine
3. Emphasis on strong ties to an extended family network, including immediate family, other relatives, and the entire tribe
4. The view that children are an asset, not a liability
5. A belief that supernatural powers exist in animate as well as in inanimate objects

6. A desire to remain Native American and avoid acculturation, thereby retaining one's own culture and language
7. A lack of materialism, lack of time consciousness, and a desire to share with others

Unless non–Native American healthcare workers are aware of these characteristics, they can easily overlook them when providing care to clients of this ethnic group. Although Anglo-American culture and Western healthcare practices have been integrated to some extent into the Native American way of life, the preceding characteristics still predominate today to set this subculture apart as a unique entity.

Native Americans see a close connection between religion and health. When a family member becomes ill, witchcraft is still perceived by some tribes as the real cause of illness. In traditional societies, witchcraft functions to supply answers to perplexing or disturbing questions. It also explains personal insecurities, intragroup tensions, fears, and anxieties.

Witches, with their supernatural powers, have served as convenient scapegoats on which to blame the misfortunes in life and provided tribes with a mechanism for social control. It is hypothesized that as the cultural practices of witchcraft were increasingly denigrated by missionaries and bureaucrats, substitutions such as compulsive drinking and frequent use of narcotics (peyote) emerged as culturally sanctioned outlets for aggressive impulses and frustrations. These behaviors were seen as less disruptive than demonstrating overt hostilities. This hypothesis has been proposed as an explanation of the high prevalence of substance abuse by Native Americans.

Some Native American tribes still practice witchcraft but tend to deny it as a reality because of the negative stereotype and stigma attached to it by outsiders. Nevertheless, the intimacy between religion and medicine persists and is exhibited in the form of "sing" prayers and ceremonial cure practices. However, few health professionals would think of providing space and privacy for several relatives to be able to conduct a ceremony for a hospitalized family member.

Some Native American tribal beliefs also require incorporating the medicine man (shaman) into the system of care given to patients. The central and formal aspects of Native American medicine are ceremonial, embracing the notion of a supernatural power. Although the ceremonies vary from tribe to tribe, the ideas of causation and cure are common to all Native Americans. The ritual performed is determined by the signs and symptoms of an illness. Sometimes rituals are conducted by family members. Cornmeal, from the sacred food of corn, is one item that is frequently used in a variety of curative ceremonies. Herbal remedies have for generations served native healers as their pharmacopoeia. The health professional must demonstrate legitimate respect for such ritualistic symbols and ceremonial activities.

To be considered really poor in the Native American world is to be devoid of relatives. The family and tribe are of utmost importance, which is a belief that children learn from infancy. It is not unusual for many family members—sometimes large groups of 10 to 15 people—to arrive at the hospital and camp out on the hospital grounds to be with their sick relative. Talking is unnecessary, but simply being there is highly important for everyone concerned. Hospital personnel have often labeled this behavior as useless and disruptive and deem the patient and family to be uncooperative.

Grandmothers, in particular, have great importance to a sick child, and they frequently must give permission for a child to be hospitalized and treated. The Native American kinship system, in fact, allows for a child to have several sets of grandparents, aunts, uncles, cousins, brothers, and sisters. Sometimes a number of women substitute as a mother figure for a child, which may cause role confusion for the non–Native American healthcare provider.

Children are given a great deal of freedom and independence to learn by their decisions and live by the consequences of their actions. Their entire childhood years consist of experiential learning to develop skills and self-confidence to function as adults. They may appear spoiled, but in fact they are taught self-care and respect for others at a very early age. Children are doted on by family members, and, in turn, they have high regard for their elders. In fact, the older adults in Native American communities are highly respected and looked to for advice and counsel. Outside of their private domain, such as in the public school system, Native American children tend not to be seen as very competitive or assertive. However, to call attention to oneself is interpreted by Native Americans as showy and inappropriate.

Another characteristic of Native Americans is that they generally are not very future oriented; they take one day at a time and do not feel they have control over their own destiny. Time is seen as being on a continuum with no beginning and no end. Native Americans tend not to live by clocks and schedules. In fact, many of their homes do not have clocks, and family members eat meals and do other activities when they please.

Members of this ethnic group tend to be more casual in their approach to life than many non–Native American people. This lack of time consciousness and pressure is a crucial factor to be remembered by healthcare providers when a prescribed regimen calls for the patient to follow a medication, exercise, or dietary schedule. This attitude or way of thinking also has proved to be a significant obstacle when health educators have attempted to provide preventive care. Inattention to time, in addition, can interfere with their keeping scheduled appointments, although lack of funds rather than time seems to be the main cause of missed appointments.

Another aspect of time is reflected in their belief that death is just a part of the life cycle—a much healthier and more accepting attitude toward dying than that held by most White Americans. Their grief process is culturally very different. Funerals are accompanied by large feasts and the sharing of gifts with relatives of the deceased. There is no belief in a life hereafter as a reward for a lifetime of good deeds while on earth. Life after death is, instead, viewed as an opportunity to join the world of long-ago ancestors. Their view of death is closely related to their opinion about the appropriate disposal of amputated limbs. Because diabetes is so prevalent in the Native American population, it is important to know that they usually want to reclaim an amputated body part for proper burial.

Sharing is another core value of Native Americans. The concept of being is fundamental, and there is little stress on achievement or the worth of material wealth. Individuals are valued much more highly than material goods. Overall, Native Americans are a proud, sensitive, cooperative, passive people, devoted to tribe and family, and willing to share possessions and self with others. They are very vulnerable when it comes to their pride and dignity. They can be easily offended by nonsensitive caregivers.

In terms of human relationships, it is important to note that Native Americans believe that to look someone in the eye is considered disrespectful. Some tribes feel that looking into the eyes of another person reveals and may even steal someone's soul. Because a friendly handshake and eye contact are acceptable and even expected in the Anglo-American culture, it must be acknowledged that these gestures do not have the same meaning for the Native American. In fact, eye contact by White American definition is interpreted to mean that someone is paying attention, is interested, or understands. Non–Native American healthcare workers, therefore, may consider lack of eye contact to mean that these patients are shiftless, shifty, uninterested in learning, or inattentive, when in fact all along they were taking in the message of instruction being given. If asked, they can often repeat verbatim what someone just said to them.

The type and incidence of health problems faced by Native Americans have undergone significant change over the years. In the first half of the 20th century, acute and infectious diseases were prevalent and were the principal cause of death. Today, as a result of increased life expectancy, Native Americans are succumbing to many lifestyle diseases and chronic conditions. Chief among the causes of morbidity and mortality are heart disease, obesity, cancer, diabetes, and drug and alcohol abuse—all of which to some extent are amenable to educational intervention (Office of Minority Health and Health Disparities, 2010).

TEACHING STRATEGIES

Health professionals in the role of educator need to focus on giving information about these diseases and risk factors, emphasize the teaching of skills related to changes in diet and exercise, and help clients to build positive coping mechanisms to deal with emotional problems. For the most part, acute and infectious diseases, with the exception of a recurrence in tuberculosis, are no longer a major cause of illness and death among Native Americans. This is the result of modern drug therapy, early case findings, improved sanitary conditions, and better provision of health education.

Another positive influence has been the greater availability of community health representatives (CHRs). These indigenous community outreach workers have played a significant role in case finding, early diagnosis, and reinforcement of patient and other health education recommendations. As Mail and others (1989) state: "Involving the CHR in patient education is an important cross-cultural consideration, because this is the individual who will reinforce behavior changes with the community and home" (p. 97).

Although all Native Americans share some of the core beliefs and practices of their culture, each tribe is unique in its customs and language. Finding the ways and means to integrate Western medicine with the traditional Native American folk medicine in caring for the varied needs of this population group presents a challenge to the health educator. It also presents a learning opportunity for the recipient of these health education services.

Preparing Health Professionals for Diversity Care

America is no longer the homogeneous melting pot society it once was. Today, myriad cultures are present in the United States, and the world faces an increasing trend toward global migration of people and globalization of health care. The delivery of appropriate health care now and in the future will depend on use of a culturally informed approach that goes beyond simple language translation and an understanding of the characteristics of different cultures. Health professionals must learn how to relate to people—clients, fellow healthcare practitioners, and students—who come from a variety of cultural backgrounds and discover the cultural meaning of various health events (Career Directory, 2005).

The various health professions must be prepared to pursue this relatively new paradigm for creating and managing diversity within their workforces as well as within the healthcare marketplace consisting of consumers and staff from multicultural backgrounds. Diversity has the potential to positively affect health practice by increasing organizational effectiveness, creating greater access to care, lifting morale of clients and staff, and enhancing productivity in the workforce (Cooper, Grywalski, Lamp, Newhouse, & Studlien, 2007; Doyle, 2008; Marquand, 2001; Sullivan Commission, 2004; Thomas & Ely, 1996).

As a result of former President Clinton's national leadership to eliminate cultural disparities in health by the year 2010, the U.S. government introduced a series of initiatives put forth in the *Healthy People 2010* document. One goal of this 10-year plan was to eliminate racial and ethnic disparities in health (USDHHS, 2000). This current initiative is lauded as "the first explicit commitment by the government to achieve equity in health outcomes" (Jones, 2000, p. 214). The health professions have embraced this goal and its objectives to eradicate discrepancies in health outcomes among minority populations.

One important step to ensure culturally competent health care in this new century is to increase minority representation in the health professions. The health professions need to recruit and retain more minority students and faculty to expand diversity within their ranks. For example, the nursing workforce comprises only 10% of people from minority groups (see **Figure 8–3**), whereas more than 28% of the total U.S. population belongs to a variety of cultural subgroups (Robinson, 2000). Lack of minority representation is not limited to nursing. Less than 10% of physicians and dentists are of minority background with even smaller percentages noted among faculty in schools of dentistry, medicine, and nursing (Sullivan Commission, 2004).

Another initiative to break down cultural barriers to health care is to strengthen multicultural perspectives in the curriculum of health professions education programs (Bond, Kardong-Edgren, & Jones, 2001; Doyle, 2008; Kelley & Fitzsimons, 2000; Shaya & Gbarayor, 2006). Innovative health professions education means incorporating social values that recognize diverse lifestyles and acknowledge multicultural and multiracial perspectives (Doyle, 2008; Rew, Becker, Cookston, Khosropour, & Martinez, 2003). As these authors point out, health professionals must not only better understand the cultural characteristics and traits of patients and families from different ethnic backgrounds, but also must improve the relationship between health professionals and clients from different cultural backgrounds.

Figure 8–3 Distribution of Registered Nurses by Racial/Ethnic Background, March 2004

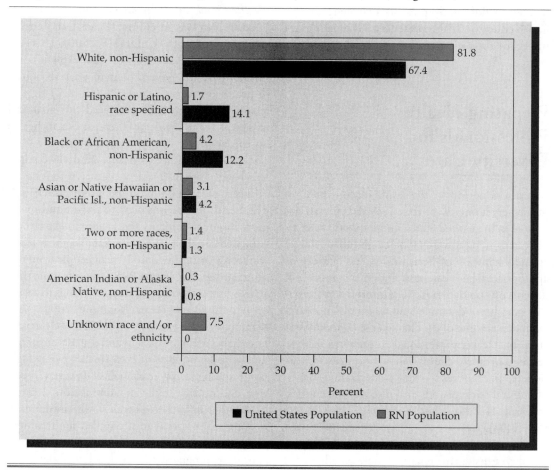

Source: U.S. Census Bureau (2006). Statistical abstract of the United States, resident population by sex, race, and Hispanic origin status: 2000 to 2004, Table 13. Retrieved from http://www.census.gov/prod/2005pubs/06statab/ pop.pdf.

Note: Census reports that, of the 293,655,000 in the U.S. population for 2004, 197,841,000 are of White race and non-Hispanic. Thus, while 67.4% of the U.S. population are White, non-Hispanic, 32.6% are non-White or Hispanic.

Health professionals must be able to create an environment in which people are encouraged to express themselves and freely describe their needs. As Dreher (1996) so aptly states, "Transcending cultural differences is more than an appreciation of cultural diversity. It is transcending one's own investment in the social and economic system as one knows it and lives it" (p. 4). Health educators must concentrate on the cultural strategies that are needed to help individuals and groups negotiate the healthcare system.

Stereotyping: Identifying the Meaning, the Risks, and the Solutions

In addressing the diversity issues of gender, socioeconomics, and culture, health professionals must acknowledge the risks of stereotyping inherent in discussing these three attributes of the learner. This chapter explicitly recognizes that differences exist in learning based on gender, socioeconomics, and culture and that these factors often require alternative approaches to teaching. It is important to realize that differences should not be equated with judgments as to what is good or bad, right or wrong; rather, educators should not ignore the need to attend to these differences in a sensitive, open, and fair manner.

Health professional educators must relate to each person as an individual. It is important to develop an awareness that although a person can be considered a member—or may identify with members—of a certain ethnic group, the individual has his or her own abilities, experiences, preferences, and practices. Learning needs, learning styles, and readiness to learn are all factors that influence lifestyle behaviors.

Nevertheless, everyone has been socialized in subtle and not so subtle ways according to their own diversity attributes, socioeconomic and political backgrounds, and other life exposures. It is imperative for health professional educators to acknowledge the prejudices, biases, and stereotypical tendencies that can come into play when they deal with others like or unlike themselves. They must consciously attempt to recognize these possible attitudes and the effect they may have on others in their care. To address the dangers of stereotyping on more than just a superficial level, this section examines examples of unacceptable forms of stereotyping, common pitfalls that can arise in dealing with diversity, and what can be done to avoid stereotypical behaviors.

Stereotyping is defined by Purnell and Paulanka (2003) as "an oversimplified conception, opinion, or belief about some aspect of an individual or group of people" (p. 357). Exaggerated generalizations are commonly made about the characteristics, behaviors, and motives associated with any person or group of people. Actually, stereotyping can be positive or negative, depending on how, where, when, why, and about whom it is applied (Satel, 2002).

For example, stereotyping can be a useful and legitimate process to organize or classify people if based on logical reasoning and accumulated facts. A system of organization and classification helps people to identify and understand information— for example, "he's Jewish," "she's Italian," or "they're Democrats." Conversely, stereotyping can be negative if it is used to place people in a mold or an artificial, unfair position based on oversimplification without true substantiation by facts. Negative stereotyping leads to disrespect, dehumanization, and denigration of others and serves as a barrier to equality and fairness toward others.

Stereotyping deserves a bad name when associated with bias or clichés. There is a huge emotional component to stereotyping. The language that people use, the attitudes that they project, the conclusions that they draw, and the context in which they employ stereotyping all determine its positive or negative quality.

Unfortunately, classification by association is often perfunctory and, therefore, laden with bias. Stereotyping in this sense is used to label someone. For example, Americans tend to think of themselves as the freedom fighters and liberty lovers of the world; in the same breath, they may describe members of other groups or nationalities as violators of human rights or terrorists. This threat of stereotyping is even greater in light of the infamous September 11, 2001, attack on this country. Simple appearance attributes, such as a beard, certain attire, or a specific form of speech, can be the basis on which broad and deep prejudices are built.

People particularly tend to use an excuse to classify individuals when they do not like or respect those whose backgrounds, attitudes, abilities, values, or beliefs are different from or opposed to their own or are misunderstood or misinterpreted. Stereotyping, conscious or subconscious, results in intolerance toward others and engenders the belief that one way of thinking or being is the only way or the right way. Corley and Goren (1998) discuss the ways in which labeling, stereotyping, and stigmatizing responses by nurses tend to marginalize clients.

Attitudes toward sex-role competencies are considered a type of stereotyping. Gender bias has produced inequality in education, employment, and other social spheres. Gender stereotypes may be relevant in health professions that are predominantly female or male. Gender stereotypes may also be a concern in client care when a client is in a nontraditional role, for example, a man who has primary responsibility for the care of the children in the family.

Research into gender stereotyping in the past 20 years documents that elementary and secondary school teachers interact more actively with boys by asking them more questions, giving them more feedback (praise and positive encouragement), and providing them with more specific and valuable comments and guidance. In these subtle ways, stereotypical expectations are reinforced (Snowman & Biehler, 2006).

Also, it used to be that an extensive list of personality differences between the sexes would be included in education and developmental psychology textbooks. However, recent psychology research has revealed that these sex-role lists are gender biased. Today, it is recognized that few personality characteristics associated with gender are consistent across cultures, except for aggression (Santrock, 2006; Snowman & Biehler, 2006; Vander Zanden et al., 2007).

As another example of gender bias, women have been labeled as attentive listeners and men as poor listeners when, in fact, listening behavior is not a measure of attentiveness but a matter of behavioral style. Men, when listening, move around and make sporadic eye contact, whereas women are likely to remain still and maintain steady eye contact with occasional nodding or smiling. As a result, the listening style of men is often misinterpreted as inattentive or rude, and the style of women is often mistaken for encouragement or agreement with what is being said (Tear, 1995).

Interruptions when engaging in dialogue also have been noted as a misinterpretation of communication differences between the sexes. Men frequently speak in a steady flow and interrupt each other to take turns, whereas women tend to speak with frequent pauses to allow others to have their say. Pause-free male speech is often misinterpreted as a device to discourage females from participating and as an attempt to be pushy. The tendency for females to pause in speaking is seen as being timid or courteous. These misinterpretations reinforce stereotypes of men as dominating, insensitive, and controlling and women as unassertive, passive, and oversensitive (Tear, 1995).

Health professionals must concentrate on treating the sexes equally when providing access to health education, delivering health and illness care, and designing health education materials that contain bias-free language. For example, they must avoid gender-specific terms and choose words that minimize ambiguity in gender identity, unless critical to the content. They should avoid using the pronouns *he* or *she* and instead use the plural pronoun *they*. If at all possible, health professionals should avoid beginning or ending words with *man* or *men*, such as *man-made*, *mankind*, and *chair-*

men. Do not specify marital status unless necessary by using *Ms.* instead of *Mrs.* Health professionals can find guidelines for nonsexist language in the *McGraw-Hill Guidelines for Bias-Free Publishing* and *The Bias-Free Word Finder.*

With respect to age, socioeconomics, culture and race, religion, and disabilities, stereotyping most definitely exists. This chapter offers many cautions against stereotyping individuals and groups. For example, just because someone belongs to a specific ethnic group does not necessarily mean that the individual adheres to all of the beliefs and practices of that particular group.

A thorough and accurate assessment of the learner is the key to determining the particular abilities, preferences, and needs of each individual. The health professional educator should choose words that are accurate, clear, and free from bias whenever speaking or writing about various individuals or groups. Health professionals should refer to someone's ethnicity, race, religion, age, and socioeconomic status only when it is essential to the content being addressed. For instance, it is more politically and socially correct to use the term *older adult* than the term *elderly* or *aged.* By using people-first language, health professionals can refrain from labeling a member of a special population as a *disabled person* but rather as a *person with a disability.* Also, it is more appropriate and more acceptable to refer to a *person with diabetes* rather than a *diabetic* or to a *person with AIDS* rather than an *AIDS victim.*

To avoid stereotyping, health professionals should ask themselves the following questions:

- Do I use neutral language when teaching clients and families?
- Do I confront bias when evidenced by other healthcare professionals?
- Do I request information equally from clients regardless of gender, socioeconomic status, age, or culture?
- Are my instructional materials free of stereotypical terminology and expressions?

- Am I an effective role model of equality for my colleagues?
- Do I treat all clients with fairness, respect, and dignity?
- Does someone's appearance influence (raise or lower) my expectations of that person's abilities or affect the quality of care I deliver?
- Do I routinely assess the educational backgrounds, experiential backgrounds, personal attributes, and economic resources of clients to ensure appropriate health teaching?
- Am I knowledgeable enough of the cultural traditions of various groups to provide sensitive care in this multicultural, pluralistic society?

It is easy to stereotype someone, not out of malice, but out of ignorance. Health professional educators have a responsibility to keep informed of the most current beliefs and facts about various gender attributes, socioeconomic influences, and cultural traditions that could positively or negatively affect teaching and learning. Every day, research in social science, psychology, and the health professions is yielding information that can assist in planning and revising appropriate health interventions to meet the needs of diverse client populations.

State of the Evidence

It is essential that health professionals base their practice on evidence from empirical studies and expert opinion to deliver the highest, most scientifically sound care to clients. Such evidence also is important as a basis for the educational preparation of staff and future members of the health professions to give them the most up-to-date knowledge and skills needed to function competently and confidently in today's healthcare environment.

With respect to gender attributes of the learner, it is evident that understanding how the human brain works and the differences between the sexes in how men and women think, feel, and respond is still in its infancy. Neuroscience is just beginning to unravel the mysteries and discover the differences and similarities in the way male and female brains are wired. In the last 5–10 years, there has been an upsurge of interest and fascination with the discoveries in the field of neurobiology. New brain imaging instruments are beginning to reveal which individual portions of the brain are responsible for cognition, emotions, and tasks, but even more important is how the different parts of the brain operate or interact with one another.

Brain research is an exciting, largely uncharted field, and some of the research findings are conflicting or inconclusive. Therefore, the challenge for health professional educators is to incorporate what is currently known to refine their approaches to teaching and learning, but not to be too quick to assume or generalize the application of preliminary research findings before the evidence is conclusive.

Further research on the impact of socioeconomics on health outcomes also needs to be conducted. For example, currently, scant information is available about IQ and socioeconomics in relation to health status and health inequalities. The research of Batty et al. (2006) shows that, although cognitive abilities are related to health, the association of socioeconomic environment, social position, educational attainment, and employment status on morbidity and mortality rates is still not altogether clear (Elstad & Krokstad, 2003; Singh-Manoux et al., 2005). Also, much more research needs to be done to understand the impact of socioeconomic position in relation to the ability, preference, and motivation for learning.

Research priorities on the influence of cultural diversity on the health of individuals and groups must be identified and defined. Knowledge gaps remain despite the increase in the number of new studies being conducted. For example, the growing multicultural nature of American society requires that health professionals understand the impact of ethnic beliefs on the epidemiology of various diseases, on the effectiveness of health promotion

efforts, on illness prevention measures, and on health maintenance and rehabilitation interventions. Bolton and colleagues (2001) pose the question: Are there ethnic variations in response to chronic illness and the performance of functional abilities of daily living? A need exists for funding to support research investigation into so many issues related to health, such as nutrition, mental status, social isolation, and prenatal to postmenopausal phases of women's lives.

Also, health professions are in the initial stages of developing instruments that can measure the cultural effects of clients' perspectives on health and responses to illness. Harris, Belyea, Mishel, and Germino (2003) call for exploration into creating as well as adopting reliable and valid instruments to measure health beliefs, attitudes, customs, and patterns of behavior in males and females of different ethnic backgrounds. It is clear that health providers lack substantial research evidence on how the context of culture affects health and illness.

Summary

This chapter explores the influence of gender characteristics, socioeconomic status, and cultural beliefs on both the ability and willingness of clients to learn healthcare measures. The in-depth examination of these three factors serves as an explanatory model for certain behaviors health professional educators might observe or encounter in teaching–learning situations. This chapter emphasizes the need to understand clients of diverse backgrounds with whom health educators interact. Health professional educators should also understand gender, socioeconomic, and cultural characteristics as useful sources of information when teaching students or staff who come with a variety of experiences and orientations.

This chapter's most important message is the care health professionals must take not to stereotype or generalize common characteristics of a group to all members associated with that particular group. For example, if health professionals do not know much about an ethnic subculture, they should ask clients about their beliefs rather than just assuming clients abide by the tenets of a certain cultural group. In that way, health professionals can avoid offending learners.

In their role as teachers, health professionals must be careful to treat each learner as an individual. They must determine the extent to which clients ascribe to, exhibit beliefs in, or adhere to ways of doing things that might affect their learning. Humans live in a double environment—an outer layer of social and cultural experiences and an inner layer of innate strengths and weaknesses—that influences how they perceive and respond to their world (Griffith, 1982).

Health professionals should constantly strive to improve the delivery of care to all people regardless of their gender orientation, ethnic origin, creed, nationality, or socioeconomic background. There is much more to know about how these three factors of gender, socioeconomics, and culture affect the teaching–learning process before health professionals can competently, confidently, and sensitively deliver care to satisfy the needs of a socially, intellectually, and culturally diverse clientele.

REVIEW QUESTIONS

1. What are five gender-related characteristics in cognitive functioning and personality behavior that affect learning?
2. How does the environment versus heredity influence gender-specific approaches to learning?
3. In what ways does SES negatively affect a person's health, and, conversely, how does illness affect an individual's socioeconomic well-being?
4. How does the SES of individuals influence the teaching–learning process?
5. What is meant by the term *poverty circle*?
6. What is the definition of each of the following terms: *assimilation*, *acculturation*, *culture*, *ethnic group*, and *ethnocentrism*?
7. How can the concept of transcultural care be applied to the assessment and teaching of clients from culturally diverse backgrounds?
8. What are the 12 cultural domains identified in Purnell's model of cultural competence that should be taken into account by health professionals when conducting a client assessment?
9. What are the four major ethnic subcultural groups in the United States?
10. What are the salient characteristics of each of these four major ethnic groups?
11. Which teaching strategies are most appropriate to meet the needs of individuals from each of the four major ethnic subcultural groups?
12. What can you do to avoid cultural stereotyping?

CASE STUDY

"They told us this might happen, but we were hoping this day would never come." Kim Hoang and her siblings crowded into the tiny conference room and were shaken to hear the news that their grandmother, Anh Hoang, a 74-year-old Vietnamese woman, was in end-stage renal failure. "My grandmother is old world. We don't know how she will cope with all of this." The healthcare team explained the treatment plan. Dialysis is required three times each week and the schedule is rigid. Mrs. Hoang's diet restrictions are also significant. New medications would be added and Mrs. Hoang needs to learn to care for her dialysis site. She would feel better once dialysis starts, but she might be fatigued and will probably require periodic blood transfusions. Kim asked to be present when her grandmother's teaching takes place. "My grandmother's English is not very good and I can help explain things to her. She doesn't respond well to strangers."

1. How would you respond to Kim's request to serve as the interpreter for her grandmother?
2. Which areas are most important for you to assess when completing Mrs. Hoang's cultural assessment?
3. If during your assessment you discover conflicts between Mrs. Hoang's cultural beliefs and treatment protocols, how will you handle them?

References

Anderson, J. M. (1987, December). The cultural context of caring. *Canadian Critical Care Nursing Journal*, 7–13.

Anderson, J. M. (1990). Health care across cultures. *Nursing Outlook*, 38(3), 136–139.

Anderson, R. M., Funnell, M. M., Arnold, M. S., Barr, P. A., Edwards, G. J., & Fitzgerald, J. T. (2000). Assessing the cultural relevance of an education program for urban African Americans with diabetes. *Diabetes Educator*, 26(2), 280–289.

Andrews, M. M., & Boyle, J. S. (1995). Transcultural nursing care. In M. M. Andrews & J. S. Boyle (Eds.), *Transcultural concepts in nursing care* (2nd ed., pp. 49–95). Philadelphia: Lippincott.

Bailey, E. J., Erwin, D. O., & Belin, P. (2000). Using cultural beliefs and patterns to improve mammography utilization among African-American women: The Witness project. *Journal of the National Medical Association*, 92(3), 136–142.

Baker, D. W., Parker, R. M., Williams, M. V., & Clark, W. S. (1998). Health literacy and the risk of hospital admission. *Journal of General Internal Medicine, 13*, 791–798.

Baker, D. W., Parker, R. M., Williams, M. V., Coates, W. C., & Pitkin, K. (1996). Use and effectiveness of interpreters in an emergency department. *Journal of the American Medical Association, 275*(10), 783–788.

Baron-Cohen, S. (2005). The essential difference: The male and female brain. *Phi Kappa Phi Forum, 85*(1), 23–26.

Batty, G. D., Deary, I. J., & Macintyre, S. (2006). Childhood IQ in relation to risk factors for premature mortality in middle-aged persons: The Aberdeen children of the 1950's study. *Journal of Epidemiology and Community Health, 61*, 241–247.

Batty, G. D., Der, G., Macintyre, S., & Deary, I. J. (2006). Does IQ explain socioeconomic inequalities in health? Evidence from a population based cohort study in the west of Scotland. *BMJ, 332*, 580–584. Retrieved July 5, 2007, from http://bmj.com/cgi/content/full/332/7541/580

Begley, S. (1996, February 19). Your child's brain. *Newsweek*, 55–62.

Begley, S., Murr, A., & Rogers, A. (1995, March 27). Gray matters. *Newsweek*, 48–54.

Bolton, L. B., Bennett, C., Richards, H., Gary, F., Harris, L., Millon-Underwood, S., et al. (2001). Nursing research priorities of the National Black Nurses Association. *Nursing Outlook, 49*(6), 258–262.

Bond, M. L., Kardong-Edgren, S., & Jones, M. E. (2001). Assessment of professional nursing students' knowledge and attitudes about patients of diverse cultures. *Journal of Professional Nursing, 17*(6), 305–312.

Borrayo, E. (2004). Where's Maria? A video to increase awareness about breast cancer and mammography screening among low-literacy Latinas. *Preventive Medicine, 39*, 99–110.

Cahill, L. (2006). Why sex matters in neuroscience. *Nature Reviews/Neuroscience.* Retrieved July 3, 2007, from http://www.nature.com/nrn/journal/v7/n6/full/nrn1909.html

Cantore, J. A. (2001, Winter). Earth, wind, fire and water. *Minority Nurse,* 24–29.

Career directory. (2005). Understanding transcultural nursing. *Nursing 2005,* 14–23.

Caudle, P. (1993). Providing culturally sensitive health care to Hispanic clients. *Nurse Practitioner, 18*(12), 40, 43–44, 46, 50–51.

Centers for Disease Control and Prevention. (2010). Lesbian, gay, bisexual and transgender health. Retrieved February 21, 2010, from http://www.cdc.gov/lgbthealth/

Chachkes, E., & Christ, G. (1996). Cross cultural issues in patient education. *Patient Education and Counseling, 27,* 13–21.

Chao, R. K. (1994). Beyond parental control and authoritarian parenting style: Understanding Chinese parenting through the cultural notion of training. *Child Development, 65,* 1111–1119.

Chideya, F. (1999). *The color of our future.* New York: William Morrow.

Chun, M. B. J., Young, K. G. M., & Jackson, D. S. (2009). Incorporating cultural competency in the general surgical residency curriculum: A preliminary assessment. *International Journal of Surgery, 7,* 368–372.

Cohen, D. (Ed.). (1991). *The circle of life: Rituals from the human family album.* New York: HarperCollins.

Cooper, M., Grywalski, M., Lamp, J., Newhouse, L., & Studlien, R. (2007). Enhancing cultural competence: A model for nurses. *Nursing for Women's Health, 11*(2), 148–159.

Core, L. (2008). Treatment across culture: Is there a model? *International Journal of Therapy and Rehabilitation, 15,* 519–525.

Corley, M. C., & Goren, S. (1998). The dark side of nursing: Impact of stigmatizing responses on patients. *Scholarly Inquiry for Nursing Practice: An International Journal, 12*(2), 99–118.

Crimmins, E. M., & Saito, Y. (2001). Trends in healthy life expectancy in the United States, 1970–1990: Gender, race, and educational differences. *Social Science & Medicine, 52,* 1629–1641.

Darling, S. (2004). Family literacy: Meeting the needs of at-risk families. *Phi Kappa Phi Forum, 84*(2), 18–21.

Davidson, K. W., Trudeau, K. J., van Roosmalen, E., Stewart, M., & Kirkland, S. (2006). Perspective: Gender as a health determinant and implications for health education. *Health Education Behavior, 33,* 731–743.

DeNavas-Walt, C., Proctor, B. D., Smith, J.C., & U.S. Census Bureau. (2009). *Income, poverty and health insurance coverage in the United States: 2008.* Current Population Reports, P60-236. Washington, DC: U.S. Government Printing Office. Retrieved September 1, 2009, from http://www.census.gov/prod/2009pubs/p60-236.pdf

Dignam, J. J. (2000). Differences in breast cancer prognosis among African-American and Caucasian women. *CA-A Cancer Journal for Clinicians, 50*(1), 50–64.

Doyle, E. (2008). Toward a culturally competent health education workforce. In M. A. Perez & R. R. Luquis (Eds.), *Cultural competence in health education and health promotion* (Chap. 9). San Francisco: Jossey Bass.

Dreher, M. C. (1996, 4th quarter). Nursing: A cultural phenomenon. *Reflections,* 4.

Duffy, M. M., & Snyder, K. (1999). Can ED patients read your education materials? *Journal of Emergency Nursing, 25*(4), 294–297.

Elstad, J. I., & Krokstad, S. (2003). Social causation, health-selective mobility, and the reproduction of socioeconomic health inequalities over time: Panel study of adult men. *Social Science and Medicine, 57,* 1475–1489.

Fadiman, A. (1997). *The spirit catches you and you fall down: A Hmong child, her American doctors and the collision of two cultures.* New York: Farrar, Straus & Giroux.

Felski, R. (2002, January 25). Why academics don't study the lower middle class. *Chronicle of Higher Education, 48*(2), B24.

Fenway Institute. (2010a). Ending invisibility: Better health for LGBT populations. Retrieved February 26, 2010, from http://www.iom.edu/Activities/SelectPops/LGBTHealthIssues.aspx

Fenway Institute. (2010b). Professional education and development for health professionals. Retrieved May 6, 2010, from http://www.fenwayhealth.org/site/PageServer?pagename=FCHC_ins_fenway_Educ Professionals

Fernandez, R. D., & Hebert, G. J. (2000). Rituals, culture, and tradition: The Puerto Rican experience. In M. L. Kelley & V. M. Fitzsimons (Eds.), *Understanding cultural diversity: Culture, curriculum, and community in nursing* (pp. 241–251). Sudbury, MA: Jones and Bartlett.

Forrester, D. A. (2000). Minority men's health: A review of the literature with special emphasis on African American men. In M. L. Kelley & V. M. Fitzsimons (Eds.), *Understanding cultural diversity: Culture, curriculum, and community in nursing* (pp. 283–305). Sudbury, MA: Jones and Bartlett.

Gage, N. L., & Berliner, D. C. (1998). *Educational psychology* (6th ed.). Boston: Houghton Mifflin.

Gates, G. J. (2010). Same sex couples: US census and the American community survey. Williams Institute of the UCLA School of Law. Retrieved February 21, 2010, from http://www.law.ucla.edu/williamsinstitute/publications/Census2010_Sponsor.html

Giorgianni, S. S. (1998). Responding to the challenge of health literacy. *Pfizer Journal, 2*(1), 1–39.

Gorman, C. (1992, January 20). Sizing up the sexes. *Time*, 42–51.

Gresenz, C. R., Rogowski, J., & Escarce, J. J. (2009). Community demographics and access to health care among U.S. Hispanics. *Health Research and Educational Trust, 44*, 1542–1562.

Griffith, S. (1982). Childbearing and the concept of culture. *Journal of Obstetrics, Gynecological, and Neonatal Nursing, 11*(3), 181–184.

Gur, R. C., Alsop, D., Glahn, D., Petty, R., Swanson, C. L., Maldjian, J. A., et al. (2000). An fMRI study of sex differences in regional activation to a verbal and a spatial task. *Brain and Language, 74*, 157–170.

Gura, T. (2005). Big plans for little brains. *Nature, 435*, 1156–1158.

Hancock, L. (1996, February 19). Why do schools flunk biology? *Newsweek*, 59.

Harding, S. (1998, June). Native healers: Part 2—The circle in practice. *Alternative and Complementary Therapies*, 173–179.

Harrigan, D. O. (Ed.). (2007). The young brain: Handle with care. *SUNY Upstate Medical University Outlook, 6*(3), 3–31.

Harris, L., Belyea, M., Mishel, M., & Germino, B. (2003). Issues in revising research instruments for use with Southern populations. *Journal of National Black Nurses Association, 14*(2), 44–50.

Hebert, G. J., & Fernandez, R. D. (2000). A challenge to the Puerto Rican community: An untold story of the AIDS epidemic. In M. L. Kelley & V. M. Fitzsimons (Eds.), *Understanding cultural diversity: Culture, curriculum, and community in nursing* (pp. 253–261). Sudbury, MA: Jones and Bartlett.

Hirsch, E. D. (2001, Summer). Overcoming the language gap. *American Educator*, 5–7.

Hisama, K. K. (2000, First quarter). Japanese theory and practice: Carrying your own lamp. *Reflections on Nursing*, 30–32.

Holt, C. L., Clark, E. M., & Kreuter, M. W. (2003). Spiritual health locus of control and breast cancer beliefs among urban African American women. *Health Psychology, 22*(3), 294–299.

Holt, C. L., Kyles, A., Wiehagen, T., & Casey, C. (2003). Development of a spiritually based breast cancer edu-

cational booklet for African American women. *Cancer Control, 10*(5), 37–44.

Horton, M., & Freire, P. (1990). *We make the road by walking*. Philadelphia: Temple University Press.

Institute of Medicine of the National Academies. (2010). Lesbian, gay, bisexual and transgender health issues and research gaps and opportunities. Retrieved February 21, 2010, from http://www.iom.edu/Activities/SelectPops/LGBTHealthIssues.aspx

Jezewski, M. A. (1993). Culture brokering as a model for advocacy. *Nursing & Health Care, 14*(2), 78–85.

Joho, K. A., & Ormsby, A. (2000). A walk in beauty: Strategies for providing culturally competent nursing care to Native Americans. In M. L. Kelley & V. M. Fitzsimons (Eds.), *Understanding cultural diversity: Culture, curriculum, and community in nursing* (pp. 209–218). Sudbury, MA: Jones and Bartlett.

Jones, C. P. (2000). Levels of racism: A theoretical framework and a gardener's tale. *American Journal of Public Health, 90*(8), 1212–1214.

Kato, P. M., & Mann, T. (1996). *Handbook of diversity issues in health psychology*. New York: Plenum Press.

Kawamura, M., Midorikawa, A., & Kezuka, M. (2000). Cerebral localization of the center for reading and writing music. *NeuroReport, 11*(14), 3299–3303.

Kelley, M. L., & Fitzsimons, V. M. (2000). *Understanding cultural diversity: Culture, curriculum, and community in nursing*. Sudbury, MA: Jones and Bartlett.

Kessels, R. P. C. (2003). Patients' memory for medical information. *Journal of the Royal Society of Medicine, 96*, 219–222.

Keyserling, T. C., Ammerman, A. S., Samuel-Hodge, C. D., Ingram, A. T., Skelly, A. H., Elasy, T. A., et al. (2000). A diabetes management program for African American women with type 2 diabetes. *Diabetes Educator, 26*(5), 796–805.

Kimura, D. (1999, Summer). The hidden mind: Sex differences in the brain. *Scientific American*, 32–37.

Kniep-Hardy, M., & Burkhardt, M. A. (1977). Nursing the Navajo. *American Journal of Nursing, 77*(1), 95–96.

Krehely, J. (2009). How to lose the LGBT health disparities gap. Center for American Progress. Retrieved February 26, 2010, from http://www.americanprogress.org/issues/2009/12/lgbt_health_disparities.html

Kroenke, C. (2007). Socioeconomic status and health: Youth development and neomaterialist and psychosocial mechanisms. *Social Science and Medicine, 66*, 31–42.

Krugman, P. (2008, February 18). Poverty is poison. *New York Times*. Retrieved February 20, 2008, from http://www.nytimes.com/2008/02/18/opinion/18krugman.html

Leininger, M. (1994). Transcultural nursing education: A worldwide imperative. *Nursing and Health Care, 15*(5), 254–257.

Lindholm, C., Burstrom, B., & Diderichsen, F. (2001). Does chronic illness cause adverse social and economic consequences among Swedes? *Scandinavian Journal of Public Health, 29*, 63–70.

Lipman, E. L., Offord, D. R., & Boyle, M. H. (1994). Relation between economic disadvantage and psychosocial morbidity in children. *Canadian Medical Association Journal, 151*(4), 431–437.

Lowe, J., & Struthers, R. (2001, Third quarter). A conceptual framework of nursing in Native American culture. *Journal of Nursing Scholarship*, 279–283.

Luciano, M., Wright, M. J., Duffy, D. L., Wainwright, M. A., Zhu, G., Evans, D. M., et al. (2006). Genome-wide scan of IQ finds significant linkage to a quantitative trait locus on 2q. *Behavioral Genetics, 36*(1) 45–55.

Mackenbach, J. P., Bos, V., Andersen, O., Cardano, M., Costa, G., Harding, S., et al. (2003). Widening socioeconomic inequalities in mortality in six Western European countries. *International Journal of Epidemiology, 32*, 830–837.

Mackenbach, J. P., Cavelaars, A. E. J. M., Kunst, A. E., Groenhof, F., & the EU Working Group on Socioeconomic Inequalities in Health. (2000). Socioeconomic inequalities in cardiovascular disease mortality: An international study. *European Heart Journal, 21*(14), 1141–1151.

Mail, P. D., McKay, R. B., & Katz, M. (1989). Expanding practice horizons: Learning from American Indian patients. *Patient Education and Counseling, 13*, 91–102.

Markides, K. S., & Coreil, J. (1986). The health of Hispanics in southwestern U.S.: An epidemiological paradox. *Public Health Reports, 101*(3), 253–265.

Marquand, B. (2001, Fall). On the front lines of diversity. *Minority Nurse*, 46–49.

Martinez-Cossio, N. (2008). Developing culturally appropriate needs assessments and planning, implementation, and evaluation for health education and promotion programs. In M. A. Perez & R. R. Luquis (Eds.), *Cultural competence in health education and health promotion* (Chap. 7). San Francisco: Jossey Bass.

Massett, H. A. (1996). Appropriateness of Hispanic print materials: A content analysis. *Health Education Research, 11*(2), 231–242.

Mattis, J. S. (2000). African American women's definitions of spirituality and religiosity. *Journal of Black Psychology, 26*(1), 101–122.

Mattis, J. S., & Jagers, R. J. (2001). A relational framework for the study of religiosity and spirituality in the lives of African Americans. *Journal of Community Psychology, 29*(5), 519–539.

Mayer, K. H., Bradford, J. B., Makadon, H. J., Stall, R., Goldhammer, H., & Landers, S. (2008). Sexual and gender minority health: What we know and what needs to be done. *American Journal of Public Health, 98*, 989–995.

McGoldrick, M. (1995). *You can go home again*. New York: W. W. Norton.

McRae, K., Ochsner, K. N., Mauss, I. B., Gabrieli, J. J. D., & Gross, J. J. (2008). Gender differences in emotion regulation: An fMRI study of cognitive reappraisal. *Group Processes and Intergroup Relations, 11*, 143–162.

Monastersky, R. (2001, November 2). Land mines in the world of mental maps. *Chronicle of Higher Education*, A20–A21.

Monden, C. W. S., van Lenthe, F. J., & Mackenbach, J. P. (2006). A simultaneous analysis of neighborhood and childhood socioeconomic environment with self-assessed health and health-related behaviors. *Health and Place, 12*, 394–403.

Mulligan, K. (2004). Chronic illness a prescription for financial distress. *Psychiatric News, 39*(23), 17. Retrieved July 3, 2007, from http://pn.psychiatryonline.org/cgi/content/full/39/23/17?eaf

Narayan, M. C. (2003). Cultural assessment. *Home Healthcare Nurse, 21*(9), 173–178.

Nash, J. M. (1997). Fertile minds. *Time, 149*(5), 48–56.

National Center for Cultural Competence. (2004). *Bridging the cultural divide in health care settings: The essential role of cultural broker programs*. Georgetown University Medical Center. Retrieved August 3, 2009, from http://www.culturalbroker.info/Cultural_Broker_EN.pdf

National Center for Education Statistics. (2006). National Assessment of Adult Literacy (NAAL): Health literacy component. Retrieved April 29, 2006, from http://nces.ed.gov/NAAL/index.asp?

National Coalition for LGBT Health. (2009). Public comments on *Healthy People 2020* development. Retrieved February 15, 2010, from http://www.lgbthealth.net/stage/documents/HP2020TestimonyFINAL.pdf

National Mental Health Information Center. (2008). Retrieved July 2, 2009, from http://mentalhealth.samhsa.gov/publications/browse.asp

Newlin, K., Knafl, K., & Melkus, G. D. (2002). African-American spirituality: A concept analysis. *Advances in Nursing Science, 25*(2), 57–70.

Office of Minority Health and Health Disparities. (2010). Racial and ethnic populations. Retrieved February 21, 2010, from http://www.cdc.gov/omhd/Populations/populations.htm

Pacquiao, D. F., Archeval, L., & Shelley, E. E. (2000). Hispanic client satisfaction with home health care: A study of cultural context of care. In M. L. Kelley & V. M. Fitzsimons (Eds.), *Understanding cultural diversity: Culture, curriculum, and community nursing* (pp. 229–240). Sudbury MA: Jones and Bartlett.

Pang, K. Y. C. (2007). The importance of cultural interpretation of religion/spirituality and depression in Korean elderly immigrant women Buddhists and Christians. *Journal of Best Practices in Health Professions Diversity: Research, Education and Policy, 1*(1), 57–89.

Parker, M., & Kiatoukaysy, L. N. (1999). Culturally responsive health care: The example of the Hmong in America. *Journal of the American Academy of Nurse Practitioners, 11*(12), 511–518.

Phan, P., Vugia, H., Wright, P., Rush-Woods, D., Chu, M., & Jones, T (2009). Teaching note: A social work program's experience in teaching about race in the curriculum. *Journal of Social Work Education, 45,* 325–333.

Poss, J. E., & Rangel, R. (1995). Working effectively with interpreters in the primary care setting. *Nurse Practitioner, 20*(12), 43–44, 46–47.

Powe, B. D., Daniels, E. C., Finnie, R., & Thompson, A. (2005). Perceptions about breast cancer among African American women: Do selected educational materials challenge them? *Patient Education and Counseling, 56,* 197–204.

Price, K. M., & Cortis, J. D. (2000). The way forward for transcultural nursing. *Nurse Education Today, 20,* 233–243.

Puchalski, C., & Romer, A. L. (2000). Taking a spiritual history allows clinicians to understand patients more fully. *Journal of Palliative Medicine, 3*(1), 129–137.

Purnell, L. D., & Paulanka, B. J. (2003). *Transcultural health care: A culturally competent approach.* Philadelphia: F. A. Davis.

Rew, L., Becker, H., Cookston, J., Khosropour, S., & Martinez, S. (2003). Measuring cultural awareness in nursing students. *Journal of Nursing Education, 42*(6), 249–257.

Reynolds, A. (2001). Multidimensional cultural competence: Providing tools for transforming psychology. *Counseling Psychologist, 29,* 833–841.

Rhem, J. (1998). Social class and student learning. *National Teaching & Learning Forum, 7*(5), 1–4.

Robinson, J. H. (2000). Increasing students' cultural sensitivity. *Nurse Educator, 25*(3), 131–135.

Rognerud, M. A., & Zahl, P-H. (2005). Social inequalities in mortality: Changes in the relative importance of income, education, and household size over a 27-year period. *European Journal of Public Health, 16*(1), 62–68.

Romero, A. P., Baumle, A., Badgett, M. V., & Gates, G. J. (2007). Census snapshot, the Williams Institute. Retrieved January 28, 2009, from http://www.law.ucla.edu/williamsinstitute/publications/uscensussnapshot.pdf

Samuel-Hodge, C. D., Keyserling, T. C., France, R., Ingram, A. F., Johnston, L. F., Davis, L. P., et al. (2006). A church-based diabetes self-management education program for African Americans with type 2 diabetes. *Preventing Chronic Disease, 3*(3), 1–16.

Santrock, J. W. (2006). *Life-span development* (10th ed.). Boston: McGraw-Hill.

Satel, S. (2002, May 26). I am a racially profiling doctor. *Post Standard,* D–6.

Scharnberg, K. (2007). Medicine men for the 21st century. *Chicago Tribune.* Retrieved June 25, 2007, from http://articles.chicagotribune.com/2007-06-04/news/0706030707_1_native-americans-american-indian-21st-century

Schenker, Y., Lo, B., Ettinger, K. M., & Fernandez, A. (2008). Navigating language barriers under difficult circumstances. *Annals of Internal Medicine, 149,* 264–269.

Schmidt, P. (2003, November 28). Academe's Hispanic future. *Chronicle of Higher Education,* B6–B9.

Severiens, S. E., & Ten Dam, G. T. M. (1994). Gender differences in learning styles: A narrative review and quantitative meta-analysis. *Higher Education, 27,* 487–501.

Sexual Minority Assessment Research Team. (2009). Best practices for asking questions about sexual orientation on surveys. Williams Institute. Retrieved January 30, 2010, from http://www.law.ucla.edu/williamsinstitute/pdf/smart_final_nov09.pdf

Shaya, F. T., & Gbarayor, C. (2006). The case for cultural competence in health professions education. *American Journal of Pharmaceutical Education, 70*(6). Retrieved February 21, 2010, from http://www.ncbi.nlm.nih.gov/pmc/articles/PMC1803701/

She, P., & Livermore, G. A. (2008). Long term poverty and disability among working age adults. *Journal of Disability Poverty Studies, 19,* 244–256.

Singh-Manoux, A., Ferrie, J. E., Lynch, J. W., & Marmot, M. (2005). The role of cognitive ability (intelligence) in explaining the association between socioeconomic position and health: Evidence from the Whitehall II prospective cohort study. *American Journal of Epidemiology, 161,* 831–839.

Smith, T. B., Constantine, M. G., Dunn, T. W., Dinehart, J. M., & Montoya, J. A. (2009). Multicultural education in the mental health professions: A meta-analytic review. *Journal of Counseling Psychology, 53*(1), 132–145.

Smolan, R., Moffitt, P., & Naythons, M. (1990). *The power to heal: Ancient arts and modern medicine.* Upper Saddle River, NJ: Prentice Hall.

Snowman, J., & Biehler, R. (2006). *Psychology applied to teaching.* Boston: Houghton Mifflin.

Speck, O., Ernst, T., Braun, J., Koch, C., Miller, E., & Chang, L. (2000). Gender differences in the functional organization of the brain for working memory. *Neuro Report*, *11*(11), 2581–2585.

Stanislav, L. (2006, October). When language gets in the way. *Modern Nurse*, 32–35.

Sue, D. W. (2001). Multiple dimensions of cultural competence. *Counseling Psychologist*, *29*, 790–821.

Sullivan, C. W., & Bristow, L. R. (2007). Summary proceedings of the National Leadership Symposium on Increasing Diversity in the Health Professions. *Sullivan Alliance*, 1–12.

Sullivan Commission. (2004). *Missing persons: Minorities in the health professions*. Retrieved February 21, 2010, from http://minorityhealth.org/pdf/Missing%20 Persons%20-%20Minorities%20in%20the%20 Health%20Professions.pdf

Tashiro, C. J. (2002). Considering the significance of ancestry through the prism of mixed-race identity. *Advances in Nursing Science*, *25*(2), 1–21.

Tear, J. (1995, November 20). They just don't understand gender dynamics. *Wall Street Journal*, A14.

Thomas, D. A., & Ely, R. J. (1996). Making differences matter: A new paradigm for managing diversity. *Harvard Business Review*, *74*(5), 79–90.

Tripp-Reimer, T., & Afifi, L. A. (1989). Cross-cultural perspectives on patient teaching. *Nursing Clinics of North America*, *24*(3), 613–619.

Turkheimer, E., Haley, A., Waldron, M., D'Onofrio, B., & Gottesman, I. I. (2003). Socioeconomic status modifies heritability of IQ in young children. *Psychological Science*, *14*(6), 623–628.

U.S. Census Bureau. (2000). Population estimates program. Washington, DC: Author.

U.S. Census Bureau. (2006). Statistical abstract of the United States. Retrieved July 9, 2007, from http://www.census.gov/compendia/statab/2006/2006edition.html

U.S. Census Bureau. (2008). An older and more diverse nation by mid-century. Retrieved August 20, 2008, from http://www.census.gov/Press-Release/www/releases/archives/population/012496.html

U.S. Department of Health and Human Services. (2000). *Healthy People 2010: Understanding and improving health, Volume 1*. Rockville, MD: Author.

U.S. Department of Health and Human Services. (2003a). *Changing demographics: Implications for physicians, nurses and other health care workers*. Retrieved August 20, 2009, from ftp://ftp.hrsa.gov/bhpr/nationalcenter/changedemo.pdf

U.S. Department of Health and Human Services. (2003b). *Communicating health: Priorities and strategies for progress*. Retrieved April 26, 2004, from http://odphp.osophs.dhhs.gov/projects/HealthComm/

U.S. Department of Health and Human Services. (2009). Death: Final data for 2006. *National Vital Statistics Reports*, *57*(14).

Uzundede, S. (2006, October). Respecting diversity: One patient at a time. *Modern Nurse*, 28–30.

Vander Zanden, J. W., Crandell, T. L., & Crandell, C. H. (2007). *Human development* (8th ed.). Boston: McGraw-Hill.

Vaughn, E. J. (2008). Cultural competence in health education. In M. A. Perez & R. R. Luquis (Eds.), *Cultural competence in health education and health promotion* (Chap. 3). San Francisco: Jossey Bass.

Villanueva, V., & Lipat, A. S. (2000). The Filipino American culture: The needs for transcultural knowledge. In M. L. Kelley & V. M. Fitzsimons (Eds.), *Understanding cultural diversity: Culture, curriculum, and community in nursing* (pp. 219–228). Sudbury, MA: Jones and Bartlett.

Vivian, C., & Dundes, L. (2004, First quarter). The crossroads of culture and health among the Roma (Gypsies). *Journal of Nursing Scholarship*, 86–91.

Weiss, B. D. (2003). *Health literacy: A manual for clinicians*. Chicago: American Medical Association and the American Medical Association Foundation.

Winkleby, M. A., Jatulis, D. E., Frank, E., & Fortmann, S. P. (1992). Socioeconomic status and health: How education, income, and occupation contribute to risk factors for cardiovascular disease. *American Journal of Public Health*, *82*(6), 816–820.

Woodiel, K., & Brindle, K. (2008). Culture and sexual orientation. In M. A. Perez & R. R. Luquis (Eds.), *Cultural competence in health education and health promotion* (Chap. 12). San Francisco: Jossey Bass.

Yanek, L. R., Becker, D. M., Moy, T. F., Gettelsohn, J., & Koffman, D. M. (2001). Project Joy: Faith based cardiovascular health promotion for African-American women. *Public Health Reports*, *116*, 68–81.

Yee, S-H., Liu, H-L., Hou, J., Pu, Y., Fox, P. T., & Gao, J-H. (2000). Detection of the brain response during a cognitive task using perfusion-based event-related functional MRI. *NeuroReport*, *11*(11), 2533–2536.

Young, H. M., McCormick, W. M., & Vitaliano, P. P. (2002). Evolving values in community-based long-term care services for Japanese Americans. *Advances in Nursing Science*, *25*(2), 40–56.

Chapter 9

Educating Learners With Disabilities

Deborah L. Sopczyk

Kay Viggiani

CHAPTER HIGHLIGHTS

KEY TERMS

OBJECTIVES

After completing this chapter, the reader will be able to

1. Compare and contrast various definitions and models of disability.
2. Describe the language that should be used when writing about, talking to, or talking about people with disabilities.
3. Describe teaching strategies that can be used when working with clients with sensory disabilities.
4. Identify the various teaching strategies that are effective when working with people who have learning or developmental disabilities.
5. Describe the different physical and mental disabilities for appropriate adaptation of the teaching–learning plan.
6. Enhance the teaching–learning process for someone with a communication disability.
7. Discuss the effects of a chronic illness on people and their families in the teaching–learning process.
8. Describe assistive technology and its application for people with disabilities.

Teaching others about health and wellness, disease and its treatment, and self-management of care is a critical and challenging role for the health professional in any setting and with any population of individuals. However, the teaching–learning process is especially demanding when working with clients whose abilities to learn are challenged by sensory, cognitive, mental health, physical, and other types of disabilities that affect their capacities to see, hear, speak, understand, remember, or process information. The educational component of practice becomes paramount in importance as the health professional's efforts are directed toward assisting these clients and their significant others to learn how to maintain already established patterns of living while addressing issues related to health or illness or to develop new patterns of living to accommodate changes in functional ability.

This chapter focuses on those clients whose sensory, cognitive, mental health, or physical conditions require health professionals to adapt their approach to client education to enable the client to learn. Although the information presented here focuses specifically on client populations, the same principles of teaching and learning can be extrapolated to apply to other categories of learners. Health professionals in the role of faculty or in-service educator may use similar strategies when working with students or staff who present learning challenges.

This chapter provides an overview of a wide range of physical, mental health, and cognitive disabilities and other issues that affect the way in which people learn. Included are the most common problems encountered by health professionals such as learning disabilities, mental illness, and stroke. Chronic illness is included because it is a situational issue that requires a change in the way the health professional approaches health education. This chapter also provides a summary of assessment, teaching, and evaluation strategies that health professional educators can use in designing and implementing teaching plans for this group of clients and their families. A resource list is provided in Appendix B as a further reference to the reader who seeks additional information about a specific disability.

Scope of the Problem

Disability is a worldwide issue. It is estimated that 650 million people, or 10% of the world's population, live with some type of disability (World Health Organization [WHO], 2010). Although as many as 80% of people with disabilities live in developing countries, about 51.2 million of these individuals live in the United States, constituting approximately 18% of the U.S. population.

Although health professionals often assume that disabilities are problems that are apparent to the casual observer, many disabilities are hidden. For example, only about 5% of people with disabilities use a wheelchair, about 5% are unable to have their speech understood, another 3% are unable to see, approximately 4% suffer from limitations in cognitive functioning, and about 2% are unable to hear (U.S. Census Bureau, 2006a). About two thirds of people with disabilities in the United States have conditions that are classified as severe (U.S. Census Bureau, 2006b). Disabilities cost about $300 billion each year (Zeller, Burke, & Glass, 2007).

For a variety of reasons, individuals with disabilities are more likely than are people without disabilities to suffer health disparities. For example, data from the National Health Interview Survey demonstrate an inverse relationship between degree of hearing loss and health status and finds that hearing loss is associated with several types of health risk behavior including cigarette smoking, alcohol consumption, sedentary lifestyle, and obesity (Shoenborn & Heyman, 2008). A study with adults who were developmentally disabled in North Carolina shows similar results (Havercamp, Scandlin, & Roth, 2004). The adults who participated in this study reported poorer health status than the general population and had significantly higher rates of chronic health conditions. Also, research shows that people with disabilities, particularly women, are less likely to have access to health care (Smith, 2008).

As the U.S. population ages, the number of individuals at risk for developing disabilities increases because the incidence of disability increases with age (Institute of Medicine, 2007). For example, U.S. Census Bureau data reveal that people between the ages of 16 and 64 years report disabilities at the rate of about 18%, whereas those older than 64 years report a disability rate of almost 42% (U.S. Department of Health and Human Services [USDHHS], 2010a). The Centers for Disease Control and Prevention and the U.S. Census Bureau monitor disability trends in the United States. The World Health Organization (WHO) tracks disability data on a worldwide basis.

Models and Definitions

Kaplan and the Center for an Accessible Society (2010) describe four models or perceptions of disabilities that influence the way in which disabilities are addressed in society:

- The moral model
- The medical model
- The rehabilitation model
- The disabilities (social) model

The moral model, which views disabilities as sin, is an old model that unfortunately still exists in some cultures. When a disability is viewed as sinful, individuals and their families not only experience guilt and shame, they may also be denied the care they require. The United Nations has established a set of Standard Rules on the Equalization of Opportunities for Persons with Disabilities that dictates that individuals with disabilities have a fundamental right of access to care, rehabilitation, and support services (WHO, 2010). The World Health Organization assists countries to comply with this United Nations ruling.

The medical and rehabilitation models are similar in that both view disabilities as problems requiring intervention, with the goal being cure or reduction of the perceived deficiency (Kaplan & The Center for an Accessible Society, 2010). The health or rehabilitation professional is central to both models. Many positive things have come out of efforts to develop medical and surgical treatment, prostheses and other equipment, and strategies to improve the quality of life of people with disabilities. However, the underlying belief associated with these two models that people with disabilities must be "fixed" has been criticized by disability advocates. The medical model, in particular, is blamed for promoting expensive procedures in an attempt to treat conditions that often cannot be cured.

The disabilities model, sometimes referred to as the social model, is the framework that has had the most influence on current thinking. The disabilities model embraces disability as a normal part of life and views social discrimination rather than the disability itself as the problem (Kaplan & The Center for an Accessible Society, 2010). Whereas the medical and rehabilitation models focus on the problem or condition of the individual, the disabilities or social model views disability as a social construct and centers around barriers in society that limit opportunities (Matthews, 2009).

The term **disability** has been defined in a number of ways, many definitions reflecting one or more of the models described by Kaplan and the Center for an Accessible Society (2010). Most definitions are broad and serve to categorize a wide variety of impairments stemming from injury, genetics, congenital anomalies, or disease. The World Health Organization defines disabilities as "a complex phenomenon, reflecting an interaction between features of a person's body and features of the society in which he or she lives" (WHO, 2010). The connection that this definition makes between an individual's ability and the expectations of society reflects the spirit of the disabilities model. WHO uses the International Classification of Functioning, Disability and Health (ICF) as a framework for measuring health and disability at the individual and population levels. Adopted in 2001, the ICF provides a framework for classifying the consequences of disease and trauma and recognizes three dimensions of disabilities: body function/impairment, activity/restrictions, and participation/restrictions (Centers for Disease Control and Prevention [CDC], 2010). The ICF identifies disability as a universal human experience and places emphasis on the impact of a disability rather than on its cause.

The Social Security Administration (SSA) defines disability in terms of an individual's ability to work. This definition and its associated criteria are designed to be used to determine eligibility for Social Security payments for individuals with severe disabilities. The criteria used by the SSA require that the individual be classified as disabled only if he or she has a condition that interferes with basic work activities. Individuals are approved for disability benefits if they are diagnosed with a condition that is severe enough to prevent them from engaging in gainful employment for an extended period of time. The Social Security Administration does not pay benefits for partial or short-term disability (SSA, 2010).

On July 26, 1990, President George H. W. Bush signed into law the Americans with Disabilities Act (ADA). The definition of disability under the ADA is "a physical or mental impairment which substantially limits one or more of the major life activities of the individual" (p. 2). A major life activity includes functions such as caring for oneself, standing, lifting, reaching, seeing, hearing, speaking, breathing, learning, and walking. This significant legislation has extended civil rights protection to millions of Americans with disabilities. The first part of the law, effective in January 1992, mandated accessibility to public accommodations. In July 1992, the second part of the law went into effect, requiring employers to make reasonable accommodations in hiring people with disabilities (Merrow & Corbett, 1994).

Although the ADA's definition of disability, with its emphasis on physical and mental impairments, may give the impression that it is steeped in the medical or rehabilitation model, the protections it provides are consistent with the disabilities perspective. The ADA legislation makes it illegal to discriminate on the basis of a disability in the areas of employment, public service, public accommodations, transportation, and telecommunications. This means that an individual cannot be denied employment or promotion because of misconceptions or biases in regard to that individual's disability.

ADA legislation provides the foundation on which all facets of society will be free of discrimination, including the healthcare system. Therefore, health professionals can expect to find people with disabilities in every setting in which they practice, such as schools, clinics, hospitals, nursing homes, workplaces, and private homes. Persons with a disability will expect healthcare professionals to provide appropriate instruction adapted to their special needs.

The Language of Disabilities

Since the 1960s, the Disability Rights Movement has worked to improve the quality of life of people with disabilities through political action. Through this effort, tremendous gains have been realized including improved access to public areas, education, and employment. The Disability Rights Movement also advocates for appropriate use of language in regard to people with disabilities, for example, use of "people-first language" (Haller, Dorries, & Rahn, 2006). As a result of this effort, the federal government uses people-first language in its legislation and many professional journals require authors to use it in their manuscripts.

The term **people-first language** refers to the practice of putting the "person first before the disability" in writing and speech and "describing what a person has, not what a person is" (Snow, 2003, p. 3). Consider the following statements.

- Justin, a 5-year-old asthmatic, has not responded well to treatment.

- Developmentally disabled people, like Marcy, do best when provided with careful direction.

In each of these statements, the emphasis is on the disability, rather than the person. Using people-first language, these statements would be reworded as follows.

- Justin is a 5-year-old boy who is diagnosed with asthma. Justin continues to have symptoms despite treatment.
- Marcy is a woman with a developmental disability. Marcy wants to learn how to care for herself and learns best when given careful directions.

Using people-first language is more than an exercise. It reflects a deliberate action on the part of the health provider to focus on the person with his or her unique qualities rather than group the individual into an impersonal category based on limitations. The words and labels health professionals use to describe people have the ability to influence the way individuals think about themselves and the way individuals are perceived by society. Therefore, it is important that health professionals be sensitive to the way in which they write about, talk about, and talk to people with disabilities. Snow (2003) offers the following suggestions for using disability-sensitive language:

- Use the phrase *congenital disability* rather than the term *birth defect*. The term *birth defect* implies that a person is defective.
- Avoid using the words *handicapped, wheelchair bound, invalid, mentally retarded, special needs*, and other labels that have negative connotations.
- Speak of the needs of people with disabilities rather than their problems. For example, an individual does not have a hearing problem but rather needs a hearing aid.
- Avoid phrases such as *suffers from* or *victim of*. Phrases like these evoke unnecessary and unwanted pity.

- When comparing people with disabilities to people without, avoid using phrases such as *normal* or *able-bodied*. Phrases such as these place the individual with a disability in a negative light.

Role of the Health Professional as Educator

The role of the health professional in teaching those who have a disability continues to evolve because more than ever before clients expect and are expected to assume greater responsibility as self-care agents. Here, the focus is on wellness and strengths—not limitations—of the individual. It is the role of the health professional to teach the individual who has a new or prior existing disability the necessary skills required to maintain or restore health and maintain independence (**habilitation**). Health professionals also work with individuals to relearn or restore skills lost through illness or injury (**rehabilitation**).

Families of individuals who have a disability are increasingly becoming involved in the individual's rehabilitation efforts, and individuals with disabilities are expecting and demanding to be a part of community life. Because of the complex needs of this population group, the health professional's role, out of necessity, must be an integral part of an interdisciplinary team effort with other providers such as nurses, physicians, physician assistants, social workers, physical therapists, psychologists, and occupational and speech therapists. In addition, the health professional as educator has the responsibility to work in concert with clients and their family members to assess learning needs, design appropriate educational interventions, and promote an environment conducive to learning (Diehl, 1989). We must become aware of the tangible barriers to learning that exist as well as the interventions and technologies that are available to help individuals with disabilities overcome those barriers (Cunningham, 2001; Edwards, 2000).

Application of the teaching–learning process is intended to promote adaptive behaviors in clients that support their optimal recovery and a return to life within the community. Emphasis on the various components of the learning process may differ depending on the disability, but it often requires changes in all three domains—cognitive, affective, and psychomotor.

Prior to teaching, assessment is always the first step in determining the needs of clients with respect to the nature of their problems, the short- and long-term consequences of their disability, the effectiveness of the coping mechanisms they employ, and the type and extent of sensorimotor, cognitive, perceptual, and communication deficits they experience. The health professional must determine the extent of the clients' knowledge with respect to their disability, the amount and types of new information needed to effect changes in behavior, and the clients' readiness to learn. At this initial stage, it is imperative that the health professional not only obtain feedback from them, but also use assessment skills of observation, testing, and interviewing of family members and significant others as well as taking into account the findings of the healthcare team.

Diehl (1989) outlines the following questions for health professional educators to ask when determining the person with a disability's readiness to learn:

1. Do the individual and family members demonstrate an interest in learning by requesting information or posing questions in an effort at problem solving or determining their needs?
2. Are there barriers to learning such as low literacy skills, vision impairments, or hearing deficits?
3. If sensory or motor differentiation exists, is the client willing and able to use supportive devices?
4. What learning style best suits the client in processing information and applying it to self-care activities?

5. Is there congruence between the goals of the client and family?
6. Is the environment conducive to learning?
7. Does the client value learning new information and skills as a means to achieve functional improvement?

Prerequisite to the role of the health professional as teacher and provider of care is the responsibility to serve as a mentor to patients and family in coordinating and facilitating the multidisciplinary services required to assist persons with a disability in attaining optimal functioning. Right from the very beginning, health professionals must invite the family and significant others, as the individual's support system in the community, to take an active part in learning information as it applies to assisting with self-care activities of their loved ones.

Types of Disabilities

Disabilities fall into two major categories: mental and physical. Physical disabilities typically are those that involve orthopedic, neuromuscular, cardiovascular, or pulmonary problems but may also include sensory conditions such as blindness. A disability is not an illness or disease but rather the result of an illness, injury, congenital anomaly, or genetics. Therefore, a physical problem such as a brain injury may result in a physical disability such as impaired ability to ambulate. Physical problems also may result in a mental disability. For example, the mental disability dementia that is associated with Alzheimer's disease is a result of physical changes in the brain. Mental disabilities include psychological, behavioral, emotional, or cognitive impairments.

Multiple subcategories of physical and mental disabilities exist. Seven subcategories of physical and mental disabilities have been chosen for discussion because they represent common conditions that the health professional is likely to encounter in practice. These subcategories also require the health professional to adapt the teaching plan to accommodate the individual's learning needs. These seven subcategories of disability include: (1) sensory disabilities, (2) learning disabilities, (3) developmental disabilities, (4) mental illness, (5) physical disabilities, (6) communication disorders, and (7) chronic illness. Included within each subcategory are the specific teaching strategies that should be used to meet the needs of the learner who has a particular disability.

Sensory Disabilities

Sensory disabilities include the spectrum of disorders that affect a person's ability to use one or more of the five senses—auditory, visual, tactile, olfactory, and gustatory. The most common sensory disabilities are those that involve the ability to hear or see. Sensory disabilities can be complex with multidimensional consequences that the health professional must address when in the role of educator. Health professionals must be prepared to attend to the physical and emotional issues that may be related or subsequent to the sensory loss. For example, age-related vision impairment is a major risk factor for depression (Centers for Disease Control and Prevention, Department of Health and Human Services Panel, 2005). Children with impaired hearing have been found to have an injury rate of twice that of children without hearing impairments (Mann, Zhou, McKee, & McDermott, 2007).

Hearing Impairments

Approximately 28 million Americans have a **hearing impairment**, a disability that is experienced by people of all ages. In the United States, almost 2% of children under the age of 18 years have some degree of hearing loss and between 0.2 and 0.3% of infants are born with this disability. The incidence of hearing loss increases with age. About 314 of every 1,000 people older than the age of 65 and 40–50% of people 75 years and older have hearing loss. Men are more likely to develop a hearing impairment than are women (National Institute on Deafness and Other Communication Disorders [NIDCD], 2005).

People with impaired hearing—both the Deaf and the hard of hearing—have a complete loss or a reduction in their sensitivity to sounds. Hearing loss is generally described according to three attributes: type of hearing loss, degree of hearing loss, and configuration of the hearing loss (American Speech-Language-Hearing Association [ASHA], 2010). The three basic types of hearing loss are the following:

1. *Conductive hearing loss:* A type of hearing loss that is usually correctable and causes reduction in the ability to hear faint noises. Conductive hearing loss occurs when the ear loses its ability to conduct sound, for example, when the ear is plugged as a result of ear wax, a foreign body, a tumor, or fluid.
2. *Sensorineural hearing loss:* A type of hearing loss that is permanent and caused by damage to the cochlea or nerve pathways that transmit sound. Sensorineural hearing loss is sometimes referred to as nerve deafness and not only results in a reduction in sound level but also in difficulty hearing certain sounds. Although they do not "cure" the hearing impairment, cochlear implants and hearing aids can improve hearing.
3. *Mixed hearing loss:* A type of hearing loss that is a combination of conductive and sensorineural losses.

People with hearing loss may have a problem with one or both ears. The degree of hearing loss experienced by people with a hearing impairment is classified on a scale ranging from slight to profound. Although health professionals may use the scale to differentiate people who are classified as being deaf or hard of hearing, clients themselves do not always agree with this classification. According to the National Association of the Deaf, how people label themselves is very personal and dependent upon a number of variables including how closely the individual identifies with the Deaf community. Therefore, some individuals with profound hearing loss may prefer to refer to themselves as hard of hearing rather than deaf (National Association of the Deaf, 2010).

When working with, writing about, or preparing printed information for individuals with hearing impairments, it is important that health professionals be sensitive to the use of language. For example, the use of people-first language is somewhat controversial in the Deaf community. There is a recognized Deaf culture with a shared identity, language, and other cultural components (Johnson & McIntosh, 2009; McLaughlin, Brown, & Young, 2004). Because of this shared culture of which they are proud, many Deaf people want to be recognized as deaf because it is a reflection of who they are as people. As with other cultural groups, health professionals as educators should take the steps necessary to know their clients and their preferences in regard to the use of this type of language. In regard to the word *deaf,* it is suggested that the word *deaf* with a lowercase *d* be used when referring to the physical condition of not being able to hear, and the word *Deaf* with an uppercase *D* be used when referring to people affiliated with the Deaf community or Deaf culture (Strong, 1996).

Communication is a primary concern for health professionals working with people who are deaf or hard of hearing. Regardless of the degree of hearing loss, any person with a hearing impairment faces communication barriers that interfere with efforts at patient teaching (Stock, 2002). Hearing loss poses a very real communication problem because some individuals who are deaf or hearing impaired also may be unable to speak or have limited verbal abilities and vocabularies. This is especially true for adults who are prelingually deaf—that is, they have been deaf since birth or early childhood. They and speakers of other languages share many of the same problems in learning English.

Problems with clients understanding health- and illness-related vocabulary also may be exacerbated with clients who are deaf. In a study of knowledge of health-related vocabulary among adults who were deaf, Pollard and Barnett (2009) found that the Deaf population is at risk for low health literacy.

In many families with children who are deaf, American Sign Language (ASL) is used in the home and is the first language children learn. For other children who are raised in an environment where Deaf culture predominates, ASL is the medium of social communication among peers, which reinforces English as a second language. Although some children who primarily use ASL have difficulty achieving fluency in English, there is some evidence to suggest that a high level of ASL proficiency is related to strong English literacy skills (Alliance for Students with Disabilities in Science, Technology, Engineering and Mathematics [AccessSTEM], 2010; Vicars, 2003).

It is clear that individuals who are deaf will have different skills and needs depending on the type of deafness and the amount of time they have been without a sense of hearing. Those who have been deaf since birth will not have had the benefit of language acquisition. As a result, they may not possess understandable speech and may have limited reading and vocabulary skills as well. Most likely, their primary modes of communication will be sign language and lipreading.

In recent years, research has inspired new hope for children with severe hearing loss to develop language skills. In 1984, the Federal Drug Administration approved marketing of the first cochlear implant, a device that restores partial hearing by sending signals directly to the auditory nerve fibers by bypassing damaged hair cells in the inner ear (American Academy of Otolaryngology-Head and Neck Surgery, 2010). Research has shown that cochlear implants have a positive effect on language development when inserted in very young children (Ertmer, Young, & Nathani, 2007; Nicho-las & Geers, 2007). However, Blume (2010) raises important ethical issues about informed consent, deafness as a social culture, and the medical model paradigm of deafness being seen as pathology when decisions are made by parents and physicians to implant an "artificial ear" in young children who are born without a sense of hearing.

If deafness has occurred after language has been acquired, Deaf people may speak quite understandably and have facility with reading and writing and some lipreading abilities. If deafness has occurred in later life, often caused by the process of aging, affected individuals will probably have poor lipreading ability, but their reading and writing skills should be within average range, depending on their educational and experiential background. If aging is the cause of hearing loss, visual impairments also may be a compounding factor. Because vision and hearing are two common sensory losses in the older adult, these deficits pose major communication problems when teaching older clients.

People with hearing impairments, like other individuals, require health care and health education information at various periods during their life. People within the Deaf community are diverse, and health professionals will encounter many differences among their Deaf clients. Therefore, assessment is a critical first step in client education. It is important to determine the extent of the client's hearing loss and the use of hearing aids, cochlear implants, or other types of assistive equipment. Individuals with hearing loss often experience social isolation and feelings of inadequacy (Fusick, 2008). These feelings may contribute to a lack of confidence when faced with health challenges. Health professionals should assess the client's prior knowledge of the issue being addressed, recognizing that people who have hearing impairments may not have been exposed to the same kinds of health information as people who can hear (Pollard, Dean, O'Hearn, & Haynes, 2009). Finally, it is important to remember that Deaf individuals will always rely on their other senses for information input, especially their sense of sight. For patient education to be effective, then, communication must be visible.

Because there are several different ways to communicate with a person who is deaf, one of the first things health professionals need to do is ask clients to identify communication preferences. Sign language, written information, lipreading, and visual aids are some of the common choices. It is true that one of the simplest ways to transfer information is through visible communication signals such as hand gestures and facial expressions. However, this method will not be adequate for any lengthy teaching sessions.

The following modes of communication are suggested as ways to decrease the barriers of communication and facilitate teaching and learning for clients with hearing impairments in any setting:

Sign Language

Many people who are deaf consider ASL to be their primary language and preferred mode of communication. ASL differs from simple finger spelling, which is a method of using different hand positions to represent letters of the alphabet. In contrast, ASL is a complex language made up of signs as well as finger spelling combined with facial expressions and body position. Eye gaze and head and body shift are also incorporated into the language (Oregon's Deaf and Hard of Hearing Services, 2010).

The health professional who does not know ASL is advised to obtain the services of a professional interpreter. Sometimes a family member or friend of the client who is skilled in signing is willing and available to act as an oral translator during teaching sessions. However, just as it is preferable to use a professional interpreter when dealing with a different spoken language, it is also preferable to use a professional interpreter for sign language (Scheier, 2009). Family members and friends may have difficulty translating medical words and phrases and may be hesitant to convey information that may be

upsetting to the client. Prior to enlisting the assistance of an interpreter, whether family member or professional, the health provider should always be certain to obtain the client's permission. Information communicated regarding health issues may be considered personal and private. If the information to be taught is sensitive or confidential, it is advised that family or friends not be enlisted as interpreters. Hiring a certified language interpreter is often the best strategy.

When a health professional is considering the services of an interpreter, he or she should consult the client. Federal law (Section 504 of the Rehabilitation Act of 1973, PL 93-112) requires that health facilities receiving federal funds secure the services of a professional interpreter upon request of a client. If the client cannot provide the names of interpreters, the health professional can contact the state Registry of Interpreters of the Deaf (RID). This registry can provide an up-to-date list of qualified sign language interpreters.

When working with an interpreter, the health professional should stand or sit next to the interpreter. He or she should talk at a normal pace and look and talk directly to the client when speaking. The interpreter will convey information to the client as well as share responses from the client. It is important to remember that ASL does not provide a word-for-word translation of the spoken or written word and misunderstandings can occur. Because client education involves the exchange of important, often very detailed information, the health professional must ascertain that the client understands the information given by asking questions, asking for demonstrations, allowing the client to ask questions, and using other appropriate assessment strategies (Scheier, 2009).

Lipreading

Lipreading is the process of interpreting speech by observing movements of the face, mouth, and tongue (Feld & Sommers, 2009). One common misconception among hearing persons is that all people who are deaf can read lips. This is a potentially dangerous assumption for the health professional to make. Not all people who are deaf read lips and even among those who do, lipreading may not be appropriate for health education or other forms of client–professional communication. Only about 40% of English sounds are visible on the lips (DiPietro, 1979). Lipreaders use context, facial expressions, and body movement as clues to augment the words they can visualize. For casual conversation, the interpretations made by the lipreader work well. However, when it is important that the client understand the details of the information being presented, lipreading may not be the best mode of communication.

When working with a client who is lipreading, it is not necessary to exaggerate lip movements because this action will distort the movements of the lips and interfere with interpretation of the words. If lipreading is preferred by the client, speakers must be sure to provide sufficient lighting on their faces and remove all barriers from around the face, such as gum, pencils, hands, and surgical masks. Beards, mustaches, and protruding teeth also present a challenge to the lipreader. Because less than half of the English language is visible on the lips, speakers should supplement this form of communication with signing or written materials.

WRITTEN MATERIALS

Written information is probably the most reliable way to communicate, especially when understanding is critical. In fact, health professionals in the role of educators should always write down the important information as a supplement to the spoken word even when the Deaf person is versed in lipreading. Written communication is the safest approach, even though it is time consuming and sometimes stressful.

Health professionals should provide printed patient education materials that match the read-ability level of the audience. The reading level of the average high school graduate who is deaf is at the fourth grade level (Holt, Hotto, & Cole, 1994). Therefore, when putting information in writing for a client who is deaf, health professionals should keep the message as simple as possible. For instance, instead of writing, "When running a fever, take two aspirin," they might revise the message to read, "For a fever of 100.5°F or more, take two aspirin." Remember that a person with limited reading skills often interprets words literally; therefore, the word *running* could be confusing because it is often used in the context of someone who is running to the store. Visual aids such as simple pictures, drawings, diagrams, models, and the like are also very useful media as a supplement to increase understanding of written materials (see Chapter 7 for guidelines on writing effective printed materials).

VERBALIZATION BY THE CLIENT

Sometimes clients who are deaf choose to communicate through speaking, especially if they have established a rapport and a trusting relationship with someone. Often the tone and inflection of the patient's voice will be different from normal speech, so educators must make time for listening carefully. They should listen without interruptions until they become accustomed to the person's particular voice intonations and speech rhythms. Those who still have trouble understanding what a client is saying might try writing down what they hear, which may help them to get the gist of the message.

SOUND AUGMENTATION

For those patients who have a hearing loss but who are not completely deaf, hearing aids are often useful devices. Clients who have already been fitted for a hearing aid should be encouraged to use it, and it should be readily accessible, fitted properly, turned on, and with the batteries in working order. If the client does not have a hearing aid, the health professional should make a referral to an auditory specialist, who can determine whether such a device is appropriate. Only one out of five people who could benefit from a hearing aid actually wear one (NIDCD, 2005). Cost contributes to this problem. Although Medicare policies vary from state to state, as a rule, Medicare does not pay for routine hearing examinations or hearing aids. Under some circumstances, Medicare will pay for diagnostic hearing tests when hearing loss is suspected as a result of illness or treatment (USDHHS, 2010b). Therefore, it is important to seek permission of the client before initiating the referral for a hearing examination and/or hearing aid.

Another means by which sounds can be augmented is by cupping the hands around the client's ear or using a stethoscope in reverse. That is, the client puts the stethoscope in his or her ears, and the health professional talks into the bell of the instrument (Babcock & Miller, 1994).

If the client can hear better out of one ear than the other, speakers should always stand or sit nearer to the good ear, using slow speech, providing adequate time for the patient to process the message and to respond, and avoiding shouting, which distorts sounds. It is not necessarily an increase in decibels that makes a difference, but it is the tone, rhythm, articulation, and pace of the words.

TELECOMMUNICATIONS

Telecommunication devices for the Deaf (TDD) are an invaluable resource for patient education. Television decoders for closed-caption programs are an important tool for further enhancing communication. Caption films for patient education are also available free of charge through Modern Talking Pictures and Services. Under federal law, these devices are considered to be reasonable accommodations for persons who are deaf or hearing impaired. However, health professionals should note that

translation of the spoken word on health-related video created for the hearing population, without the tone of voice, voice level, and other strategies speakers use to emphasize a point, may alter the message that is conveyed to Deaf clients (Pollard & Dean, et al., 2009; Wallhagen, Pettengill, & Whiteside, 2006). In summary, health professionals can apply the following guidelines when using any of the aforementioned modes of communication (McConnell, 2002; Navarro & Lacour, 1980):

- Health professionals as educators should:
  - Be natural, not rigid, stiff, or attempt to overarticulate speech
  - Use simple sentences
  - Be sure to get the client's attention by a light touch on the arm before beginning to talk
  - Face the patient and stand no more than 6 feet away when trying to communicate
  - Ask the client's permission to eliminate environmental noise by lowering the television, closing the door, and so forth
  - Make sure the client's hearing aid is turned on and the client's glasses are clean and in place
- Professionals in the role of health educators must refrain from doing the following:
  - Talking and walking at the same time
  - Bobbing their heads excessively
  - Talking from another room or turning away from the person with hearing loss while communicating
  - Standing directly in front of a bright light, which may cast shadows across their faces or glare directly into the client's eyes
  - Placing an IV in the hand the client will need for sign language
  - Joking, using slang or other language the client might misunderstand

No matter which methods of communication for teaching health professionals choose, they must confirm that clients have received health messages and understand. It is essential to validate patient comprehension in a nonthreatening manner. In attempts to avoid embarrassing or offending one another, clients as well as healthcare providers will often acknowledge with a smile or a nod in response to what either one is trying to communicate when, in fact, the message is not understood at all. To ensure that the health education requirements of clients with hearing impairments are being met, the health professional must find effective strategies to communicate the intended message clearly and precisely while at the same time demonstrating acceptance of individuals by making accommodations to suit their needs (Harrison, 1990). Clients who have lived with a hearing impairment for a while usually can indicate which modes of communication work best for them.

Visual Impairments

The American Foundation for the Blind (AFB) estimates that there are more than 25 million people in the United States who are blind or visually impaired. About 5.5 million of these people are older than the age of 65. Visual impairment is not a problem that is restricted to adults; more than half a million children in the United States have issues with vision. About 1.3 million Americans have vision problems severe enough to classify them as legally blind, and about 60,000 of them are children (American Foundation for the Blind [AFB], 2007). Approximately 100 million Americans require corrective lenses and almost 3 million people are color blind (University of Washington Department of Ophthalmology, 2004; Vitale, Cotch & Sperduto, 2006).

There are many causes of blindness and visual impairment. (See **Figure 9–1**.) Disease is the major cause of loss of vision, with trauma accounting for less than 4% of all cases (University of Washington Department of Ophthalmology, 2004). The four major causes of vision loss are age-related macular degeneration, glaucoma, diabetic retinopathy, and age-related cataracts (Braille Institute, 2010).

Although severe vision loss provides the greatest challenge to the health professional as educator, it is important to note that mild to moderate vision loss is commonplace. The most prevalent condition that results in some degree of visual impairment is myopia (nearsightedness). This refractive error usually can be corrected with eyeglasses or contact lenses. As the population ages and is becoming more racially and ethnically diverse, the rates of myopia have increased in the United States and in the population worldwide. Improving the vision of those individuals with myopia through refractive correction is considered to be an important public health initiative. Correction of this common visual impairment has implications for safety and quality of life by reducing falls, fractures, depression, and car accidents.

A **visual impairment** is defined as some form and degree of visual difficulty and includes a wide spectrum ranging from partial vision to total blindness. In the United States, a person is determined to be legally blind if vision is 20/200 or less in the better eye with correction or if visual field limits in both eyes are within 20° in diameter. About 90% of people who are legally blind have some degree of vision (Braille Institute, 2010). Typically, a person who is legally blind is unable to read the largest letter on the eye chart with corrective lenses (Braille Institute, 2010). In comparison, total blindness is defined as an inability to perceive any light or movement (Braille Institute, 2010).

Clients who seem to be legally blind but who have not been evaluated by a low-vision specialist should be provided with contact information for these sources: the local Blind Association and the local Commission for the Blind and Visually Handicapped. Clients may require assistance in negotiating the complex system and in obtaining services.

Fortunately, many devices are available to help legally blind persons maximize their remaining vision. Clients who are without sight most likely have had services and are familiar with those

Figure 9–1 Photo Essay on Partial Sight (Low Vision)

Major diseases causing serious vision impairment that cannot be corrected with conventional spectacles or lenses are cataract, macular degeneration, glaucoma, and diabetic retinopathy. People who have advanced stages of these diseases have difficulty performing ordinary visual tasks, like reading.

MACULAR DEGENERATION—The deterioration of the macula, the central area of the retina, results in an area of decreased central vision. Peripheral, or side, vision remains unaffected. This is the most prevalent eye disease.

CATARACT—An opacity of the lens results in diminished acuity but does not affect the field of vision. There are no blind spots, but the person's vision is hazy overall, particularly in glaring light.

GLAUCOMA—Chronic elevated eye pressure in susceptible individuals may cause atrophy of the optic nerve and loss of peripheral vision. Early detection and close medical monitoring can help reduce complications.

DIABETIC RETINOPATHY—Leaking of retinal blood vessels in advanced or long-term diabetes can affect the macula or the entire retina and vitreous, producing blinding areas.

The Lighthouse Inc.

Reprinted courtesy of The Lighthouse Inc., New York, New York.

adaptations that work best for them. However, depending on patients' situations and the circumstances, the health professional may want to investigate the clients' background further to ensure that they use the most appropriate format and tools for communicating with clients with visual impairment.

Healthcare encounters present challenges for both the client with low vision or blindness and for the professionals who care for them. In a series of focus groups with people with blindness or low vision, O'Day, Killeen, and Iezonni (2004) identified four barriers encountered in healthcare settings. These barriers include the following:

- Lack of respect
- Communication problems
- Physical barriers
- Information barriers

Lack of respect was the basis for many of the negative healthcare encounters described by the participants. For example, participants felt that healthcare providers often made assumptions that clients would be unable to participate in their own care and recovery. Directing comments to a sighted companion rather than to the client was another common complaint. In terms of education, participants expressed concern that many health providers are not prepared to care for clients with visual impairments. Without Braille versions of information sheets, audiotaped instructions, and other assistive strategies, clients with visual impairments left teaching sessions feeling anxious and, most important, without the information required.

The following are some tips health professionals might find helpful when teaching a client who is blind or visually impaired:

- A low-vision specialist can prescribe optical devices such as a magnifying lens (with or without a light), a telescope, a closed-circuit TV, or a pair of sun shields, any of which can enable health professionals to adapt their teaching material to meet the needs of their clients.

- Persons who have long-standing blindness have learned to develop a heightened acuity of their other senses of hearing, taste, touch, and smell. When conveying messages, they rely on their auditory and tactile senses as a means to help them assimilate information from their environment. Usually their listening skills are particularly acute. When teaching, the health professional should speak in a normal tone of voice.

Unlike sighted people, people who are blind cannot attend to nonverbal cues such as hand gestures, facial expressions, and other body language. Those who approach a person with visual impairment should always announce their presence, identify themselves, and explain clearly why they are there and what they are doing. Because the memory and recall of people who are blind are better than the abilities of most sighted persons, educators can use this talent to maximize learning (Babcock & Miller, 1994).

- When explaining procedures, educators should be as descriptive as possible. They should expound on what they are doing and explain any noises associated with treatments or the use of equipment. The client should be allowed to touch, handle, and manipulate equipment. Instructors should use the client's sense of touch in the process of teaching psychomotor skills as well as when the client is learning to return demonstrate.

- Because people who are blind are unable to see shapes, sizes, and the placement of objects, tactile learning is an important technique to use when teaching. For example, such clients can identify their medications by feeling the shape, size, and texture of tablets and capsules. Gluing pills to the tops of bottle caps and putting medications in different-sized or -shaped containers aids them in identifying various medications (Boyd, Gleit, Graham, & Whitman, 1998). This strategy enables the person with a vision deficit to be more self-sufficient in following a prescribed regimen. Also, keeping items in the same place at all times helps clients to locate their belongings independently. When teaching tasks that must be accomplished in an orderly step-by-step manner, health professionals should arrange the required materials in a clockwise fashion (McConnell, 1996).

- When using printed or handwritten materials, enlarging the print (font size) is an important first step for those who have diminished sight.

- Color is a key factor in whether a person with visual impairment can distinguish objects. Assessment should be done on the medium in which the client sees better—black ink on white paper or white ink on black paper. Older persons with vision problems find it more difficult to discriminate colors and varying hues of color other than black and white.

- Proper lighting is of utmost importance in assisting clients who are visually impaired to read the printed word. Regardless of the print size and the color of the type and paper used, if the light is insufficient, clients with visual impairments will have a great deal of difficulty reading print or working with objects.

- Providing contrast is a very helpful technique. For example, using a dark placemat with white dishes or serving black coffee in a white cup will allow persons with visual problems to better see items in front of them. Likewise, clients with visual impairment should be taught to place pills, equipment, or other materials they are using on a contrasting background to help them to visualize the material they are working with.

- Health professionals often teach clients to perform treatments or take medications that must be done on a timed schedule. Clients whose vision impairment is new should be encouraged to get large-print watches or clocks with either black or white backgrounds. This equipment is available through a local chapter for people with visual impairments.

- Audiotapes and cassette recorders are very useful tools. Today, many health education texts as well as other printed health information materials are available as talking books and can be obtained through the National Library Service (see Appendix B) or through the state library for persons who are blind and visually handicapped. Also, these services are available for people with other disabilities.

- Oral instructions can be audiotaped so that clients can listen to information as necessary at another time and place. Repetition allows the opportunity for memorization to reinforce learning.

- The computer is a popular and useful tool for this population of learners. Although they are costly, some computers have synthetic speech as well as Braille keyboards.

- Most blind associations have a Braille library, or clients can access appropriate resources for information, such as the National Braille Press (see Appendix B). Local blind associations might print client education materials in Braille so that they can be used by learners with visual impairments.

- When assisting the person who is blind to ambulate, helpers should always use the sighted guide technique; that is, the guide should allow the person to grasp his or her forearm while the guide walks about one half step ahead of the person who is blind. Another resource person to help with ambulation is an orientation and mobility instructor. These specialists are available in most school districts and local associations for the blind.

- Whenever possible, teaching sessions should be held in a quiet, private space where the client can focus on what is being taught without distraction. Allow adequate time so that the instruction can be delivered in an unhurried manner.

Diabetes education consumes a great deal of a nurse, physician, pharmacist, and other health professionals' teaching time and presents unique challenges. Because of the high incidence of this disease in the American population, diabetic retinopathy is a major cause of blindness. Persons who have lost their sight as a result of diabetic retinopathy probably have already mastered some of the necessary skills to care for themselves but need continued assistance. However, it is also possible for persons with visual impairments to be diagnosed at a later time with diabetes. In either case, at some point in the course of their lives, these persons will need to learn how to use appropriate adaptive equipment.

In 1993, a task force consisting of representatives from groups of diabetes educators and rehabilitation specialists for the blind developed a document titled *Adaptive Diabetes Education for Visually Impaired Persons (ADEVIP). ADEVIP* provides consistent practice guidelines for the care of people with diabetes who have visual handicaps (Visually Impaired Persons Specialty Practice Group, 1994).

Fortunately, there also has been continuous improvement in the equipment used for self-monitoring of blood glucose levels. Easy-to-use monitors with large display screens or voice instructions are available now. Just as several devices for monitoring blood glucose levels have been developed, several nonvisual adaptive devices for measuring insulin are also available. It is evident that the teamwork among these health professionals has led to the development of a variety of useful mechanisms that allow clients who have diabetes and are blind the opportunity to care for themselves and achieve both a successful medical outcome and a good rehabilitation outcome (Baker, 1993).

Learning Disabilities

Over the past 30 years, learning disabilities have emerged as a major issue in the United States (CDC, 2008). Although often associated with school-aged children, these neurologically based disorders begin in childhood and persist through adulthood (National Institute for Literacy, 2008). Learning disorders are complex conditions that are frequently hidden and vary from individual to individual. As a result, they are often misunderstood and underestimated (Bridges to Practice, 2004).

A definitive definition of the term learning disability (LD) has been the subject of a great deal of controversy over the years (Santrock, 2006; Snowman & Biehler, 2006; Vander Zanden, Crandell, & Crandell, 2007; Ysseldyke & Allgozzine, 1983). Because of the multidisciplinary nature of the field, experts continue to discuss the issue. However, despite the debate, professionals agree on some common components. First, the experts agree that learning disabilities involve learning problems and uneven patterns of development in children and adults. Second, there is consensus that learning disabilities are caused by factors other than environmental disadvantage, mental retardation, and emotional disturbance (Child Development Institute, 2010). Instead, learning disabilities are the result of a different wiring of the human brain that influences the way in which information is received, processed, and communicated (LDOnline, 2010).

A number of definitions of learning disabilities can be found in the literature. The Individuals with Disabilities Education Improvement Act (1997) defines **learning disability** as a "disorder in one or more of the basic psychological processes involved in understanding or in using language, spoken or written, that may manifest itself in an imperfect ability to listen, think, speak, read, write, spell or do mathematical calculations" (Learning Disabilities Roundtable, 2005). This definition stands as the accepted working definition for purposes of assessment, diagnosis, and categorization of an array of learning disabilities.

Learning disabilities is an umbrella term that includes such conditions as dyslexia, dyscalculia, and auditory processing disorder. The statistics on learning disabilities are sobering. As many as one out of every five people in the United States has a learning disability (U.S. Department of Education, 2006). Almost 3 million children in the United States receive special education services to address learning disabilities (National Center for Learning Disabilities, 2009), and educators and pediatricians continue to report significant increases in the number of children with learning disorders being seen in the classroom and healthcare facilities (CDC, 2008). About 27% of high school students with learning disabilities drop out of school, and only 14% of high school students with learning disabilities go on to postsecondary education programs (U.S. Department of Education, 2006). Among the adult population with learning disabilities, 48% are out of the workforce and approximately 43% are living at or below the poverty level (Bridges to Practice, 2004). Estimates of the number of inmates and parolees with learning disabilities are as high as 65% (Learning Disabilities Association of America, 2010).

About three to four times as many boys as girls are identified as having a learning disability, but this gender difference is thought to be caused by referral bias—more boys are referred for treatment because of their behavior (Santrock, 2006; Vander Zanden et al., 2007). Most children with LD receive special education in school (National Dissemination Center for Children With Disabilities, 2004), which accounts for about 14% of the total federal education budget of more than $360 billion (Vander Zanden et al., 2007).

In the past, a learning disability was thought to be a problem involving only children. Now, however, evidence supports the belief that most individuals do not outgrow the problem (Vander Zanden et al., 2007). Indeed, the rate of learning disabilities in adults is probably similar to the rate in children. However, because awareness of learning disabilities was not widespread in years past, many adults with learning disabilities remain undiagnosed. The majority of people with learning disabilities have language and/or memory deficits. If the problem is compounded with the stresses and anxieties caused by illness and subsequent hospitalization or the pressures of having to perform in an academic setting, people with learning disabilities find themselves in a situation that is not at all conducive to learning.

The causes of learning disabilities are varied and often unclear. Genetics plays a role in approximately 50% of cases. It is also suspected that a number of factors that affect the brain, especially during gestation, delivery, and the early years of life, can result in a learning disability. For example, the use of alcohol during pregnancy, difficulties during delivery, and exposure to toxins such as lead paint can all result in learning disabilities (Learning Disabilities Association of America, 2010).

Despite the statistics that reveal the lifelong challenges of individuals with learning disabilities, these individuals have been found to have at least average, if not superior (gifted), intelligence. In fact, learning disabilities are often labeled the invisible handicap because they do not necessarily result in low achievement. Some very famous and successful people in world history are thought to have had some type of learning disability—artists (Leonardo da Vinci), political leaders (Woodrow Wilson, Winston Churchill, and Nelson Rockefeller), military figures (George Patton), and scientists (Albert Einstein and Thomas Edison) (Vander Zanden et al., 2007).

Even though there is a large discrepancy between the intellectual abilities of a person with a learning disability and his or her performance levels, no cause-and-effect relationship exists. Those who exhibit this discrepancy are not necessarily learning disabled (Santrock, 2006; Vander Zanden et al., 2007). **Table 9–1** lists common myths and corresponding facts about learning disabilities. A person can be of average or above average intelligence, not have any major sensory problems, and still struggle to keep up with people the same age in learning.

Table 9–1 Myths and Facts About Learning Disabilities

Myth:	Children are labeled "learning disabled" because they can't learn.
Fact:	They can learn, but their preferred learning modality must be identified.
Myth:	Children who have a learning disability must be spoken to more slowly.
Fact:	Those who learn auditorily may become impatient with slower speech and stop listening; those who learn visually would benefit more from seeing the information.
Myth:	Children who are learning disabled just have to try harder.
Fact:	Telling these children to try harder is a turnoff. They already do try hard.
Myth:	Children outgrow their disabilities.
Fact:	Children do not outgrow their disabilities. They develop strategies to compensate for and minimize their disabilities.
Myth:	Children with learning disabilities should be treated like everyone else.
Fact:	That treatment would be unfair; they would not get what they need.
Myth:	Nearly all children with learning disabilities are boys.
Fact:	Boys are more often referred for proper identification of learning disabilities because they are more overt in acting out their frustrations.

Reprinted from Greenberg, L. A. (1991, September/October). Teaching children who are learning disabled about illness and hospitalization. *MCN: American Journal of Maternal Child Nursing, 16*(5), 260–263. Used with permission.

Although these problems and their associated characteristics are frequently identified in reference to children with disabilities in particular, many of the characteristics of these problems can apply equally well to an older person who has not been diagnosed as learning disabled until later in adulthood. It is important to remember that an individual with a learning disability can experience one type of learning disability or a combination thereof.

The most common learning disorders are discussed in the following subsections.

Dyslexia

Dyslexia is a learning disability that affects approximately 10–15% of the U.S. population (Dyslexia Research Institute, 2010). Dyslexia accounts for the largest percentage of the LD population (Vander Zanden et al., 2007). Often associated with reading difficulty, dyslexia is actually a language disorder that results in a wide array of symptoms including reading difficulty, problems with writing and spelling, and delays in speech (Dyslexia Research Institute, 2010; International Dyslexia Association, 2010). Individuals with dyslexia often have other learning disabilities including attention deficit hyperactivity disorder (Dyslexia Research Institute, 2010).

The exact cause of dyslexia is unclear, although several theories exist. Dyslexia has been found to run in families, so a hereditary component is theorized. Dyslexia also is associated with early hearing loss, and it is suggested that this hearing loss results in a failure of the brain to make the necessary connections between sounds and letters. A combination of factors is also suspected (Dyslexia Research Institute, 2010; International Dyslexia Association, 2010).

It is a common misconception that people with dyslexia simply see letters in reverse order. The problem of dyslexia is much more complex. Recent research indicates there are several subtypes of dyslexia, each with a different neurologic deficit (Heim et al., 2008; Menghini et al., 2010). These subtypes are made up of a combination of problems including the ability to break down words into individual sounds, difficulty distinguishing letters visually, and an inability to associate sounds with letters (Heim et al., 2008; Hultquist, 2006; PBS, 2010). Furthermore, people with dyslexia have been shown to have a deficit in "working" or "short-term memory," making it difficult for them to process complex sentences (Vander Zanden et al., 2007; Wiseheart, Altmann, Park, & Lombardino, 2008). Levine (2002) has created a Web site, Misunderstood Minds, that includes exercises that simulate the reading difficulties of someone with dyslexia. Dr. Levine's site can be accessed at http://www.pbs.org/wgbh/misunderstoodminds.

Although people with dyslexia can learn to read, the challenges they face can result in self-esteem issues. Young children experience school problems (Ingesson, 2007), and older adults who were never diagnosed or who did not receive reading intervention are at greatest risk. The health professional must be sensitive to these issues when engaged in teaching.

People with visual perception problems such as dyslexia face a number of other challenges. For example, they may experience a figure ground problem so that the person is unable to attend to a specific object within a group of objects, such as finding a cup of juice on a food tray. Furthermore, judging distances or positions in space or dealing with spatial relationships may prove difficult, resulting in the person's bumping into things, being confused about left and right or up and down, or being unable to throw a ball or do a puzzle.

Health professionals face a number of issues when teaching clients with dyslexia and other types of perceptual deficits. Assessment is a critical first step. A discussion with the client is advisable to determine the extent of the client's abilities and disabilities and the manner in which the client learns best. For example, many people with visual perceptual deficits tend to be auditory learners. With auditory learners visual stimulation should be kept to a minimum. Visual materials such as pamphlets and books are ineffective unless the content is explained orally or the information is read aloud. If visual items are used, health professional educators should give only one item at a time, with a sufficient period in between times to allow for the client to focus on and master the information. It may also be helpful to add pictures to written material wherever possible to help convey information. CDs and audiotapes (with or without earphones) and verbal instruction may also be helpful.

Some clients with dyslexia have difficulty with the spoken word and may struggle to express themselves or understand what is being said to them (International Dyslexia Association, 2010). For these clients, it is important to proceed in an unhurried manner, presenting small amounts of information over a period of time with frequent assessment of learning. If a client has difficulty with spoken as well as written words, a combined approach using both oral instruction and visual information may be effective. Health professional educators can assess recall and retention of information by oral questioning, allowing learners to express orally what they understand and remember about the content that has been presented.

Finally, when teaching motor skills, it is important that educators remember that people with dyslexia may have impaired left–right discrimination and may get confused during instruction and coaching if the health professional makes reference to a "left hand" or "right foot." Health professional educators can tape an *X* on the appropriate hand or reference the "arm with the watch" to help.

Auditory Perceptual Disorders

Under usual conditions, sound vibrations are converted to electrical impulses in the ear and then transmitted by the auditory nerves to the brain where they are interpreted. Auditory perceptual disorders, also known as central processing disorders, occur when the brain fails to process or interpret these sound impulses effectively (NIDCD, 2010). This type of disability affects about 5% of children (KidsHealth, 2007), and although the cause is usually unknown, the condition is associated with head trauma in both adults and children (Musiek, Barran, & Shinn, 2004). Central processing disorders may also be present in children and adults with other types of learning disabilities such as dyslexia and autism (NIDCD, 2010).

Central processing disorders are characterized by an inability to distinguish subtle differences in sounds—for example, *blue* and *blow* or *ball* and *bell*. There also may be a problem with auditory figure ground such that the sound of someone speaking cannot be identified clearly when others are speaking or when there is noise in the same room. Auditory lags may occur whereby sound input cannot be processed at a normal rate. Parts of conversations may be missed unless speakers speak at a speed that allows the client enough time to process the information.

During instruction, it is important to limit the noise level and eliminate background distractions. Using as few words as possible and repeating them when necessary (using the same words to avoid confusion) are useful strategies. Health professionals should work with the client to determine the volume and rate of speech that are best understood. For example, some clients find that speech that is a little slower and a little louder works well (Musiek et al., 2004). Direct eye contact helps keep the learner focused on the task at hand.

Visual teaching methods such as demonstration–return demonstration, gaming (e.g., puppetry), role modeling, and role-playing, as well as provision of visual instructional tools such as written materials, pictures, charts, films, books, puzzles, printed handouts, and the computer are the best ways to communicate information. Using hand signs for key words when giving verbal instructions and allowing the learner to have hands-on experiences and opportunities for observation are useful techniques. Individuals with auditory perceptual problems often rely on tactile learning as well. They enjoy doing things with their hands, want to touch everything, prefer writing and drawing, engage in physical exploration, and enjoy physical movement through sports activities.

Individuals with auditory perceptual disorders may rely on vision to help them learn. The visual learner may intently watch the instructor's face for the formation of words, expressions, eye movements, and hand gestures. Awareness of these details may have developed as a compensatory strategy to aid comprehension. If the learner does not understand something being taught, he or she may exhibit frustration in the form of irritability and inattentiveness. Clients may desire to audiotape instruction so that they can replay it as needed. For example, if a client has questions after leaving the hospital or clinic, the audiotape may help a spouse or caregiver clarify the instructions that were given.

Dyscalculia

Dyscalculia is a learning disability that impairs those parts of the brain involved in mathematical processing (Shalev & Gross, 2001). Dyscalculia can be developmental, that is, acquired at birth, or the result of injury to the brain. The developmental form of this condition is present in about 5–6% of school-aged children and persists for some individuals into adulthood (Wilson, 2010). Acquired dyscalculia can occur at any time. Individuals with dyscalculia often have other learning or developmental disabilities such as dyslexia or attention deficit hyperactivity disorder (Lindsay, Tomazic, Levine, & Accardo, 2001).

It is important for health professionals to recognize that the impact of dyscalculia on a client extends beyond his or her ability to calculate an insulin dose or count the correct number of pills. These individuals may also have a number of the following issues (Dyscalculia.org, 2010):

- Difficulty grasping the abstract concept of time. As a result, these clients may be unable to read a clock, follow a schedule, or understand the sequence of past and future events.
- Inability to differentiate between right and left.
- Problems learning specific activities that require sequential processing, that is, any activity that has steps that must be followed.
- Problems reading numbers, such as on a prescription bottle.
- Confusion when schedules or routines change.

The approach to working with a client with dyscalculia varies depending on the age of the client and the client's experience with this disorder. A teenager or adult who has lived with dyscalculia for a number of years may have developed strategies for addressing issues such as time, schedules, and numbers. It is important that assessment be done prior to teaching to determine the extent of the disability and the strategies that have been successful for the client. As with any client who has a learning disability, teaching should be done in an environment that is as free from distraction as possible and conducted in an unhurried manner. Health professionals may find it helpful to begin with the concrete when teaching and move to the abstract slowly and carefully. Pictures and diagrams may help the client grasp more abstract concepts. Assessment to determine that the client has learned the content or skills presented is vital, and reinforcement of learning is critical.

Developmental Disabilities

Child development is a "progressive process that follows along a course of expected outcomes" (Quinn, 2000, p. 17). The standards that are used to measure these outcomes incorporate the variability in development that is expected to occur within the general population. Built into developmental standards are a series of milestones that measure the child's ability to demonstrate age-expected skills in areas such as language, cognition, gross and fine motor control, and social and emotional behavior.

Children who do not meet developmental milestones are considered to have a developmental delay. Approximately 6–8% of preschool children demonstrate delays in one or more areas of development (Tervo, 2003). Many of these children are simply developing at a slower than normal rate and, with intervention, will eventually achieve developmental milestones (Quinn, 2000). Others have more significant problems.

A **developmental disability** is a condition resulting from an alternation in the pattern or nature of a child's development. "Children with developmental disabilities are not traveling at a slower pace; they are traveling a different route altogether [sic]" (Quinn, 2000, p. 22). Although children with developmental disorders may find alternative paths to meeting developmental milestones, many are left with deficits that are present in adulthood. Examples of developmental disorders include attention deficit hyperactivity disorder (ADHD) and Down syndrome.

Another group of developmental disorders is classified as pervasive developmental disorders. Pervasive developmental disorders are those that involve impairment in the development of socialization and communication skills (National Institute of Neurological Disorders and Stroke, 2009). Because socialization and communication are keys to an individual's connectedness to the world, impairments in these areas tend to *pervade* over all areas of development (Quinn, 2000). Examples of pervasive developmental disorders include autism, Rett syndrome, and Asperger syndrome.

Public policy has been enacted to protect the 3 to 4 million people in the United States with developmental disabilities. The Developmental Disabilities Assistance and Bill of Rights Act of 2000 defines developmental disabilities in broad terms as those chronic mental or physical conditions present before 22 years of age that are likely to continue indefinitely and result in substantial limitations in at least three of the following major life activities: self-care, receptive and expressive language learning, mobility, self-direction, capacity for independent living, and economic self-sufficiency (USDHHS, 2000a). This legislation establishes state councils on developmental disabilities; university centers for excellence in disability education, research, and service; and national initiatives to collect data and provide assistance as needed.

In 1975, Public Law (PL) 94-142, the Education of All Handicapped Children Act, mandated state grant money be made available to provide all children with disabilities with a free and appropriate public education. In 1986, PL 99-457 amended the earlier law to provide special funding for educating all eligible preschool children with disabilities, ages 3 through 5 years, to help states develop early intervention programs for infants and toddlers (birth through age 2), and to require states to use qualified providers of special education and related services. In 1990, PL 101-476 made additional changes to the law, including a name change to Individuals with Disabilities Education Act (IDEA). In 1997, IDEA was again amended to entitle all eligible preschool and school-aged children with disabilities to receive a free and appropriate education, including special education and related services (Snowman & Biehler, 2006). In the latest update of IDEA, which took effect in 2004, regulations include more specific clas-sifications of developmental disabilities such as autism, emotional disturbance, hearing and visual impairment, traumatic brain injuries, learning disabilities, and mental retardation (Vander Zanden et al., 2007).

Many health professionals are limited in their ability to provide holistic care for this population because they lack prior experience and often feel uncomfortable caring for those with developmental disabilities, particularly severe ones. This problem becomes acute when the health professional is faced with trying to help the clients understand particular treatments or tasks. The real experts in caring and working with children who are developmentally disabled are their parents. It is a wise health professional who invites these parents to participate and assist the staff during their child's hospitalization and works with them in the home. Likewise, when caring for an adult with a developmental disability, caregivers are often the people who know the client best. However, the health professional needs to be sensitive to the arduous schedule involved in caring for a child or adult with a severe developmental disability in the home. During times of illness, parents and family members are often stressed and fatigued.

Managing the treatment of persons with developmental disabilities accounts for an increasing portion of healthcare practice today. Because developmental disabilities usually are diagnosed during infancy and are likely to last a lifetime, health professionals must acquire sensitivity to family issues and learn to be flexible in their approaches to meet the intellectual, emotional, and medical concerns of clients with special needs (Webb, Tittle, & Van-Cott, 2000). Several of the common developmental disabilities are described in detail in the following subsections.

Attention Deficit Hyperactivity Disorder

The many controversies surrounding the diagnosis and treatment of **attention deficit hyperactivity disorder** have made this developmental disability a household word. However, despite the debate about diagnosis, treatment, and unnecessary labeling of children, attention deficit hyperactivity disorder (ADHD) is recognized as a legitimate medical condition by the American Medical Association, the American Psychiatric Association, and multiple other major professional and health organizations. Health professionals who work with adults and children with ADHD must be prepared to deal with the stigma resulting from the many misconceptions that exist regarding this condition and its treatment (Nauert, 2007).

ADHD is a developmental condition that manifests in three forms (American Psychiatric Association, 2000; Sensory Processing Disorder Resource Center, 2010; Fundukian & Wilson, 2007):

1. ADHD, Predominantly Inattentive Type, a form of ADHD that is characterized by inability to attend to tasks, forgetfulness, and distraction.
2. ADHD, Predominantly Hyperactive Impulsive Type, a type of ADHD that results in restlessness and a lack of control. Individuals with this form of ADHD are hyperactive and exhibit impulsive behavior.
3. ADHD, Combined Type, a combination of Types 1 and 2.

Although all three types are referred to as ADHD, hyperactivity is not present in all cases. Heredity plays a role in ADHD, making individuals susceptible to certain environmental factors that are associated with the condition. These environmental risk factors include but are not limited to low birth weight, traumatic brain injury, and maternal smoking (Kessler, 2006).

ADHD is a common and growing problem. Approximately 2 million children between the ages of 6 and 11 years are diagnosed with ADHD (Vander Zanden et al., 2007). The number of children being diagnosed with ADHD has been shown to be increasing at a rate of about 3% per year (Pastor & Reuben, 2008). Boys outnumber girls by at least

three to one in incidence of this disorder (Snowman & Biehler, 2006). Although some children outgrow symptoms of ADHD, many do not. Research on the incidence of ADHD in the adult population is inconclusive; however, estimates range from 4 to 5% (Davidson, 2008).

ADHD affects individuals at all levels of intellect and is often compounded with other learning disabilities (Davidson, 2008). The classic symptoms of ADHD include inattention, hyperactivity, and impulsivity. These symptoms present numerous challenges for adults and children and as a result people with ADHD often struggle in school, at work, and in society. Often, medication therapy in combination with psychological interventions is the treatment of choice for both children and adults with ADHD.

Before embarking on any educational intervention with adults or children with ADHD, health professional educators should conduct a careful assessment. Educators should have an open discussion with the client, including parents if the client is a child, to determine how the client learns best. If the client is unable to articulate strategies that have worked well in school or work, the health professional must assess the client's response to various techniques and make accommodations as necessary. The educator can then develop an individualized education plan (IEP) to promote learning through use of teaching and learning strategies that compensate for or minimize the effect of the disability (Greenberg, 1991; Vander Zanden et al., 2007).

Health professionals should consider the following strategies when working with adults and children with ADHD:

- Provide encouragement during teaching. Both adults and children with ADHD are likely to have experienced failure in school and in work settings and may lack confidence in their abilities to manage their health care.
- Consider the learning style of the client. For visual learners, use colorful handouts and slides;

for kinesthetic learners, incorporate movement and activity; and for auditory learners, have them read out loud and consider the use of a recorder so that teaching sessions can be replayed. Clients with ADHD may have difficulty maintaining appropriate attention levels, and strategies such as these may attract and hold their attention. Break content to be taught into small, focused sessions whenever possible. If clients have multiple care-related tasks to accomplish on their own, teach them to break their care into smaller tasks.

- Structure the environment to eliminate unnecessary distraction.
- Consider using stress reduction techniques prior to teaching. Helping clients who may be anxious about teaching to relax may result in better learning.

Intellectual Disabilities

Intellectual disabilities are among the most common developmental disabilities in the United States, affecting about 3% of the population (CDC, 2005; National Dissemination Center for Children with Disabilities, 2010). An intellectual disability is a condition that originates before the age of 18 and results in impaired reasoning, learning, problem solving, and adaptive behavior (American Association on Intellectual and Developmental Disabilities, 2010). A score below 75 on an IQ test is one of the major indicators of intellectual disability and is typically supplemented with tests to assess limitations in conceptual, practical, and social skills (National Dissemination Center for Children with Disabilities, 2010).

There are multiple causes of intellectual disabilities. First, intellectual disability is a major characteristic of several syndromes such as Down syndrome, Fragile X syndrome, and fetal alcohol syndrome. Second, any factor that affects the developing neurologic system of the fetus can result in intellectual disability. These factors include drugs, disease, and trauma. Third, birth trauma, low birth weight, disease, and other factors that negatively affect the newborn or young child can cause intellectual disability (Harris, 2005). Finally, intellectual disability can occur as a result of social factors such as lack of education and stimulation or adult responsiveness to infants and young children (National Dissemination Center for Children with Disabilities, 2010).

When planning a teaching intervention with a client who has an intellectual disability, health professionals must keep in mind the client's developmental stage, not his or her chronological age. If the client does not communicate verbally, the health professional should note whether the client uses certain nonverbal cues, such as gestures, signing, or other symbols, for communication purposes. Most clients with intellectual disabilities are incapable of abstract thinking. Although the majority can comprehend simple explanations, educators must give concrete examples. For example, instead of saying, "Lunch will be here in a few minutes," the health professional could show a clock and point to the time. For children scheduled to have surgery, giving them a surgical mask to play with will help dispel fears they may have when entering the operating room. Likewise, adults with intellectual disabilities benefit from simple explanations and demonstrations prior to treatments. Lack of explanation can result in misunderstanding and unnecessary anxiety.

Health professionals must always remember that facial expression and voice tone are more important than words spoken. They should be sure the family members or caregivers of individuals with severe intellectual disabilities explain any nonverbal cues for a "yes" or "no" response, and then try to ask questions in a manner requiring a "yes" or "no" answer. Health professionals should lavish any positive behavior with great praise. They should keep the information simple, concrete, and repetitive, and they should be consistent, but firm, setting appropriate limits. They should be careful not to dominate any teaching session, but let the client actively participate and have a sense of accomplishment. Health professionals in the role of educators must assign simple tasks with simple directions and show what is to be done, rather than relying on verbal commands. They should give only one direction at a time. A reward system often works very well with such clients. For children, stickers with familiar childhood characters placed on a bed or pajamas can remind a child of a job well done. For adults, rewards that are important to that individual will work as well.

Asperger Syndrome

Asperger syndrome is a pervasive developmental disability that falls at the high end of the autism spectrum (Atwood, 2006). It is estimated that 2 out of every 10,000 children in the United States are diagnosed with Asperger syndrome every year (National Institute of Neurological Disorders and Stroke, 2009). Asperger syndrome is caused by a brain dysfunction that is typically genetic in origin (Atwood, 2006).

Children with Asperger syndrome exhibit a variety of symptoms including impairment in language and communication skills, impaired social interaction, repetitive rituals, clumsiness, and limited areas of interest (National Institute of Neurological Disorders and Stroke, 2009). Asperger syndrome cannot be cured, but with treatment, children with Asperger syndrome can learn to grow into functioning adults. However, adults with Asperger syndrome may continue to display subtle symptoms of the disorder, particularly in relation to social interactions (Bauer, 2008).

Teaching the child with Asperger syndrome presents many challenges. Although intellectual disability is usually not present, the communication and social problems associated with the disorder make it difficult for the child to attend to the instruction and difficult for the educator to assess response. For example, research shows that children with Asperger syndrome have significantly more difficulty following verbal instructions than do other children (Saalasti et al., 2008). The health professional should provide multiple cues and a lot of repetition when teaching. Like other individuals with autism, "Aspergers patients do not use the human face as a source of important clues in social interactions and avoid eye contact" (Topel & Lachmann, 2008, p. 603). Therefore, it is important that the health professional pay close attention to other cues when assessing how the individual is responding to the interaction.

Creative strategies are often helpful in teaching the child with Asperger syndrome. Because these children often have difficulty generalizing to other situations what they are taught, it may be helpful to teach the child skills in context. For example, Hayhurst (2008) suggests that if working on motor skills, practice climbing the steps on the bus or using equipment in the playground.

As with other developmental disabilities, parents are often a valuable resource for suggestions on how to relate to their child with Asperger syndrome. Most children will have a treatment plan in place, and parents are taught how to help their children overcome their challenges in communicating, interacting with others, and learning. It is important that the health professional talk about the child's plan with the family and implement strategies that have proved effective.

Mental Illness

In the United States, mental disorders are determined based on the *Diagnostic and Statistical Manual of Mental Disorders (DSM-IV)*. According to the National Institute of Mental Health (NIMH, 2007) and based on the data provided by its large global burden of disease study, mental illness, including suicide, accounts for more than 15% of the burden of disease in established market economies, such as the United States. This is more than that caused by all cancers.

In the United States, mental disorders affect an estimated 26.2% of Americans ages 18 and older. That is, about one in four adults suffer from a diagnosable mental disorder in any given year. When applied to the U.S. Census Bureau's (2006b) residential population estimates for ages 18 and older, this figure translates to 57.7 million people. Mental disorders are the leading cause of disability in the United States and Canada for people ages 15–44 years, and many suffer from more than one type at a given time (NIMH, 2007). These statistics reveal the relative prevalence of mental illness in U.S. society and indicate that health professionals will often work with clients with a psychiatric problem as a primary or secondary diagnosis.

Until about 1886, individuals with mental illness were restrained in iron manacles. With the advent of pharmacotherapy in the 1950s, the lives of persons with mental illness began to change. The discovery of the various neuroleptic and antidepressant drugs was a major contribution to the improved quality of life for these individuals. Previously dependent clients were able to live outside of an institution. For the last 25 years, the care of people with mental illness has been moving into community health centers, and clients are spending less time confined to a mental health facility and more time in the community, at work, and at home (Haber, Krainovich-Miller, McMahon, & Price-Hoskins, 1997). The quality of treatments and, therefore, the quality of life for those with mental illness can only improve. It is incumbent upon health professionals to examine their own feelings about mental illness so that they can enter into a viable teaching–learning relationship.

Although educating clients with mental disorders requires the same basic principles of patient teaching, educators can consider some specific teaching strategies. As with any other intervention by a health professional, the first step is a comprehensive assessment. In this case, it is wise to determine whether the client has any cognitive impairment or inappropriate behavior as well as to assess the patient's level of anxiety. The emotional threat that a person perceives as a result of a psychiatric disorder may result in an increased anxiety level and subsequently begin a chain of physiological reactions that then decrease his or her readiness to learn (Haber et al., 1997). High anxiety can make learning nearly impossible (Kessels, 2003; Stephenson, 2006). Despite the health professional's best efforts, clients with a mental disorder may not be able to identify their need to learn and may not be sufficiently ready to learn. However, the health professional may not be able to wait for readiness to happen. Therein lies the challenge.

Although persons with mental disorders are able to learn given the right circumstances and strategies, it is important to remember that at times people with mental illness can experience difficulty in processing information and verbally communicating information. In addition, they may experience decreased concentration and become easily distracted, which can limit their ability to stay on task. These symptoms of their disease can be compounded by the medications used to treat mental illness, which can cause drowsiness, difficulty concentrating, blurred vision, or agitation.

It is important that care, including education, of the client with mental illness build upon the client's strengths and skills (Jackson, 2009). The health professional must enter into a partnership with the client and, when appropriate, the client's family or caregiver. Also, because the client's behavior can be unpredictable, it is very important that the family or significant other participate in the health education of the client. Therefore, they should be included in teaching sessions (Haber et al., 1997).

The following is a summary of three essential strategies that have been successful when teaching people with mental illness (Haber et al., 1997):

1. Teach by using small and brief words, repeating information over and over—use mnemonics (**Table 9–2**), write down important information

Table 9–2 MNEMONICS

P	artner
R	esponsible
E	nthusiastic
C	oach
E	valuation
P	atience
T	eacher
O	pen minded
R	ole model

on index cards, and use simple drawings or symbols. Be creative.

2. Keep sessions short and frequent. For instance, instead of a 1-hour session, break the learning period into four 15-minute sessions.
3. Involve all possible resources, including the client and his or her family. Actively engage them to help determine the client's learning styles as well as the best way to reinforce content. Consider using computer-assisted instruction, videotapes, and role modeling with clients.

As with any teaching program, it is important to set goals and determine outcomes with the client (Jackson, 2009). The specific behavioral objectives depend on individual learning needs as well as overall learning outcomes. These would include empowering clients to take as much control over their health as possible.

Despite all the great strides made in the treatment of acute mental illness, the person who is mentally ill still faces the problem of being stigmatized and misunderstood. Assumptions sometimes are made that people who are mentally ill are incapable of and not interested in learning to care for themselves. Their needs for learning are great, but they are often not given the same op-

portunities for educational programs as are those persons with physical disabilities.

Motivating the patient with a chronic mental illness can be challenging. Educators can give a certificate of recognition to each patient when he or she completes a program, which can be a powerful motivator. To have a positive effect on the quality of life of the chronically mentally ill, educators must provide useful information. Independence and self-management remain goals for this special population, as with all other populations.

Physical Disabilities

Traumatic Brain Injury

A fall, car accident, gunshot wound, or blow to the head are just a few potential causes of traumatic brain injury. In the United States, approximately 1.4 million people sustain a traumatic brain injury (TBI) each year. Of these, 235,000 are hospitalized and 1.1 million are treated and released from the emergency department (CDC, 2006). TBI includes two specific types: closed head injury, which refers to nonpenetrating injury, and open head injury, which refers to penetrating injury resulting in brain tissue exposure and disruption of normal protective barriers.

Males are about 1.5 times as likely to sustain a TBI. The two age groups at highest risk for the injury are 0–4-year-olds and 15–19-year-olds. Of course, military duty increases the risk of sustaining a TBI (Marchione, 2007). The Centers for Disease Control and Prevention estimates that at least 5.3 million Americans currently have a long-term or lifelong need for help to perform activities of daily living as a result of a TBI (CDC, 2006).

The cognitive deficits that occur as a result of TBI depend on the severity and location of the injury. Cognitive deficits may include poor attention span, slowness in thinking, confusion, difficulty with short-term and long-term memory, distractibility, impulsive and socially inappropriate behaviors, poor judgment, mental fatigue, and difficulty with organization, problem solving, reading, and writing. Communication skills will more than likely be an issue. Cognitive deficits may persist for an extended period of time.

The treatment of people with severe brain injury is most often divided into three stages:

1. Acute care (in an intensive care unit)
2. Acute rehabilitation (in an inpatient brain-injury rehabilitation unit)
3. Long-term rehabilitation after discharge (at home or in a long-term care facility)

At every stage of treatment, there are many hurdles to conquer. Once the injured person's life is ensured and the physical condition improves, the patient is discharged from the acute care unit. It is at this point that someone not familiar with traumatic brain injuries might wonder why a person who looks healthy and independent still needs rehabilitation. For this reason, families need to be kept up-to-date on their loved one's prognosis and progress from the very beginning. Throughout the rehabilitation process, family teaching must be consistent and thoughtful because most of the residual impairments are not visible, with the exception of the sensorimotor deficits.

The communication, cognitive-perceptual, and behavioral changes associated with TBI may be dramatic. However, the most difficult problem for the family is the recognition that their relative will probably never be the same person again. In fact, personality changes present the biggest burden for the family. Studies have shown that the level of family stress is directly related to personality changes and the relative's own perception of the symptoms arising from the head injury (Grinspun, 1987).

Although most of the literature deals with the importance of family inclusion during the reha-

bilitation period, it is clear that persons with brain injury will always need the involvement of their family. Again, the benefits of participation in family groups are immeasurable. Considerable strength is gained from group participation, and learning is accomplished through a friendly, informal approach. Of particular importance for persons with brain injury is the need for unconditional acceptance from their friends and family.

Clients recovering from TBI face many challenges. Just as the family needs to adjust to the changes in their injured family member, clients themselves must cope with loss of identity. The significant physical and cognitive changes caused by the brain injury often result in changes to the client and how he or she interacts with the world (Fraas & Calvert, 2009). Clients not only face recovery from physical injury, they must face an uncertain future.

Learning needs for this population center on the issues of client safety and family and client coping. Safety issues are related to cognitive and behavioral capabilities. Clients and their families are faced with a life-changing event and require ongoing support and encouragement to take care of themselves. Recovery may require several years, and most often the person is left with some form of impairment.

According to the National Center for Injury Prevention and Control (1999), 40% of those hospitalized with a TBI have at least one unmet need for services 1 year after the injury. The most frequent are managing stress and emotional upsets, controlling one's temper, improving one's job skills, and regaining memory and problem-solving skills.

Table 9–3 lists some dos and don'ts for effective teaching of the person with a brain injury.

Memory Disorders

Memory is a complex process that allows people to retrieve information that has been encoded and stored in the brain (Cherry, 2010). Typically, most

Table 9–3 GUIDELINES FOR EFFECTIVE TEACHING OF THE BRAIN-INJURED PATIENT

DO	DON'T
Use simple rather than complex statements.	Stop talking or trying to communicate.
Use gestures to complement what you are saying.	Speak too fast.
Give step-by-step directions.	Talk down to the person.
Allow time for responses.	Talk in the person's presence as though he or she is not there.
Recognize and praise all efforts to communicate.	Give up (instead, seek the assistance of a speech-language pathologist).
Ensure the use of listening devices.	
Keep written instructions simple, with a small amount of information on each page.	

people can retrieve information fairly quickly and without much effort from either their short-term or long-term memories. Short-term memory refers to information that is remembered as long as one is attending to it—for example, being able to complete the steps of a procedure in a return demonstration immediately following a presentation. Individuals with short-term memory deficits may be unable to recall what they learned an hour before, but they may be able to recall the information at a later point in time. Long-term memory consists of information that has been repeated and stored and becomes available whenever the individual thinks about it, such as being able to remember a telephone number (including one's own) over a long period of time. Brain injury, a wide range of diseases, and medical disorders can all result in mild to severe memory disorder.

Brain injury often results in a memory disorder referred to as amnesia. Individuals with antero-grade amnesia have memory up until the brain injury but are unable to form memories in the present. Individuals with retrograde amnesia have memory loss for a period of time prior to the brain injury. Most people with brain injury have a combination of both types of amnesia. Memories lost through retrograde amnesia cannot be restored (Memory Disorders Project, 2010).

Alzheimer's disease, multiple sclerosis, Parkinson's disease, brain tumors, and depression are just a few of the conditions that can result in some degree of memory disorder. In some conditions, such as Alzheimer's disease, memory loss increases as the disease progresses. In other conditions, memory impairment is more of a nuisance than a life-altering disability.

The following strategies may be helpful when working with clients who have difficulty with memory. Each of the strategies must be assessed in terms of the level of memory impairment experienced by the client.

- Clients with memory loss need to relearn the memory process. Encouraging memory techniques such as the need for attention and the benefit of repeating information and practicing retrieval assist the client to grasp the information being taught (Thomas, 2009).
- If the client has intact communication skills, encourage him or her to take notes during teaching sessions. If the client is unable to take notes, audiotaping the session can provide the client and his or her family with a resource for referral.
- If a client has minor memory problems, assist him or her to create a system of reminders, for example, use of a personal digital assistant (PDA), calendar, or sticky notes.

- Incorporate visualization into teaching. By helping clients attach a vivid picture to a concept, they are more likely to remember (Wadsley, 2010).
- Teach clients to "chunk information." When chunking, they decrease the number of items to be remembered by increasing the size of each chunk. For example, rather than remembering the seven numbers in a phone number, they can think about a phone number in double digits. For example, 7-45-86-42 (Wadsley, 2010). The same principle can be applied to any procedure that has multiple steps.
- Structure teaching sessions to allow for brief, frequent repetitive sessions that provide constant reinforcement of learning.

Communication Disorders

"Communication is a universal process by which human beings exchange ideas, impart feelings and express needs" (Adkins, 1991, p. 74). Communication occurs in a variety of ways, including drama, music, literature, and art. It is verbal and nonverbal, and there are both sending and receiving components.

Stroke, or cerebrovascular accident, is the most common cause of impaired communication. As is true with the other disabilities discussed in this chapter, a stroke is a major crisis for both the person and the family. This discussion covers some useful strategies appropriate for working with an individual with impaired communication such as aphasia.

In the United States, almost 800,000 people have a stroke every year; about 600,000 of these people are experiencing their first attack (Stroke Center, 2010). Women make up more than 60% of stroke deaths. African Americans and Native Americans are at greatest risk (American Heart Association, 2010). Stroke is the number one cause of long-term disability (American Heart Association,

2010). More than 4 million Americans are living with the effects of stroke. About one third have mild impairments, another third are moderately impaired, and the remainder are severely impaired (National Stroke Association, 2003).

One of the most common residual deficits of a stroke is a problem with language. Aphasia is a language disorder resulting from damage to the language center of the brain. Primary signs of the aphasia include difficulty in expression, trouble understanding speech, and difficulty reading and writing. Although seen commonly in adults who have suffered a stroke, aphasia can also result from a brain tumor, infection, head injury, or dementia.

It is estimated that about 1 million people in the United States today suffer from aphasia. The type and severity of the language dysfunction depends on the precise location and the extent of the damaged brain tissue (National Institute for Neurological Disorders and Stroke, 2007). Health professionals preparing to work with clients with aphasia must determine which type it is—expressive or receptive. If the health professional's involvement with the client occurs during the early stage of rehabilitation, the speech-language pathologist is a good teammate.

The function of language primarily resides in the left hemisphere of the brain. About three quarters of the overall population has a dominant left hemisphere. Most often when an injury affects the dominant cerebral hemisphere, which is usually the left, the result is **expressive aphasia**. Expressive aphasia occurs when an injury damages the inferior frontal gyrus, just anterior to the facial and lingual areas of the motor cortex, known as Broca's area. Because Broca's area is so near the left motor area, the stroke often leaves the person with right-sided paralysis as well. Clients with expressive aphasia understand what is being said to them, but they have difficulty conveying their thoughts.

Wernicke's area of the brain is located in the temporal lobe and is needed for auditory and reading comprehension. When this area is affected, persons are left with **receptive aphasia**. Although their hearing is unimpaired, individuals with receptive aphasia are nevertheless unable to understand the significance of the spoken or written word. See **Table 9–4** for different types of aphasia.

Although persons with both types of aphasia are unable to communicate verbally or have difficulty doing so, it does not mean they are intellectually impaired. The inability to communicate verbally is a highly frustrating experience for the patient and caregivers. Speech therapy should be one of the earliest interventions, and the health professional needs to incorporate those strategies into the teaching–learning plan. Every effort must be made to establish communication at some level. Remember, regardless of how severe the communication deficit, it is almost always possible to have stroke patients communicate in some manner and to some extent.

Expressive Aphasia

Most clients with expressive aphasia receive speech therapy. However, health professionals in inpatient and outpatient settings encounter these clients in a variety of ways. Health professionals are called on to provide explanation and instruction while providing care and services to these clients. Therefore, it is important that they understand how to communicate effectively with clients with aphasia. It is also important that they support efforts to assist clients to learn how to care for themselves with their disability.

Patience is critical when working with a client with expressive aphasia. These clients need time to express themselves and to make themselves understood. When explaining something to a client with expressive aphasia, it is important not to talk down to the client. Communication should be kept simple and be enhanced, when possible, with pictures and other forms of visual support. When using pictures with clients with severe aphasia, the health professional should use personally relevant, contextualized photographs whenever possible (McKelvey, Hux, Dietz, & Beukelman, 2010). Health professionals who have difficulty understanding clients with expressive aphasia should try asking simple, direct yes/no questions to help the clients make themselves understood.

Health professionals can support clients' speech therapy programs by having them recall word images, first by naming commonly used objects (e.g., spoons, knives, forks) and then those objects in the immediate environment (e.g., bed, table). Another strategy is to have the person repeat the words spoken by the health professional. It is wise to begin with simple terms and work progressively to the more complex.

These exercises may be carried out frequently during the day, keeping the sessions short. Most people become tired when sessions are longer than 30 minutes. Often, their speech will become slurred, and they will experience mental fatigue. A subsequent section of this chapter provides helpful information regarding assistive technology. Computers are a wonderful tool to assist patients with expressive aphasia in their efforts to communicate.

Receptive Aphasia

Patients who have receptive aphasia need help establishing a means for nonverbal communication. Facial expressions, gestures, and even pantomime are effective in conveying messages. Most often, patients are unaware of their impairment and speak in what seems to them like a correct statement, but on examination the words do not make sense. Health professionals should speak more slowly and slightly louder to the person with receptive aphasia because auditory stimulation seems to be effective. When comprehension and memory span increase, the person can begin to respond appropriately.

Also, persons with aphasia have trouble with retention and recall. It seems that old personal memories return first and that recent events take longer to reappear. "It is a lonely, isolated world for

Table 9-4 CLINICAL FEATURES OF APHASIA

Type	Involved Anatomy	Expression	Auditory Comprehension	Written Comprehension	Naming	Word/Phrase Repetition	Ability to Write
Broca's (motor, expressive)	Precental gyrus, Broca's area	Nonfluent, telegraphic, may be mute	Subtle deficits	Subtle deficits	Impaired	Impaired	Impaired
Wernicke's (receptive, sensory)	Superior temporal gyrus	Fluent but content inappropriate	Impaired	Impaired	Severely impaired	Impaired	Impaired
Global (mixed)	Frontal-temporal area	Nonfluent	Severely impaired	Impaired	Severely impaired	Impaired	Severely impaired
Conductive (central)	Arcuate fasciculus	Fluent	Intact	Intact	Impaired	Severely impaired	Impaired
Anomic (amnesic)	Angular gyrus	Fluent	Intact	Intact	Severely impaired	Intact	Subtle deficits
Transcortical sensory (TCSA)	Periphery of Broca's and Wernicke's areas (watershed zone)	Fluent	Impaired	Impaired	Impaired	Intact	Severely impaired
Transcortical motor (TCMA)	Anterior, superior, or lateral to Broca's area	Nonfluent, speech initiation difficult	Intact	Subtle Deficits	Impaired	Intact	Impaired

Source: Reprinted by permission from Bronstein, S., Popvich, J. M., & Stewart-Amidei, C. (1991). *Promoting stroke recovery: A research-based approach for nursing.* St. Louis, MO: Mosby-Year Book, Table 11-1.

those who cannot communicate with other human beings" (Jennings, 1981, p. 39). As health professionals attempt to work with and engage persons with aphasia in a teaching–learning intervention, they must be aware of their own attitudes. The effort to communicate with someone without using usual speech and language is one of the more frustrating experiences. Health professionals should be sure to take time out and reflect on the rewards of assisting the client and family in overcoming this barrier.

Encouragement and explanation when teaching people with aphasia go a long way in ensuring client participation and recovery. Educators should be sure their teaching sessions are filled with praise and acknowledgment of the client's frustration. They should keep distractions to a minimum by turning off the radio and television so that they have the full attention of the client.

Usually, extra effort is required by people with aphasia to understand spoken messages. To them it is as if they are trying to comprehend a foreign language. The person may need extra time to process and understand what is being said. It may be especially hard to follow very fast speech like that heard on the radio or television news. Also, the subtleties of language can be easily misinterpreted (e.g., taking the literal meaning for sarcasm or a figure of speech such as, "He kicked the bucket").

Difficulty with one or more of these skills may lead to communication breakdowns and frustrating communication for both the person with aphasia and the listener (ASHA, 2007a). Sometimes health professionals can help the person develop stronger language skills to express himself or herself, such as by using gestures and writing rather than speaking. Also, group sessions for teaching and learning allow the patient to practice conversation, as well as listen to others in the group.

Dysarthria

Many people with degenerative disorders, such as Parkinson's disease, multiple sclerosis, and myas-

thenia gravis, also have dysarthria. **Dysarthria** is a problem with the voluntary muscle control of speech. It occurs as a consequence of damage to the central or peripheral nervous system and affects the same muscles used in eating and speaking. The result is unintelligible speech. The type and severity of dysarthria depend on which area of the nervous system is affected (ASHA, 2007b).

Several types of dysarthria exist, including flaccid, spastic, ataxic, hypokinetic, and mixed. Although the incidence of the various types is unknown, this category of communication problems will certainly increase as the medical treatments for the various brain diseases improve and people live longer. Those who do survive need help in overcoming all the residual social and communication problems.

Currently, Parkinson's disease is managed very well with medication, and there is ongoing research in the medical management of multiple sclerosis and myasthenia gravis. The intervention of a speech-language pathologist may help improve the function of various muscles used for speech. There are also some helpful mechanical devices, such as a prosthetic palate, which is used to control hypernasality.

Another useful tool is sign language, which may be used if the person's arm and hand muscles are unaffected. The health professional should work with the speech-language pathologist to determine whether any of the other nonverbal aids would be appropriate, such as communication boards or a portable electronic voice synthesizer. With the advent of adaptive technologies, the possibilities are limitless.

To improve communication with people with dysarthria, Yorkston et al. (2001) make the following suggestions:

- Listeners should control the communication environment by reducing distractions.
- Listeners should pay attention to the speaker and watch him or her as he or she talks.

- Listeners should be honest and let the speaker know they have difficulty understanding him or her.
- Listeners should convey the part of the message that they don't understand so that the patient does not have to repeat the entire message.
- If listeners are unable to get the gist of the message after repeated attempts, they can ask questions that require a yes or no answer or have the patient write his or her message.

Chronic Illness

Chronic illness is the leading cause of death in the United States, accounting for approximately 70% of deaths each year. Chronic illness also is a major cause of disability resulting in blindness, amputations, stroke, and other cognitive, sensory, and physical impairments (CDC, 2009). Unlike acute illnesses, which usually have a clearly defined beginning and end, chronic illness is permanent. It is never completely cured and requires the full involvement of its victims. Every aspect of life is affected—physical, psychological, social, economic, and spiritual. Because successful management of a chronic illness is a lifelong process, the development of good learning skills is a matter of survival. Because it is impossible within the confines of this chapter to cover specific teaching strategies for each chronic illness, some general teaching and learning principles are suggested in the following pages.

The learning process for individuals with a chronic illness is fraught with hills and valleys. There is no cure, little predictability, and much uncertainty. Most illnesses have several phases that affect the educational needs of both the ill person and his or her family. Therefore, no one approach fits each teaching–learning situation.

It is important to be aware of the timing, acuity, and severity of the disease progression. The family's reaction and perception of the chronic illness are also important influences on the teaching–learning process (Miller, 2009). Families need information and education to deal with the limitations and changes in their loved one's lifestyle.

People who are chronically ill often experience conflict between feelings of dependence and the need to be independent. Sometimes the energy and focus of maintaining independence are overwhelming, both physically and emotionally. Often, living with a chronic illness includes a loss and/or change in roles. When people suffer from loss of role (e.g., a father who is no longer able to keep his job), their self-esteem also may be affected. If there are lingering issues surrounding the individual's role loss and self-esteem, these need to be addressed because they are obstacles to readiness to learn.

Controlling symptoms is a major time-consuming activity for those with chronic illnesses. Strauss and others (1984) identify the following eight key problem areas experienced by chronically ill patients and their families:

1. Prevention of medical crises and the management of problems once they occur
2. Control of symptoms
3. Carrying out prescribed regimens and the management of problems attendant with adhering to self-care
4. Prevention of, or living with, social isolation that decreases contact with others
5. Adjustment to changes in the course of the disease, whether it exacerbates or enters remission
6. Normalizing both interactions with others and one's lifestyle
7. Funding (finding the necessary money to pay for treatments or to survive despite partial or complete loss of employment)
8. Confronting attendant psychological, marital, and family problems

When working with a person who is chronically ill who must manage a complex therapeutic regimen, it is easy to see how the label of noncompliance might enter the assessment. The truth is, the person with a chronic illness requires more than just new information and psychomotor skills to deal with the problems of everyday life. Self-care is a complex concept when it is applied to what it takes for people with chronic illnesses to successfully control and manage their own health successfully. Hertz (2009) explores self-care frameworks as they relate to activities for health maintenance, disease prevention, and health promotion in chronic illness. Lubkin and Larsen (2009) describe the chronic illness experience in totality and the numerous factors that enhance learning and mediate responses in chronic illness to assist health professionals in developing appropriate teaching interventions.

The Family's Role in Chronic Illness or Disability

Families' reactions to and perceptions of the impact of chronic illness or disability, rather than the illness or disability itself, influence all aspects of adjustment. Families are usually the care providers and the support system for the person who is disabled, and they need to be included in all the teaching–learning interactions. The literature documents that family participation does have a profound influence on the success of a client's rehabilitation program (Turner et al., 2007; Lubkin & Larsen, 2009).

When assessing the client and family, it is important to note what the family considers high-priority learning needs. Most often, these will be related to the caregiver's perceived lifestyle change. A caregiver might ask, "Can I continue working outside the home?" or "Will I be able to maintain my relationships with friends?" It is important that the health professional assist the client and family to identify problems and develop mutually agreed-upon goals. Adaptation is key. Communication between and among family members is crucial. If a family has open communication, the health professional is in a good position to help the family mobilize so as to obtain needed educational and emotional support.

Also the educational process needs to take into consideration the family's strategies for coping with their relative's disability. Without a doubt, the overwhelming nature of chronic illness affects the quality of life not only for the chronically ill person, but for all the family members (Lubkin & Larsen, 2009). In their role as caregivers, they have their own anxieties and fears.

A chronic illness or disability can either destroy or strengthen family unity. Siblings and children of the person with a disability may be at different stages of acceptance. Denial may be present during the initial diagnosis of an illness or disability. Later, as the client and his or her family realize the permanency and the consequences of the situation, the health professional may witness periods of anger, guilt, depression, fear, and hostility. As these feelings dissipate, the health professional can readjust teaching lessons to fit the new circumstances. Flexibility is vital to attaining successful outcomes. Health professionals should be sure to treat each family member as unique and recognize that some family members may never fully adjust. **Table 9–5** lists some of the most common sources of tension in client and family education.

Health professionals need to value their teaching role when they work with the family of a person with disabilities. Unlike families dealing with an acutely ill member, families with permanently disabled members have intermittent contact with the healthcare system throughout their lives. Therefore, whenever teaching sessions are required, the families' availability should be a primary consideration. Given adequate support and resources, families with a chronically ill family member can adapt, make adjustments, and live healthy, happy, full lives.

Assistive Technologies

The growth of modern technology has pervaded all areas of people's lives. Without a doubt, the personal computer has become the technology that has had the greatest impact. Until recently,

Table 9–5 Relieving External Tensions in Client and Family Education

Problem	Response
FAMILY DYNAMICS	
Client or family member feels overwhelmed	Goal setting: Help family refocus on tasks at hand. Review goals that have been attained to boost morale.
Anxiety and fear of performing complex procedures	Establish an atmosphere of acceptance. Don't be in a hurry. Offer opportunities for talk and questions. Reassure client and family that they have made the right treatment choice.
Emotions associated with chronic or terminal conditions	Provide opportunities to express feelings. Offer referrals to community resources.
Caregiver burnout and illness	Simplify client management where possible (e.g., scheduling drug doses to reduce nighttime treatment). Remain accessible. Remember: When caregiver needs are not being met, resentments increase. Provide information on respite care.
Client fatigue, especially with chronic illness	Help the client identify individual tolerance for tiredness in planning for as much active participation in the family life as possible.
Young clients are frequently overwhelmed by complex emotions about their illness and therapy	Encourage both children and adolescents to use artwork to express their feelings. Suggest support groups. Offer support to parents and siblings who must alter their family lifestyle.
GERIATRIC CONSIDERATIONS	
An increase in the number of drugs taken daily (on average four or more per day) increases the potential for adverse reactions	Use only one pharmacy so that one source keeps track of medications. Continually evaluate all drugs taken for need, safety, compatibility, potential adverse reactions, and expiration dates.
Decreased visual acuity	Use teaching materials with large, bold type. Encourage the use of a magnifying glass.

Source: Adapted by permission from LaRocca, J. C. (1994). *Mosby's home health nursing pocket consultant.* St. Louis, MO: Mosby–Year Book.

however, computers have been inaccessible to individuals with a disability. Yet, when assistive technology is made available, individuals with disabilities can experience dramatic changes in their lives. Computers with the appropriate adaptations have liberated people from social isolation and feelings of helplessness and have instilled feelings of self-worth and independence.

Since the enactment of the ADA in 1990, the diversity of the client population that health professionals care for and serve has grown to include more individuals with disabilities in every practice setting. As health professionals' understanding of assistive technology is enhanced, so is their ability to advocate for, recommend, and assist persons with disabilities to attain the appropriate equipment and training (Reed & Bowser, 1999). **Assistive technology** is defined as technological tools (computers and communication devices) available for people with disabilities that provide access to education, employment, recreation, and communication opportunities that allow them to live as independently as possible (Alliance for Technology Access [ATA], n.d.). Some examples of assistive technology include, but are not limited to, talking word processors, specialized keyboards, communication devices, arm and wrist supports, amplified telephone handsets, screen magnifiers, and environmental controls (ATA, n.d.).

Assistive technology plays an ever increasing role in people's work and daily living activities. Today the possibilities are endless. For instance, the *Journal of Visual Impairment and Blindness*, published by the American Foundation for the Blind and available at http://www. afb.org, advertises several products available to persons with disabilities, such as those that read aloud from the computer screen in either human or synthetic speech and a glow-in-the-dark print Braille rubber wristband for children who are visually impaired. These adaptations are very helpful to anyone who has vision, learning, or cognitive disabilities.

Most people use a combination of systems or devices depending on their needs. The good news is that the mainstream technology is moving in the direction of universal design, which means that it will be available to almost anyone. Technology has the potential to improve the lives of people with disabilities by giving them the tools to become more independent, more productive, and better able to participate in a wide range of life experiences.

People with communication problems, especially those who are unable to speak or whose speech is difficult to understand, can use **augmentative and alternative communication** devices, such as the computer, to add a whole new dimension or quality to their lives. Technology has already made much of the previously impossible possible and even greater advances can be expected in the future. It is incumbent upon health professionals to know how to help individuals with disabilities locate and access whatever assistive technology is needed to convey health information. This technology might include software programs with closed captioning built in for people with hearing impairments or on-screen keyboards that can be accessed with a mouse, trackball, or an illuminated pointer device for those with fine or gross motor deficits.

Every computer-based solution is the result of a carefully planned, individually determined process. Individuals with a disability are the experts on what works best for them. However, some guidelines should be considered when selecting the best adaptive computer. The best computer solution for individuals with disabilities allows for independent and effective use. Other criteria include affordability, portability, flexibility, and simplicity of learning. If these criteria are met, then the adaptive computer is probably in compliance with the ADA's reasonable accommodations.

Scherer, Say, Vanbiervleit, Cashman, and Scherer (2005) point out that as available options of assistive technologies have increased, their use has been more widely considered and recommended. It remains a challenging and sometimes complex process to match a person with the right technology. Those with physical, sensory, and/or cognitive impairments that affect their ability to use a computer may benefit from a host of adaptive devices (McKinley et al., 2004).

Assistive technology is here to stay. Although assistive technology will probably be forever changing, the process for ensuring individualized computer solutions will remain much the same, and the benefits are enormous. It is exciting to reflect on the positive, possibly life-changing effects the personal computer and other telecommunication devices can have on the lives of individuals with a disability. They have the potential of changing what it means to be disabled.

The role of health professional educators includes a client advocacy component. As client advocate, the health professional can work with the multidisciplinary team, including the assistive technology specialist, to enable special populations to participate in all of life's experiences. Thanks to what assistive technologies will be able to do, more people with disabilities will enjoy greater independence and fulfillment.

State of the Evidence

The current debate on health care and healthcare reform has created a growing awareness of the rising cost of health care. The national spotlight has been focused on obesity, tobacco and alcohol use, and other risk factors for chronic illness and disability. Healthcare research and government funding for programs designed to cut costs by preventing these costly health conditions are beginning to emerge. Unfortunately, the problems associated with chronic illness and disability in the United States continues to grow. Health education remains a viable solution for teaching people to reduce risk factors and to manage their health and health care when illness and disability strike.

As previously noted, for the first time, the U.S. Surgeon General's Report on Health Promotion and Disease Prevention, *Healthy People 2010*, includes data and health objectives for people with disabilities. This national report is a reflection of almost all accommodations and services, especially health services, available to people with disabilities. This is particularly notable in the area of patient education. The *Healthy People 2010* report identifies 207 objectives of care for people with disabilities; however, data regarding those objectives are only available for 88 of the 207 objectives (CDC, 2006).

In a recent search of the literature, one reference (Ravesloot, 2003) provides specific recommendations for teaching clients with disabilities based on a study of Medicaid beneficiaries. Although the primary goal of the study was not centered on teaching strategies, it nonetheless identifies barriers to increased participation in health promotion programs. The investigators determined that the two most problematic barriers to health promotion activities were pain and fatigue. Certainly, this is useful information for health professionals when trying to implement a successful teaching plan.

In a recent review of the Cochrane Database of Systematic Reviews (2007), there was a notable lack of research on the topic of disabilities. This review found little or no data on teaching people with disabilities. It is encouraging that there is an emerging base of research for some of the more common disabilities such as traumatic brain injury, learning disabilities, and spinal cord injuries. However, it is apparent that an area in need of further investigation is patient education for people with mental health and other chronic illnesses. One recent review of education for those with schizophrenia, titled "Psychoeducation for Schizophrenia," by Pekkala and Merinder (2002) concludes that there seems to be some suggestion that psychoeducation may improve compliance with medication, although the extent of improvement remains unclear. However, the study shows a possibility that psychoeducation has positive effects on a person's overall well-being. This type of study may have implications for health professional educators managing patients with other chronic mental illnesses. Yet, as the review on patients with schizophrenia concludes, "The scarcity of studies made the comparison between efficacy of different formats weak" (Pekkala & Merinder, 2002). Clearly, this is true of the evidence to support and identify specific teaching strategies that would help health professional educators work with a variety of special populations.

Summary

This chapter covers some of the most common disabilities faced by millions of Americans as a result of disease, injury, heredity, aging, and congenital defects. These conditions affect physical, cognitive, or sensory capacities and require behavioral change in one or more of these domains of learning. The health professional in the role of educator must be creative, innovative, flexible, and persistent when applying the principles of teaching and learning to meet the needs of these special populations of individuals, their families, and others.

The shock of any disability, whether it occurs at the beginning of life or toward the end, has a tremendous impact on individuals and their families. At the onset and all through the transition and recovery processes, the patient and family are met with new information to be learned because successful habilitation or rehabilitation means acquiring knowledge and applying it to their situation. Inner strength and courage are attributes needed to face each new day because the effort to live a normal life never ends. The physical, social, emotional, and vocational implications of living with a disability necessitate that health professionals be well prepared to meet any client with a disability right where they are in their struggle to live independently.

REVIEW QUESTIONS

1. What is the disabilities model and how does it differ from the moral model, medical model, and rehabilitation model?
2. What is people-first language, and why should health professionals incorporate it into their writing and speech?
3. What questions should the health professional ask when assessing readiness to learn in a person with a disability or chronic illness?
4. How can the health professional enhance communication with a client who has a hearing impairment?
5. What strategies can the health professional use when teaching a client who has a visual impairment?
6. What are six myths regarding learning disabilities?
7. How can the health professional adapt teaching strategies to meet the needs of a client with dyslexia?
8. What are the characteristic behaviors of persons with ADHD and the educational interventions that should be used with them for effective teaching and learning?
9. How is the term *developmental disability* defined, and what laws have been enacted to protect children with mental and/or physical impairments?
10. What are the key problem areas experienced by chronically ill patients and their families?
11. How can assistive technology devices improve the quality of life for a person with a disability?

CASE STUDY

It is early morning on the Pediatric Unit and the staff are conducting morning rounds. They are discussing 10-year-old Matthew Yoakum, who was transferred to the unit yesterday evening from the ICU. Matt had a below-the-elbow amputation of his right arm following an accident on his family farm. The following conversation takes place.

Jose Garcia, MSW: "Matt and his family are having a very hard time. Apparently Matt was helping his father when he started fooling around, slipped, and fell into the hay elevator. His lower arm was so badly mangled that the surgeon couldn't save it."

Kristen Stryker, PT: "I've met with the family. They are feeling very guilty. Matt has ADHD and has had a lot of behavior problems at school. His dad told me that he should have been watching Matt more carefully because he knows that his son has a hard time concentrating on what he is doing."

Usha Gupta, RN: "We have seen some behavior problems here as well. Last night one of the staff went into his room to ask him to lower his radio and he refused. When she turned the radio off, Matt began spitting and swearing at her."

Carly Thomas, OTR: "I think he and his family are very frightened. We need to develop a teaching plan. Maybe if they have a better sense of what is going to happen, they will begin to feel more in control."

Develop a teaching plan for the Yoakum family by responding to the following questions.

1. What information should be collected as part of the assessment of this family?
2. Which factors in this situation might interfere with the client's readiness to learn?
3. Which strategies would you use to facilitate learning?

References

Adkins, E. R. H. (1991). Nursing care of the client with impaired communication. *Rehabilitation Nursing, 16*(2), 74–76.

Alliance for Students with Disabilities in Science, Technology, Engineering and Mathematics (AccessSTEM). (2010). How can I work with a student who is deaf and speaks ASL but struggles with written English. Retrieved April 6, 2010, from http://www.washington.edu/doit/Stem/articles?77

Alliance for Technology Access. (n.d.). Services. Retrieved June 28, 2007, from http://www.ataccess.org/about/services.html

American Academy of Otolaryngology-Head and Neck Surgery. (2010). Cochlear implants. Retrieved April 6, 2010, from http://www.entnet.org/HealthInformation/cochlearImplants.cfm

American Association on Intellectual and Developmental Disabilities. (2010). FAQ on intellectual disability.

Retrieved April 21, 2010, from http://www.aamr.org/content_104.cfm

American Foundation for the Blind. (2007). Home page. Retrieved May 21, 2007, from http://www.afb.org

American Heart Association. (2010). Stroke statistics. Retrieved April 25, 2010, from http://www.americanheart.org/presenter.jhtml?identifier=4725

American Psychiatric Association. (2000). *Diagnostic and statistical manual of mental disorders* (4th ed.). Washington DC: Author.

American Speech-Language-Hearing Association. (2007a). Aphasia. Retrieved June 28, 2007, from http://www.asha.org/public/speech/disorders/aphasia.htm

American Speech-Language-Hearing Association. (2007b). Dysarthria. Retrieved June 28, 2007, from http://www.asha.org/public/speech/disorders/dysarthria.htm

American Speech-Language-Hearing Association. (2010). Type, degree, and configuration of hearing loss. Retrieved April 4, 2010, from http://www.asha. org/public/hearing/disorders/types.htm

Atwood, T. (2006). *The complete guide to Aspergers syndrome.* London: Jessica Kingsley.

Babcock, D. E., & Miller, M. A. (1994). *Client education: Theory and practice.* St. Louis, MO: Mosby.

Baker, S. S. (1993). Teamwork between the health care community and the blind rehabilitation system. *Journal of Visual Impairment and Blindness, 87*(9), 349–352.

Bauer, S. (2008). Aspergers syndrome: General information across the lifespan. Retrieved February 6, 2010, from http://www.education.com/reference/article/ Ref_Asperger_Long/

Blume, S. (2010, January). *The artificial ear.* Piscataway, NJ: Rutgers University Press.

Boyd, M. D., Gleit, C. J., Graham, B. A., & Whitman, N. I. (1998). *Health teaching in nursing practice* (3rd ed.). Stamford, CT: Appleton & Lange.

Braille Institute. (2010). Facts about sight loss and definitions of blindness. Retrieved April 9, 2010, from http:// www.brailleinstitute.org/facts_about_sight_loss

Bridges to Practice. (2004). Florida's focus on adults with learning disabilities. Retrieved April 14, 2010, from http://www.floridatechnet.org/bridges/

Centers for Disease Control and Prevention. (2005). Intellectual disability. Retrieved April 21, 2010, from http:// www.cdc.gov/ncbddd/dd/ddmr.htm

Centers for Disease Control and Prevention. (2006). Monitoring developmental disabilities. Retrieved June 19, 2007, from http://www.cdc.gov/ncbddd/dd/ddsurv. htm

Centers for Disease Control and Prevention. (2008). Diagnosed attention deficit hyperactivity disorder and learning disability: 2004–2006. *Vital and Health Statistics, 10*(237), 1–15.

Centers for Disease Control and Prevention. (2009). Chronic disease and health promotion. Retrieved April 25, 2010, from http://www.cdc.gov/chronicdisease/ overview/index.htm

Centers for Disease Control and Prevention. (2010). International Classification of Functioning, Disability and Health (ICF). Retrieved March 20, 2010, from http:// www.cdc.gov/nchs/icd/icf.htm

Centers for Disease Control and Prevention, Department of Health and Human Services Panel. (2005). Sensory and communication disorders: Crosscutting breakout session. *Neurorehabilitation and Neural Repair, 19,* 73S–77S.

Cherry, K. (2010). Memory. Retrieved April 25, 2010, from http://psychology.about.com/od/cognitive psychology/a/memory.htm

Child Development Institute. (2010). About learning disabilities. Retrieved April 9, 2010, from http:// www.childdevelopmentinfo.com/learning/learning_ disabilities.shtml

Cunningham, C. (2001, February). Breaking the barriers to math and science for students with disabilities. *Syllabus,* 41–42.

Davidson, M. A. (2008). ADHD in adults: A review of the literature. *Journal of Attention Disorders, 11,* 628–641.

Diehl, L. N. (1989). Client and family learning in the rehabilitation setting. *Nursing Clinics of North America, 24*(1), 257–264.

DiPietro, L. (1979). *Deaf patients, special needs, special responses.* Washington, DC: National Academy of Gallaudet College.

Dyscalculia.org. (2010). Dyscalculia symptoms. Retrieved April 22, 2010, from http://www.dyscalculia.org/calc. html

Dyslexia Research Institute. (2010). Dyslexia. Retrieved April 18, 2010, from http://www.dyslexia-add.org/ issues.html

Edwards, P. A. (2000). *The specialty practice of rehabilitation: A core curriculum* (4th ed.). Glenville, IL: Association of Rehabilitation Nurses.

Ertmer, D., Young, N., & Nathani, S. (2007). Profiles of vocal development in young cochlear implant recipients. *Journal of Speech, Language and Hearing Research, 50,* 393–407.

Feld, J. E., & Sommers, M. S. (2009). Lipreading, processing speed, and working memory in younger and older adults. *Journal of Speech, Language and Hearing Research, 52,* 155–156.

Fraas, M., & Calvert, M. (2009). The use of narratives to identify characteristics leading to a productive life following acquired brain injury. *American Journal of Speech-Language Pathology, 18,* 315–328.

Fundukian, L., & Wilson, J. (2007). *The Gale encyclopedia of mental disorders.* Florence, KY: GACL.

Fusick, L. (2008). Serving clients with hearing loss: Best practices in mental health counseling. *Journal of Counseling and Development, 86*(1), 102–111.

Greenberg, L. A. (1991). Teaching children who are learning disabled about illness and hospitalization. *MCN: American Journal of Maternal Child Nursing, 16*(5), 260–263.

Grinspun, D. (1987). Teaching families of traumatic brain-injured adults. *Critical Care Nursing Quarterly, 10*(3), 61–72.

Haber, J., Krainovich-Miller, B., McMahon, A. L., & Price-Hoskins, P. (1997). *Comprehensive psychiatric nursing.* St. Louis, MO: Mosby.

Haller, B., Dorries, B., & Rahn, J. (2006). Media labeling versus the US disability community identity. A study of shifting cultural language. *Disability and Society, 21*(1), 61–75.

Harris, J. (2005). *Intellectual disability: Understanding its development, causes, classification, evaluation and treatment*. New York: Oxford University Press.

Harrison, L. L. (1990). Minimizing barriers when teaching hearing-impaired clients. *MCN: American Journal of Maternal Child Nursing, 15*(2), 113.

Havercamp, S., Scandlin, D., & Roth M. (2004). Health disparities among adults with developmental disabilities, adults with other disabilities, and adults not reporting disabilities in North Carolina. *Public Health Reports, 119*, 418–426.

Hayhurst, C. (2008). Treating kids with autism. *PT Magazine, 16*, 20–27.

Heim, S., Tschierse, J., Amunts, K., Wilms, M., Vossel, S., Willmes, K., et al. (2008). Cognitive subtypes of dyslexia. *Acta Neurobiologiae Experimentalis, 68*(1), 73–82.

Hertz, J. E. (2009). Self-care. In I. M. Lubkin & P. D. Larsen (Eds.). *Chronic illness: Impact and interventions* (7th ed., pp. 299-315). Sudbury, MA: Jones and Bartlett.

Holt, J., Hotto, S., & Cole, K. (1994). *Demographic aspects of hearing impairments: Questions and answers* (3rd. ed.). Retrieved April 4, 2010, from http://gri.gallaudet.edu/ Demographics/factsheet.html

Hultquist, A. (2006). *Introduction to dyslexia for parents and professionals*. London: Jessica Kingsely.

Ingesson, S. G. (2007). Growing up with dyslexia: Interviews with teenagers and young adults. *School Psychology International, 28*, 574–590.

Institute of Medicine. (2007). *Future of disability in America*. Washington, DC: National Academies Press.

International Dyslexia Association. (2010). IDA Fact sheets on dyslexia and related language-based learning differences. Retrieved April 14, 2010, from http://www. interdys.org/FactSheets.htm

Jackson, C. (2009). Keys to unlocking better care. *Mental Health Practice, 12*(9), 6–7.

Jennings, S. (1981). Communicating with your aphasic patients. *Journal of Practical Nursing, 31*, 22–23.

Johnson, J. R., & McIntosh, A. (2009). Toward a cultural perspective and understanding of the disability and deaf experience in special and multicultural education. *Remedial and Special Education, 30*(2), 67–83.

Kaplan, D., & The Center for an Accessible Society. (2010). The definition of disability. Retrieved March 3, 2010, from http://www.accessiblesociety.org/topics/ demographics-identity/dkaplanpaper.htm

KidsHealth. (2007). Auditory processing disorders. Retrieved April 15, 2010, from http://kidshealth.org/ parent/medical/ears/central_auditory.html#

Kessels, R. P. C. (2003). Patients' memory for medical information. *Journal of the Royal Society of Medicine, 96*, 212–222.

Kessler, R. C. (2006). The prevalence and correlates of ADHD in the United States: Results for the national comorbidity survey replication. *American Journal of Psychiatry, 163*, 716–723.

LDOnline. (2010). What is a learning disability? Retrieved April 9, 2010, from http://www.ldonline.org/ldbasics/ whatisld

Learning Disabilities Association of America. (2010). Adults with learning disabilities: An overview. Retrieved April 14, 2010, from http://www.ldaamerica. org/aboutld/adults/special_pop/adult_ld.asp

Learning Disabilities Roundtable. (2005, February). Comments and recommendations on regulatory issues under the Individuals with Disabilities Education Improvement Act of 2004. Public Law 108-446, 1–12. Retrieved May 21, 2007, from http://www.cec.sped.org/ pdfs/Appendix2004LDRoundtableRecs.pdf

Levine, M. (2002). Misunderstood minds. Retrieved April, 14, 2010, from http://www.pbs.org/wgbh/ misunderstoodminds

Lindsay, R. L., Tomazic, T., Levine, M., & Accardo, P. (2001). Attentional function as measured by a continuous performance task in children with dyscalculia. *Journal of Developmental and Behavioral Pediatrics, 22*, 287–292.

Lubkin, I. M., & Larsen, P. (2009). *Chronic illness* (7th ed.). Sudbury, MA: Jones and Bartlett.

Mann, J. R., Zhou, L., McKee, M., & McDermott, S. (2007). Children with hearing loss and increased risk of injury. *Annals of Family Medicine, 5*, 528–530.

Marchione, M. (2007, September 9). Thousands of GIs cope with brain damage. Retrieved September 10, 2007, from http://www.washingtonpost.com/wp-dyn/ content/article/2007/09/09/AR2007090900905.html

Matthews, N. (2009). Contesting representations of disabled children in picturebooks: Visibility, the body, and the social model of disability. *Children's Geographies, 7*(1), 37–49.

McConnell, E. A. (1996). Clinical do's & don'ts: Caring for a patient with a vision impairment. *Nursing, 26*(5), 28.

McConnell, E. A. (2002). How to converse with a hearing-impaired patient. *Nursing, 32*(8), 20.

McKelvey, M., Hux, K., Dietz, A., & Beukelman, D. (2010). Impact of personal relevance and contextualization on word-picture matching by people with aphasia. *American Journal of Speech Language Pathology, 19*, 22–33.

McKinley, W., Tewksbury, M., Sitter, P., Reed, J., & Floyd, S. (2004). Assistive technology and computer adaptations for individuals with spinal cord injury. *Neuro Rehabilitation, 19*, 141–146. Retrieved from EBSCOhost, June 15, 2007.

McLaughlin, H., Brown, D., & Young, A. M. (2004). Consultation, community and empowerment—lessons from the Deaf community. *Journal of Social Work, 4*(2), 153–166.

Memory Disorders Project. (2010). Frequently asked questions. Retrieved April 24, 2010, from http://www.gluck.edu/memory/faqs.html

Menghini, D., et al. (2010). Different underlying neurocognitive deficits in developmental dyslexia: A comparative study. *Neuropsychologia, 48*(i4), 863–873.

Merrow, S. L., & Corbett, C. (1994). Adaptive computing for people with disabilities. *Computers in Nursing, 12*(4), 201–209.

Miller, E. T. (2009). Client and family education. In I. M. Lubkin & P. Larsen (Eds.), *Chronic illness: Impact and interventions* (7th ed., pp. 319–343). Sudbury, MA: Jones and Bartlett.

Musiek, F., Barran, J., & Shinn, J. (2004). Assessment and remediation of an auditory processing disorder associated with head trauma. *Journal of the American Academy of Audiology, 15*, 117–132.

National Association of the Deaf. (2010). Community and culture. Retrieved April 4, 2010, from http://www.nad.org/issues/american-sign-language/community-and-culture-faq

National Center for Injury Prevention and Control. (1999, December). Traumatic brain injury in the United States: A report to Congress. Retrieved May 8, 2007, from http://www.cdc.gov/NCIPC/tbi/ tbi_congress/tbi_congress.htm

National Center for Learning Disabilities. (2009). LD fast facts. Retrieved April 14, 2010, from http://www.ncld.org/ld-basics/ld-explained/basic-facts/ld-fast-facts

National Dissemination Center for Children with Disabilities. (2004). Twenty-fourth annual report to Congress. U.S. Department of Education. Retrieved May 21, 2007, from http://www.nichcy.org/IDEA.htm

National Dissemination Center for Children with Disabilities. (2010). Intellectual disability (formerly mental retardation). Retrieved April 22, 2010, from http://www.nichcy.org/Disabilities/Specific/Pages/IntellectualDisability.aspx

National Institute on Deafness and Other Communication Disorders. (2005, August 18). Fact sheets. Retrieved May 21, 2007, from http://www.nidcd.nih.gov

National Institute on Deafness and Other Communication Disorders. (2010). Auditory processing disorder in children. Retrieved April 14, 2010, from http://www.nidcd.nih.gov/health/voice/auditory.asp

National Institute for Literacy. (2008). *Learning to achieve: A review of the research literature on serving adults with learning disabilities.* Washington, DC. Retrieved April 14, 2010, from http://www.nifl.gov/publications/pdf/L2ALiteratureReview09.pdf

National Institute of Mental Health. (2007). Statistics. Retrieved May 21, 2007, from http:// www.nimh.nih.gov/healthinformation/statisticsmenu.cfm

National Institute of Neurological Disorders and Stroke. (2003). Aspergers syndrome fact sheet. Retrieved September 18, 2009, from http://www.ninds.nih.gov/disorders/asperger/detail_asperger.htm

National Institute of Neurological Disorders and Stroke. (2007). NNDS aphasia information. Retrieved June 17, 2007, from http://www.ninds.nih.gov/disorders/aphasia/aphasia.htm

National Institute of Neurological Disorders and Stroke. (2009). NINDS pervasive developmental disorders information page. Retrieved April 22, 2010, from http://www.ninds.nih.gov/disorders/pdd/pdd.htm

National Stroke Association. (2003). What is a stroke/brain attack? Retrieved May 28, 2007, from http://www.stroke.org/site/DocServer/NSA_complete_guide.pdf

Nauert, R. (2007). Social stigma awaits kids with ADHD. *Psych Central News.* Retrieved April 14, 2010, from http://psychcentral.com/news/2007/05/01/social-stigma-awaits-kids-with-adhd/789.html

Navarro, M. R., & Lacour, G. (1980). Helping hints for use with deaf patients. *Journal of Emergency Nursing, 6*(6), 26–28.

Nicholas, J. G., & Geers, A. E. (2007). Will they catch up? The role of age at cochlear implantation in the role of spoken language development of children with severe to profound hearing loss. *Language and Hearing Research, 50*, 1048–1062.

O'Day, B. L., Killeen, M., & Iezonni, L. (2004). Improving healthcare experiences for persons who are blind or low vision: Suggestions from focus groups. *American Journal of Medical Quality, 19*(5), 193–200.

Oregon's Deaf and Hard of Hearing Services. (2010). ASL: A distinct culturally rich language. Retrieved April 4, 2010, from http://www.oregon.gov/DHS/odhhs/tadoc/deaf5a.shtml

Pastor, P. N., & Reuben, C. A. (2008). Diagnosed attention deficit hyperactivity disorder and learning disability, United States, 2004–2006: Data from the National Health Interview Survey. (DHHS publication no. (PHS) 2008-1565). *Vital and Health Statistics, 10*(237). Retrieved April 14, 2010, from http://www.cdc.gov/nchs/data/series/sr_10/Sr10_237.pdf

PBS. (2010). A primer on dyslexia. Retrieved April 14, 2010, from http://www.pbs.org/parents/readinglanguage/articles/dyslexia/main.html

Pekkala, E., & Merinder, L. (2002). Psychoeducation for schizophrenia. Cochrane Database of Systematic Reviews. Retrieved September 26, 2007, from http://www2.cochrane.org/reviews/en/ab002831.html

Pollard, R. Q., & Barnett, S. (2009). Health-related vocabulary knowledge among deaf adults. *Rehabilitation Psychology, 54*(2), 182–185.

Pollard, R. Q., Dean, R. K., O'Hearn, A., & Haynes, S. L. (2009). Adapting health education materials for Deaf audiences. *Rehabilitation Psychology, 54*, 232–238.

Quinn, B. (2000). *Pervasive developmental disorder.* London: Jessica Kingsley.

Ravesloot, C. (2003). *Marketing health promotion for people with disabilities rural disability and rehabilitation research progress report #18.* Retrieved September 26, 2007, from http://rtc.ruralinstitute.umt.edu/health/marketing.htm

Reed, P., & Bowser, G. (1999, November). Assistive technology and the IDEA. *Exceptional Parent*, 54–55, 57–58.

Rehabilitation Act of 1973, PL 93-112, Section 504. Retrieved September 26, 2007, from http://www.dol.gov/oasam/regs/statutes/sec504.htm

Saalasti, S., et al., (2008). Language abilities of children with Aspergers syndrome. *Journal of Autism and Developmental Disorders, 38*. 1574–1580.

Santrock, J. W. (2006). *Lifespan development* (10th ed.). Boston: McGraw-Hill.

Scheier, D. B. (2009, Spring/Summer). Barriers to health care for people with hearing loss: A review of the literature. *Journal of the American Nurses Association*, 4–10.

Scherer, M., Say, C., Vanbiervleit, A., Cashman, L., & Scherer, J. (2005). Prediction of assistive technology use: The importance of personal and psychosocial factors. *Disability & Rehabilitation, 27*(21), 1321–1331. Retrieved through EBSCOhost June 15, 2007.

Sensory Processing Disorder Resource Center. (2010). Sensory processing disorder checklist: Signs and symptoms of dysfunction. Retrieved April 14, 2010, from http://www.sensory-processing-disorder.com/sensory-processing-disorder-checklist.html

Shalev, R., & Gross, T. (2001). Developmental dyscalculia. *Pediatric Neurology, 24*, 337–342.

Shoenborn, C. A., & Heyman, K. (2008, May). Health disparities among adults with hearing loss: United States 2000–2006. Health E-Stats. Retrieved March 22, 2010, from http://www.cdc.gov/nchs/data/hestat/hearing00-06/hearing00-06.htm

Smith, D. L. (2008). Disparities in health care access for women with disabilities in the United States from the 2006 National Health Interview Survey. *Disability and Health Journal, 1*(2), 79–88.

Snow, K. (2003). *People first language.* Retrieved March 21, 2010, from http://pages.towson.edu/cholmes/similarities/peoplefirst.pdf

Snowman, J., & Biehler, R. (2006). *Psychology of applied teaching* (11th ed.). Boston: Houghton Mifflin.

Social Security Administration. (2010). What we mean by disability. Retrieved February 28, 2010, from http://www.ssa.gov/dibplan/dqualify4.htm

Stephenson, P. L. (2006). Before teaching begins: Managing patient anxiety prior to providing education. *Clinical Journal of Oncology Nursing, 10*(2), 241–245.

Stock, S. (2002, January 21). When science isn't golden. *Advance for Nurses*, 28–29.

Strauss, A. L., Corbin, J., Fagerhaugh, S., et al. (1984). *Chronic illness and quality of life* (2nd ed.). St. Louis, MO: Mosby.

Stroke Center. (2010). Stroke statistics. Retrieved April 25, 2010, from http://www.strokecenter.org/patients/stats.htm

Strong, M. (1996). *Language learning and deafness.* New York: Cambridge University Press.

Tervo, R. (2003). Identifying patterns of developmental delays can help diagnose neurodevelopmental disorders. A Pediatric Perspective. *Gillette Children's Specialty Healthcare, 12*(3), 1–6.

Thomas, D. (2009). The journey back to effective cognitive function after brain injury: A patient perspective. *International Journal of Therapy and Rehabilitation, 16*, 497–501.

Topel, E., & Lachmann, F. M. (2008). Life begins on an ant farm for two patients with Aspergers syndrome. *Psychoanalytic Psychology, 25*, 602–617.

Turner, B., et al. (2007). A qualitative study of the transition from hospital to home for individuals with acquired brain injury and their family caregivers. *Brain Injury, 21*, 1119–1130.

University of Washington Department of Ophthalmology. (2004). Statistics on blindness and blinding disease in the United States. Retrieved April 8, 2010, from http://depts.washington.edu/ophthweb/statistics.html

U.S. Census Bureau. (2006a). Facts: Americans with Disabilities Act: July 26. Retrieved February 26, 2010, from http://www.census.gov/newsroom/releases/archives/facts_for_features_special_editions/cb10-ff13.html

U.S. Census Bureau. (2006b). The 2006 statistical abstract. Resident population by sex and age: 2005–2050. Retrieved May 28, 2010, from https://www.census.gov/compendia/statab/2006/2006edition.html

U.S. Department of Education. (2006). Twenty-sixth annual report to Congress on the implementation of the Individuals with Disabilities Education Act. Retrieved April 14, 2010, from http://www2.ed.gov/about/reports/annual/osep/2004/index.html

U.S. Department of Health and Human Services. (2000a). The Developmental Disabilities Assistance and Bill of Rights Act of 2000. Retrieved April 23, 2010, from http://www.acf.hhs.gov/programs/add/ddact/DDACT2.html

U.S. Department of Health and Human Services. (2000b). *Healthy People 2010: Understanding and Improving Health* (2nd ed.). Washington, DC: U.S. Government Printing Office.

U.S. Department of Health and Human Services. (2010a). Office on Disability. Retrieved March 20, 2010, from http://www.hhs.gov/od/about/fact_sheets/whatisdisability.html

U.S. Department of Health and Human Services. (2010b). Your Medicare coverage. Retrieved April 4, 2010, from http://www.medicare.gov/coverage/Home.asp

Vander Zanden, J. W., Crandell, T. L., & Crandell, C. H. (2007). *Human development* (8th ed.). Boston: McGraw-Hill.

Vicars, M. (2003). The relationship between literacy and ASL. Retrieved April 6, 2010, from http://www.lifeprint.com/asl101/pages-layout/literacy1.htm

Visually Impaired Persons Specialty Practice Group. (1994). Guidelines for the practice of adaptive diabetes education for visually impaired persons (ADEVIP). *Diabetes Educator, 20,* 111–118.

Vitale, S., Cotch, M. F., & Sperduto, R. D. (2006). Prevalence of visual impairment in the United States. *Journal of the American Medical Association, 295*(18), 2158–2163.

Wadsley, P. (2010, Spring). Healthy living: Memory loss. *Momentum,* 38–41.

Wallhagen, M. I., Pettengill, E., & Whiteside, M. (2006). Sensory hearing impairment in older adults. *American Journal of Nursing, 106*(10), 40–48.

Webb, M., Tittle, M., & VanCott, M. (2000). Increasing students' sensitivity to families of children with disabilities. *Nurse Educator, 25*(1), 43–47.

Wilson, A. J. (2010). Dyscalculia primer and resource guide. Retrieved April 22, 2010, from http://www.oecd.org/document/8/0,3343,en_2649_35845581_34495560_1_1_1_1,00.html

Wiseheart, R., Altmann, L. J. P., Park, H., & Lombardino, L. J. (2008). Sentence comprehension in young adults with developmental dyslexia. *Annals of Dyslexia, 59,* 151–167.

World Health Organization. (2010). Health topics: Disability. Retrieved February 28, 2010, from http://www.who.int/topics/disabilities/en/

Yorkston, K. M., Spencer, K. A., Duffy, J. R., Beukelman, D. R., Golper, L. A., Miller, R. M., et al. (2001). Evidence-based practice guidelines for dysarthria: Management of velopharyngeal function. *Journal of Medical Speech-Language Pathology, 9*(4), 257–273.

Ysseldyke, J., & Allgozzine, B. (1983). LD or not LD: That's not the question! *Journal of Learning Disabilities, 16*(1), 29–31.

Zeller, J. L., Burke, A. E., & Glass, R. M. (2007) Assessing disabilities. *Journal of the American Medical Association, 298*(17), 2096.

Part Three

Techniques and Strategies for Teaching and Learning

Chapter 10

Behavioral Objectives

Susan B. Bastable

Julie A. Doody

CHAPTER HIGHLIGHTS

KEY TERMS

OBJECTIVES

After completing this chapter, the reader will be able to

1. Identify the differences between goals and objectives.
2. Recognize opposing viewpoints regarding the use of behavioral objectives in education.
3. Demonstrate the ability to write behavioral objectives accurately and concisely using the four components of condition, performance, criterion, and who will do the performing.
4. Cite the most frequent errors made in writing objectives.
5. Distinguish among the three domains of learning.
6. Explain the instructional methods appropriate for teaching in the cognitive, affective, and psychomotor domains.
7. Develop teaching plans that reflect internal consistency between elements.
8. Recognize the role of the health professional in formulating objectives for the planning, implementation, and evaluation of teaching and learning.
9. Describe the importance of learning contracts as an alternative approach to structuring a learning experience.
10. Identify the potential application of the learning curve concept to the development of psychomotor skills.

Previous chapters address the characteristics and attributes of the learner with respect to learning needs, readiness to learn, and learning styles. Clearly, assessment of the learner is an essential first step in the teaching–learning process. Assessment determines what the learner needs to know, when and under what conditions the learner is most receptive to learning, and how the learner actually learns best or prefers to learn.

Before a decision can be made about selecting the content to be taught or choosing the instructional methods and materials to be used to change learner behavior, the educator must first decide what the learner is expected to accomplish. Client needs are determined by identifying the gaps in the learner's knowledge, attitudes, or skills. Identification of needs is a prerequisite to formulating behavioral objectives that serve as a "road map" (Nothwehr, Dennis, & Wu, 2007, p.794) guiding subsequent planning, implementation, and evaluation of teaching and learning.

Historically, noted educators and education psychologists in the 20th century developed approaches to writing and classifying behavioral objectives that offer teachers assistance in organizing instructional content for learners functioning at various levels of ability. Mager (1997) has been the primary educator credited with developing a system for writing behavioral objectives that serves to help teachers make appropriate instructional decisions as well as to assist learners in understanding what they need and are expected to know. The underlying principle has been, if one does not know where he or she is going, how will the person know when he or she has arrived?

In addition, the taxonomic system devised by Bloom, Englehart, Furst, Hill, and Krathwohl (1956) for categorizing learning objectives according to a hierarchy of behaviors has been the cornerstone of teaching for almost a half century. This concept of **taxonomy**, that is, the ordering of these behaviors according to their type and complexity, pertains to the nature of the knowledge to be learned, the behaviors most relevant and attainable for a particular learner or group of learners, and the sequencing of knowledge and experiences for learning.

The skill in preparing and classifying behavioral objectives is a necessary function of the educator's role, whether teaching patients and their families in healthcare settings, teaching staff in in-service and continuing education programs, or teaching health profession's students in academic institutions. The importance of understanding the systems of writing and categorizing behavioral objectives for the purpose of specifying learner outcomes is imperative if data yielded from educational efforts are to be consistent and measurable. Additionally, the knowledge and use of these techniques are becoming essential because of the need to quantify and justify the costs of teaching others in an environment characterized by ever-increasing cost-containment pressures.

This chapter examines the importance of behavioral objectives for effective teaching; describes how to write clear and precise behavioral objectives; explores the levels of achievement in the taxonomic hierarchy of cognitive, affective, and psychomotor domains; and outlines the development of teaching plans and learning contracts. All of these elements provide a framework for the successful instruction of the learner.

Types of Objectives

It is important to clarify the meaning of the terms **educational objectives**, **instructional objectives**, and **behavioral** or **learning objectives**. Although often used synonymously, these terms can be distinguished from one another. Educational objectives are used to identify the intended outcomes of the education process, whether in reference to an aspect of a program or a total program of study, that guide the design of curriculum units. Instructional objectives describe the teaching activities

and resources used to facilitate effective learning (Morrison, Ross, & Kemp, 2004). Behavioral objectives, also referred to as learning objectives, on the other hand, make use of the modifier *behavioral* or *learning* to denote that this type of objective is action oriented rather than content oriented, learner centered rather than teacher centered, and short-term outcome focused rather than process focused. Behavioral objectives describe precisely what the learner will be able to do following a learning situation.

Characteristics of Goals and Objectives

The terms *goal* and *objective* are often used interchangeably—albeit incorrectly. A real difference exists between the two terms. Health professionals must clearly understand this distinction when in the role of educator. Time span and specificity are the two factors that differentiate goals from objectives (Haggard, 1989).

A **goal** is the final outcome of what is achieved at the end of the teaching–learning process. A goal is a statement that describes the ideal or ultimate state of being at some future point in time. Goals are global and broad in nature; they serve as long-term targets for both the learner and the teacher. Goals are the desired outcomes of learning that are realistically achievable usually in weeks or months. They are considered multidimensional in that a number of objectives are subsumed under or incorporated into an overall goal.

An **objective**, in contrast, is a specific, single, unidimensional behavior. As stated by Anderson et al. (2001), "When we teach, we want our students to learn. What we want them to learn as a result of our teaching are our objectives" (p. 3). Objectives are short term in nature and should be achievable at the conclusion of one teaching session or usually within a matter of days following a series of teaching sessions. According to Mager (1997), an objective describes a performance that learners should be able to exhibit before they are considered competent. A behavioral objective is the intended result of instruction, not the process or means of instruction itself. Objectives are statements of specific or short-term behaviors that lead step by step to the more general, overall long-term goal.

Subobjectives also may be written and reflect aspects of a main objective. They, too, are specific statements of short-term behaviors that lead to the achievement of the primary objective. Objectives and subobjectives specify what the learner will be able to do as a result of being exposed to one or more learning experiences.

Objectives must be achieved before the goal can be reached. They must be observable and measurable to be able to determine whether they have been met by the learner. Objectives can be thought of as advance organizers, statements that inform the learner of what is expected from a cognitive, affective, or psychomotor perspective prior to meeting the goal, which is the intended outcome (Babcock & Miller, 1994). Objectives are derived from a goal and must be consistent with and related to that goal. As an analogy, a goal can be thought of as an entire pie, the objectives as individual portions of the pie that make up the goal, and the subobjectives as bite-sized pieces of a single portion of the pie.

Together, objectives and goals form a map that provides directions (objectives) as to how to arrive at a particular destination (goal). For example, a goal might be that a patient with diabetes will learn to manage his disease. To accomplish this goal, which both the health provider and the patient have agreed on, specific objectives must be outlined to address changes in behavior such as the need to learn diet therapy, insulin administration, exercise regimens, stress management, and glucose monitoring. The objectives to accomplish the goal become the blueprint for attaining the desired outcomes of learning.

The successful achievement of predetermined objectives is, in part, the result of appropriate instruction. Certainly, many other factors, such as learner motivation and ability to perform, are also key factors to the successful demonstration of specific behaviors before overall competence by the learner can be declared.

If the teaching–learning process is to be successful, the setting of goals and objectives must be a mutual decision on the part of both the teacher and the learner. Both parties must participate in the decision-making process and buy into the immediate objectives and ultimate goals. Involving the learner right from the start in creating goals and objectives is absolutely crucial. Otherwise, time and effort on the part of the educator and the learner may be wasted because the learner may choose to reject the content if it is deemed from his or her perspective to be unimportant, irrelevant, impractical, or something already known.

Goal and objective setting for any educational experience should be as much a responsibility of the learner as it is of the teacher. Blending what the learner wants to learn with what the teacher has determined that the learner needs to know into a common set of objectives and goals provides for an educational experience that is mutually accountable, respectful, developmental, and fulfilling (Reilly & Oermann, 1990).

Objectives and goals must also be clearly written, realistic, and learner centered. If they do not precisely state what the learner is expected to do in the short and long term, then there are no clear guideposts to follow or an obvious end result for which to strive in the learning process. Likewise, if goals and objectives are unrealistic in that they are too difficult to achieve, the learner can become discouraged, which dampens motivation and interferes with the ability to comply. For instance, a goal that a patient will maintain a salt-free diet is likely to be impossible to accomplish or to adhere to over an extended period of time. Establishing a goal of maintaining a low-salt diet, with the objectives of learning to avoid eating and preparing high-sodium foods, is a much more realistic and achievable expectation of the learner.

Also, goals and objectives must be directed to what the learner is expected to be able to do, not what the teacher is expected to teach. Educators must be sure not only that their teaching remains objectives oriented but also that the objectives are learner centered. This approach keeps educators targeted on results, not on the act of teaching. Educators must remember, as Anderson et al. (2001) emphasizes, not all learners will take away the same thing from the same instruction, unless objectives are focused and precisely expressive.

The Debate About Using Behavioral Objectives

Educators have made strong arguments for and against the use of behavioral objectives for teaching and learning. Certainly, behavioral objectives are not a panacea for all the problems encountered in the planning, implementation, and evaluation of education (Reilly & Oermann, 1990). The following list, based on the contributions by Arends (1994); Reilly and Oermann (1990); Haggard (1989); Durbach, Goodall, and Wilkinson (1987); Brottman (2009); and Morrison et al. (2004), presents some common arguments by educators against using behavioral objectives:

- The understanding by experienced educators of learners' needs is so sophisticated that the exercise of writing behavioral objectives is superfluous.
- The practice of writing specific behavioral objectives leads to reductionism, a format that reduces behavioral processes into equivalents that do not reflect the sum total of the parts.
- Objectives writing is a time-consuming task, requiring more effort for development than is

warranted by their effect on an instructional program. That is, the cost benefit does not justify the amount of time required to formulate them.

- The preparation of objectives is merely a pedagogic exercise often expressing the teacher's expectations of the outcome of teaching and precluding the opportunity for learners to seek their own objectives.
- Predetermined objectives, with their emphasis on precise and observable learner behaviors, force teachers and learners to attend only to specific areas, which stifle creativity and interfere with the freedom to learn and to teach.
- The writing of specific objectives is incompatible with the many complex fields of study in health care because an infinite number of objectives are possible for almost any subject or topic.
- Behavioral objectives are unable to capture the more intricate cognitive processes that are not readily observable and measurable.

The rationale for using behavioral objectives, however, far outweighs the arguments against their use. The following considerations justify the need for writing behavioral objectives (Ferguson, 1998; Morrison et al., 2004). Careful construction of objectives

- Helps to keep educators' thinking on target and learner centered.
- Communicates to others, both learners and healthcare team members alike, what is planned for teaching and learning.
- Helps learners understand what is expected of them so that they can keep track of their progress.
- Forces the educator to organize educational materials so as not to get lost in content and forget the learner's role in the process.
- Encourages educators to question their own motives—to think deliberately about why they

are doing things and analyze what positive results will be attained from accomplishing specific objectives.

- Tailors teaching to the learner's particular circumstances and needs.
- Creates guideposts for teacher evaluation and documentation of success or failure.
- Focuses attention not on what is taught but on what the learner will come away with once the teaching–learning process is completed.
- Orients both teacher and learner to the specific end results of instruction.
- Makes it easier for the learner to visualize performing the required actions.

Robert Mager (1997), a recognized authority on preparing behavioral objectives, points out three other major advantages to writing explicit objective statements:

1. They provide a sound basis for the selection or design of instructional content, methods, and materials.
2. They provide learners with the means to organize their efforts and activities toward accomplishing the intent of instruction.
3. They allow for a determination as to whether an objective has, in fact, been accomplished.

As Mager (1997) asks, "If you don't know where you're going, how will you know which road to take to get there?" (p. 14). That is, before the educator prepares instruction, before materials and teaching methods are selected and implemented, before the means to evaluate learning is chosen, it is important to clearly and concisely state just what the intended results of instruction are to be. To paraphrase Mager's thinking, mechanics do not select repair tools until they know what has to be fixed; surgeons do not choose instruments until they know what operation is to be performed; and builders do not buy construction materials before drafting a blueprint.

Haggard (1989) summarizes the following questions that arise if objectives are not always written:

- How will anyone else know what objectives have been set?
- How will the educator evaluate and document success or failure?
- How will learners keep track of their progress?

The writing of objectives is not merely a mechanical task but a synthesizing process. The process of developing behavioral objectives not only helps educators explore their own knowledge, values, and beliefs about the entire spectrum of teaching and learning, but it also encourages them to examine the experiences, values, motivations, and knowledge of the learner. The time and effort expended in writing objectives represent a thoughtful deliberation about the knowledge, attitude, and skill requirements needed by the learner in meeting the desired level of competency.

The educator and learner should work together to compose objectives and goals that focus on what is to be accomplished in the short and long run. This process provides direction that helps the educator and learner identify

- The time that will be needed for teaching and learning
- The clues as to how the learner best acquires information
- The teaching methods that will work most effectively
- The best ways to evaluate the learner's progress

In addition, the process of stating well-written objectives encourages the educator to seriously contemplate what is worth teaching and what is worth spending time to accomplish. Also, the process can serve to highlight the value of an existing instructional program and provide the basis for improving a current teaching plan. Thus, the mutual setting of objectives and goals is considered by many educators to be the initial, most important consideration in the education process (Haggard, 1989; Mager, 1997).

Writing Behavioral Objectives and Goals

Well-written behavioral objectives give learners very clear statements about what is expected of them and assist teachers in being able to measure learner progress toward achieving outcomes of learning. Over the past 3 decades, Robert Mager's (1997) approach to writing behavioral objectives has been widely accepted among educators. His message to educators is that for objectives to be meaningful, they must precisely, clearly, and very specifically communicate the teacher's instructional intent (Arends, 1994).

According to Mager (1997), the format for writing concise and useful behavioral objectives includes the following three important characteristics:

1. *Performance:* Describes what the learner is expected to be able to do or perform to demonstrate the kinds of behaviors the teacher will accept as evidence that objectives have been achieved. Activities performed by the learner may be visible, such as writing or listing, or invisible, such as identifying or recalling.
2. *Condition:* Describes the testing situation, resources, assistance, or constraints under which the behavior will occur, will be observed, or will be completed.
3. *Criterion:* Describes how well, with what accuracy, or within what time frame the learner must be able to perform for the behavior to be considered acceptable; the standard, quality level, or amount of performance defined as satisfactorily demonstrating mastery. It is the level of competence that a learner must achieve.

The aforementioned three characteristics translate into the following questions: (1) What should the learner be able to do? (2) Under what conditions should the learner be able to do it? (3) How well must the learner be able to do it?

A fourth component must also be included; it should describe the "who" to ensure that the behavioral objective is learner centered. For education in health care, the learner may be the patient, family members or significant others of the patient, professional staff, or health professions students.

Thus, behavioral objectives are statements that communicate who will do what under what conditions and how well (Cummings, 1994). The more complete the statements of objectives, the better the objectives will serve to communicate exactly what is expected of the learner and what is the intent of instruction. An easy way to remember the four elements that should be in a behavioral objective is to follow the ABCD rule proposed by Heinich, Molenda, Russell, and Smaldino (2001):

A—audience (who)
B—behavior (what)
C—condition (under what circumstance)
D—degree (how much; how well; to what extent)

To link the behavioral objectives together, the following four steps are recommended:

1. Identify the testing situation (condition).
2. Identify who will perform (learner).
3. State what the learner will demonstrate (performance).
4. State how well the learner will perform (criterion).

For example: "Following a 20-minute teaching session on relaxation techniques (condition), Mrs. Smith (learner) will be able to identify (performance) three distinct techniques for lowering her stress level (criterion)."

Table 10–1 outlines the four-part method of objective writing. **Table 10–2** gives samples of well-written and poorly written objectives.

Table 10–1 THE FOUR-PART METHOD OF OBJECTIVE WRITING

Condition (Testing Situation)	Who (Identify Learner)	Performance (Learner Behavior)	Criterion (Quality or Quantity of Mastery)
Without using a calculator	the student	will solve	5 out of 6 math problems
Using the computer	the new employee	will demonstrate	the correct procedure for entering patient assessment data
Following group discussion	the patient	will list	at least two reasons for losing weight
After watching a video	the caregiver	will describe	the correct procedure for transferring the patient from bed to chair

Table 10–2 SAMPLES OF WRITTEN OBJECTIVES

WELL-WRITTEN OBJECTIVES

After watching a video on the Heimlich maneuver, the staff member will be able to demonstrate the correct procedure for intervening with a client who is choking.

Following a class on hypertension, the patient will be able to state three out of four causes of high blood pressure.

On completing the reading materials provided on the care of a newborn, the mother will be able to express any concerns she has about caring for her baby after discharge.

POORLY WRITTEN OBJECTIVES

The patient will be able to prepare a menu using low-salt foods (*condition and criterion missing*).

Given a list of exercises to relieve low back pain, the patient will understand how to control low back pain (*performance not stated in measurable terms, criterion missing*).

The physical therapist will demonstrate crutch walking postoperatively to the patient (*teacher-centered*).

It is important to note, however, that there are really two accepted approaches to writing behavioral objectives, depending on the audience of learners. Reilly and Oermann (1990) distinguish between what are known as specific behavioral objectives and general behavioral objectives. With both types of objectives, the learners and the behaviors to be learned must be clearly stated. The difference between the two types of objectives lies in the desirability of including the conditions of learning and the criteria for the level of performance expected.

Specific behavioral objectives are closed-ended statements that incorporate the condition and criterion for learning, which make them more prescriptive and predictive for the measurement of outcomes. This relatively linear format for writing specific behavioral objectives is an asset to help focus the learning process on a step-by-step basis, especially when a low-level skill is the intended outcome. For example, when teaching a patient to test blood glucose levels or teaching a staff member a new procedural protocol for documenting teaching using the electronic medical record, the writing of specific behavioral objectives is preferred.

General behavioral objectives, which do not include the condition or criterion for learning, are open-ended statements that lend themselves to be used in evaluating higher cognitive skills. This format is more appropriate for stating outcomes of an academic program, when knowledge of the learner is not expected to be just an accumulation of designated parts, but rather an integration and synthesis of broader concepts and theories over time. As such, the writing of general behavioral objectives is more compatible when teaching employees in a staff development program or students in a course within a professional program of study. It allows teachers to be more creative in teaching and accommodates acceptable variations in the learner that foster the creative expression of ideas and knowledge. Also, it allows the educator to assign grades, which distinguishes high achievers from moderate to lower achievers.

It is important to recognize the existence of and distinction between these two types of behavioral objectives. In this chapter, however, the focus is on writing specific behavioral objectives appropriate for the learning of particular skill sets by patients and staff.

In contrast to writing behavioral objectives, formulating well-written goals also is an important skill for the educator to acquire. In particular, a goal statement should clearly express the intended outcome the learner is expected to achieve in the long run after a series of specific behavioral objectives has been met. A goal represents the anticipated end result of an aggregate of behavior changes in the learner that are predicted to occur. A goal should reflect the final destination that the learner, in partnership with the educator, is striving to reach. A goal statement needs to be a succinctly written sentence that is learner centered, future oriented, realistic, and achievable within a reasonable time frame. Unlike behavioral objectives, a goal statement does not contain the characteristics of condition and criterion. A goal is a broad statement of behavior that identifies the learner, uses a future tense verb, and includes the overall outcome of learning to be achieved. Examples of well-written goal statements are in Appendix C.

Performance Words With Many or Few Interpretations

When writing behavioral objectives using the format suggested by Mager (1997), the recommendation is to use precise action words (verbs as labels, known as verbals) that are open to few interpretations when describing learner performance. An objective is considered useful only when it clearly states what a learner must demonstrate for mastery in a knowledge, attitude, or skill area. A performance verb (verbal) describes what the learner is expected to do. A performance may be overt, visible, or audible—for example, the learner is able *to list, to write, to state,* or *to walk.* These performances are directly observable. A performance also may be invisible—for example, the learner is able *to identify, to solve, to recall,* or *to recognize.* Any performance, visible/audible or invisible, described by a "doing" word is measurable.

If a word is used to describe something a learner can be, then it is not a doing word but rather a being word. Examples of being words, known also as abstractions, are *to understand, to know, to enjoy,* or *to appreciate* (Mager, 1997). Understanding, knowing, enjoying, and appreciating are considered abstract states of being and cannot be directly measured but merely inferred from performances. Therefore, verbs that signify an internal state of thinking, feeling, or believing should be avoided because they are difficult to measure or observe.

It is impossible to identify all behavioral terms that may be used in objective writing. The important thing to remember in selecting verbs (verbals) to describe performance is that they must be specific, observable or measurable, and action oriented. As stated by Anderson et al. (2001), if the teacher is able to describe the behavior to be attained, it will be easily recognized when the learning has occurred. The lists in **Table 10–3** give examples of verbals that, on the one hand, are too broad, ambiguous, and imprecise to evaluate and, on the other hand, are specific and relatively easy to measure (Gronlund, 1985, 2004).

Common Mistakes When Writing Objectives

In formulating behavioral objectives, there are a number of common pitfalls that can easily be made by the novice as well as by the seasoned educator. The most frequent errors in writing objectives are these:

- To describe what the instructor rather than the learner is expected to do
- To include more than one expected behavior in a single objective (avoid using the compound word *and* to connect two verbs—e.g., the learner will select *and* prepare)
- To forget to identify all four components of condition, performance, criterion, and the learner
- To use terms for performance that are subject to many interpretations, not action oriented, and difficult to measure
- To write an objective that is unattainable given the ability level of the learner
- To write objectives that do not relate to the stated goal
- To clutter an objective by including unnecessary information

- To be too general so as not to specify clearly the expected behavior to be achieved

In summary, if you use the SMART rule, it is easy to create effective objectives for different audiences in diverse settings. This objective-setting process is shown in **Table 10–4**.

Taxonomy of Objectives According to Learning Domains

A taxonomy is a mechanism used to categorize things according to how they are related to one another. "A taxonomy is a special kind of framework in which categories lie along a continuum" (Anderson et al., 2001, p. 4). For example, biologists use taxonomies to classify plants and animals based on their natural characteristics.

In the late 1940s, psychologists and educators became concerned about the need to develop a system for defining and ordering levels of behavior according to their type and complexity (Reilly & Oermann, 1990). Bloom et al. (1956) and Krathwohl, Bloom, and Masia (1964) developed a very useful taxonomy, known as the taxonomy of educational objectives, as a tool for systematically and logically classifying behavioral objectives. This taxonomy, which became widely accepted as a standard aid for planning as well as evaluating learning, is divided into three broad categories or domains—cognitive, affective, and psychomotor.

Inherent in the concept of taxonomy is the notion that although these three domains of cognitive, affective, and psychomotor learning are described as existing as separate entities, they are, in fact, interdependent and can be experienced simultaneously. Humans do not possess thoughts, feelings, and actions in isolation of one another and typically do not compartmentalize learning. For example, the affective domain influences the cognitive domain and vice versa; the processes of

Table 10–3 VERBALS WITH MANY OR FEW INTERPRETATIONS

Terms With Many Interpretations (Not Recommended)	Terms With Few Interpretations (Recommended)	
to know	to apply	to explain
to understand	to choose	to identify
to appreciate	to classify	to list
to realize	to compare	to order
to be familiar with	to contrast	to predict
to enjoy	to construct	to recall
to value	to define	to recognize
to be interested in	to describe	to select
to feel	to demonstrate	to state
to think	to differentiate	to verbalize
to learn	to distinguish	to write

Source: Adapted from Gronlund, N. E. (1985). *Stating objectives for classroom instruction* (3rd ed.). New York: Macmillan; and Gronlund, N. E. (2004). *Writing instructional objectives for teaching and assessment* (7th ed.). Upper Saddle River, NJ: Pearson Merrill, Prentice Hall.

Table 10–4 WRITING SMART OBJECTIVES

Specific	Be specific about what is to be achieved (i.e., use strong action verbs, be concrete).
Measurable	Quantify or qualify objectives by including numeric, cost, or percentage amounts or the degree/level of mastery expected.
Achievable	Are the objectives attainable?
Realistic	Are resources available to achieve objectives (i.e., personnel, facilities, equipment)?
Timely	When will the objectives be achieved (i.e., within a week, a month, by the day of patient discharge, before a new staff member completes orientation)?

Source: Adapted from Glenn M. Parker Associates, Inc. (2000). *Team workout.* Amherst, MA: HRD Products.

thinking and feeling influence psychomotor performance and vice versa (Menix, 1996).

In the taxonomy of educational objectives, the objectives in each domain are ordered in a taxonomic form of hierarchy. Behavioral objectives are classified into low, medium, and high levels with simple behaviors listed first (designated by numbers 1.0 or 2.0), followed by behaviors of moderate difficulty (designated by numbers 3.0 and 4.0), and the more complex behaviors listed last (designated by numbers 5.0, 6.0, or 7.0). Subobjectives are listed under the main objective and are designated by numbers that range between whole numbers (e.g., an objective will have subobjectives identified as 2.1, 2.2, 2.3). Inherent in the concept of hierarchy is the serial structure that learners must successfully achieve behaviors at lower levels of the domains (1.0 or 2.0) before they are able to adequately learn behaviors at higher levels of the domains (3.0 to 7.0).

The Cognitive Domain

The **cognitive domain** is known as the "thinking" domain. Learning in this domain involves the acquisition of information and addresses the development of the learner's intellectual abilities, mental capacities, understanding, and thinking processes (Eggen & Kauchak, 2001). Objectives in this domain are divided into six levels, each specifying cognitive processes ranging from the simple (knowledge) to the more complex (evaluation), as listed and described by Bloom et al. (1956) in **Table 10–5**.

EXAMPLES OF BEHAVIORAL OBJECTIVES IN THE COGNITIVE DOMAIN

Analysis level: After reading handouts provided by the educator, the family member will calculate the correct number of total grams of protein included on average per day in the family diet.

Synthesis level: Given a sample list of foods, the patient will devise a menu to include foods from the four food groups (dairy, meat, vegetables and fruits, and grains) in the recommended amounts for daily intake.

Table 10–6 lists verbs commonly used in writing cognitive-level behavioral objectives.

Table 10–5 Levels of Cognitive Behavior

Knowledge (1.00–1.99): Ability of the learner to memorize, recall, define, recognize, or identify specific information, such as facts, rules, principles, conditions, and terms, presented during instruction.

Comprehension (2.00–2.99): Ability of the learner to demonstrate an understanding or appreciation of what is being communicated by translating it into a different form or recognizing it in a translated form, such as grasping an idea by defining it or summarizing it in his or her own words (knowledge is a prerequisite behavior).

Application (3.00–3.99): Ability of the learner to use ideas, principles, abstractions, or theories in particular and concrete situations, such as figuring, writing, reading, or handling equipment (knowledge and comprehension are prerequisite behaviors).

Analysis (4.00–4.99): Ability of the learner to recognize and structure information by breaking it down into its constituent parts and specifying the relationship between parts (knowledge, comprehension, and application are prerequisite behaviors).

Synthesis (5.00–5.99): Ability of the learner to put together parts and elements into a unified whole by creating a unique product that is written, oral, pictorial, and so on (knowledge, comprehension, application, and analysis are prerequisite behaviors).

Evaluation (6.00–6.99): Ability of the learner to judge the value of something, such as an essay, design, or action, by applying appropriate standards or criteria (knowledge, comprehension, application, analysis, and synthesis are prerequisite behaviors).

Table 10–6 Commonly Used Verbs According to Domain Classification

COGNITIVE DOMAIN

Knowledge: choose, circle, define, identify, label, list, match, name, outline, recall, report, select, state

Comprehension: describe, discuss, distinguish, estimate, explain, generalize, give example, locate, recognize, summarize

Application: apply, demonstrate, illustrate, implement, interpret, modify, order, revise, solve, use

Analysis: analyze, arrange, calculate, classify, compare, conclude, contrast, determine, differentiate, discriminate

Synthesis: categorize, combine, compile, correlate, design, devise, generate, integrate, reorganize, revise, summarize

Evaluation: appraise, assess, conclude, criticize, debate, defend, judge, justify

AFFECTIVE DOMAIN

Receiving: accept, admit, ask, attend, focus, listen, observe, pay attention

Responding: agree, answer, conform, discuss, express, participate, recall, relate, report, state willingness, try, verbalize

Valuing: assert, assist, attempt, choose, complete, disagree, follow, help, initiate, join, propose, volunteer

Organization: adhere, alter, arrange, combine, defend, explain, express, generalize, integrate, resolve

Characterization: assert, commit, discriminate, display, influence, propose, qualify, solve, verify

PSYCHOMOTOR DOMAIN

Perception: attend, choose, describe, detect, differentiate, distinguish, identify, isolate, perceive, relate, select, separate

Set: attempt, begin, develop, display, position, prepare, proceed, reach, respond, show, start, try

Guided response mechanism and complex overt response: align, arrange, assemble, attach, build, change, choose, clean, compile, complete, construct, demonstrate, discriminate, dismantle, dissect, examine, find, grasp, hold, insert, lift, locate, maintain, manipulate, measure, mix, open, operate, organize, perform, pour, practice, reassemble, remove, repair, replace, separate, shake, suction, turn, transfer, walk, wash, wipe

Adaptation: adapt, alter, change, convert, correct, rearrange, reorganize, replace, revise, shift, substitute, switch

Origination: arrange, combine, compose, construct, create, design, exchange, reformulate

Source: Adapted from Gronlund, N. E. (1985). *Stating objectives for classroom instruction* (3rd ed.). New York: Macmillan; and Gronlund, N. E. (2004). *Writing instructional objectives for teaching and assessment* (7th ed.). Upper Saddle River, NJ: Pearson Merrill, Prentice Hall.

TEACHING IN THE COGNITIVE DOMAIN

A variety of teaching methods and tools exists for the primary purpose of developing cognitive abilities. The methods most often used to stimulate learning in the cognitive domain include lecture, one-to-one instruction, and self-instruction activities such as computer-assisted instruction (see Chapter 11). Verbal, written, and visual tools are all particularly successful in supplementing the teaching methods (see Chapter 12) to help learners master cognitive content. For example, research has shown computer-assisted instruction to be effective in teaching clients about HIV prevention and students about musculoskeletal testing (Evans, Edmunson-Drane, & Harris, 2000; Ford, Mazzone, & Taylor, 2005).

Cognitive skills can be gained by exposure to all types of educational experiences, including the instructional methods used primarily for affective and psychomotor learning. Cognitive knowledge, however, is an essential prerequisite for the learner to engage in other educational activities such as group discussion or role-playing. Otherwise, what results is pooled ignorance. For example, clients cannot adequately learn through group discussion if they do not possess an accurate and at least basic knowledge level of the subject at hand to draw on for purposes of discourse. Participating in a group discussion experience is not the same thing as engaging in a brainstorming session. Brainstorming does not necessarily require prior knowledge of information about issues or problems to be explored.

Cognitive domain learning is the traditional focus of most teaching. In education of patients, staff, and students, emphasis remains on the sharing of facts, theories, concepts, and the like. Cognitive processing—that is, the means through which knowledge is acquired—often takes precedence over psychomotor skill development and the learning of affective behaviors (Ellis, 1993). Perhaps this emphasis has occurred because educators typically feel more confident and more skilled in being the giver of information rather than being the facilitator and coordinator of learning. Lecture and one-to-one instruction are the most often used methods of teaching. Both of these instructional approaches, when taught in a typical fashion, are directed almost exclusively at the cognitive domain.

With respect to cognitive learning, how much time for practice is necessary to influence the short-term and long-term retention of factual information? Cognitive scientists have been exploring the allocation of practice time to the learning of new material. Generally, research findings indicate that learning distributed over several sessions leads to better memory than information learned in a single session.

This phenomenon has been described by Willingham (2002) as the "spacing effect." That is, learning information all at once on one day, which is known as **massed practice**, is much less effective for remembering facts than learning information over successive periods of time, which is known as **distributed practice**. Massed practice, similar to what is commonly identified as cramming, might allow the recall of information for a short time, but evidence strongly supports that distributed practice is very important in forging memories that last for years.

The effect of spreading out learning over time is very clear. The average person exposed to distributed practice remembers 67% better than people getting massed training. That is, spacing the time allocated for learning significantly increases memory. The longer the delays between practice sessions, the greater and more permanent is the learning. In fact, if learning is distributed over time, not only does this spacing effect hold, but it becomes even more robust (Willingham, 2002).

This evidence, when applied to the education of patients, staff, or students, strongly suggests the need to allocate time for the acquisition of knowledge. Such scientific findings explain, for example, why teaching a patient on the day of discharge from the hospital is ineffective.

The Affective Domain

The **affective domain** is known as the "feeling" domain. Learning in this domain involves an increasing internalization or commitment to feelings expressed as emotions, interests, beliefs, attitudes, values, and appreciations. Whereas the cognitive domain is ordered in terms of complexity of behaviors, the affective domain is divided into categories that specify the degree of a person's depth of emotional responses to tasks. The affective domain includes emotional and social development goals.

As stated by Eggen and Kauchak (2001), educators use the affective domain to help learners realize their own attitudes and values.

Although educators recognize the need for individuals to learn in the affective domain, constructs such as attitudes, beliefs, and values cannot be directly observed but can only be inferred from words and actions (Maier-Lorentz, 1999). Educators tend to be less confident and more challenged in writing behavioral objectives for the affective domain because it is difficult to develop easily measurable objectives and evaluation of learning outcomes is based on inferences of someone's observed behavior (Goulet & Owen-Smith, 2005; Morrison et al., 2004).

Competencies in the affective domain relate to the development of a value system. Behavior is guided by notions held by an individual and society as to what is considered good and right. Thus, affective competencies involve moral reasoning and ethical decision making. For professional staff, competency in the affective domain is required to intervene with clients in a humanistic and caring manner.

Reilly and Oermann (1990) differentiate among the terms *beliefs*, *attitudes*, and *values*. Beliefs are what an individual perceives as reality; attitudes represent feelings about an object, person, or event; and values are operational beliefs that guide actions and ways of living. Although writing and measuring specific objectives in the affective domain is challenging, educators have been successful in identifying strategies for measuring beliefs, attitudes, and values, particularly of students in the health professions. For example, Hayward, Blackmer, and Markowski (2006) developed an assessment rubric for evaluating clinical and professional core values among their physical therapy students.

Objectives in the affective domain are divided into five categories, each specifying the associated level of affective responses as listed and described by Krathwohl et al. (1964) in **Table 10–7**.

EXAMPLES OF BEHAVIORAL OBJECTIVES IN THE AFFECTIVE DOMAIN

> *Receiving level:* During a group discussion session, the patient will admit to any fears he may have about needing to undergo a repeat angioplasty.
>
> *Responding level:* At the end of one-to-one instruction, the child will verbalize feelings of confidence in managing her asthma using the peak flow tracking chart.
>
> *Characterization level:* Following a series of inservice education sessions, the staff members will display consistent interest in maintaining strict hand-washing technique to control the spread of nosocomial infections to patients in the hospital.

Table 10–6 lists verbs commonly used in writing affective-level behavioral objectives.

TEACHING IN THE AFFECTIVE DOMAIN

A variety of teaching methods has been found to be powerful and reliable in helping the learner acquire elements of the affective domain. Role modeling, role-playing, simulation gaming, and group discussion sessions are examples of instructional methods that can be used to prepare staff and students as well as patients and their families to incorporate values and to explore attitudes, interests, and feelings in the process of developing affective behaviors.

Health professionals have been encouraged to attend to the needs of the whole person by recognizing that learning is subjective and values driven (Schoenly, 1994). For practicing health professionals, affective learning is especially important because they are constantly faced with ethical issues and value conflicts (Tong, 2007). In addition, this increasingly pluralistic society requires health professionals to respect the racial and ethnic diversity in the population groups they serve (Marks, 2009). Advancing technology also places health

---

Table 10–7 Levels of Affective Behavior

Receiving (1.00–1.99): Ability of the learner to show awareness of an idea or fact or a consciousness of a situation or event in the environment. This level represents a willingness to selectively attend to or focus on data or to receive a stimulus.

Responding (2.00–2.99): Ability of the learner to respond to an experience, at first obediently and later willingly and with satisfaction. This level indicates a movement beyond denial and toward voluntary acceptance, which can lead to feelings of pleasure or enjoyment as a result of some new experience (receiving is a prerequisite behavior).

Valuing (3.00–3.99): Ability of the learner to regard or accept the worth of a theory, idea, or event, demonstrating sufficient commitment or preference to be identified with some experience seen as having value. At this level, there is a definite willingness and desire to act to further that value (receiving and responding are prerequisite behaviors).

Organization (4.00–4.99): Ability of the learner to organize, classify, and prioritize values by integrating a new value into a general set of values, to determine interrelationships of values, and to harmoniously establish some values as dominant and pervasive (receiving, responding, and valuing are prerequisite behaviors).

Characterization (5.00–5.99): Ability of the learner to integrate values into a total philosophy or worldview, showing firm commitment and consistency of responses to the values by generalizing certain experiences into a value system or attitude cluster (receiving, responding, valuing, and organization are prerequisite behaviors).

Source: Krathwohl, D. R., Bloom, B. J., & Masia, B. B. (1964). *Taxonomy of educational objectives: The classification of educational goals. Handbook II: The affective domain.* New York: David McKay.

professionals in advocacy positions when patients, families, and other healthcare professionals are constantly grappling with treatment decisions. In turn, patients and family members are faced with making moral and ethical choices as well as learning to internalize the value of complying with prescribed treatment regimens and incorporating health promotion and disease prevention practices into their daily lives.

The environment in which teaching and learning take place is important to the successful achievement of affective behavioral outcomes. A trusting relationship and an open, empathetic, accepting attitude by the educator toward clients are necessary to secure client interest and involvement in learning. Staff beliefs, attitudes, and values significantly influence their affective behavior and, thus, the quality of care they deliver. A health professional who is teaching students must have a personal value

system that coincides with the values of their profession. The health professions each have a code of ethics that sets forth the values and principles with which its members practice (see Chapter 2, Table 2–1).

Unfortunately, adequate weight is not usually given to teaching in the affective domain. The educator's focus more often emphasizes cognitive processing and psychomotor functioning with little time set aside for exploration and clarification of learner feelings, emotions, and attitudes (Ellis, 1993; Morrison et al., 2004; Rinne, 1987; Zimmerman & Phillips, 2000).

Schoenly (1994) examined affective teaching strategies that can be used to assist learners in acquiring affective domain behaviors. Once appropriate objectives and an accepting climate have been established, the following educational interventions can be selected and implemented:

Questioning: Although the lecture method is usually identified with helping the learner gain cognitive skills, the technique of careful questioning during the lecture process can assist in meeting objectives in the affective domain. Affective questioning increases interest and motivation to learn about feelings, values, beliefs, and attitudes regarding a topic under study. Low-level affective questions are directed at stimulating learner awareness and responsiveness to a topic, midlevel affective questioning assists in determining the strength of a belief or the internalization of a value, and high-level affective questioning probes for information about the depth of integration of a value.

Case study: This method can assist the learner in developing problem-solving and critical-thinking skills through exploration of participant attitudes, beliefs, and values. Using learning groups with the reader assuming the role of a key player in the situation (healthcare provider, family member, patient) rather than as a neutral observer can help in eliciting affective behavioral responses.

Role-playing: This method provides an excellent opportunity to practice new behaviors and explore feelings, attitudes, and values; to problem solve; and to resolve personal problems associated with human circumstances. Role-playing allows the learner to walk in someone else's shoes, but without the actual risk, thereby gaining empathy for the reality of another's situation. Being an observer during role-playing can sensitize the learner to the phenomenon, while active participation in role-playing energizes the learner to attend and respond to the phenomenon under consideration. Medicine, physical therapy, and other health fields have adapted the concept of role-playing to include the use of standardized patients, that is, individuals who have been taught to play a certain role in a learning or assessment interaction with a student (Coplan, Essary, Lohenry, & Stoehr, 2008; Hayward et al., 2006; Lee et al., 2008). Because the standardized patient can be programmed to introduce a moral, ethical, or other type of dilemma into the interaction, this approach works well when teaching or evaluating within the affective domain.

Gaming: Games that are controlled by the participants and have flexible rules are more appropriate for accomplishing affective behavioral objectives than are games that are characterized by structured roles and have specific rules, which are better for cognitive learning. Gaming promotes active involvement of the learner in goal-directed, but not necessarily competitive, activities. Debriefing following gaming is an important aspect of the technique to provide an opportunity for learners to understand how attitudes, beliefs, and values from the gaming experience can be applied and incorporated into everyday life.

Group discussion: This method provides an opportunity for clarifying personal values as well as exploring social values and moral issues. Value clarification involves identifying and sharing personal values for the purpose of increasing self-awareness and self-discovery. Values inquiry involves investigating the value systems of various ethnic groups. Both approaches provide the chance for in-depth learning of affective behaviors.

The affective domain encompasses three levels (Menix, 1996) that govern attitudes and feelings:

- The intrapersonal level includes personal perceptions of one's own self, such as self-concept, self-awareness, and self-acceptance.
- The interpersonal level includes the perspective of self in relation to other individuals.
- The extrapersonal level involves the perception of others as established groups.

All three levels are important in affective skill development and can be taught through a variety of methods specifically geared to affective domain learning.

Affective learning is a part of every educational experience, even though the primary focus for learning may be on either the cognitive or the psychomotor domain. Learner feelings or emotions cannot help but be aroused to some extent when the learner is exposed to new and different educational experiences (Bucher, 1991). In fact, Morrison et al. (2004) suggest that attitudinal development, such as receptivity, cooperation, and motivation, can even precede successful learning in other domains.

Without a doubt, learning is a multidimensional process that can occur in all three domains simultaneously, formally or informally, and in structured or unstructured settings. Evaluation of learning is just as complex a process. However, evaluation of affective behavior is more difficult than determining cognitive and psychomotor skill acquisition because affective behaviors are not usually overt and clearly observable. Rather, these behaviors are less tangible and more challenging to measure. Bucher (1991) and Maier-Lorentz (1999) suggest using the Likert scale as a means of discovering learner attitudes relative to particular learning experiences.

The Psychomotor Domain

The **psychomotor domain** is known as the "skills" domain. Learning in this domain involves acquiring fine and gross motor abilities with increasing complexity of neuromuscular coordination to carry out physical movement such as walking, handwriting, manipulation of equipment, or performing a procedure. Psychomotor skill learning, according to Reilly and Oermann (1990), "is a complex process demanding far more knowledge than suggested by the simple mechanistic behavioral approach" (p. 81). However, according to Eggen and Kauchak (2001), "while intellectual abilities enter into each of the psychomotor tasks, the primary focus is on the development of manipulative skills rather than on the growth of intellectual capability" (p. 17).

Thus, for development of psychomotor skills to take place, there must be integration of the other two domains of learning as well. The affective component conveys recognition of the value or worth of the skill being learned; the cognitive component relates to knowing the principles, relationships, and processes in carrying out the overt physical movement. Although all three domains are involved in demonstrating a psychomotor competency, the psychomotor domain can be examined separately and requires different teaching approaches and evaluation strategies (Reilly & Oermann, 1990). In contrast to the cognitive and affective domains, psychomotor skills are easy to identify and measure because they include primarily overt movement-oriented activities that are relatively easy to observe.

Psychomotor learning, including perceptual-motor tasks, can be classified in a variety of ways (Dave, 1970; Harrow, 1972; Moore, 1970; Simpson, 1972). Simpson's system seems to be the most widely recognized as relevant to client teaching. Objectives in this domain, according to Simpson (1972), are divided into seven levels as listed and described in **Table 10–8**.

EXAMPLES OF BEHAVIORAL OBJECTIVES IN THE PSYCHOMOTOR DOMAIN

Guided response level: After watching a 15-minute video on the procedure for self-examination of the breast, the client will perform the exam on a model with 100% accuracy.

Set level: Following demonstration of proper crutch walking, the patient will attempt to crutch walk using the correct three-point gait technique.

Table 10–6 lists verbs commonly used in writing psychomotor-level behavioral objectives.

Table 10–8 LEVELS OF PSYCHOMOTOR BEHAVIOR

Perception (1.00–1.99): Ability of the client to show sensory awareness of objects or cues associated with some task to be performed. Cues relevant to a situation are attended to, symbolically translated, and selected to guide action, gain insight, and receive feedback. This level involves reading directions or observing a process with attention to steps or techniques inherent in a process.

Set (2.00–2.99): Ability of the learner to exhibit readiness to take a particular kind of action, such as following directions, through expressions of willingness, sensory attending, or body language favorable to performing a motor act (perception is a prerequisite behavior).

Guided response (3.00–3.99): Ability of the learner to exert effort via overt actions under the guidance of an instructor to imitate an observed behavior with conscious awareness of effort. Imitating may be performed hesitantly but with compliance to directions and coaching (perception and set are prerequisite behaviors).

Mechanism (4.00–4.99): Ability of the learner to repeatedly perform steps of a desired skill with a certain degree of confidence, indicating mastery to the extent that some or all aspects of the process become habitual. The steps are blended into a meaningful whole and are performed smoothly with little conscious effort (perception, set, and guided response are prerequisite behaviors).

Complex overt response (5.00–5.99): Ability of the learner to automatically perform a complex motor act with independence and a high degree of skill, without hesitation and with minimum expenditure of time and energy; performance of an entire sequence of a complex behavior without the need to attend to details (perception, set, guided response, and mechanism are prerequisite behaviors).

Adaptation (6.00–6.99): Ability of the learner to modify or adapt a motor process to suit the individual or various situations, indicating mastery of highly developed movements that can be suited to a variety of conditions (perception, set, guided response, mechanism, and complex overt response are prerequisite behaviors).

Origination (7.00–7.99): Ability of the learner to create new motor acts, such as novel ways of manipulating objects or materials, as a result of an understanding of a skill and developed ability to perform skills (perception, set, guided response, mechanism, complex overt response, and adaptation are prerequisite behaviors).

Source: Simpson, E. J. (1972). The classification of educational objectives in the psychomotor domain. In M. T. Rainer (Ed.), *Contributions of behavioral science to instructional technology: The psychomotor domain* (3rd ed.). Englewood Cliffs, NJ: Gryphon Press, Prentice Hall.

Another taxonomic system for psychomotor learning proposed by Dave (1970) is also based on behaviors that include muscular action and neuromuscular coordination. Reilly and Oermann (1990) suggest that this taxonomy allows teachers to acknowledge the multivariant characteristics of psychomotor behavior and to focus on the orderly process of neuromuscular development over time of students in academic programs. They support this taxonomy to measure competence in perfor-mance within educational programs because it stresses accuracy over speed. Also, Dave's system recognizes that levels of skill attainment can be achieved and refined over a period of months as a result of the infrequency of students using certain skills in practice. Objectives in this domain, according to Dave (1970), are divided into five levels, as shown in **Table 10–9**.

These taxonomic criteria for the development of psychomotor skill competency suggest

---

Table 10–9 Dave's Levels of Psychomotor Learning

Imitation (1.0–1.99): At this level, observed actions are followed. The learner's movements are gross, coordination lacks smoothness, and errors occur. Time and speed required to perform are based on learner needs.

Manipulation (2.0–2.99): At this level, written instructions are followed. The learner's coordinated movements are variable, and accuracy is measured based on the skill of using written procedures as a guide. Time and speed required to perform vary.

Precision (3.0–3.99): At this level, a logical sequence of actions is carried out. The learner's movements are coordinated at a higher level, errors are minimal and relatively minor. Time and speed required to perform remain variable.

Articulation (4.0–4.99): At this level, a logical sequence of actions is carried out. The learner's movements are coordinated at a high level, and errors are limited. Time and speed required to perform are within reasonable expectations.

Naturalization (5.0–5.99): At this level, the sequence of actions is automatic. The learner's movements are coordinated at a consistently high level, and errors are almost nonexistent. Time and speed required to perform are within realistic limits, and performance reflects professional competence.

---

that accuracy should be stressed before the speed at which a skill is acquired (Reilly & Oermann, 1990). The levels of psychomotor behavior, no matter which taxonomic system is used, require the general and orderly steps of observing, imitating, practicing, and adapting.

Teaching of Psychomotor Skills

When teaching psychomotor skills, it is important for the educator to remember to keep skill instruction separate from a discussion of principles underlying the skill (cognitive component) or a discussion of how the learner feels about carrying out the skill (affective component). Psychomotor skill development is very egocentric and usually requires a great deal of concentration as the learner works toward mastery of a skill.

It is easy to interfere with psychomotor learning if the teacher asks a knowledge (cognitive) question while the learner is trying to focus on the performance (psychomotor response) of a skill.

For example, while a staff member is learning to perform massage therapy, it is not unusual for the teacher to ask, "Can you give me an explanation of how this therapy will benefit the client?" or "How often should massage be done for this particular patient?" As another example, while the patient is learning to self-administer parenteral medication, the teacher may simultaneously ask the patient to respond cognitively to the question, "What are the actions or side effects of this medication?" or "How do you feel about injecting yourself?" These questions demand cognitive and affective responses during psychomotor performance.

Although a teacher frequently intervenes with questions in the midst of a learner's performing, it is definitely an inappropriate teaching technique. What the educator is doing, in fact, is asking the learner to demonstrate at least two different behaviors at the same time. This technique can result in frustration and confusion, and ultimately it may result in failure to achieve any of the behaviors successfully. Questions related to the cognitive or affective domain should be posed only before or after the learner practices a psychomotor skill (Oermann, 1990).

In psychomotor skill development, the ability to perform a skill is not equivalent to having learned or mastered a skill. Performance is a transitory action, while learning is a more permanent behavior that follows from repeated practice and experience (Oermann, 1990). The actual mastery of a skill requires practice to allow the individual to repeat the performance time and again with accuracy, coordination, confidence, and out of habit. Practice does make perfect, so repetition leads to perfection and reinforcement of the behavior.

The riding of a bicycle is a perfect example of the difference between being able to perform a skill and having mastered or learned that skill. When one first attempts to ride a bicycle, movements tend to be very jerky, and the performance requires a great deal of concentration. Once the skill is learned, bicycle riding becomes a smooth, automatic operation that requires minimal attention to the details of fine and gross motor movements acting in concert to allow the learner to achieve the skill of riding a bicycle.

Some behaviors that are mastered do not require much reinforcement, even over a long period of disuse, whereas other behaviors, once mastered, need to be rehearsed or relearned for the learner to perform them at the level of skill once achieved. The amount of practice required to acquire any new skill varies with the individual, depending on many factors. Oermann (1990) and Bell (1991) have addressed some of the more important variables:

Readiness to learn: The motivation to learn affects the degree of perseverance exhibited by the learner in working toward mastery of a skill.

Past experience: If the learner is familiar with equipment or techniques similar to those needed to learn a new skill, then mastery of the new skill may be achieved at a faster rate.

The effects of learning one skill on the subsequent performance of another related skill is known as **transfer of learning** (Gomez & Gomez, 1984). For example, if someone already has experience with downhill skiing, then learning cross-country skiing should come more easily and with more confidence because the required coordination and equipment are similar. To use an example in teaching healthcare skills, if a family member already has experience transferring a client from bed to chair, then learning to assist the client into the shower should not take as much time to master.

Health status: Illness state or other physical or emotional impairments in the learner may affect the time it takes to acquire or successfully master a skill.

Environmental stimuli: Depending on the type and level of stimuli as well as the learning style (degree of tolerance for certain stimuli), distractions in the immediate surroundings may interfere with skill acquisition.

Anxiety level: The ability to concentrate can be dramatically affected by how anxious someone feels. Nervousness about performing in front of someone is particularly a key factor in psychomotor skill development. High anxiety levels interfere with coordination, steadiness, fine muscle movements, and concentration levels when performing complex psychomotor skills. It is important to reassure learners that they are not necessarily being tested during psychomotor skill performance. Reassurance and support reduce anxiety levels related to the fear of not meeting expectations of themselves or of the teacher.

Developmental stage: Physical, cognitive, and psychosocial stages of development all influence an individual's ability to master a movement-oriented task. Certainly, a young child's fine and gross motor skills as well as cognitive abilities are at a different level from those of an adult. The older adult, too, likely exhibits slower cognitive processing and increased response time (needing longer time to perform an activity) compared to younger clients.

Practice session length: During the beginning stages of learning a motor skill, short and carefully planned practice sessions and frequent rest periods are valuable techniques to help increase the rate and success of learning. These techniques are thought to be effective because they help prevent physical fatigue and restore the learner's attention to the task at hand.

Performing motor skills is not done in a vacuum. The learner is immersed in a particular environmental context full of stimuli. Learners must select those environmental influences that will assist them in achieving the behavior (relevant stimuli) and ignore those that interfere with a specific performance (irrelevant stimuli). This process of recognizing and selecting appropriate and inappropriate stimuli is called **selective attention** (Gomez & Gomez, 1984).

Motor skills should be practiced first in a laboratory setting to provide a safe and nonthreatening environment for the novice learner. Gomez and Gomez (1987) suggest also arranging for practice sessions to be done in the clinical or home setting to expose the learner to actual environmental conditions. This technique is known as open skills performance learned under changing and unstable environments.

In addition, research findings indicate that progress in mastery of a psychomotor skill can be accomplished just as effectively through self-directed study as with teaching in a structured laboratory situation (Love, McAdams, Patton, Rankin, & Roberts, 1989). Yoder (1993) found that computer-assisted interactive video instruction (CAIVI) resulted in a greater amount of transfer of cognitive learning than did linear video for the performance of psychomotor skills in a clinical setting. Yoder reports that the following three types of transfer learning occur: (1) self-transfer (repetition of learning), (2) near transfer (occurs in situations that are very similar), and (3) far transfer (occurs in situations that are very different). Application of psychomotor skills in the clinical arena is a type of far transfer.

Research on educational strategies using computer simulation for teaching psychomotor skills in the health professions is limited. Although a number of studies have been conducted in medicine on the use of simulators to teach invasive procedures to physicians, further research is warranted in other areas of healthcare education (Damewood, Cadigan, & Jeanmonod, 2009; Shirai et al., 2008). In any event, contact with the teacher during practice sessions is an important element for successful psychomotor learning. Although educator workload necessitates finding cost-effective and time-efficient ways to teach skill development, mediated instruction should not be used as a substitute, only a supplement, for instructor input (Baldwin, Hill, & Hanson, 1991).

In addition to using demonstration and return demonstration, mediated instruction, and self-directed study as teaching methods for psychomotor learning, mental imaging (also known as mental practice) has surfaced as a viable alternative for teaching motor skills, particularly for patients who have suffered a stroke (Page, Levine, & Khourey, 2009; Page, Levine, Sisto, & Johnston, 2001). Research indicates that learning psychomotor skills can be enhanced through use of imagery. Mental practice is similar to the type of practice athletes use when preparing to perform in a sports competition (Bachman, 1990; Doheny, 1993; Eaton & Evans, 1986; Miracle, 1999).

Another hallmark of psychomotor learning is the type and timing of the feedback given to learners.

Psychomotor skill development allows for immediate feedback such that learners have an immediate idea of the results of their performance. During skill practice, learners receive **intrinsic feedback** that is generated from within the self, giving them a sense of or a feel for how they have performed. They may sense that they either did quite well or that they felt awkward and need more practice. In addition, the teacher has the opportunity to provide **augmented feedback** by sharing with learners an opinion or conveying a message through body language about how well they performed (Oermann, 1990). The immediacy of the feedback, together with the self-generated and teacher-supplemented feedback, makes this a unique feature of psychomotor learning. Performance checklists, which can serve as guides for teaching and learning, are also an effective tool for evaluating the level of skill performance.

An important point to remember is that it is all right to make mistakes in the process of teaching or learning a psychomotor skill. If the teacher makes an error when demonstrating a skill or the learner makes an error during return demonstration, this is the perfect teaching opportunity to offer anticipatory guidance: "Oops, I made a mistake. Now what do I do?" Unlike cognitive skill development, where errorless learning is the objective, in psychomotor skill development a mistake made represents an opportunity to demonstrate how to correct an error and to learn from the not-so-perfect initial attempts at performance. The old saying "You learn by your mistakes" is most applicable to psychomotor skill mastery.

The spacing of practice time, which has been found to improve the likelihood that learners will remember new facts as described by Willingham (2002) in the cognitive domain section of this chapter, seems to apply to the learning of simple motor skills as well. However, to what degree this spacing effect positively influences the acquisition of complex skills is still not well understood. Will-

ingham (2004) also addresses the value of sustained practice when learning a new psychomotor skill. In fact, he describes the necessity for practice to be repeated beyond the point of perfection if skill learning is to be long lasting, automatic, and achieved with a high level of competence.

Thus, learning is a very complex phenomenon. It is clear that the cognitive, affective, and psychomotor domains, although representing separate behaviors, are to some extent interrelated. Movement-oriented activities require an integration of related knowledge and values (Morrison et al., 2004; Oermann, 1990). For example, the performance of a psychomotor skill requires a certain degree of cognitive knowledge or understanding of information, such as the scientific principles underlying a practice or why a skill is important to carry out. Also, there is an affective component to performing the movement dimension for the psychomotor behavior to be integrated as part of the learner's overall experience and ability to attain the ultimate goal of independence in self-care or practice delivery.

Development of Teaching Plans

After mutually agreed-upon goals and objectives have been written, it should be clear what the learner is to learn and what the teacher is to teach. A predetermined goal and related objectives serve as a basis for developing a teaching plan.

Organizing and presenting information in the format of an internally consistent teaching plan require skill by the educator. A **teaching plan** is a blueprint for action to achieve the goal and the objectives that have been agreed upon by the educator and the learner. In addition to the goal and objectives, it also should include purpose, content, methods and tools, timing, and evaluation of instruction. The teaching plan should clearly and concisely identify the sequencing of these various elements of the education process.

The three major reasons for constructing teaching plans are as follows:

1. To force the teacher to examine the relationship among the steps of the teaching process to ensure that a logical approach to teaching is taken, which can serve as a map for organizing and keeping instruction on target.
2. To communicate in writing and in an outline format exactly what is being taught, how it is being taught and evaluated, and the time allotted for accomplishment of the behavioral objectives. If this is done, not only is the learner aware of and able to follow the action plan, but, just as important, other healthcare team members are informed and can contribute to the teaching effort with a consistent approach.
3. To legally document that an individual plan for each learner is in place and is being properly implemented. Also, the existence of current teaching plans is essential evidence required by healthcare agencies and organizations to satisfy mandates for institutional accreditation.

Teaching plans can be presented in a number of different formats to meet institutional requirements or the preference of the user, but all parts must be included for the teaching plan to be considered comprehensive and complete. A teaching plan should consist of the following eight basic elements (Ryan & Marinelli, 1990):

1. The purpose
2. A statement of the overall goal
3. A list of objectives (and subobjectives, if necessary)
4. An outline of the related content
5. The instructional method(s) used for teaching the related content
6. The time allotted for the teaching of each objective

7. The instructional resources (materials/tools and equipment) needed
8. The method(s) used to evaluate learning

A sample teaching plan format is shown in **Figure 10–1**. This format is highly recommended because the use of columns allows the educator, as well as anyone else who is using it, to see all the parts of the teaching plan at one time. Also, this format provides the best structure for determining whether a relationship is apparent among all the elements of a plan. Internal consistency is the major criterion for judging the integrity of a teaching plan.

When constructing a teaching plan, the educator must be certain that, above all else, internal consistency exists within the plan (Ryan & Marinelli, 1990). A teaching plan is said to be internally consistent when all of its eight parts are related to one another. Adherence to the concept of internal consistency requires that the domain of learning of each objective must be consistently reflected across each of the elements of the teaching plan, from the purpose all the way through to the end process of evaluation. The following example is adapted from Ryan and Marinelli's self-study module, "Developing a Teaching Plan":

If the educator has decided to teach to the psychomotor domain, then the goal, objectives and subobjectives, related content, and so on should be reflective of the psychomotor domain.

Purpose: To provide the client with the information necessary for monitoring blood glucose

Goal: The client will demonstrate the ability to test for blood glucose on a regular basis.

Objective: Following a 20-minute teaching session, the client will be able to use a reagent strip, Chemstrip bG, to determine blood glucose level with 100% accuracy.

Subobjective: The client will be able to assemble all equipment necessary to test for blood

Figure 10–1 Sample Teaching Plan

Objectives and Subobjectives	Content Outline	Method of Instruction	Time Allotted (in min.)	Resources	Method of Evaluation

PURPOSE:
GOAL:

glucose using a reagent strip without assistance.

In the example, the purpose, goal, objective, and subobjective are reflective of the psychomotor domain, and, thus, the content, instructional method(s), instructional resource(s), time allotment, and evaluation method(s) should be appropriate to the psychomotor domain as well. This ensures internal consistency of the plan.

The decision about the number and types of objectives (reflecting one or more domains of learning) that should be included in a teaching plan must be made prior to developing the plan. If the purpose and goal are written for the accomplishment of a skill set that includes more than one domain, then the teaching plan should include one or more objectives for each domain. Important also is that the content, method(s) of teaching, and method(s) of evaluation should flow across the plan in parallel with each objective and be appropriate for accomplishing the domain of learning in each objective (see **Figure 10–2**). Thus, in the overall design of the teaching plan, internal consistency requires that all elements must match whichever domain(s) of learning has/have been selected.

In addition to determining the type (domain) of the objective to be achieved, another aspect of internal consistency identified by Ryan and Marinelli (1990) that must be considered is related to the complexity of each objective. The educator must determine the detail of the content to be taught depending on the data obtained during assessment of the learner. The client's readiness to learn, learning needs, and learning style must be taken into consideration when deciding the amount and depth of information to be taught. For example, the focus for teaching a low-level learner would be to concentrate on the need to know information. This would ensure that a skill can be performed safely without overwhelming the learner. By comparison, a high-level learner can

handle and may desire additional nice-to-know information.

Whomever the client may be, the content to be taught for each objective must be directly related to the type and complexity of that objective. If subobjectives are included in the plan, then the same rule applies; that is, the content to be taught for each subobjective must be directly related to that subobjective.

The method of instruction chosen also should be appropriate for the type and level of content being taught. If, for example, the purpose is to teach a client to clean and reassemble the continuous positive airway pressure (CPAP) device he will use to treat his sleep apnea (psychomotor domain), then the primary method of teaching that best helps with psychomotor skill development should be chosen, such as demonstration and return demonstration. Conversely, if the objective is to impart knowledge of what constitutes a low-fat diet (cognitive domain), then lecture and programmed instruction are appropriate teaching methods.

The time set aside for the teaching and learning of each objective and subobjective also must be specified. How much time is needed for instruction and acquisition of a skill depends on learner attributes, the type and complexity of the behavior, the depth of content, and the resources to be used to supplement teaching and assist with learning. Ideally, each patient teaching session should be no more than 15 to 20 minutes in length and certainly no more than 30 minutes. Audiences of staff and students can tolerate longer sessions. In this period of time, one or more objectives may be accomplished or partially accomplished. Additional teaching sessions may be required for the learner to attain expected outcomes.

The resources to be used, which refer to instructional materials and equipment needed for teaching, should appropriately match the content and teaching methodology. If the purpose is to teach breast self-examination, for example, then written

Figure 10–2 Completed Teaching Plan for Self-Administration of Insulin

PURPOSE: To provide patient with information necessary for self-administration of insulin as prescribed

GOAL: The patient will be able to perform insulin injections independently according to treatment regimen

Objectives	Content Outline	Method of Instruction	Time Allotted (in min.)	Resources	Method of Evaluation
Following a 20-minute teaching session, the patient will be able to:					
Identify the five sites for insulin injection with 100% accuracy (cognitive)	Location of five anatomical sites Rotation of sites	1:1 instruction	2	Anatomical chart	Post-testing
Demonstrate proper techniques according to procedure for drawing up insulin from a multidose vial (psychomotor)	Accepted technique according to procedure

Reading syringe unit dose markings | Demonstration Return demonstration | 5 | Alcohol sponges Sterile SQ needles and insulin syringes Multidose vial of sterile water | Observation of return demonstration |
| Give insulin to self in thigh area with 100% accuracy (psychomotor) | Procedure for injecting insulin SQ at 90° angle using aseptic technique | Demonstration Return demonstration | 10 | Human model SQ needle and syringe Multidose vial of sterile water Alcohol sponges | Observation of return demonstration |
| Express any concerns about self-administration of insulin (affective) | Summarize common concerns Exploration of feelings | Discussion | 3 | Video Written handouts | Question and answer |

or audiovisual materials or an anatomic model of the breast would be useful instructional tools. It is also important for the educator to keep in mind which resources would be an appealing, comfortable, and convenient medium for the learner. A variety of resources may be necessary to maintain the learner's attention and to serve as reinforcers of information. An important consideration is the literacy level of the learner. Giving a low-literate person technical reading materials can merely frustrate and confuse the learner and defeat the plan for teaching.

Finally, the method of evaluation should match the type and complexity of learning that are to be achieved. For example, if the learner is expected to be able to state, list, or circle (or some other low-level cognitive performance term) the three most important symptoms of a heart attack, then the evaluation method that appropriately tests that knowledge must be chosen. Evaluation methods must measure the desired learning outcomes to determine if and to what extent the learner achieved the expectations for learning.

In summary, just as with a client's care plan, all elements of a teaching plan need to hang together. Figure 10–2 is a good example of a plan that adheres to all the rules of construction. The goal is reflective of the purpose, the objectives depend on and are derived from the goal, the instructional content depends on and is appropriate to meet the objectives, the teaching methodology depends on and is related to the content, and so forth.

If, for instance, content outlined in a teaching plan is not related to any of the objectives, then the content is either unnecessary or another objective must be written as a basis for including the extra content. Likewise, if a teaching plan has no content relative to a particular stated objective or subobjective, then either additional content must be included or the objective or subobjective eliminated.

Also, during the teaching process, if the learner indicates in some way an interest in or demon-

strates a need for knowing more than an original plan addressed, then the plan should be revised accordingly. Whether a plan is adhered to or revised, it must, above all else, reflect internal consistency (see Appendix C for additional samples of completed teaching plans).

Use of Learning Contracts

The concept of learning contracts is a relatively new but increasingly popular approach to teaching and learning that can be implemented with any audience of learners—patients and their families, staff, or students. Learning contracts are "based on the principle of the learners being active partners in the teaching–learning system, rather than passive recipients of whatever it is that the teacher thinks is good for them" (Atherton, 2005, p. 1).

In the strictest sense, a contract is a formal legal agreement governing the terms of a transaction over a specified period of time between two or more parties (O'Reilly, 1994). In education, a **learning contract** is defined as a written (formal) or verbal (informal) agreement between the teacher and the learner that delineates specific teaching and learning activities that are to occur within a certain time frame. A learning contract is a mutually negotiated agreement, usually in the form of a written document drawn up by the teacher and the learner, that specifies what the learner will learn, the resources needed, how learning will be achieved and within what time allotment, and the criteria for measuring the success of the venture (Jones-Boggs, 2008; Keyzer, 1986; Knowles, Holton, & Swanson, 1998; Matheson, 2003; McAllister, 1996).

Inherent in the learning contract is the existence of some type of reward for upholding the contractual agreement (Wallace & Mundie, 1987). For patients and families, the reward may be recognition of their success in mastery of a task that facilitates moving closer to independence in self-care and a higher quality of life. For staff, the reward might be having the privilege granted to practice in a chosen setting or at an advanced level. For students, the reward might result in being allowed continued progression through a program of study. Rewards may be tangible, such as a certificate or award in recognition of successful attainment of an outcome, or intangible, such as outward praise from the teacher or an intrinsic sense of satisfaction in accomplishing a predetermined goal.

Contract learning has been introduced in education as an alternative, innovative approach to structuring a learning experience that embodies the principles of adult learning (Knowles et al., 1998). The origin of contract learning is derived from humanistic theory that acknowledges the person as an autonomous being whose efforts are continuously aimed at self-determination and self-actualization. The central view of the humanistic educational theory is that knowledge is a process, not a product (Mazhindu, 1990). As such, according to Kreider and Barry (1993), contract learning emphasizes how a body of knowledge will be acquired (process plan), not how a body of knowledge will be transmitted (content plan).

Learning contracts are considered to be an effective teaching strategy for empowering the learner because they emphasize self-direction, mutual negotiation, and mutual evaluation of established competency levels (Jones-Boggs, 2008). A number of terms have been used to describe this approach, such as independent learning, self-directed learning, and learner-centered or project-oriented learning (Chan & Chien, 2000; Lowry, 1997; Waddell & Stephens, 2000).

Knowles and colleagues (1998) describe the purpose of using learning contracts, the steps to developing a learning contract, and the guidelines for the implementation of learning contracts. He and his colleagues observed that years of research on adult learners reveal time and again that "what adults learn on their own initiative, they learn more deeply and permanently than what they learn by being taught" (p. 211).

The imposed structure of traditional education—that is, telling learners the objectives they need to work toward, what resources they are to use, how and when to use those resources, and how their accomplishments will be evaluated—conflicts with the psychological need by adults to be self-directing. Being told what, how, and when to learn something may lead to resistance, apathy, or withdrawal by the learner. This does not mean that adult learners do not need guidance or that they do not want structure or specifics, but rather that they often desire flexibility for learning and they want to be involved in decision making when it comes to planning, implementation, and evaluation of their learning.

Learning contracts stress shared accountability for learning between the teacher and the learner. The method of contract learning actively involves the learner at all stages of the teaching–learning process, from assessment of learning needs and identification of learning resources to the planning, implementation, and evaluation of learning activities.

Because learning contracts are a unique way of presenting information to the learner and are the essence of an equal and cooperative partnership, they challenge the traditional teacher–client relationship through a redistribution of power and control. Allowing learners to negotiate a contract for learning shifts the control and emphasis of the learning experience from a traditionally teacher-centered focus to a learner-centered focus. Active involvement of the learner increases feelings of commitment and fosters accountability for self-directed learning (Knowles et al., 1998; Wallace & Mundie, 1987).

The purpose of learning contracts is to encourage active participation by the learner, improve teacher–client communication, and enhance learner expressiveness and creativity. Learning contracts, whether formal or informal, can be used to facilitate personal development of the learner.

In the case of staff and students, this approach to learning can enhance professional development as well. As stated by Waddell (1998), "The use of learning contracts empowers the students to learn on their own, reflect on their strengths and weaknesses, choose learning activities which best match their learning styles, use resources effectively to promote their learning, and self-evaluate" (p. 1). Jones-Boggs (2008) goes on to say that the use of learning contracts "assists students in developing life-long learning behaviors" (p. 1480).

Learning contracts serve as a vehicle for fulfilling the internal needs of the learner and the external needs of an organization (Keyzer, 1986; Knowles, 1990). Learners have an opportunity to change behavior and reach their human potential through an approach that fosters choice and growth-promoting independence and allows for self-paced learning. Clearly defined expectations reduce learner anxiety, decrease frustration, increase levels of personal satisfaction, encourage the development of self-directed learning habits, increase the rate and quality of learning, and provide a defined basis for evaluation of the learner (Waddell, 1998).

Learning contracts also can be used to facilitate discharge of patients to the home setting. In complex cases involving the care of a patient by a large number of multidisciplinary team members, a contract provides cohesion and an excellent communication tool between the patient, family caretakers, and the healthcare team (Cady & Yoshioka, 1991).

Components of the Learning Contract

A complete learning contract includes the following four major components (Knowles, 1990; Wallace & Mundie, 1987):

1. *Content*—specifies the precise behavioral objectives to be achieved. Objectives must clearly state the desired outcomes of learning activities. Negotiation between the educator and the learner determines the content, level, and sequencing of objectives according to learner needs, abilities, and readiness.

2. *Performance expectations*—specify the conditions under which learning activities will be facilitated, such as instructional strategies and resources.

3. *Evaluation*—specifies the criteria used to evaluate achievement of objectives, such as skills checklists, care standards or protocols, and agency policies and procedures of care that identify the levels of competency expected of the learner.

4. *Time frame*—specifies the length of time needed for successful completion of the objectives. The target date for completion should reflect a reasonable period in which to achieve expected outcomes depending on the learner's abilities and circumstances.

In addition to these four components, it is important to include the terms of the contract. Role definitions describe the teacher–learner relationship with respect to clarifying the expectations and assumptions about the roles each will play. The educator is responsible for coordinating and facilitating all phases of the contract process. In the case of staff and student learning, the educator plays a major role in the selection and preparation of preceptors and acts as a resource person for both the learner and the preceptor. (See **Figure 10–3** for a sample learning contract.)

Steps to Implement the Learning Contract

Knowles and colleagues (1998) and Knowles (1990) described the steps involved in developing a learning contract with any adult learner. Wallace and Mundie (1987) also outline the steps to implement a learning contract, although they specifically address the implementation of contract learning with regard to the orientation of new staff nurses. The following steps apply to establishing and carrying out a learning contract for any type of learner:

Figure 10–3 Sample Learning Contract

| Name of Learner: _____ |
| Name of Educator: _____ |
| Name of Preceptor (if applicable): _____ |
| Date of Contract Negotiated: _____ |
| Terms of Contract: _____ |

Objectives	Activities	Evaluation	Target Date	Completion Date
Lists cognitive, affective, and psychomotor behaviors mutually agreed on and intended to be achieved	Lists teaching–learning strategies and resources to be used to achieve the objectives	Lists the criteria to be used to measure learning demonstrated	Lists a realistic time frame for achievement of expected outcome(s)	Specifies the dates that each objective is accomplished

Signatures: _____ (Learner) _____ (Educator) _____ (Preceptor)

Step 1 *Determine specific learning objectives.* Encourage the learner to identify his or her learning needs and what the learner wants to be able to do within an allotted time frame.

Step 2 *Review the contracting process.* It is vital that learners have a complete understanding of what contract learning is all about as well as their role in the process. Because learning contracts have not been widely used until recently, most people are unfamiliar with this teaching–learning strategy.

Step 3 *Identify the learning resources.* Introduce the learner to instructional resources available, such as self-study materials and audiovisual tools.

Step 4 *Assess the learner's competency level and learning needs.* The entire process of negotiation of a contract is based on the learner's current abilities and learning needs. The educator initiates the assessment of the learner and collects data primarily through interview, observation, and pretesting to formulate objectives.

Step 5 *Define roles.* Before planning learning experiences and negotiating a contract, the roles of the learner and the educator must be clearly established regarding expectations of each.

Step 6 *Plan the learning experiences.* Determine the content, learning resources to be used, the skills that must be demonstrated, and the amount of time to pursue learning through assisted study or self-study to meet the predetermined objectives.

Step 7 *Negotiate the time frame.* Based on appropriate sequencing of behaviors, from simplest to most complex, establish a target date for completion of each objective.

Step 8 *Implement the learning experience.* Take into consideration individual variations in the level of ability to do self-directed study and any other variables that may play a factor in completion of the specified learning activities. For patients, progress in learning may be influenced by changes in their health status. For staff, the constant pressures of providing patient care services may place constraints on the time available for educational activities. For any learner, the education process is influenced by readiness to learn and how well the information to be learned is organized and communicated.

Step 9 *Renegotiate.* The type and level of complexity of behavioral objectives and the target dates set forth for accomplishing these objectives may be renegotiated at any point along the continuum of the learning experience to meet the needs of the learner. Adults may change their notions about what they want to learn, how they want to learn it, and how long it will take to achieve objectives, so they should be encouraged to revise their contract as it is being carried out.

Step 10 *Evaluate.* Periodic (formative) and final (summative) evaluation of the learner's progress and the actual learning experience itself is a shared responsibility between the learner and the educator. Preestablished performance criteria, agreed on prior to the initiation of the learning process, serve as the means to ascertain achievement of outcomes based on predetermined and prenegotiated behavioral objectives.

Step 11 *Document.* Evidence of achievement of learning objectives is determined jointly by the learner and the educator (and preceptors if used for staff and students). When an objective is satisfactorily met according to written performance expectations, each party signs the date completed in the appropriate column. (See **Figure 10–4** for an example of a completed learning contract.)

The Concept of Learning Curve

Learning is an active process in which learners attempt to make sense of information that ultimately results in a change in behavior. Specifically, the concept of the **learning curve** has historically been used only to describe how long it takes for a learner to acquire a psychomotor skill. As such, it also implies the level of difficulty in achieving an outcome related to simple and complex motor skill development.

Recently, the term *learning curve* has been applied more loosely, albeit incorrectly from a theoretical perspective, to the time it takes someone to learn anything new, including cognitive and affective behaviors. It is a misnomer to use the term in describing learning of any behavior other than psychomotor. Research findings only support the use of this term in relation to psychomotor learning.

Although the learning curve concept has great potential for understanding psychomotor skill development when teaching patients, staff, or students, a thorough search of the health professions literature reveals little documentation that this concept has been applied to skill practice. Only in the last few years has reference been found in the medical literature to describe the application of this concept to the learning of surgical and other invasive techniques (Gawande, 2002). Medicine is just beginning to realize the usefulness of the

Figure 10–4 Completed Learning Contract

| Name of Learner: _____ |
| Name of Educator: _____ |
| Name of Preceptor (if applicable): _____ |
| Date of Contract Negotiated: _____ |
| Terms of Contract: Employee will increase work efficiency at place of employment by 20% within 2 months |

Objectives	Activities	Evaluation	Target Date	Completion Date
Improve time management and organizational skills to increase productivity by 20%	Read articles and books on topic Interview three managers on how to organize work and manage time Observe a productive colleague for one day, noting techniques used	Report on knowledge acquired Performance of productivity observed with feedback from observer		

Source: Adapted from Knowles, N. S., Holton, E. F., & Swanson, R. A. (1998). *The definitive classic in adult education and human resource development* (3rd ed., p. 245). Houston, TX: Gulf Publishing.

learning curve concept in determining how long it takes for physicians to become competent in performing procedures using new technologies, such as simulators, laparoscopes, or robotic instruments (Eversbusch & Grantcharov, 2004; Flamme, Stukenborg-Colsman, & Wirth, 2006; Hernandez et al., 2004; Savoldi et al., 2009).

To understand the learning curve concept as it relates to the process of teaching and learning, one must refer to educational psychology literature. Cronbach (1963) defines the learning curve, specifically related to psychomotor skill development, as "a record of an individual's improvement made by measuring his ability at different stages of practice and plotting his scores" (p. 297).

The learning curve (also sometimes referred to as the experience curve) is a phenomenon that can be applied to the analysis of learning that occurs by any individual or groups of individuals. The concept of learning curve has been adopted by business and industry to measure employee productivity. It has a direct effect on cost of labor, the time it takes to manufacture a product or deliver a service, the quality of the product or service, and the pricing of goods and services. The concept has been broadened to be used in other fields of activities because the cost of doing repetitive tasks generally decreases as experience is gained. For example, Kratzer (1995) reports on a study measuring the effectiveness of mentoring beginning teachers in their first year of practice. She concludes that the mentorship model offers a way to accelerate the learning curve of new teachers as well as to increase their longevity in the profession.

McCray and Blakemore (1985) note that the learning curve "is basically nothing more than a graphic depiction of changes in performance or output during a specified time period" (p. 5). A learning curve shows the relationship between practice and performance of a psychomotor skill and provides a concrete measure of the rate at which one or more people learn a task. In many situations, evidence of learning (improvement) follows a very productive and predictable pattern.

The theoretical learning curve is a schematic used to summarize many features of psychomotor skill acquisition, which, according to Cronbach (1963), is divided into six stages (see **Figure 10–5**):

1. *Negligible progress:* Initially very little improvement in score is detected. This prereadiness period is when the learner is not ready to perform the entire task, but relevant learning is taking place, such as developing attention, manipulation, and perceptual skills. This period can be relatively long in young children who are developing physical and cognitive abilities, as well as in older adults who may have difficulty in making key discriminations.

2. *Increasing gains:* The rate of learning increases as the learner grasps the essentials of the task. Scores rise rapidly as the learner becomes aware of cues to attend to, goals to attain, or ways to organize responses effectively. Motivation may account for rapid gains when the learner has interest in the task, receives approval from others, or experiences a sense of pride in discovering the ability to perform.

Figure 10–5 A Schematic Learning Curve

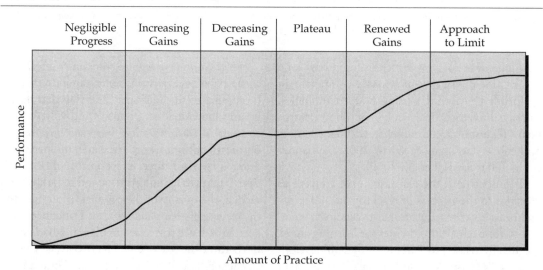

Source: Adapted from Cronbach, L. J. (1963). *Educational psychology* (2nd ed., p. 299). New York: Harcourt, Brace, & World.

3. *Decreasing gains:* The rate of improvement slows. In this period of refinement, the slowing of task mastery is inevitable because practice does not produce such steep gains. Learning occurs in smaller increments of response as the learner incorporates changes by using cues to smooth out performance.

4. *Plateau:* No substantial gains are made. This leveling off period is characterized by a negligible rate of progress in level of performance, but further gains are possible. During this stage, the learner is making small adjustments, such as modifying subskills, reducing dependence on mediators, and correcting responses to more remote cues. Plateaus are not observed in all instances, and the very idea of a period of no progress is considered false. Gains in skills can occur even though overall performance scores remain stable.

5. *Renewed gains:* The rate of performance again rises if further gains are possible. If additional progress can be made after the plateau period has ended, it usually is to the result of growth in physical development, renewed interest in the task, a response to challenge, or the drive for perfection.

6. *Approach to limit:* Progress at this point becomes negligible. The ability to perform has reached its potential. That is, no matter how much more someone practices a skill, he or she is incapable of doing any better. The limit is a hypothetical stage only because there is never certainty that a learner cannot improve further. Just as with an Olympic athlete who has broken a world record or achieved a personal best level of performance, he or she may at some point be able to exceed his or her top score.

Individual learning curves are characterized by irregularity (see **Figure 10–6**) and are often unlike the smooth theoretical curve. Fluctuations in performance can be attributed to changes in such factors as focus, interest, energy, ability, situational circumstances, or favorable/unfavorable conditions for learning (Barker, 1994; Cronbach, 1963; Gage & Berliner, 1998). The learning curve can be skewed by the reliability of the performance. As stated by Atherton (2005), "Any novice can get it right occasionally (beginner's luck), but it is consistency which counts and the progress of learning is often assessed on this basis" (p. 1). As Atherton further elaborates, it is incorrect to use the cliché "steep learning curve" to imply that something is difficult to learn. In fact, just the opposite is true. As a learner practices a difficult skill, in almost all cases, the line rises slowly, not quickly, over time. This means the steepness of the curve actually refers to the demands of the task—how many trials it takes as well as, in reality, how long it takes to master a skill—rather than the description of the process itself. In other words, a steep, short learning curve indicates that the learner was able to master a skill rapidly and easily.

Health professions research on application of the learning curve concept to the teaching and learning of psychomotor skills by patients, staff, and students must be expanded beyond medicine to other healthcare practice disciplines. Such studies would help educators to improve their understanding of the normal or expected pattern and pace of learning, assist them in recognizing the multitude of variables that affect the length of time and the ease or difficulty for any given learner to achieve an intended outcome, and aid them in choosing appropriate educational interventions based on evidence of the different stages of practice required by the learner for improvement in skill development. Research could answer such questions in patient, student, and staff education as the following:

- Can a learning curve be shortened given the characteristics of the learner, the situation, or the task at hand?
- Why is the learning curve steeper, more drawn out, or more irregular for some learners than for others?

Figure 10–6 Learning Curve During One Year of Typing Practice

Source: Adapted from Cronbach, L. J. (1963). *Educational psychology* (2nd ed., p. 303). New York: Harcourt, Brace, & World.

- Can we predict the learning curves of our patients or healthcare staff and students depending on their educational or experiential backgrounds?
- How many times on average does a particular skill need to be practiced to improve competency and ensure consistency of performance?
- What can we do from an educational standpoint to influence the pace and pattern of learning that may result in earlier or more complete achievement of expected outcomes?
- How can the learning curve concept be applied to improve staff performance, thereby increasing work satisfaction and productivity, decreasing costs of care, and improving the quality and safety of care?

These are just a few of the questions that research could attempt to answer to provide evidence as a basis for practice changes in approaches to teaching and learning by the educator in the health professions.

The implications of applying the learning curve concept to patient teaching and staff and student education are many. Perhaps one key benefit to understanding this concept is to realize that the pattern and pace of learning is irregular, not linear and even as once supposed. The learning of any task is often rapid after an initial slow start, inevitably decreases, reaches a plateau, and then increases again, until a limit is reached when likely no more significant improvement in mastery of a skill can be achieved. Understanding this phenomenon can help educators adjust their expectations or deal with their frustrations when different paces and patterns of learning occur in individuals as they attempt to master any psychomotor skill.

Awareness that learning is not linear and that the amount of practice needed to improve performance is variable can also be shared with learners to reduce their expectations and frustrations when mastering a skill. For example, a patient who is undergoing rehabilitation to learn how to walk again following a stroke or injury may easily become discouraged with the progress she is making toward the achievement of a goal. This may happen because the pace of learning may slow down or the patient may experience a time at the beginning or in the middle of the curve when she seems not to be learning at all. Educators can realistically support the learner if they understand the pace and pattern of skill development.

State of the Evidence

Educators in health care require not only knowledge and experience to teach various audiences of learners effectively, but they also need the clinical evidence to prove their teaching methods and interventions are actually effective. Evidence should be based on up-to-date research to help guide the health professional in the delivery of evidence-based care. Health professionals should identify the types of information needed in particular situations and be competent in accessing the appropriate databases to obtain the information and research necessary to carry out all aspects of the educator role. "This leads to an increased awareness for the need for appropriate information to provide best care, solve an identified clinical problem, or facilitate a change in practice" (Pierce, 2005, p. 236).

Plenty of evidence establishes the value and utility of behavioral objectives for teaching and learning. Also, numerous research studies in the psychology literature have substantiated the framework, known as the taxonomic hierarchy, for categorizing behaviors (cognitive, affective, and psychomotor) according to type (domain) and complexity (level of difficulty). Furthermore,

a body of knowledge on how to develop internally consistent teaching plans using these behavioral objectives for the purpose of legally documenting and properly implementing individual plans of care for patient education is available. These plans are mandated according to expectations set forth by accrediting bodies of healthcare agencies and organizations.

Although the use of learning contracts is a relatively new concept, evidence has been forthcoming by educational psychologists based on developmental research indicating the needs of adult learners for independent, self-directed, problem-centered, and participatory learning. However, the concept of the learning curve, although a term superficially and widely adopted by educators, has not been well defined or well explored for its theoretical application to teaching and learning in the health professions. Little evidence exists on its reliability and validity in patient, staff, and student education for psychomotor skill acquisition. It is clearly apparent more research needs to be conducted to prove that the learning curve concept is a useful principle for educators to incorporate into the process of teaching and learning.

Summary

The major portion of this chapter focuses on differentiating goals from objectives, preparing accurate and concise objectives, classifying objectives according to the three domains of learning, and the teaching of cognitive, affective, and psychomotor skills using appropriate instructional interventions. The writing of behavioral objectives as to type and complexity is fundamental to the education process. Goals and objectives serve as a guide to the educator in the planning, implementation, and evaluation of teaching and learning.

Assessment of the learner is a prerequisite to formulating objectives. Prior to selecting the content to be taught and the methods and materials to be used for instruction, there must be a clear understanding of what the learner is expected to be able to do. Appraisal should be based on a mutual determination between the educator and the client as to what needs to be learned, under what conditions learning can best occur, and the teaching and evaluation methods most preferred. Objectives setting must be a partnership effort by the learner and the educator for any learning experience to be successful and rewarding in the achievement of expected outcomes.

This chapter also outlines the development of teaching plans and learning contracts. Teaching plans provide the blueprint for organizing and presenting information in a coherent manner. Above all else, a teaching plan must reflect inter-nal consistency of its parts. Learning contracts are an innovative and unique alternative to structuring a learning experience based on adult learning principles. Contracts are designed to provide for self-directed study, thereby encouraging active involvement and accountability on the part of the learner. The communication of desired behavioral outcomes and the mechanisms for accomplishing behavioral changes in the learner are essential elements in the decision-making process with respect to both teaching and learning.

The concept of learning curve is applicable to the process of teaching and learning. It must be explored from a research perspective to yield findings for the practice of evidence-based teaching.

REVIEW QUESTIONS

1. What is the difference between the terms *educational, instructional,* and *behavioral* or *learning objectives*?
2. What two major factors distinguish goals and objectives from one another?
3. What are the definitions of the terms *goal* and *objective*?
4. Why do some educators argue against the use of behavioral objectives?
5. What five reasons justify the importance of writing clear and concise statements of expected behaviors?
6. What are the four components that should be included in every written behavioral objective?
7. What eight mistakes are commonly made when writing behavioral objectives?
8. What are the three domains of learning?
9. Which levels of behavior, according to the taxonomic form of hierarchy, are considered the most simple and the most complex in the cognitive, affective, and psychomotor domains?
10. Why is it important for the educator to remember to keep psychomotor skill instruction separate from the cognitive and affective components of skill development?
11. What five factors or variables influence the amount of practice required to learn any new skill?
12. What are the eight basic components of a teaching plan?
13. Why are learning contracts an increasingly popular approach to teaching and learning?
14. What are the four major components of a learning contract?
15. Why is the concept of the learning curve an important consideration in teaching and learning for psychomotor skill development?

CASE STUDY

Mark Vincenzo, director of the Outpatient Clinics at Lakeview Medical Center, is meeting with the members of the staff development team in the hope of gaining approval for a new class on writing behavioral objectives. "Teaching is such an important part of what we do in the clinics that it is vital that all staff are able to develop and implement well-written teaching plans." He has found that many of the staff need more detailed instruction than what currently exists in the new staff orientation, particularly in the area of constructing clear, concise, and realistic behavioral objectives. "We can't measure and document the outcomes of our teaching very well if the staff aren't writing good behavioral objectives to guide their patient teaching."

You have been asked to develop two 1-hour classes on writing behavioral objectives that will be offered to all new and current employees of the Lakeview Medical Center. The first class will cover basic information about how to formulate good objective statements. During the second class, participants will apply what they have learned by writing objectives based on case scenarios and enter them into sample teaching plans in the electronic medical record.

1. What is the goal of your new two-class program on behavioral objectives?
2. What is one objective and the related subobjectives for the first class?
3. What is one behavioral objective for the second class from each of the following domains: cognitive, affective, and psychomotor?
4. How would you classify the behavioral objectives written in question 3 according to the level of cognitive, affective, and psychomotor behavior identified?

References

Anderson, L. W., Krathwohl, D. R., Airasian, P. W., Cruikshank, K. A., Mayer, R. E., Pintrich, P. R., et al. (2001). *A taxonomy for learning, teaching, and assessing* (Rev. ed.). New York: Longman.

Arends, R. I. (1994). *Learning to teach* (3rd ed.). New York: McGraw-Hill.

Atherton, J. S. (2005). Learning contracts. Retrieved October 31, 2006, from http://www.learningandteaching.info/teaching/learningcontracts.htm

Babcock, D. E., & Miller, M. A. (1994). *Client education: Theory and practice*. St. Louis: Mosby–Year Book.

Bachman, K. (1990). Using mental imagery to practice a specific psychomotor skill. *Journal of Continuing Education in Nursing, 21*(3), 125–128.

Baldwin, D., Hill, P., & Hanson, G. (1991). Performance of psychomotor skills: A comparison of two teaching strategies. *Journal of Nursing Education, 30*(8), 367–370.

Barker, L. M. (1994). *Learning and behavior: A psychobiological perspective*. New York: Macmillan College Publishing Company.

Bell, M. L. (1991). Learning a complex nursing skill: Student anxiety and the effect of preclinical skill evaluation. *Journal of Nursing Education, 30*(5), 222–226.

Bloom, B. J., Englehart, M. S., Furst, E. J., Hill, W. H., & Krathwohl, D. R. (1956). *Taxonomy of educational objectives: The classification of educational goals. Handbook 1: Cognitive domain*. New York: David McKay.

Brottman, M. (2009, December 13). Learning to hate learning objectives. *Chronicle of Higher Education*. Retrieved December 15, 2009, from http://chronicle.com/article/Learning-to-Hate-Learning/49399/

Bucher, L. (1991). Evaluating the affective domain. *Journal of Nursing Staff Development, 7*(5), 234–238.

Cady, C., & Yoshioka, R. S. (1991). Using a learning contract to successfully discharge an infant on home total parenteral nutrition. *Pediatric Nursing, 17*(1), 67–70, 74.

Chan, S. W., & Chien, W.-T. (2000). Implementing contract learning in a clinical context: Report on a study. *Journal of Advanced Nursing, 31*(2), 298–305.

Coplan, B., Essary, A. C., Lohenry, K., & Stoehr, J. D. (2008). An update on the utilization of standardized patients in physician assistant programs. *Journal of Physician Assistant Education, 19*(4), 14–19.

Cronbach, L. J. (1963). *Educational psychology* (2nd ed.). New York: Harcourt, Brace, & World.

Cummings, C. (1994). Tips for writing behavioral objectives. *Nursing Staff Development Insider, 3*(4), 6, 8.

Damewood, S., Cadigan, B., & Jeanmonod, D. (2009). Teaching the focused assessment with sonography in trauma exam: Is the ultrasound mannequin simulator better or as good as using live models for practical training? *Annals of Emergency Medicine, 54*(3), s70.

Dave, R. (1970). *Psychomotor levels in developing and writing objectives*. Tucson, AZ: Educational Innovators Press.

Doheny, M. O. (1993). Mental practice: An alternative approach to teaching motor skills. *Journal of Nursing Education, 32*(6), 260–264.

Durbach, E., Goodall, R., & Wilkinson, K. (1987). Instructional objectives in patient education. *Nursing Outlook, 35*(2), 82–83, 88.

Eaton, S. L., & Evans, S. B. (1986). The effect of nonspecific imaging practice on the mental imagery ability of nursing students. *Journal of Nursing Education, 25*(5), 193–196.

Eggen, P. D., & Kauchak, D. P. (2001). *Strategies for teachers teaching content and thinking skills* (4th ed.). Boston: Allyn and Bacon.

Ellis, C. (1993). Incorporating the affective domain into staff development programs. *Journal of Nursing Staff Development, 9*(3), 127–130.

Evans, A. E., Edmunson-Drane, E. W., & Harris, K. K. (2000). Computer-assisted instruction: An effective instructional method for HIV prevention? *Journal of Adolescent Health, 26,* 244–251.

Eversbusch, A., & Grantcharov, T. P. (2004). Learning curves and impact of psychomotor training on performance in simulated colonoscopy: A randomized trial using virtual reality endoscopy trainer. *Surgical Endoscopy, 18*(10), 1514–1518.

Ferguson, L. M. (1998). Writing learning objectives. *Journal of Nursing Staff Development, 14*(2), 87–94.

Flamme, C. H., Stukenborg-Colsman, C., & Wirth, C. J. (2006). Evaluation of the learning curves associated with uncemented primary total hip arthroplasty depending on the experience of the surgeon. *HIP International, 16*(3), 191–197.

Ford, G. S., Mazzone, M. A., & Taylor, K. (2005). Effects of computer-assisted instruction versus traditional modes of instruction on student learning of musculoskeletal tests. *Journal of Physical Therapy Education, 19*(2), 22–30.

Gage, N. L., & Berliner, D. C. (1998). *Educational psychology* (6th ed.). Boston: Houghton Mifflin.

Gawande, A. (2002, January 28). The learning curve. Annals of medicine. *The New Yorker,* 52–61.

Gomez, G. E., & Gomez, E. A. (1984). The teaching of psychomotor skills in nursing. *Nurse Educator, 9*(4), 35–39.

Gomez, G. E., & Gomez, E. A. (1987). Learning of psychomotor skills: Laboratory versus patient care setting. *Journal of Nursing Education, 26*(1), 20–24.

Goulet, C., & Owen-Smith, P. (2005). Cognitive-affective learning in physical therapy education: From implicit to explicit. *Journal of Physical Therapy Education, 19*(3), 67–72.

Gronlund, N. E. (1985). *Stating objectives for classroom instruction* (3rd ed.). New York: Macmillan.

Gronlund, N. E. (2004). *Writing instructional objectives for teaching and assessment.* (7th ed.). Upper Saddle River, NJ: Pearson Merrill Prentice Hall.

Haggard, A. (1989). *Handbook of patient education.* Rockville, MD: Aspen.

Harrow, A. J. (1972). *A taxonomy of the psychomotor domain: A guide for developing behavioral objectives.* New York: David McKay.

Hayward, L., Blackmer, B., & Markowski, A. (2006). Standardized patients and communities of practice: A realistic strategy for integrating core values in a physical therapist education program. *Journal of Physical Therapy Education, 20*(2), 29–37.

Heinich, R., Molenda, M., Russell, J., & Smaldino, S. (2001). *Instructional methods and technologies for learning* (7th ed.). Upper Saddle River, NJ: Prentice Hall.

Hernandez, J. D., Bann, S. D., Munz, Y., Moorthy, K., Datta, V., Martin, S., et al. (2004). Qualitative and quantitative analysis of the learning curve of a simulated surgical task on the da Vinci system. *Surgical Endoscopy, 18*(3), 372–378.

Jones-Boggs, K. (2008). Perceived benefits of the use of learning contracts to guide clinical education in respiratory care students. *Respiratory Care, 53,* 1475–1481.

Keyzer, D. (1986). Using learning contracts to support change in nursing organizations. *Nurse Education Today, 6*(8), 103–108.

Knowles, M. (1990). *The adult learner: A neglected species* (4th ed.). Houston, TX: Gulf.

Knowles, M. S., Holton, E. F., & Swanson, R. A. (1998). *The definitive classic in adult education and human resource development* (3rd ed.). Houston, TX: Gulf.

Krathwohl, D. R., Bloom, B. J., & Masia, B. B. (1964). *Taxonomy of educational objectives: The classification of educational goals. Handbook II: The affective domain.* New York: David McKay.

Kratzer, C. C. (1995, April). *Reflective practice in a community of beginning teachers: Implementing the STEP program.* Paper presented at the annual meeting of the American Educational Research Association, San Francisco, CA.

Kreider, M. C., & Barry, M. (1993). Clinical ladder development: Implementing contract learning. *Journal of Continuing Education in Nursing, 24*(4), 166–169.

Lee, J., Triola, M., Gillespie, C., Gourevitch, M. N., Hanley, K., Truncali, A., et al. (2008). Working with patients with alcohol problems: A controlled trial of the impact of rich media Web module on medical student performance. *Journal of Medical and Internal Medicine, 23,* 1006–1009.

Love, B., McAdams, C., Patton, D. M., Rankin, E. J., & Roberts, J. (1989). Teaching psychomotor skills in nursing: A randomized controlled trial. *Journal of Advanced Nursing, 14*(11), 970–975.

Lowry, M. (1997). Using learning contracts in clinical practice. *Professional Nurse, 12*(4), 280–283.

Mager, R. F. (1997). *Preparing instructional objectives* (3rd ed.). Atlanta, GA: Center for Effective Performance.

Maier-Lorentz, M. M. (1999). Writing objectives and evaluating learning in the affective domain. *Journal for Nurses in Staff Development, 15*(4), 167–171.

Marks, R. (2009). Ethics and patient education: Health literacy and cultural dilemmas. *Health Promotion Practice, 10,* 328–332.

Matheson, R. (2003). Promoting the integration of theory and practice by the use of a learning contract. *International Journal of Therapy and Rehabilitation, 10*(6), 264–270.

Mazhindu, G. N. (1990). Contract learning reconsidered: A critical examination of implications for application in nurse education. *Journal of Advanced Nursing, 15*(1), 101–109.

McAllister, M. (1996). Learning contracts: An Australian experience. *Nurse Education Today, 16*(3), 199–205.

McCray, P., & Blakemore, T. (1985). *A guide to learning curve technology to enhance performance prediction in vocational evaluation.* Menomonie, WI: Research and Training Center, Stout Vocational and Rehabilitation Institute, School of Education and Human Services, University of Wisconsin–Stout.

Menix, K. D. (1996). Domains of learning: Interdependent components of achievable learning outcomes. *Journal of Continuing Education in Nursing, 27*(5), 200–208.

Miracle, D. J. (1999). Teaching psychomotor skills in simulated learning labs. In K. R. Stevens and V. R. Cassidy (Eds.), *Evidence-based teaching: Current research in nursing education* (pp. 71–103). Sudbury, MA: Jones and Bartlett.

Moore, M. R. (1970). The perceptual-motor domain and a proposed taxonomy of perception. *Audio Communications Review, 18,* 379–413.

Morrison, G. R., Ross, S. M., & Kemp, J. E. (2004). *Designing effective instruction* (4th ed.). Hoboken, NJ: Wiley.

Nothwehr, F., Dennis, L., & Wu, H. (2007). Measurement of behavioral objectives for weight management. *Health Education and Behavior, 34,* 793–807.

Oermann, M. H. (1990). Psychomotor skill development. *Journal of Continuing Education in Nursing, 21*(5), 202–204.

O'Reilly, D. (1994). Communication and effective learning: Negotiated study and learning contracts. *Nursing Times, 90*(9), i–viii.

Page, S. J., Levine, P., & Khourey, J. (2009). Modified constraint induced therapy combined with mental practice: Think through better motor outcomes. *Stroke, 40*(2), 551–554.

Page, S. J., Levine, P., Sisto, S. A., & Johnston, M. V. (2001). Mental practice with physical practice for upper-limb motor deficit in subacute stroke. *Physical Therapy, 81,* 1455–1462.

Pierce, S. T. (2005). Integrating evidence-based practice into nursing curricula. In M. H. Oermann and K. T. Heinrich (Eds.), *Annual review of nursing education strategies for teaching, assessment, and program planning* (3rd ed., pp. 233–248). New York: Springer.

Reilly, D. E., & Oermann, M. H. (1990). *Behavioral objectives: Evaluation in nursing* (3rd ed.). Pub. No. 15–2367. New York: National League for Nursing.

Rinne, C. (1987). The affective domain: Equal opportunity in nursing education. *Journal of Continuing Education in Nursing, 18*(2), 40–43.

Ryan, M., & Marinelli, T. (1990). Developing a teaching plan. Unpublished self-study module, College of Nursing, State University of New York Health Science Center at Syracuse.

Savoldi, G. L., Schiffer, E., Abegg, C., Baeriswyl, V., Clerique, F., & Weber, J. (2009). Learning curves of the Glidescope, the McGrath, and the Airtraq laryngoscopes: A manekin study. *European Journal of Anaesthesiology, 26,* 554–558.

Schoenly, L. (1994). Teaching in the affective domain. *Journal of Continuing Education in Nursing, 25*(5), 209–212.

Shirai, Y., Shiraishi, R., Okamoto, T., Nakamura, H., Harada, T., Nishikawa, J., & Sakaida, I. (2008). Prospective randomized study on the use of computer based endoscopy simulator for training in esophogastroduodenoscopy. *Journal of Gastroenterology and Hepatology, 23,* 1046–1050.

Simpson, E. J. (1972). The classification of educational objectives in the psychomotor domain. In M. T. Rainier

(Ed.), *Contributions of behavioral science to instructional technology: The psychomotor domain* (3rd ed.). Englewood Cliffs, NJ: Gryphon Press, Prentice Hall.

Tong, R. (2007). *New perspectives in health care ethics: An interdisciplinary and crosscultural approach.* Upper Saddle River, NJ: Pearson Education.

Waddell, D. L. (1998). Facilitating independent study through learning contracts. *National Student Nurses' Association Dean's Notes, 19*(5), 1–3.

Waddell, D. L., & Stephens, S. (2000). Use of learning contracts in a RN-to-BSN leadership course. *Journal of Continuing Education in Nursing, 31*(4), 179–184.

Wallace, P. L., & Mundie, G. E. (1987). Contract learning in orientation. *Journal of Nursing Staff Development, 3*(4), 143–149.

Willingham, D. T. (2002, Summer). Allocating student study time: "Massed" versus "distributed" practice. *American Educator,* 37–39, 47.

Willingham, D. T. (2004, Spring). Practice makes perfect—but only if you practice beyond the point of perfection. *American Educator,* 31–33, 38.

Yoder, M. E. (1993). Computer use and nursing research: Transfer of cognitive learning to a clinical skill: Linear versus interactive video. *Western Journal of Nursing Research, 15*(1), 115–117.

Zimmerman, B. J., & Phillips, C. Y. (2000). Affective learning: Stimulus to critical thinking and caring practice. *Journal of Nursing Education, 39*(9), 422–425.

Chapter 11

Instructional Methods and Settings

Kathleen Fitzgerald

CHAPTER HIGHLIGHTS

Instructional Methods
    Lecture
    Group Discussion
    One-to-One Instruction
    Demonstration and Return Demonstration
    Gaming
    Simulation
    Role-Playing
    Role Modeling
    Self-Instruction

Selection of Instructional Methods
Evaluation of Instructional Methods
Increasing Effectiveness of Teaching
    Techniques to Enhance the Effectiveness of
    Verbal Presentations
    General Principles for Teaching Across
    Methodologies
Instructional Settings
    Sharing Resources Among Settings
State of the Evidence

KEY TERMS

- ❏ instructional strategy
- ❏ instructional method
- ❏ lecture
- ❏ group discussion
- ❏ one-to-one instruction
- ❏ demonstration
- ❏ return demonstration
- ❏ gaming
- ❏ simulation

- ❏ role-playing
- ❏ role modeling
- ❏ self-instruction
- ❏ skill inoculation
- ❏ pacing
- ❏ instructional setting
- ❏ healthcare setting
- ❏ healthcare-related setting
- ❏ non-healthcare setting

The information on instructional settings in this chapter was taken directly from Virginia E. O'Halloran's Chapter 14, Instructional Settings, in S. B. Bastable (2003), *Nurse as educator: Principles of teaching and learning for nursing practice* (2nd ed., pp. 465–492). Sudbury, MA: Jones and Bartlett.

OBJECTIVES

After completing this chapter, the reader will be able to

1. Define the term *instructional method*.
2. Explain the various types of instructional methods.
3. Describe how to use each method effectively.
4. Identify the advantages and limitations of each method.
5. Discuss the variables that influence the selection of the various methods.
6. Recognize techniques to enhance teaching effectiveness.
7. Explain how to evaluate instructional methods.
8. Classify instructional settings according to the primary purpose of the organization or agency in which the health professional functions as educator.

After an excellent presentation, you might have heard someone comment, "Now, there is a born teacher!" This comment would seem to indicate that effective teaching comes automatically. In reality, teaching effectively is a learned skill. Development of this skill requires knowledge of the educational process, including the instructional methods to use with different audiences in a variety of settings.

Stimulating and effective educational experiences are designed, not accidental. **Instructional strategy** is the overall plan for a teaching–learning experience that involves the use of one or several methods of instruction to achieve the desired learning outcomes (Rothwell & Kazanas, 2004).

An **instructional method** is the way information is taught that brings the learner into contact with what is to be learned. Some examples of methods are lecture, group discussion, one-to-one instruction, demonstration and return demonstration, gaming, simulation, role-playing, role modeling, and self-instruction modules. As the use of technology evolves, these methods may be incorporated into Internet-based courses (Cook et al., 2008).

Instructional materials or tools, on the other hand, are the objects or vehicles to transmit information that supplement the act of teaching. An audience response system (ARS), books, videos, and posters are examples of materials and tools used as adjuncts to communicate information (see Chapter 12). It is important to draw this distinction between the terms *instructional methods* and *instructional materials* because they often are used interchangeably by educators and not dealt with as distinctly separate entities, which they should be when planning an educational activity.

This chapter reviews the types of instructional methods available and considers how to choose and use them most efficiently and effectively. In doing so, the advantages and limitations of each method, the variables influencing the selection of various methods, and the approaches for evaluating the methods are identified to improve the delivery of instruction. Because the health professional is expected to teach many different audiences in all types of situations and circumstances, this chapter provides examples throughout in the application of these instructional methods to enhance teaching and learning experiences. Settings in which the health professional educator functions also are highlighted.

Instructional Methods

There is no one perfect method for teaching all learners in all settings. Also, no one method is necessarily more effective for changing behavior in any of the three learning domains (see Chaper 10). Whatever the method chosen, to optimize learning it usually is most effective if used in conjunction with other instructional techniques and tools.

Employing a variety of instructional methods and materials improves retention rates and positively affects learner outcomes (Ridley, 2007). The importance of selecting appropriate methods to meet the needs of learners should not be underestimated. The popular Chinese proverb "Tell me, I forget. Show me, I remember. Involve me, I understand." (author unknown) clearly implies that information retention rates vary with different teaching methods and that using alternative approaches for interactive teaching has the potential to improve learning outcomes (Ridley, 2007).

The health professional as educator functions in a vital role of facilitator by providing guidance and support for learning (Musinski, 1999). Even though a teacher may rely on one teaching method predominantly, the teacher rarely adheres to that single method in a pure fashion and often uses it in combination with various methods. For example, a teacher may use the lecture as the primary format and intersperse opportunities for question and answer periods and short discussion sessions throughout the lecture.

Decisions about which methods to use must be based on a consideration of such major factors as the following:

- Audience characteristics (size, diversity, learning style preferences)
- Educator's expertise
- Objectives of learning

- Potential for achieving learning outcomes
- Cost effectiveness
- Instructional setting
- Evolving technology

These many variables are addressed in the following review of the instructional methods available for teaching and learning.

Lecture

Lecture can be defined as a highly structured method by which the teacher verbally transmits information directly to a group of learners for the purpose of instruction. It is one of the oldest and most often used approaches to teaching.

The word *lecture* comes from the Latin term *lectura*, which means "to read." The lecture method has been much maligned in recent years because in its purest form, the lecture format allows for only minimal exchange between the teacher and the learner. Also, critics of the lecture method have expressed particular concern about the passive role of learners (DeYoung, 2003). However, as Brookfield (2006) points out, "An abused method calls into question the expertise of those abusing it, not the validity of the method itself" (p. 99).

Thus, if a lecture is well organized and delivered effectively, it can be a very useful method of instruction (Bain, 2004; Bartlett, 2003; Brookfield, 2006; Woodring & Woodring, 2007). The lecture format can demonstrate patterns, highlight main ideas, or present unique ways of viewing information, such as introducing an agency's mission statement to new health professional staff orientees or explaining diabetes mellitus to a group of lay people. The lecture should not be employed, however, to give people the same information that they could read independently at another time and place. It is the lecturer's expertise, both in theory and experience, that can substantially contribute to the learner's understanding of a subject.

The lecture is an ideal way to provide foundational background information as a basis for subsequent group discussions. Also, it is a means to summarize data and current research findings not available elsewhere (Boyd, Gleit, Graham, & Whitman, 1998; Brookfield, 2006). In addition, the health professional educator can easily supplement the lecture with handout materials and other audiovisual aids. **Table 11–1** summarizes the main advantages and limitations of the lecture method of instruction.

Lecturing is an acquired skill learned over time, and it is a more complex task than commonly thought (Young & Diekelmann, 2002). Specific strategies exist to strengthen the effectiveness of a lecture (Cantillon, 2003).

According to Silberman (1990), five approaches to the effective transfer of knowledge during a lecture are the following:

- *Use an opening summary.* At the beginning of the lecture, present major points and conclusions to help students organize their listening.

- *Present key terms.* Reduce the major points in the lecture to key words that act as verbal subheadings or memory aids.
- *Offer examples.* When possible, provide real-life illustrations of the ideas in the lecture.
- *Use analogies.* If possible, make a comparison between the content of the lecture and knowledge the students already have.
- *Use visual backups.* Use a variety of media to enable students to see as well as hear what is being said.

Each lecture should include three main parts: introduction, body, and conclusion. These three parts are described as follows (Miller & Stoeckel, 2011; Woodring & Woodring, 2007).

INTRODUCTION

During the introduction phase of a lecture, the lecturer should present learners with an overview

---

Table 11–1 MAJOR ADVANTAGES AND LIMITATIONS OF LECTURE

ADVANTAGES

- An efficient, cost-effective means for transmitting large amounts of information to a large number of people at the same time and within a relatively reasonable time frame.
- Useful to demonstrate patterns, highlight main ideas, summarize data, and present unique ways of viewing information.
- An effective approach for cognitive learning, especially at lower levels of the cognitive domain.
- Useful in providing foundational background information as a basis for subsequent learning, such as group discussion.
- Easily supplemented with handout materials and other audiovisual aids to enhance learning.

LIMITATIONS

- Largely ineffective in influencing affective and psychomotor behaviors.
- Does not provide for much stimulation or participatory involvement of learners.
- Very instructor centered, and thus the most active participant is frequently the most knowledgeable one—the teacher.
- Does not account for individual differences in background, attention span, or learning style.
- All learners are exposed to the same information regardless of their cognitive abilities, learning needs, or stages of coping.
- The diversity within groups makes it challenging, if not impossible, for the teacher to reach all learners equally.

of the behavioral objectives pertinent to the lecture topic, along with an explanation as to why these objectives are significant. The use of set, the opening to a presentation, can engage attention and focus the group on the speaker, which gets learners ready to listen. This technique of set captures attention, clarifies goals and objectives, motivates the learner, and demonstrates the relevance of the content in a way that can stimulate the interest of learners in the subject. For example, prior to a lecture on creative problem solving, the speaker can ask each member of the audience to solve a puzzle that requires them to think in a different manner (Kowalski, 2004). Lecturers can also engage learners' attention by conducting an informal survey or stating the objectives as questions that will be answered during the body of the lecture.

If the occasion is one of a series of lectures, the lecturer needs to make a connection with the overall subject and the topic being presented as well as its relationship to previous topics covered and the lectures that will follow. And lastly, the lecturer should establish a rapport with the audience by letting his or her personality shine through and by using humor, if appropriate.

Body

The next portion of the lecture involves the actual delivery of the content related to the topic being addressed. Careful preparation is needed so that the important aspects are covered in an organized, accurate, logical, cohesive, and interesting manner. Examples should be used throughout to enhance the salient points, but extraneous facts and redundant examples should be avoided so as not to reduce the impact of the message. Because the lecture format tends to be a passive approach to learning, the instructor can enhance the effectiveness of the presentation by combining it with other instructional methods, such as discussion or question and answer sessions, to enhance active learner participation.

Conclusion

The instructor should always include a wrap-up with every lecture. This final section of the lecture format is reserved to summarize the information provided in the presentation. At this juncture, the speaker can review the major concepts presented. Try to leave some leeway for questions and answers. Lecturers who use a microphone in a large group should be sure to repeat the questions asked so that the rest of the audience can hear them and understand the response. If time runs short, the instructor can answer only a few queries, but he or she should invite immediate follow-up by meeting with interested individuals alone or in a smaller group or by suggesting relevant readings.

The educator's speaking skills also are important to the delivery of a lecture. According to Jacobs (2009), the following variables of speech need to be considered:

Volume
Rate
Pitch/tone
Pronunciation
Enunciation
Proper grammar
Avoid annoying habits such as the use of "ums"

Not only are speaking skills important, but body language should be considered. Presentation skills that lecturers can employ are the following:

Demonstrate enthusiasm
Make frequent eye contact with audience
Use posture and movement
• Convey self-confidence
• Convey professionalism
Use gestures
• Avoid repetitive movement
• Rely on head and hands to emphasize points and to keep the audience's attention

Nervous or inexperienced educators should practice first before a mirror, a video camera, or a colleague (Germano, 2003). They should outline just the key points of their presentation on index cards, overhead projections, or PowerPoint slides. They can use this summary information to elaborate on the topic by giving examples and further explanations. Reading a printed copy of the entire presentation word for word is exceedingly boring and is a sure way to turn off the audience. Speakers should address a large audience as if speaking to an individual listener (Woodring & Woodring, 2007). Also, instructors should move around the stage or room and vary their presentation style and tone of voice to avoid monotony. Demonstrating enthusiasm, expertise, and interest in the topic captures and holds the group's attention. Finally, instructors should be sure to keep within the time allotted. Lectures of long duration can result in loss of attention and boredom on the part of the learners.

The use of audiovisual materials, such as a video, a podcast, or PowerPoint slides, can also add variety to a lecture. The widespread availability of technology makes it easy to enhance a presentation. When developing PowerPoint slides educators should adhere to the following general guidelines (Evans, 2000):

- Do not put all content on slides, but include only the key concepts to supplement the presentation.
- Use the largest font possible.
- Do not exceed 25 words per slide.
- Choose colors that provide a high level of contrast between background and text if presenting in a large room with bright lights.
- Use graphics for presenting large amounts of numerical data.
- Do not overdo the use of animation, which can be very distracting to the audience.

Overall, it is important to keep the following in mind: Make sure that the visual aids are large enough and positioned well enough for all to see, and keep them simple and easy to understand (Jacobs, 2009).

With technology, lectures are being delivered to an even wider variety of learners in locations remote from one another. Distance learning is an ideal way to maximize resources and to transmit current information to people separated by space and time. The cost, time, and inconvenience of travel no longer can keep an audience from meeting face-to-face with an expert (Cook et al., 2008).

Although the lecture method is considered efficient and cost effective, the effort put into design and delivery should not be determined just by calculating the teacher–learner ratio of contact hours. Educators must take into consideration other factors, such as teacher preparation time, how often the same material needs to be repeated to different audiences, and follow-up time required to individualize learning and evaluate outcomes.

Group Discussion

Group discussion, by definition, is a method of teaching whereby learners get together to exchange information, feelings, and opinions with one another and with the teacher. Also known as guided, collaborative, small-group, or cooperative learning, the benefits of group discussion are that it leads to a deeper understanding and a longer retention of information, increased social support, greater transfer of learning from one situation to another, more positive interpersonal relationships, more favorable attitudes toward learning, and more active learner participation (Brookfield, 2006; Johnson, Johnson, & Smith, 2007; Oakley & Brent, 2004; Springer, Stanne, & Donovan, 1999). As a commonly employed instructional technique, this method is learner centered as well as subject centered. Group discussion is an effective method for teaching in both the affective and cognitive domains (Springer et al., 1999).

Group size, a major consideration in group teaching, should be determined by the purpose or task to be accomplished (Boyd et al., 1998). Group size can vary somewhat but discussion is most effective with relatively small groups because more learners can take an active role (DeYoung, 2003). For client education, 2–20 members with an average of 10 has been recommended as the most desirable size (Tang, Funnell, & Anderson, 2006).

Preset behavioral objectives should be the focus when using this method. These objectives guide the achievement of the learning outcomes for the interaction and should be presented at the beginning of each session. Careful adherence to them will prevent the discussion from becoming an aimless wandering of ideas or a forum for the strongest group member to expound on his or her opinions and feelings (Billings & Halstead, 2009). The group, functioning as a "dynamic whole," motivates its members to move toward accomplishing one or more common goals (Johnson et al., 2007). The teacher's role is to act as a facilitator to keep the discussion focused and to tie important points together. The instructor must be well versed in the subject matter to field questions, to move the discussion along in the direction intended, and to give appropriate feedback (Miller & Stoeckel, 2011).

Teacher involvement and control of the process vary with the needs of the group members. Group discussion requires the teacher to be able to tolerate less structure and organization than other methods such as lecture or one-to-one instruction. The group must have some knowledge of the content before this method can be effective (Billings & Halstead, 2009); otherwise, the discussion will be based on pooled ignorance. For example, a group of staff with a significant amount of practical knowledge and expertise may need little input while they work out a complex client problem. A new group of clients or family members with little

understanding of a topic will need to access information directly from the teacher or another source before they can meaningfully participate in problem solving integral to the discussion process.

The teacher's responsibility is to make sure that every member of the group has interpreted information correctly, because failure to do so will lead to conclusions based on faulty data. For this reason, client groups need to be prescreened. While diversity within a group is beneficial, a large range in literacy skills, states of anxiety, and experiences with acute and chronic conditions may lead to difficulty in meeting any one member's needs.

Abruzzese (1996) suggests some learning techniques as good vehicles for active learning that require preparation by staff prior to the group discussion activity. For example, debates offer teams with opposing views the opportunity to present each side of an issue and help staff consider others' perspectives. Seminars can be designed so that each member reads an assignment and considers questions prior to the discussion so that all learners can actively participate. The case study approach offers an opportunity to thoroughly become acquainted with a client situation before discussing client needs and identifying health-related problems. Another example of the creative use of this teaching method with staff is arranging a panel presentation by clients coping with a specific disease or problem. Following the panel, a group session is most beneficial, in particular, for affective learning. This was found to be a useful approach for some healthcare workers to break down their negative stereotypes of persons living with AIDS (Peters & Connell, 1991).

Carkhuff (1996), Musolino and Mostrom (2005), and Wainwright, Shepard, Harman, and Stephens (2010) address the reflection-on-action technique for work groups as learning groups to develop the critical thinking skills of health professional staff in the workplace. The educator facilitates staff to critically analyze their actions and determine whether there is an alternative to their action. It is an approach that helps learners learn to learn.

It is important for the teacher to maintain the trust of the group. Everyone must feel safe and comfortable enough to express his or her point of view. Harsh or sarcastic treatment resulting in insults breaks down the relationship between the teacher and the learners as well as relationships among learners, which creates an environment unsuitable for learning. One helpful approach is for the educator to tell the group at the beginning of the session that the goal is to hear from all members by asking for their input and points of view during the discussion period. Persons who digress should be requested to hold questions that can be handled privately until the end of class because these inquiries are important but unique to their circumstances.

Respectful attention and tolerance toward others should be modeled by the teacher and required of all group members. Of course, this consideration does not preclude correcting errors or disagreements. A clear message must be given stating that while personal opinions may be debatable, the inherent value of what each member has to say and the member's right to participate are guaranteed (Ridley, 2007).

Teaching people in groups rather than individually allows the teacher to reach a number of learners at the same time. The group discussion method is economically beneficial from a time-efficiency perspective when compared with educating each learner individually. With healthcare costs rising, this method should be considered as an efficient and effective method to teach simultaneously a number of individuals who have similar learning needs, such as information to prepare for childbirth or cardiac bypass surgery. Oermann (2003) reports that a group of clients in a waiting room of an ambulatory care center were educated via a videotape about glaucoma, which was then followed by group interaction with a patient educator to discuss key points and answer questions. This approach led to higher satisfaction with the education received during their visit.

Discussion is effective in assisting learners to identify resources and to internalize the topic being discussed by helping them to reflect on its personal meaning (Brookfield & Preskill, 1999). Through group work, members share common concerns and receive reinforcement from one another. The idea that "everyone is in the same boat" or "if one person can do it, so can the others" serves to stimulate motivation for learning as a result of peer support.

Group discussion has proved particularly helpful to clients and families dealing with chronic illness. This method is most effective during the accommodation stage of psychological adjustment to chronic illness, because the interactions reduce isolation and foster identification with others who are in similar circumstances (Fredette, 1990). Discussion in a group offers members a forum in which to share information for cognitive growth as well as an opportunity to learn self-efficacy. This increase in confidence levels of clients and families enhances their ability to handle an illness (Lorig & Gonzalez, 1993).

Group process informs people about how to respond to situations, improve their coping mechanisms, and explore ways to incorporate needed changes into their lives. Group self-management education for people with diabetes has been found in some instances to be not only more cost effective but to result in greater treatment satisfaction and to be slightly better in supporting lifestyle changes (Tang et al., 2006). **Table 11–2** highlights the main advantages and limitations of group discussion as a method of instruction.

It must be noted that third-party reimbursement for some types of group client education programs may be difficult to obtain when the traditional fee-for-service payment system is not in place. However, these programs may be economically valuable in preventing hospitalization or reducing time in acute care. Documenting these

Table 11–2 Major Advantages and Limitations of Group Discussion

ADVANTAGES

- Enhances learning in both the affective and cognitive domains.
- Is both learner centered and subject centered.
- Stimulates learners to think about issues and problems.
- Encourages members to exchange their own experiences, thereby making learning more active and less isolating.
- Provides opportunities for sharing of ideas and concerns.
- Fosters positive peer support and feelings of belonging.
- Reinforces previous learning.

LIMITATIONS

- One or more members may dominate the discussion.
- Easy to digress from the topic, which interferes with achievement of the objectives.
- Shy learners may refuse to become involved or may need a great deal of encouragement to participate.
- Requires skill to tactfully redirect learners who digress or dominate without losing their trust and that of other group members.
- Particularly challenging for the novice teacher when members do not easily interact.
- More time consuming for transmission of information than other methods such as lecture.
- Requires teacher's presence at all sessions to act as facilitator and resource person.

benefits based on measurable outcomes can justify the importance of group discussion as a cost-effective method of instruction.

One-to-One Instruction

One-to-one instruction, given formally, or informally, involves face-to-face delivery of information specifically designed to meet the needs of an individual learner. It is the most common method used for client education (Haggard, 1989). Formal one-to-one instruction is a planned activity whereas informal one-to-one instruction is an unplanned interaction, such as a "teachable moment," that occurs unexpectedly when the client demonstrates a readiness to learn (Miller & Stoeckel, 2011). It is an opportunity for both the teacher and the learner to communicate knowledge, ideas, and feelings primarily through oral exchange, although nonverbal messages can be conveyed as well. Thus, this method of teaching is a process of mutual inter-

change between the client and the health professional. It requires interpersonal skill and sensitivity on the part of the educator and the ability to establish rapport with the learner (Falvo, 2004). This method should never be a lecture delivered to an audience of one to meet the teacher's goals. Instead, the experience should actively involve the learner and be based on his or her unique learning needs. Ideally, a one-to-one teaching session should be about 15 to 20 minutes in length, and educators should offer information in small, bite-sized portions to allow time for processing (Haggard, 1989). Research shows that the more information given at any one time, the less it is remembered and correctly recalled. Thus effective communication depends more on the quality of the information presented than the quantity to increase adherence to and client participation with a recommended plan of care (Kessels, 2003).

One-to-one instruction can be tailored to meet objectives in all three domains of learning.

It begins with an assessment of the learner and the mutual setting of objectives to be accomplished (Burkhart, 2008). As part of the assessment process, it is very important to determine whether any problem behaviors exist, such as smoking, and at which stage of change the person is with respect to dealing with such behaviors. Once this information is determined, the educator can tailor educational interventions to that stage (Prochaska, DiClemente, Velicer, & Rossi, 1993). The stages of change model (as described in Chapter 6) is generalizable across a broad range of behaviors, including but not limited to smoking cessation, weight control, avoidance of high-fat diets, safer sex, and exercise initiation (Prochaska et al., 1994). The following describes how health professional educators can focus their interactions to help a learner through the stages of change (Saarmann, Daugherty, & Riegel, 2000):

- *Precontemplation stage*—provide information in a nonthreatening manner so that the learner becomes aware of the negative aspects or consequences of his or her behavior.
- *Contemplation stage*—support decision making for change by identifying benefits, considering barriers to the change, and making suggestions for dealing with these obstacles.
- *Preparation stage*—support a move to action by contracting with the learner in establishing small, realistic, and measurable goals; providing information on effective ways to achieve the desired change; and giving positive reinforcement.
- *Action stage*—encourage constant practice of the new behavior to instill commitment to change by pointing out the benefits of each step achieved, providing rewards and incentives, and assisting the learner to monitor his or her behavior through the implementation of such strategies as keeping a food diary.
- *Maintenance stage*—continue encouragement and support to consolidate the new behavior and prevent relapses.

For example, the client with a chronic problem such as obesity must consider the options available for weight control and then an action plan he thinks can be accomplished can be designed. His confidence level can be assessed by asking on a scale of 0–10 how certain he is of achieving this goal. A score of 7 or higher makes it more likely he will be successful (Lorig, 2003).

Mutual goal setting is a very important first step to be undertaken between the teacher and the learner. Contracting, which clearly spells out the roles and expectations of both teacher and learner, is one effective way to facilitate mutual goal setting. Contracts should be written in specific terms and evaluated by both participants. (See an explanation of learning contracts in Chapter 10.)

Whenever teaching is done on a one-to-one basis, instructions should be specific and time should be given for an immediate response from the learner followed by direct feedback from the teacher. Allowing learners the opportunity to state their understanding of information gives the teacher an opportunity to evaluate the extent of learning. Also, communicating to learners what further information is forthcoming allows them to connect what they have just learned with what they will be learning (Falvo, 2004). For example, the health professional teaching a client about hypoglycemia might say, "Now that you understand what causes low blood sugar, we will talk about how to tell when you have it and what to do if you experience it after discharge."

The process of one-to-one instruction involves moving learners from repeating the information that was shared to applying what they have just learned. In the preceding example regarding hypoglycemia, the health professional might offer the learner a hypothetical situation similar to what the client might experience given his lifestyle and have him work through how to respond to it. In this type of one-to-one exchange, a potentially threatening situation can be presented in a nonthreatening manner (Boyd et al., 1998).

For instance, the instructor might ask a busy executive who has diabetes how he would respond to feeling shaky and sweaty at 2:00 p.m. on a day when a meeting runs late and he misses lunch.

Educators should be sure to clearly state that scenarios like this are not a test but rather a "dress rehearsal" for life situations. They can change the scenarios with further questioning to help learners plan how they could prevent such occurrences in the future. This technique gives learners a chance to use the information at a higher cognitive level and provides an opportunity for the health professional as educator to evaluate the client's learning in a safe environment.

With the one-to-one method of instruction, questioning is an excellent technique. It encourages learners to be active participants in the learning process and gives the instructor important feedback on their progress (Falvo, 2004). Questions can be matched with the behavioral objectives to be achieved. For example, to determine a client's knowledge level in the cognitive domain, the instructor might ask "What is the next step that you should take?" For the higher level of synthesis in the cognitive domain, the health professional educator might ask a staff member to plan for how he or she would respond to an angry family member (Abruzzese, 1996).

Questioning should not be interpreted by the learner as a test of knowledge but rather as a way to exchange information and stimulate thinking. However, two problems can occur with questioning. Questions can be so ambiguous that the learner does not know what the question is, or they can contain too many facts to process effectively (House, Chassie, & Spohn, 1990). Instructors should watch the learner's nonverbal reactions and rephrase the question if he or she detects either of these problems. If the learner seems confused, it is helpful to state that perhaps the question was not clear. This technique guards against the learner feeling guilty or becoming discouraged if he answers a question incorrectly (Falvo, 2004).

Also, it is important to give learners time to process information and respond to your questions. Sometimes teachers are uncomfortable waiting in silence for an answer or are impatient and attempt to correct an answer before learners complete their responses. Questioning is ineffective as a technique when educators do not give learners enough time to process information. Preliminary interruption may further interfere with a learner's thinking abilities and create a tense atmosphere.

Many health professional educators conduct individualized teaching of other health professionals or student learners in the skills laboratory and clinical setting. Clinical instruction is not a discrete instructional method but rather can be an extension of one-to-one teaching in a very complex setting for experiential learning. Educators can use a variety of methods other than one-to-one instruction, such as role modeling, demonstration, return demonstration, and group discussion. However, one-to-one instruction very well may be involved as a teaching approach during new employee orientation, student preceptorship, or a continuing staff education activity. The learner is singularly guided in the actual practice setting and each learning experience requires specific objectives, known to both the instructor and the learner, that are tailored to meet the individual's needs (Emerson, 2007; Gaberson & Oermann, 2007; O'Connor, 2006).

Preceptors who assume clinical teaching roles are usually expert clinicians but may not necessarily be expert teachers. If this is the case, to carry out their roles effectively, they need to be taught how to be educators through workshops and coaching sessions. One-to-one instruction has many strengths as a teaching method, but it also has its drawbacks. **Table 11–3** summarizes the major advantages and limitations of this method.

From an economic standpoint, one-to-one instruction is a very labor-intensive method and should be well tailored to make the expense worthwhile in terms of achieving learner outcomes.

Table 11–3 Major Advantages and Limitations of One-to-One Instruction

ADVANTAGES

- The pace and content of teaching can be tailored to meet individual needs.
- Ideal as an intervention for initial assessment and ongoing evaluation of the learner.
- Effective for teaching behaviors in all three domains of learning.
- Especially suitable for teaching those who are learning disabled, low literate, or educationally disadvantaged.
- Provides opportunity for immediate feedback to be shared between the teacher and the learner.

LIMITATIONS

- The learner is isolated from others who have similar needs or concerns.
- Deprives learners of the opportunity to identify with others and share information, ideas, and feelings with those in like circumstances.
- Can put learners on the spot because they are the sole focus of the teacher's attention.
- Questioning may be interpreted by the learner as a technique to test their knowledge and skills.
- The learner may feel overwhelmed and anxious if the educator makes the mistake of cramming too much information into each session.

One-to-one teaching of clients and families is often considered an inefficient approach to learning because the educator is reaching only one person at a time. Clinical teaching of students and continuing education for staff are vital for professional development, but they are costly endeavors when carried out on a one-to-one basis. Also, orientation of new staff is a significant expense to an institution or agency in terms of payroll dollars and short-term nonproductivity of the employee being oriented (del Bueno, Griffin, Burke, & Foley, 1990).

Demonstration and Return Demonstration

It is imperative to begin this discussion by making a clear distinction between demonstration and return demonstration. **Demonstration** is done by the teacher to show the learner how to perform a particular skill. **Return demonstration** is carried out by the learner in an attempt to establish competence by performing a task with cues from the teacher as needed. These two methods require dif-

ferent abilities by both the teacher and the learner. In particular, they are effective in teaching psychomotor domain skills (see Chapter 3 for a discussion on motor learning principles). However, both also may be used to enhance cognitive and affective learning, such as when helping a staff member develop interactive skills for crisis intervention or assertiveness training.

Prior to giving a demonstration, the teacher should inform learners of the purpose of the procedure, the sequential steps involved, the equipment needed, and the actions expected of them. Equipment should be tested before use to ensure that it is complete and in working order. For the demonstration method to be employed effectively, the learners must be able to clearly see and hear the steps being taught. Therefore, the demonstration method is best suited to teaching individuals or small groups. A large screen or multiple screens for video presentations of demonstrations can allow larger groups to participate.

Watching a demonstration can be a passive activity for learners, whose role is to observe the teacher presenting an exact performance of a required skill. The demonstration can be enhanced if the teacher slows down the pace of performing the demonstration, exaggerates some of the steps (de Tornyay & Thompson, 1987), or breaks lengthy procedures into a series of shorter steps. This incremental approach to sequencing discrete steps of a procedure is known as *scaffolding* and provides the learner with a clear and exacting image of each stage of skill development (Brookfield, 2006). In the process of demonstrating a skill to either health professionals or clients, it is important to explain why each step needs to be carried out in a certain manner to prevent bad habits from being integrated prior to the learner performing a new skill set (Brookfield, 2006; DeYoung, 2003; Lorig, 2003). Demonstration as a teaching method provides educators with the opportunity to model their commitment to a learning activity, builds teacher credibility, and inspires learners to achieve a level of excellence (Brookfield, 2006).

Demonstration allows for mental rehearsal of procedures (Haggard, 1989). The performance should be flawless, but it is important that the educator take advantage of a mistake to show how errors can be handled. If an error does occur, it may serve to increase rapport with the learners and allow them to relax and not be intimidated, knowing mistakes do happen and can be corrected (Brookfield, 2006). However, too many mistakes disrupt the mental image that the learners are forming.

When demonstrating a psychomotor skill, if possible, the health professional educator should work with the exact equipment that the learner is expected to use. This consideration is particularly important for novice learners. For instance, the client or family member who is learning to carry out an activity of daily living at home will be anxious and frustrated if taught with one type of assistive device, such as a wheelchair or shower seat in the hospital, when another type is used after discharge. Often the learner is too inexperienced to see the skill pattern and instead will be confused

in using one device versus another. The seasoned health professional, on the other hand, might find it easier to transfer what is already known about a type of assistive device if called on to learn to use a newly purchased piece of equipment from a different manufacturer.

Return demonstration should be planned to occur as close as possible to when the demonstration was given. Learners may need reassurance to reduce their anxiety prior to beginning the performance because the opportunity for return demonstration may be viewed by them as a test. This may lead them to believe they are expected to carry out a perfect performance the very first time around. Once a learner recognizes that the teacher is a coach and not an evaluator, the climate will be less tense and the learner will be more comfortable in attempting to practice a new skill. Educators can stress the fact that it is expected that the initial performance will not be perfect.

In addition, allowing the learner to manipulate the equipment before being expected to use it may help to reduce anxiety levels. Some clients, however, may experience an increased sense of unease when faced with learning a new skill because they identify the need to learn a skill in relation to their illness. For example, a young woman learning to care for a venous access device may be very anxious because her diagnosis of cancer has necessitated the need for this device.

When the learner is giving a return demonstration, the teacher should remain silent except for offering cues when necessary or briefly answering questions. Learners may be prompted by a series of pictures or coached by a partner with a checklist. The first time clients return a demonstration they may need a significant amount of coaching. Instructors should limit their help to coaching and not doing the task for the clients. The next time they practice, the instructor should observe and coach only if needed (Lorig, 2003). Also, instructors should avoid casual conversations or asking questions because they merely serve to interrupt the learner's thought processes and interfere with efforts to focus on mentally imprinting the procedure while performing the task.

Breaking the steps of the procedure into small increments will give the learner the opportunity to master one sequence before attempting the next. Praising the learner along the way for each step correctly performed reinforces behavior and gives the learner confidence in being able to successfully accomplish the task in its entirety. Emphasis should be on what to do, rather than on what not to do.

Practice should be supervised until the learner is competent enough to perform steps accurately. It is important that the initial skill pattern be correct before allowing for independent practice. To ensure safety, high-risk skills should be performed first on a model prior to actual clinical application.

Different learners need different amounts of practice to become competent, but once they have acquired the skill, they can then practice on their own to increase speed and proficiency. The value of practice should not be underestimated. For a new skill to become automatic and long lasting, repeated practice beyond the point of mastery is essential (Willingham, 2004). However, if a task is similar to one performed before, the time required to master a skill will be less. For example, a mother who has already learned to use sterile technique at home to change the dressing on her son's abdominal wound will likely learn more quickly and with much more ease how to properly use aseptic measures when managing home IV therapy.

Return demonstration sessions should be planned close enough together so that the learner does not lose the benefit of the most recent practice session. As with demonstration, the equipment for return demonstration needs to exactly match that used by the instructor and expected to be used by the learner. Learners also will require help in compensating for individual differences. For instance, if you are right-handed and the learner is left-handed, sitting across from each

other during instruction would be more helpful than sitting adjacent to one another. The person with difficulty seeing the increments on a syringe may need a magnifying device to facilitate accurate performance of a skill.

A summary of the advantages and limitations of demonstration and return demonstration can be found in **Table 11–4**.

Perhaps the biggest drawbacks to demonstration and return demonstration are the expenses associated with these methods. Group size must be kept small to ensure that each learner is able to visualize the procedures being performed and to have the opportunity for practice. Individual supervision is required during follow-up practices. Furthermore, the cost of obtaining, maintaining, and replacing equipment is significant and also must be calculated.

There are some ways, however, to reduce the cost of these methods. If, for example, the audience is composed of a homogeneous group of health professionals who need yearly CPR review, demonstration can be done via videotape. Also, return demonstration can initially be performed with a partner supervising the competency of the skill. Nevertheless, the final evaluation of staff competency must be carried out by an expert to ensure the accuracy of learning. In addition, expenses can be reduced by reusing equipment if it will not interfere with the accuracy, safety, or completeness of the demonstration/return demonstration.

Gaming

Gaming is an instructional method requiring the learner to participate in a competitive activity with preset rules (Allery, 2004). The goal is for the learners to win a game by applying knowledge and rehearsing skills previously learned. Games can be simple or they can be more complex to challenge the learner's ability to use higher order problem-solving and critical-thinking strategies. These activities do not have to reflect reality, but they are

---

Table 11–4 MAJOR ADVANTAGES AND LIMITATIONS OF DEMONSTRATION AND RETURN DEMONSTRATION

ADVANTAGES

- Especially effective for learning in the psychomotor domain.
- Actively engages the learner through stimulation of visual, auditory, and tactile senses.
- Repetition of movement and constant reinforcement increases confidence, competence, and skill retention.
- Provides opportunity for overlearning to achieve the goal.

LIMITATIONS

- Requires plenty of time to be set aside for teaching as well as learning.
- Size of audience must be kept small to ensure opportunity for practice and close supervision.
- Equipment can be expensive to purchase and replace.
- Extra space and equipment is needed for practicing certain skills.
- Competency evaluation requires 1:1 teacher–learner ratio.

---

designed to accomplish educational objectives. This instructional method is primarily effective for improving cognitive functioning but can also be used to enhance skills in the psychomotor domain and to influence affective behavior through increased social interaction (Berbiglia, Goddard, Littlefield, 1997; Beylefield & Struwig, 2007; Robinson, Lewis, & Robinson, 1990). Games connect theory to experience for health professionals without any risk to client safety (Henry, 1997).

In comparison with other didactic methods, gaming is an interactive teaching strategy that creates a dynamic environment for learning. As an experiential approach to learning, the use of games has been found to stimulate enjoyment of learning, increase active participation and engagement of learners, provide variety from a teaching/learning perspective, enhance skill acquisition, and improve problem-solving and clinical reasoning processes (Raines, 2010). Also, evidence suggests that gaming may improve recall and long-term retention of information (Allery, 2004; Beylefield & Strewig, 2007; Blakely, Skirton, Cooper, Allum, & Nelmes, 2008; O'Leary, Diepenhorst, Churley-Strom, & Magrane, 2005).

Games can be placed anywhere in the sequence of a learning activity (Joos, 1984)—as a device to conduct a needs assessment, introduce a topic, check learner progress, or summarize information. However, some games may require prerequisite knowledge for the learner to participate effectively and, therefore, may require a prior session of teaching before the game can be played (Henry, 1997). For purposes of a needs assessment, Rowell and Spielvogle (1996) used an infection-control game to determine whether a knowledge deficit among staff was contributing to rising rates of methicillin–resistant *Staphylococcus aureus* (MRSA). The staff members were asked to identify violations of infection-control practices in a mock isolation room. Participants completed and turned in an answer sheet, and then proceeded to an answer station. Not only did staff have an opportunity to test themselves and correct wrong information, but participants also provided information that was helpful in planning future education programs.

Games can be designed for a single individual, such as puzzles, or for a group of players, such as Bingo or Jeopardy. For gaming activities that involve multiple participants, the teacher's role is that of a facilitator. At the beginning of a game, the educator tells learners the objectives and the rules, distributes any materials required to play the game, and assigns the various teams. Once the game starts, the teacher needs to keep the flow going and interpret the rules. The game should be interrupted as seldom or as briefly as possible so as not to disturb the pace (Joos, 1984).

When the game is completed, winners should be rewarded. Prizes do not have to be expensive because their main purpose is to acknowledge achievement of learners in a public manner (Robinson et al., 1990). At the finish of the game, the teacher should conduct a debriefing session focusing on educational content and evaluating the gaming experience. Learners should be given a chance to discuss what they learned, ask questions, receive feedback regarding the outcome of the game, and offer suggestions for improving the process.

Games may be either purchased or designed. Well-known commercial games such as Trivial Pursuit, Bingo, Monopoly, and Jeopardy have the advantage in that their formats can be modified, the equipment is reusable for different topics, and many players already have familiarity with the rules of the games (Bender & Randall, 2006). Word searches, crossword puzzles, treasure hunts, and card and board games also are flexible in format and can be developed inexpensively and with relative ease. Educators should be sure to test any games prior to widespread use. Some examples of games are: a word search puzzle for foods (**Figure 11–1**) known to elevate serum potassium that is appropriate for use by patients with end-stage renal disease (Robinson et al., 1990) and Emergency Pursuit, which has content related to emergency situations that staff might encounter on a medical-surgical unit (Schmitz, MacLean, & Shidler, 1991).

Computer games, although much more expensive, are becoming increasingly available and are a popular option for many learners (Begg, 2008). Computer games, also referred to as edutainment (educational software disguised in a game format),

introduce content or involve the process of competition in the application of strategies for decision making toward attaining a goal. They are an enjoyable and effective way to teach specific cognitive, psychomotor, and affective skills. The Game Show Presenter, software that is now available to educators to create many types of games, can be accessed at http://www.almorale.com.

Gaming is a method particularly attractive to children, who enjoy the challenge of learning through play-like activity. Lieberman (2001) describes an interactive video game designed for clients ages 8–16 years with type 1 diabetes. This game modeled the daily challenges of self-care, and participants were told to play the game as much or as little as they wished. By the end of the 6-month trial, there was a 77% drop in diabetes-related urgent care as well as an increase in self-efficacy in communication with parents about diabetes and in self-care related to diabetes.

Lewis, Saydak, Mierzwa, and Robinson (1989) designed a game suitability checklist that remains relevant today in determining whether gaming is a viable alternative to meet the objectives for learning (**Figure 11–2**). It is particularly important to remember that games, whether purchased or self-developed, must serve the purpose of helping the learner accomplish the predetermined behavioral objectives. Are people learning while they are having fun? Bays and Hermann (1997) tested students who learned the same content but through two different methods. One group was taught with gaming and the other with lecture. A posttest showed no significant difference in scores between the two groups. Lieberman (2001) reports that children and adolescents improved their self-care after engaging in interactive games related to smoking prevention, asthma, and diabetes. Research indicates that electronic games as a tool for client education have the potential to improve health outcomes (Editorial, 2009).

The advantages and limitations of the gaming method are outlined in **Table 11–5**.

Figure 11–1 Sample Word Search Game for Clients

Source: Robinson, K. J., Lewis, D. J., & Robinson, J. A. (1990, August). Games: A way to give laboratory values meaning. *ANNA Journal, 17*(4), 307. Reprinted with permission of the American Nephrology Nurses Association, publisher.

Economic considerations include either the cost of purchasing a game or the time taken by the instructor to design, test, and update the gaming material. Also, some types of games require the educator to be present as facilitator each time that they are played.

Simulation

Simulation is a trial-and-error method of teaching whereby an artificial or hypothetical experience is created that engages the learner in an activity that reflects real-life conditions but without the risk-taking consequences of an actual situation. Simu-

lation is a highly innovative instructional method to teach health professionals the complex world of health care in their respective disciplines in an effective, efficient, safe, and high quality fashion. As Gaba (2004) explains, "Simulation is a technique—not a technology—to replace or amplify real experiences with guided experiences that evoke or replicate substantial aspects of the real world in a fully interactive manner" (p. i2). Over the past 20 years, and especially in the last few years, interest in simulation has grown rapidly as a way to hone the knowledge and practice skills of the healthcare workforce for the ultimate purpose of improving patient safety and patient care outcomes (Beaubien

Figure 11–2 Game Suitability Checklist

GAME SUITABILITY CHECKLIST		
Criteria	**Yes**	**No**
• Does the game meet the program objectives?	_____	_____
• Can the game be completed within the time allotted?	_____	_____
• Is the size and layout of the room conducive to the game?	_____	_____
• Will the available participants meet the minimum number required for the game?	_____	_____
• Do staff members have the time and interest to design or adapt games? If not, are funds available to purchase games?	_____	_____
• If the game requires equipment or supplies, are they readily available?	_____	_____
a. Are resources or funds available to design or purchase needed materials?	_____	_____
b. Does the game require replacement of materials following each use?	_____	_____
• Does the game require preparation or cleanup time?	_____	_____

Source: Lewis, D. J., Sayjack, S. J., Mierzwa, I. P., & Robinson, J. A. (1989). Gaming: A teaching strategy for adult learners. *Journal of Continuing Education in Nursing, 20,* 80–84. Reprinted with permission from SLACK Incorporated.

& Baker, 2004; Gaba, 2004). No longer seen as a technological toy for learning basic skills, simulation is now used to teach critical thinking and high level decision-making skills (Gaba, 2009). It is also a means to foster collaborative interdisciplinary education to improve teamwork, communication, and role valuing among the healthcare disciplines (Dillon, Noble, & Kaplan 2009).

To some extent, an overlap exists between the methods of gaming, simulation, and role-playing because all three instructional approaches require learners to engage in experiential learning (Allery, 2004). Simulation allows participants to make decisions in a safe and controlled environment, witness the consequences, and evaluate the effectiveness of their actions (Beaubien & Baker, 2004; Corbridge et al., 2008; DeYoung, 2003).

A follow-up discussion with learners after use of these experiential methods is important to facilitate their analysis of the experience. Simulation should always be followed by a debriefing session that includes a discussion of events that happened during the experience, the decisions made, the actions taken, the consequences of the choices, the possible alternatives, and suggestions for improvement in skill performance. Simulations provide

Table 11–5 Major Advantages and Limitations of Gaming

ADVANTAGES

- Games are fun with a purpose.
- Retention of information is promoted by stimulating learner enthusiasm and increasing learner involvement.
- Easy to devise or modify for individual or group learning.
- Adds variety to the learning experience.
- Excellent for dull or repetitious content that must be periodically reviewed.

LIMITATIONS

- Creates a competitive environment that may be threatening to some learners.
- Group size may need to be kept small for participation by all learners.
- Requires more flexible space for teamwork than a traditional conference room or classroom.
- Potentially higher noise level may require special space accommodations.
- Requirements may be more physically demanding than many other methods.
- Some learners may not be able to participate if they are restricted by a disability.

the opportunity for anticipatory learning (Allery, 2004; Jeffries, 2005).

When planning a simulation, it is most effective if the educators make the learning experience resemble real life as much as possible but in a nonthreatening way. The activity should challenge the decision-making ability of the learner by imposing time constraints, providing realistic levels of tension, and using actual equipment or other important features of the environment in which the specific skill will be performed. For example, a scenario could be developed to help parents prevent sudden infant death syndrome (SIDS) by working through a situation in which a monitor signals respiratory difficulty in their baby. As another example, a health professional along with other staff team members are expected to make a rapid assessment and intervene with accuracy, coordination, and speed in caring for a chest trauma victim in a simulated emergency room setting. These simulations can be created for the purpose of determining whether the learner has the necessary skills to perform the activity correctly.

There are many types of simulations, including the following (Beaubien & Baker, 2004; Childs &

Sepples, 2006; Epstein, 2007; Gaba, 2004; Jeffries, 2005; Turner, 2007; Yoo & Yoo, 2003):

- Written simulations that use case studies about real or fictitious situations and the learner must respond to these scenarios. Health professionals, for example, are asked to describe how they would handle a personnel communication problem on a unit or manage a physiologically complex patient in the critical care environment.
- Clinical simulations can be set up to replicate complex care situations, such as a mock cardiac arrest. An experienced staff member is a buddy or a coach for the inexperienced staff member who is running the code. This simulation allows the novice to practice these skills in a nonthreatening situation with immediate feedback. Participants reported that this simulation helped validate their thinking and allowed for ongoing thinking out loud in formulating questions they might otherwise not have asked.
- Model simulations are frequently used to teach a variety of health professional audiences. An effective and economical method to teach certain

noninvasive skills is to ask a peer, instructor, or trained individual to act as a patient. Standard patients—people trained to act as patients— were found to be a more effective method of simulation to teach students than were lectures and laboratory practice with a model.

An exciting new technology is high-fidelity whole-body patient simulators, such as Sim-Man, that reproduce in a sophisticated, lifelike manner the cardiovascular, respiratory, urinary, and neurological systems. The more sophisticated models (SimMan 3G) have the ability to respond to selected drugs; mimic heart, lung, and bowel sounds; and give oximeter and vital sign readings that respond to a variety of interventions (Epstein, 2007). However, widespread use of this resource is still limited by the high cost of this technology.

• Computer simulations are in use in learning laboratories to mimic situations whereby information as well as feedback is given to learners in helping them to develop decision-making skills.

Although the learning laboratory is a commonplace teaching environment for health professional students on college campuses and has been used in the last 15 years to update the skills of health professionals reentering the workforce, these simulated experiences are not yet widely available to train patients or family providers in self-care skills because of lack of space and the high cost of simulators. In the future, simulation with high-tech, portable equipment could revolutionize client education.

Simulated experiences for the learner should be followed with actual experiences as soon as possible. Simulation is never exactly the same as the real thing to prepare the learner. Therefore, the learner will need help with the transfer of skills acquired in a simulated experience to the actual situation. Virtual reality technology, still in its infancy in healthcare settings, has the potential to narrow the distance even more between simulation and real life for the education of clients, health professional students, and staff (Gaba, 2009; Kaphingst, 2009; Turner, 2007).

Simulation can be made more cost effective by reuse of supplies and the interdisciplinary sharing of simulation equipment. Given the shortage of healthcare faculty, the diminishing number of clinical sites available for practice teaching, and the growing knowledge base and skills needed to produce competent and confident care providers, simulation offers a cost-effective approach to student teaching, staff orientation, and continuing staff development (Jeffries 2005). **Table 11–6** summarizes the main strengths and drawbacks of the simulation method of instruction.

Role-Playing

Role-playing is an instructional method by which learners actively participate in an unrehearsed dramatization. They are asked to play assigned parts of a character as they think the character would act in reality. This method is a technique to arouse feelings and elicit emotional responses in the learners. It is used primarily to achieve behavioral objectives in the affective domain. Unlike high fidelity simulation, which teaches learners mastery of skills for application to their own real-life situations, role-playing, a form of simulation, is a method that teaches learners real-life situations to develop understanding of other people and why they behave the way they do (Lowenstein 2007; Redman, 2007). For example, a recreational or occupational therapist attending an education program on sensory disabilities will be given the experience of wearing special glasses to see how it feels to function with impaired vision.

Role-playing is a technique that, according to Comer (2005), can be used to substitute for or supplement the more costly high tech simulations to teach students various skills and develop clinical judgment at varying levels of difficulty. Role-play as

Table 11–6 Major Advantages and Limitations of Simulation

ADVANTAGES

- Excellent for psychomotor skill development.
- Enhances higher level problem-solving and interactive abilities in the cognitive and affective domains.
- Provides for active learner involvement in a real-life situation with consequences determined by variables inherent in the situation.
- Guarantees a safe, nonthreatening environment for learning.

LIMITATIONS

- Can be expensive.
- Very labor intensive in many cases.
- Not readily available to all learners yet.

an instructional method is of particular usefulness because it serves multiple functions: It helps learners to explore their own and others' feelings; gain insight into their values, attitudes, and beliefs; develop problem-solving and decision-making skills; explore a topic in more depth; and develop a better understanding of interpersonal relationships (Billings & Halstead, 2009; Lowenstein, 2007).

The responsibility of the teacher is to design a situation with enough information for learners to be able to assume the role of someone else without actually giving them a script to follow. Occasionally, people are assigned to play themselves to rehearse desired behavior, or the educator takes a part to act as a positive role model for the learners. Most often, however, the teacher acts as the facilitator and designates members in a group to play particular characters. They then pretend to be these people for the duration of the exercise. Participants do and say things that they perceive actual persons would do, say, and feel.

The purpose is to help learners see and understand a problem through the eyes of others. In other words, it gives them a chance to walk in someone else's shoes. For example, children may use role-playing with puppets to explore their responses to such illnesses as asthma (Ramsey & Siroky, 1988). Role-playing also has been used

to teach cultural competence by having a learner assume the role of a client from another culture. This "client" interacts with another learner who models a health professional displaying potentially inappropriate cultural responses. After the role-play, a third learner can then explain the important cultural characteristics and why the "health professional's" responses were inappropriate and insensitive (Shearer & Davidhizar, 2003). When professional caregivers take the place of clients, this role reversal helps to sensitize staff to the care they deliver.

For role-playing to be employed effectively, the teacher must be sure that the group has attained a comfort level that allows each member to feel secure enough to participate in a dramatization. This method should never be used with learners in the beginning of a group session encounter. Members need time to establish a rapport with one another as well as with the instructor, or else learners may feel embarrassed or self-conscious about playing a part. All members of the group should be given an assignment to ensure that they are actively involved in the teaching–learning experience (Haggard, 1989). Those who are actual participants need to be informed about the role they are to portray so that they can effectively develop the appropriate actions. Those who are designated as observers require specific instructions about what to attend to during the role-playing session.

The actual length of a role-playing session can be as little as 5 minutes, but should not exceed 15 to 20 minutes (Lowenstein, 2007). Role-playing is best done in small groups so that all learners can serve as either players or as observers. Active participation by learners is particularly important during a postactivity discussion or debriefing session. Because this method is most effective for learning in the affective domain, all participants need to discuss how they felt and share what they observed to gain insight into their understanding of interpersonal relationships and their reactions to role expectations or conflicts (Comer, 2005).

Role-playing can be used in conjunction with other instructional methods, but such a combination requires careful planning as to the sequential placement of this strategy and the important points to be captured during the dramatization period. See **Table 11–7** for a summary of the main advantages and limitations of role-playing.

Role Modeling

The use of self as a role model is often overlooked as an instructional method. Learning from **role modeling** is called identification and emanates from learning and developmental theories such as Bandura's social learning theory and Erickson's psychosocial stages of development, which explain how people acquire new behaviors and social roles (Snowman & Biehler, 2006; Vander Zanden, Crandell, & Crandell, 2007). This method primarily achieves behavior change in the affective domain.

Preceptors and mentors are excellent examples of experienced health professionals who, through role modeling, guide, support, and socialize students and novice practitioners in their transition to a new level of functioning. Preceptors help bridge the gap between theory and practice. Role modeling is an instructional technique that helps new

health professionals develop psychomotor skills, critical thinking competencies, and interpersonal skills, as well as assists them to assume the responsibilities and values of the profession with which they identify (Sorenson & Yankech, 2008).

Health professional educators have many opportunities to demonstrate behaviors they would like to instill in learners, whether they be clients, healthcare staff, or students. The competency with which the educator performs a skill, the way he or she interacts with others, the personal example he or she sets, and the enthusiasm and interest he or she conveys about a subject or problem all can influence learners' motivation levels and the extent to which they successfully perform a desired behavior.

Behavior is regulated by the social norms and professional expectations that specify what is considered to be appropriate and inappropriate behavior. Role conflict can arise when a learner's past behavior patterns are incompatible or different from another role that person must assume (Vander Zanden et al., 2007). Health professionals can teach students and staff new behaviors by consistently setting examples and living the standards of the health profession. "Actions speak louder than words" is a popular saying relevant to the use of self as a role model (de Tornyay & Thompson, 1987).

See **Table 11–8** for a summary of the advantages and limitations of this method of instruction.

Self-Instruction

Self-instruction is a method used by the teacher to provide or design instructional activities that guide the learner in independently achieving the objectives of learning. Each self-study module usually focuses on one topic, and the hallmark of this format is independent study. The self-instruction method is effective for learning in the cognitive and psychomotor domains, where the goal is to master information and apply it to practice. Self-

---

Table 11–7 MAJOR ADVANTAGES AND LIMITATIONS OF ROLE-PLAYING

ADVANTAGES

- Opportunity to explore feelings and attitudes.
- Potential for bridging the gap between understanding and feeling.
- Narrows the role distance between and among clients and professionals.

LIMITATIONS

- Limited to small groups.
- Tendency by some participants to overly exaggerate their assigned roles.
- A role part loses its realism and credibility if played too dramatically.
- Some participants may be uncomfortable in their roles or unable to develop them sufficiently.

Table 11–8 MAJOR ADVANTAGES AND LIMITATIONS OF ROLE MODELING

ADVANTAGES

- Influences attitudes to achieve behavior change in the affective domain.
- Positive role models have the potential to instill socially desired behaviors.

LIMITATIONS

- Requires rapport between the role model and the learner.
- Negative role models have the potential to instill unacceptable behaviors.

---

study also can be an effective adjunct for introducing principles and step-by-step guidelines prior to demonstration of a psychomotor skill.

This method is sometimes difficult to identify as a singular entity because of the variety of terms used to describe it, such as *mini-course, self-instructional package, individualized learning activities*, and *programmed instruction*. For the purposes of this discussion, the term *self-instruction* is used, and it is defined as a self-contained instructional activity that allows learners to progress by themselves at their own pace (Abruzzese, 1996).

Self-instruction modules come in a variety of forms including, but not limited to, work books, study guides, work stations, videotapes, Internet modules, and computer programs. They are specifically designed to be used independently. The teacher serves as a facilitator/resource person to provide motivation and reinforcement for learning. This method requires less teacher time to give information, and each session with the learner is intended to meet individual needs.

Some learners and teachers resist the self-instructional method because it appears to depersonalize the teaching–learning process. This is not necessarily true. Communication can still occur between the teacher and the learner, but the focus of instruction is different. The amount of time for direct interaction is more limited than with other methods of teaching such as lecture, group discussion, and one-to-one instruction. This method adheres to the principles of adult education whereby the learner assumes responsibility for learning and is self-directed (Knowles, Holton, & Swanson, 1998).

A self-instruction module is carefully designed to achieve preset objectives by bringing learners from diverse knowledge and skill backgrounds to a similar level of achievement prior to undertaking the next step in a series of learning activities. For example, a self-instructional activity can be made available to educate all staff on new infection-control practices in an agency, and clients can learn breast self-examination or cardiopulmonary resuscitation techniques by using specifically prepared self-study materials.

Modules can be made readily accessible to learners along with any resources that are needed to complete the self-study program. Each self-instruction module needs to contain the following elements:

- An introduction and statement of purpose, which generally include a table of contents, the terminal objectives, the intent of the module, and directions for its use.
- A list of prerequisite skills that the learner needs to have to use the module.
- A list of behavioral objectives, which are clear and measurable statements describing which skills the learner is expected to acquire on completion of the unit.
- A pretest to determine diagnostically whether the learner needs to proceed with the module. Some learners may demonstrate mastery in the pretest and can move on to the next module. Other learners can get a sharper focus on their areas of weakness and may decide to seek additional preparation prior to beginning the module.
- An identification of resources and learning activities, which specifies the equipment needed, such as videotapes, slides, or written materials, and outlines the actual learning activities that will be presented. Objectives are given to direct the learner, followed by material presented in small units of discrete information called frames. The total length of a well-designed module is kept relatively short so as not to dampen the motivation to learn.

How the material is presented varies with the objectives and the resources available. For exam-

ple, information may be given via programmed instruction or through a series of readings. This can be followed by a video presentation of a relevant case study with the requirement that the learner write a response to what has been read and observed.

- Periodic self-assessments to provide feedback to the learner throughout the module. The user is frequently able to do periodic self-assessments prior to moving on to the next unit. This allows the learner to decide whether the previous information has been processed sufficiently enough to progress further.
- A posttest to evaluate the learner's level of mastery in achieving the objectives. If learners are aware that a posttest needs to be completed, this requirement encourages them to pay attention to the information. Keeping a record of final outcomes is helpful in both staff and client education as documentation of competency, as proof that standards were met, and for the purpose of planning for continuing education.

Self-instruction represents an attractive alternative to traditional classroom and group learning methods in the rapidly changing healthcare environment. Hospitals and community agencies are not able to release staff in large numbers for continuing education programs that are rigidly timed. This constraint conflicts with the need to share information on the newest advances and documentation of continuing competence of staff. Self-instruction modules are excellent choices for annual training updates in selected topics or skills that require periodic review to determine competency (Markiewicz & Wells, 1997; O'Very, 1999).

The Internet also offers a myriad of continuing education self-instruction modules. Health practitioners have the advantage of being educated about numerous problems and issues in primary care with interactive, realistic case studies. E-mail to and from faculty can facilitate communication (Hayes, Huckstadt, & Gibson, 2000).

The information explosion coupled with the rapidly advancing technology of computers has made Web-based teaching and learning available for client education, staff development, and student instruction. See Chapter 13 on technology in education for an in-depth description of synchronous and asynchronous options for teaching and learning. See **Table 11–9** for a list of major advantages and limitations of this method of instruction.

Self-instruction modules have been found to be cost effective because they are designed to be used by large numbers of individuals with minimal and infrequent revisions. It may be less time consuming and more efficient to purchase, rather than produce, a self-instruction module if the information presented in a commercial product is appropriate for the target audience.

Computer-assisted instruction (CAI) is an individualized method of self-study using technology to deliver an educational activity. CAI allows learners to proceed at their own pace with immediate and continuous feedback on their progress as they respond to a software program. Most computer programs assist the learner in achieving cognitive domain skills (DeYoung, 2003), but psychomotor skills can be effectively taught through a Web-

enhanced approach (Salyers, 2007). CAIs offer consistent presentation of material and around-the-clock accessibility. This instructional method not only saves time but also accommodates different types of learners. It allows slow learners to repeat lessons as many times as necessary, while learners familiar with material can skip ahead to more advanced material (DeYoung, 2003).

There is concern that computer instruction depersonalizes the learning process (DeYoung, 2003). However, the use of CAIs does not preclude the teacher's availability for guidance in learning. Even though this technology simply delivers content, it allows more time for the health professional educator to concentrate on the personal aspects of individual reinforcement and ongoing assessments of learning. For example, CAIs have been used with good client acceptance for precolposcopy education (Martin, Hoffman, & Kaminski, 2005). Recently, computer programs, known as Interactive Health Communication Applications (IHCAs), have been used by people with chronic disease. Research findings indicate that IHCAs have improved user knowledge, have had a positive effect on social support, have led to better clinical outcomes, and have increased self-efficacy (a person's

---

Table 11–9 MAJOR ADVANTAGES AND LIMITATIONS OF SELF-INSTRUCTION

ADVANTAGES

- Allows for self-pacing.
- Stimulates active learning.
- Provides opportunity to review and reflect on information.
- Frequent feedback is built in.
- Indicates mastery of material accomplished in a particular time frame.

LIMITATIONS

- Limited with learners who have low literacy skills.
- Not ideal for learners with visual and hearing impairments.
- Requires high levels of motivation.
- Not ideal for learners who tend to procrastinate.
- May induce boredom if this method is overused with a population with no variation in the activity design.

belief in his or her capacity to take specific action) when compared to non-users of IHCAs (Murray, Burns, Tai, Lai, & Nazareth, 2005).

Selection of Instructional Methods

The process of selecting an instructional method requires a prior determination of the behavioral objectives to be accomplished and an assessment of the learners who will be involved in achieving the objectives. Also, consideration must be given to available resources such as time, money, space, and materials to support learning activities. The teacher is also an important variable in the selection and effectiveness of a method. **Table 11–10** summarizes the general characteristics of instructional methods.

Teachers are at different levels on the novice-to-expert continuum, and how seasoned they are influences their choices of instructional methods. An expert skilled at facilitating small-group discussion may be a novice in the design and selection of games. A health professional may be an expert clinician but have only limited education and experience to be effective in the teaching role. Health professionals are expected to teach but may not have adequate time, inclination, energy, or capability for developing the quality and variety of instruction necessary. Teaching is a skill that can be developed in formal academic settings, in continuing education programs, or through guidance by an expert peer mentor.

Teachers are likely to focus on a particular method because it is the one they feel most comfortable using without considering all the criteria for selection. There is no one right method, because the best approach depends on many variables, such as the audience, the content to be taught, the setting in which teaching and learning are to take place, and the resources available. For so long it has been thought that the ideal method for any given situation is the one that best suits the learner's needs, not the teacher's. However, Glenn (2009) recently pointed out that no strong scientific evidence exists to support the idea that a teaching method should match the learning style(s) of the audience. Instead, learners should be challenged with a variety of learning experiences and "teachers should worry about matching their instruction with the content they are teaching. Some concepts are best taught through hands-on work, some are best taught through lectures, and some are best taught through group discussion" (Glenn, 2009).

A novice should begin instruction with very familiar content so that he or she can focus on the teaching process itself and feel more confident in trying out different techniques and instructional materials. He or she should ask questions of learners and peers in the evaluation process to ascertain whether the method chosen was appropriate for accomplishing the behavioral objectives and meeting the needs of different learners in terms of their learning styles and readiness to learn.

Narrow (1979) emphasizes the importance of educators periodically examining their role as teachers and assessing the factors of energy, attitudes, knowledge, and skills, which influence the priority they assign to teaching and the ability to teach effectively. The following is a summary of her suggestions that after many years still remain very relevant to the teaching role.

At any given point in time, the teacher's energy level is influenced by both psychological and physical factors, such as the amount of satisfaction derived from work, the demands and responsibilities of his or her professional and personal life, and the teacher's state of health. Feelings toward the learner also influence the enthusiasm the teacher brings to the teaching–learning situation. Health professionals as educators who feel drawn to learners because they find them interesting or are concerned or anxious about their situation will find teaching to be a satisfying experience. If, on the other hand, the learners are demanding or display inappropriate

Table 11–10 GENERAL CHARACTERISTICS OF INSTRUCTIONAL METHODS

Methods	Domain	Learner Role	Teacher Role	Advantages	Limitations
Lecture	Cognitive	Passive	Presents information	Cost effective Targets large groups	Not individualized
Group discussion	Affective Cognitive	Active—if learner participates	Guides and focuses discussion	Stimulates sharing ideas and emotions	Shy or dominant member High levels of diversity
One-to-one instruction	Cognitive Affective Psychomotor	Active	Presents information and facilitates individualized learning	Tailored to individual's needs and goals	Labor intensive Isolates learner
Demonstration	Psychomotor Cognitive	Passive	Models skill or behavior	Preview of exact skill/ behavior	Small groups needed to facilitate visualization
Return demonstration	Psychomotor	Active	Individualizes feedback to refine performance	Immediate individual guidance	Labor intensive to view individual performance
Gaming	Cognitive Affective	Active—if learner participates	Oversees pacing Referees Debriefs	Captures learner enthusiasm	Environment too competitive for some learners
Simulation	Cognitive Psychomotor	Active	Designs environment Facilitates process Debriefs	Practice reality in safe setting	Labor intensive Equipment costs
Role-playing	Affective	Active	Designs format Debriefs	Develops understanding of others	Exaggeration or underdevelopment of role
Role modeling	Affective Cognitive	Passive	Models skill or behavior	Helps with socialization to role	Requires rapport
Self-instruction	Cognitive Psychomotor	Active	Designs package Gives individual feedback	Self-paced Cost effective Consistent	Procrastination Requires literacy

behavior, teachers may feel negatively about them and find the teaching–learning encounter more difficult and less fulfilling. Educators can develop the ability to accept individuals without necessarily approving of their behavior.

Another factor to consider is the teacher's comfort with and confidence in the nature of the subject matter to be taught. Those who find certain content to be stressful to teach because of a lack of relevant knowledge or skills can increase their understanding of the subject and relieve their stress and apprehension with additional study and practice. This allows them to function more effectively in the teaching role.

Those who have difficulty communicating with learners about what they may consider sensitive material, such as sexual behavior, mental illness, abortion, birth defects, disfigurement, terminal illness, and the like, should examine their own feelings, seek support from colleagues, and use resources to help create an effective teaching approach. If the teaching–learning process is to be a partnership, not only is it crucial to assess the learner but it is equally important that health professional educators assess themselves as teachers. Often teachers fail to take into account their own circumstances and needs.

Evaluation of Instructional Methods

An important aspect of evaluating any instructional program is to assess the effectiveness of the method. Was the choice selected as effective, efficient, and appropriately used as possible? Educators should ask five major questions to help decide which method to choose or whether the method selected should be revised or rejected:

1. **Does the method help the learners to achieve the stated objectives?**

    This question is the most important criterion for evaluation—if the method does not facili-

tate accomplishing the objectives, then all the other criteria are unimportant. Examine how well matched the method is to the learning domain of the predetermined objectives. Will the method expose learners to the necessary information and training to learn the desired behaviors?

2. **Is the learning activity accessible to the learners who have been targeted?**

    Accessibility includes such issues as when information is presented, the location and setting in which teaching takes place, and the availability of resources and equipment to deliver the message. Clients and their family members need programs to be offered at suitable times and accessible locations. For example, childbirth preparation classes scheduled during the daytime hours likely would not be convenient for expectant couples who are working.

3. **Is the method efficient given the time, energy, and resources available in relation to the number of learners the educator is trying to reach?**

    To teach large numbers of learners, educators have to choose a method that can accommodate groups, such as lecture, discussion sessions, or role-playing, or a method that can reach many individuals at one time, such as the use of various self-instructional formats.

4. **To what extent does the method allow for active participation to accommodate the needs, abilities, and style of the learner?**

    Active participation has been well documented as a way to increase interest in learning and the retention of information. Evaluate how active learners want to be or are able to be in the process of gaining knowledge and skills. No one method can satisfy all learners, but adhering to one method exclusively addresses the preferred style of only a segment of the audience.

5. **Is the method cost effective?**

    It is vital to examine the cost of educational programs to determine whether similar outcomes might be achieved by using less costly methodologies. In this era of cost containment, employers and insurers want their money invested in client programs that yield the best possible outcomes at the lowest price as measured in terms of preventing illness and injury, minimizing the severity and extent of illness, and reducing the length of hospital stays and readmissions. Healthcare agencies want the best staff performance with the most reasonable use of resources and the least amount of time taken away from actual practice.

Increasing Effectiveness of Teaching

Excellent teachers have one thing in common—a passion to keep improving their abilities. One does not arrive at being an expert teacher. The drive toward excellence is an ongoing process that continues throughout the teacher's entire professional life. What constitutes creative teaching? The following are techniques, not listed in any particular order, that health professionals as educators can use to enhance the effectiveness of verbal presentations. In addition, some general principles for teaching are put forth that can be applied when using almost any instructional methodology (Bradshaw & Lowenstein, 2007; Brookfield, 2006; Caputi, 2010; Cunningham & Baker, 1986; Freitas, Lantz, & Reed, 1991; Irvin, 1996; Musinski, 1999; Narrow, 1979; Parrott, 1994; Phillips, 1999).

Techniques to Enhance the Effectiveness of Verbal Presentations

PRESENT INFORMATION ENTHUSIASTICALLY

The teacher who comes across as invested in the material excites the learner to identify with the subject at hand. No matter how well a lesson is planned or how clearly it is presented, if it is delivered in a dry and dull monotone, it will likely fall on deaf ears.

The teacher should try to vary the quality and pitch of his or her voice, use a variety of gestures and facial expressions, change position if necessary to make direct and frequent eye contact with everyone in the group, and demonstrate an ardent interest in the topic to attract and fascinate an audience. The enthusiastic teacher is aware that an energetic attitude is contagious and enticing. However, one must exercise caution in overusing body language and overt actions because mannerisms can be distracting and can adversely affect learning.

INCLUDE HUMOR

Many teachers use humor as a technique to grab, arouse, and maintain the attention of the learner. Appropriate humor can help establish a rapport with learners by humanizing the teacher. Humor does not necessarily require the teacher to tell jokes, and joke telling should not be attempted if this is not a skill a teacher possesses. Furthermore, the teacher should avoid making someone the object of humor if it results in a put-down.

Humor establishes an atmosphere that allows for human error without embarrassment and encourages freedom and comfort to explore alternatives in the learning situations. Humor is a means to reduce anxiety when dealing with sensitive material, to provide poignant examples of everyday life experiences, and to reinforce information.

EXHIBIT RISK-TAKING BEHAVIOR

Effective teachers are willing to develop exercises in which many variables can lead to any number of possible outcomes. They use this technique to encourage learners to reach their own conclusions about controversial issues. Regardless of the outcome, teachers should be prepared to deal with uncertainty. Exercises that allow learners freedom to experiment and express their ideas focus more on the process than on the result.

Deliver Material Dramatically

Effective teachers seek ways to engage the learner emotionally by using surprise, controlled tension, or ploys. The teacher uses strategies that connect the educational material directly to the learner's life experiences so that information is made more understandable and relevant. Learners may be asked to participate in simulations, games, or role-playing to act out a part, live an experience, or test their capacities. These activities involve the learner and can leave a profound, lasting impression that can be recalled vividly and can be drawn upon when faced with a real situation. This technique engages learners by arousing their emotions.

Choose Problem-Solving Activities

Whether the learners are staff members or clients, the health professional as educator must recognize that learners need to be immersed in activities to help them develop problem-solving skills. In today's world, professionals must have the ability to identify both client and system needs by searching and sorting data, uncovering problems, and finding solutions. Increasingly, they are expected to work with interdisciplinary teams to determine and implement solutions to healthcare problems. Learning activities must be designed to help these healthcare staff members and students develop critical-thinking and collaborative skills.

Clients, especially those with chronic conditions, also need problem-solving skills to know how to respond to changes demanded by their condition. What should they do differently on a sick day, or what constitutes an emergency? Clients and their families need more than just low-level cognitive information to make adjustments in their lives. The teacher must therefore devise and orchestrate opportunities that challenge learners to

critically analyze situations as well as support the learner in exploring possible alternative solutions to meet their needs.

Serve as a Role Model

Educators should constantly seek new information by keeping abreast of current research, theories, and issues in clinical practice for application relevant to the teaching situation. By expanding their own knowledge base, teachers give credence to what they teach and gain the confidence of learners in the teacher's expertise. A commitment to lifelong learning transmits an important value to others of their need for continuous personal or professional development.

Educators are seen as credible role models when they are actively engaged in scholarly activities, are experienced in the field, and have advanced credentials to teach complex skills. The believability of a role model is greatly affected by the values displayed and the congruence demonstrated between what the teacher says and does (Babcock & Miller, 1994). If the learners regard the behavior of the creative teacher as desirable, they will likely imitate that behavior, which they perceive as eliciting positive effects.

Use Anecdotes and Examples

The creative teacher uses stories and examples of incidences and episodes to illustrate points. Anecdotes, whether amusing, alarming, sad, or anger provoking, are valuable in driving a point home, clarifying a topic under discussion, or helping someone better relate to an issue. The teacher can reinforce the learning principle that simple representations can assist the learner to grasp complex ideas by using examples relevant to past experiences and the knowledge base of learners that help them identify and connect in a concrete way with the material being taught. For example, using the analogy of police cells (lymphocytes) fighting against outlaw cells (bacteria) can help a child with a serious infection understand in concrete terms how his body is working to heal itself.

Use Technology

Innovative teachers use technology to broaden and add variety to the opportunities for teaching and learning. They continue to increase the level of their own skills by taking advantage of the advances in technology to introduce and coach others in new ways of learning. They recognize that the sophisticated use of technology is a primary skill that will be needed for educational programs of the future.

The use of different types of technology assists the teacher in helping learners meet their individual needs and styles of learning. Technology has the potential for making the teaching–learning process more convenient, accessible, and stimulating. Effective teachers must be future oriented. A mastery of technological skills ensures that they possess the ability to teach in innovative and eclectic ways to prepare students for learning in the 21st century.

General Principles for Teaching Across Methodologies

Give Positive Reinforcement

Educational research is replete with examples of the effects of positive reinforcement on learning. Acknowledging ideas, actions, and opinions of others by using words of praise or approval, such as "That's a good answer," "I agree with you," and "You have a very good point," or using nonverbal expressions of acceptance, such as smiling, nodding, or a reassuring pat on the back, encourages learners to participate more readily or try harder to improve their performance. Rewarding even a small success can instill satisfaction in the learner. Reproval, on the other hand, dampens motivation and causes learners to withdraw. Positive reinforcers, in the form of recognition, tangible rewards,

or opportunities, should closely follow the desired behavior. The clearer the correlation between the desired behavior and the reward, the more meaningful the reinforcement is (see Chapter 3 on learning theories).

A powerful incentive is to ask learners to share their experiences with others. In a group, it is important to recognize the contributions of each member rather than focus primarily on the more aggressive learner or high achiever. What constitutes positive reinforcement for one individual may not suffice for another because rewards are closely tied to value systems.

The quantity of reinforcement also varies in its effectiveness from one individual to another. A small amount of praise can have a strong effect on the learner who is not used to succeeding, whereas significant praise may be relatively ineffective for a consistently high achiever. In addition, the effects of reinforcement are transitory. An incentive that works for a learner at one time may not work well at another time.

Project an Attitude of Acceptance and Sensitivity

The ease with which teachers conduct themselves, the willingness to receive and answer questions, the simple courtesies extended, and the responsiveness demonstrated toward an audience are all actions that set the tone for a friendly, warm, and receptive atmosphere for learning. If the teacher exhibits self-confidence and self-respect, the learner in turn will feel comfortable, confident, and secure in the learning environment. If the teacher comes across as believable, trustworthy, considerate and competent, he or she helps to put the audience at ease, which serves as an invitation for them to learn. When teachers exercise patience and sensitivity with respect to age, race, culture, and gender, this projects an acceptance of others, which serves to establish a rapport and opens up the avenues of communication for the sharing of ideas and concerns.

People learn better in a comfortable and supportive environment. Not only is it important that the physical environment be conducive to learning, but the psychological climate should also be respectful of learners and focused on their need for an atmosphere of support and acceptance. Educators must have a clear view of their role as facilitators and expert coaches and avoid acting as controlling disseminators of information.

BE ORGANIZED AND GIVE DIRECTION

Excellent discussions, meaningful experiences in role-playing, and successful attempts at self-study are examples of teaching that do not happen by accident. They are the result of hours of skilled preparation, careful planning, and organization, which allow the learner to stay focused on the objectives. Material should be logically organized, objectives clearly defined and presented up front, and directions given in a straightforward, specific, and easily understood manner.

Instructional sessions should be relatively brief so as not to overload the learner with too much detail and extraneous content. Need-to-know information should take precedence over the nice-to-know information to ensure that enough time is allotted for the essentials. As Kessels (2003) has clearly documented, "40–80% of medical information provided by healthcare practitioners is forgotten immediately. The greater the amount of information presented, the lower the proportion correctly recalled; furthermore, almost half of the information that is remembered is incorrect" (p. 219).

Regardless of the method of instruction used, the attention span of the learner waxes and wanes over time, and what is learned first and last is retained the most (Ley, 1972). Audiovisual materials selected to supplement various methods of teaching should clarify or enhance a message. Advance organizers, topic headings that clue the learner into what is going to be presented and help focus the learner's attention on the message, should be used

to structure information. These headers assist the learner in identifying the subject to be addressed and anticipating in what order the information will be presented.

ELICIT AND GIVE FEEDBACK

Feedback should be a reciprocal process. It is a strategy to give information to the learner as well as to receive information from the learner. Both the teacher and the learner need to seek information about the quality of their performance. Feedback should be encouraged during and at the end of each teaching–learning encounter as well as at the completion of an educational program. It can take the form of either verbal or nonverbal responses to a situation.

Feedback that learners receive can be subjective or objective. Subjective data, whether physiological or psychological, come from within the learners themselves. People sense how they are reacting to a situation. Internally, they usually know how well they performed or how they feel by their own responses, such as fatigue, anxiety, disinterest, or satisfaction. Learners are able to compare their own performance to what they expect of themselves or what they think others expect of them.

Objective data come to the learners from the teacher, who measures their behavior based on a set of standards or criteria and who gives them an opinion on the progress they have made. To get feedback, the learner might ask, "How well did I do?" "Am I on track?" "Did I do all right?" or "What do you think?"

Feedback to the teacher is equally important because the effectiveness of teaching depends to a great extent on the learners' reactions. Whether positive or negative, verbal or nonverbal, feedback enables the teacher to determine whether he or she should maintain or modify his or her approach to teaching. Feedback indicates whether to proceed, take time to review or explain, or cease instruction altogether for the moment.

The teacher should be direct in eliciting feedback from the learners by asking questions such as "Did I answer your questions?" "Is this clear?" "Do you need me to explain it further?" or "What more can I help you with?" The teacher should also be sensitive to nonverbal expressions such as a nod, a smile, a look of bewilderment, or a frown indicating an understanding or lack thereof.

Feedback is neutral unless it is compared with established norms, preset criteria, or past behavior. How much someone learned, for example, is meaningless unless compared to what the person knew previously or how the person stacks up against other learners under similar conditions.

Feedback, either positive or negative, is needed by both the learner and the teacher. Praise reinforces behavior and increases the likelihood the behavior will continue. Constructive criticism tends to redirect behavior to conform with expected norms. Labeling someone's personality as cooperative, smart, stubborn, unmotivated, or uncaring is harmful, but it is helpful to label someone's performance to give that person specific information for improving, correcting, or continuing the behavior.

Use Questions

Questioning is one of the means for both the teacher and the learner to elicit feedback about performance. If the educator is skillful in the use of questioning, it serves multiple purposes in the teaching–learning process. Questions help to clarify or substantiate concepts, assess what the learner already knows about the topic, stimulate interest in a new subject, or evaluate the learner's mastery of the predetermined objectives.

Babcock and Miller (1994) identified three types of questions that can be used to elicit different types of answers:

1. Factual or descriptive questions begin with words such as *who, what, which, where,* or *when* and ask for recall-type responses from the learner.

Factual questions such as "Which foods are high in fat?" or "Whom should you call if you run out of medication?" elicit straightforward facts. Descriptive questions take a more open-ended approach, such as "What kinds of exercise do you get daily?" "What problems do you have with activities of daily living?" or "What are the signs and symptoms of infection?" These questions require a more detailed and organized response from the learner.

2. Clarifying questions ask for more information and help the learner to convey thoughts and feelings. Such questions might include "What do you mean when you say …?" or "When do you feel most anxious?"

3. High-order questions require more than memory or perception to answer. They ask the learner to make inferences, establish cause and effect, or compare and contrast concepts. Examples include "Why does a low-salt diet help to control blood pressure?" or "What do you think will happen if you don't take your medication?" or "What do you see as the advantages and disadvantages in following the treatment plan?"

After asking questions, a period of silence may occur. This can be uncomfortable for both the teacher and the learner. Teachers can reduce anxiety over silence by encouraging the learner to think about the answer before responding. In a group, this strategy also allows all participants to have a chance to think through their responses to the questions, which gives them the opportunity to make more thoughtful and deliberate responses. How long a teacher should wait for a response is dependent on many variables, such as the complexity of the questions, who the learners are, and what they are expected to know. Wait time is a matter of judgment on the part of the educator.

Questioning helps the teacher appropriately pace the material being presented. Also, answers to questions allow the educator to arrive at an evaluative judgment as to the progress the learner is making in the achievement of the behavioral objectives.

KNOW THE AUDIENCE

The effectiveness of teaching can be severely limited when the choice of instructional method is based on the interest and comfort level of the teacher and not on the assessed needs of the learner. Teachers must use methods that match the topic rather than their personality (Glenn, 2009).

Most teachers have a preferred style of teaching and tend to rely on that approach regardless of the content to be taught. Skilled teachers adapt themselves to a teaching style appropriate to the subject matter, setting, and various styles of the learners. Flexibility is their hallmark in tailoring the instructional design to the unique needs of each population of learners. They should be willing to use a variety of teaching methods to provide the best possible experience for achievement of objectives.

USE REPETITION AND PACING

Repetition, if used with discretion, is a technique that strengthens learning. It reinforces learning by aiding in the retention of information (Willingham, 2004). If overused, repetition can lead to boredom and frustration because the teacher is repeating what is already understood and remembered. If used deliberately, it can assist the learner in focusing on important points and keep the learner on track.

Repetition is especially important when presenting new or difficult material. The opportunity for repeated practice of behavioral tasks is called **skill inoculation**. Repetition can take the form of a simple reminder, a review of previously learned material, or the continued practice of a skill. Assessing the learner's understanding helps educators use repetition effectively.

Pacing refers to the speed at which information is presented. Some self-instruction methods of teach-

ing, such as programmed instruction, allow for individualized pacing so that learners can proceed at their own speed, depending on their abilities and style of learning. Other methods, such as group learning, require the teacher to take command of the rate at which information is presented and processed.

Many factors determine the optimal rate of teaching, such as the following:

- Previous history with learning
- Attention span
- The domain in which learning is to take place
- The learner's eagerness and determination to obtain a reward or attain a goal
- The degree of progress in learning
- The learner's ability to cope with frustration and discomfort

Keeping in touch with the audience helps teachers pace their teaching. It should be slow enough for assimilation of information, yet fast enough to maintain interest and enthusiasm.

SUMMARIZE IMPORTANT POINTS

Summarizing information at the completion of the teaching–learning encounter gives a perspective on what has been covered, how it relates to the objectives, and what the educator expects the learner to have achieved. Summarizing also reviews key ideas to instill information in the mind and helps the learner to see the parts of a whole. Closure should be used at the end of one lesson before proceeding to a new topic. Summary reinforces retention of information. It provides feedback as to the progress made, thereby leaving the learner with a feeling of satisfaction with what has been accomplished.

Instructional Settings

Traditionally, the primary focus of healthcare practice has been on the delivery of acute care in hospital settings. In recent years, however, the practice of health professionals in community-based settings has experienced tremendous growth. The reasons for the shift in orientation of healthcare practice from inpatient care sites to outpatient sites relate to the trends affecting the nation's healthcare system as a whole. These trends include public and private reimbursement policies, changing population demographics, advances in healthcare technology, an emphasis on wellness care, and increased consumer interest in health. In response to these trends, the domains of healthcare practice have broadened to include a greater emphasis on the delivery of care in community settings such as homes, clinics, health maintenance organizations (HMOs), physicians' offices, public schools, and the workplace.

With the increased focus on prevention, promotion, and independence in self-care activities, today's newly emerging healthcare system mandates the education of consumers to a greater extent than ever before. Opportunities for client teaching have become increasingly more varied in terms of the types of clients encountered, their particular learning needs, and the settings in which healthcare teaching occurs. Because health education has become an increasingly important responsibility of health professionals in all practice environments, it is important to acknowledge the various settings where clients, well or ill, are consumers of health care.

Instructional settings are classified according to the relationship health education has to the primary purpose of the organization or agency that provides health instruction. An **instructional setting** is defined as any place where health professionals engage in teaching for disease prevention, health promotion, and health maintenance and rehabilitation. An instructional setting is any environment in which health education takes place to provide individuals with learning experiences for the purpose of improving their health or reducing their risk for illness and injury. O'Halloran (2003) identified three types of settings for the education of clients:

1. A **healthcare setting** is one in which the delivery of health care is the primary or sole func-

tion of the institution, organization, or agency. Hospitals, home care associations, public health departments, outpatient clinics, extended-care facilities, health maintenance organizations, physician's offices, and therapist owned and managed centers are some examples of organizations whose primary purpose is to deliver health care. Health education is an integral aspect of the overall care delivered within these settings. Health practitioners function to provide direct client care, and their role encompasses the teaching of clients as part of that care.

2. A **healthcare-related setting** is one in which healthcare-related services are offered as a complementary function of the agency. Examples of this type of setting include the American Heart Association, the American Cancer Society, the American Arthritis Association, and the Muscular Dystrophy Association. These organizations provide client advocacy, conduct health screenings and self-help groups, distribute health education information and materials, and support research on disease and lifestyle issues for the benefit of consumers within the community. Education on health promotion, disease prevention, and improving the quality of life for those who live with a particular illness or disability is the key function of health professionals within these agencies.

3. A **non-healthcare setting** is one in which health care is an incidental or supportive function of an organization. Examples of this type of setting include businesses, industries, schools, and military and penal institutions. The primary purpose of these organizations is to produce a manufactured product or offer a non-health-related service to the public. Industries, for example, are involved in health care only to the extent of providing health screenings and nonemergent health coverage to their employees through a health office within their place of employment, making available instruction in job-related health and safety issues to meet Occupational Safety and Health

Administration (OSHA) regulations, or providing opportunities for health education through wellness programs to reduce absenteeism or improve employee morale.

Classifying instructional settings in which the health professional functions as teacher provides a frame of reference through which to better understand the interrelationship between the components of the organizational climate, the target audience, and the resources within the environment influencing the educational tasks to be accomplished. The role and functioning of the health professional are affected differently by these components in each of the identified settings.

Health professionals must recognize the numerous opportunities available for the teaching of those who are currently or potentially consumers of health care. Given that teaching is an important aspect of healthcare delivery and given the fact that health professionals are functioning as teachers in a multitude of settings, they encounter clients of differing ages and at various stages along the wellness-to-illness continuum. Wherever and whenever teaching takes place, health professionals need to recognize the importance of consciously applying the principles of teaching and learning to these encounters for maximum effectiveness in helping clients to attain and maintain optimal health.

Sharing Resources Among Settings

Health professionals involved in client health education should use available opportunities to share resources among the three identified settings (**Figure 11–3**). Many already perform this service as printed or audiovisual materials are borrowed, rented, or purchased for small fees from area institutions, organizations, or agencies; health professional educators from healthcare or health care-related settings are contracted for or voluntarily provide health education programs to small and large groups in other healthcare, healthcare-related, or non-healthcare settings; and health professionals from each category of setting collaborate on individual client situations or on major community health projects.

The health professionals from each of these settings can establish a health education committee in their community to coordinate health education programming, ensure effective use of all resources, and reduce duplication of efforts. The members of this committee can develop standardized health education content, delineate roles and services for each of the instructional settings, and share resources to provide a well-planned, comprehensive community program of health education for a wide spectrum of clients.

State of the Evidence

Client education is very complex. Clients present with a wide variety of chronic and acute illnesses, financial resources, developmental stages, cultural values, reading abilities, learning styles, motivation levels, and social support. Health professional students and staff differ widely on their educational and experiential backgrounds and are also influenced by generation gaps. This reality makes it difficult to generalize the results of research studies. Also it is difficult in some of the literature to analyze the cause and effect relationship between the instructional method used and the outcomes achieved. This, in turn, becomes more challenging when the goal is to compare studies.

Cooper, Booth, Fear, and Gill (2001) critically reviewed 12 meta-analysis studies concerning client education for people with chronic diseases where the treatment regime required behavior change. The question they asked concerned what type of educational interventions can actually produce the most benefit for these clients. The determination of effects by type of educational intervention was hampered by inadequate descriptions of the interventions. Another problem was the fact that the

Figure 11–3 Types of Instructional Settings for Health Education

EXAMPLES OF INSTRUCTIONAL SETTINGS

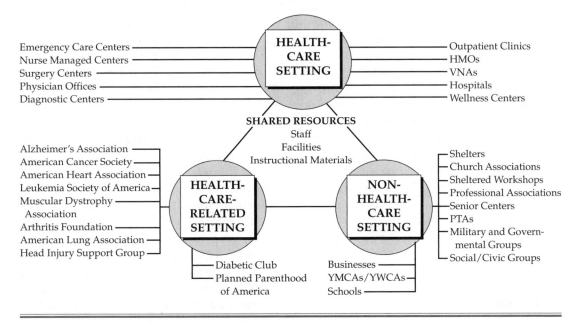

Emergency Care Centers
Nurse Managed Centers
Surgery Centers
Physician Offices
Diagnostic Centers

HEALTH-CARE SETTING

Outpatient Clinics
HMOs
VNAs
Hospitals
Wellness Centers

SHARED RESOURCES
Staff
Facilities
Instructional Materials

Alzheimer's Association
American Cancer Society
American Heart Association
Leukemia Society of America
Muscular Dystrophy
 Association
Arthritis Foundation
American Lung Association
Head Injury Support Group

HEALTH-CARE-RELATED SETTING

NON-HEALTH-CARE SETTING

Shelters
Church Associations
Sheltered Workshops
Professional Associations
Senior Centers
PTAs
Military and Governmental Groups
Social/Civic Groups

Diabetic Club
Planned Parenthood
 of America

Businesses
YMCAs/YWCAs
Schools

Source: O'Halloran, V. E. (2003). Instructional settings. In S. B. Bastable, *Nurse as educator: Principles of teaching and learning for nursing practice* (2nd ed., p. 468). Sudbury, MA: Jones and Bartlett.

interventions comprised more than one educational method. Their findings were that effect by educational approach could not be differentiated. Some evidence suggested that didactic and psychosocial strategies produced smaller outcome effects than a combination of behavioral, cognitive, and affective therapies.

Deakin, McShane, Cade, and Williams (2005) systematically reviewed 11 studies of group-based, patient-centered educational programs for people with type 2 diabetes to assess the effects on clinical, lifestyle, and psychosocial outcomes. This review provided evidence that group-based diabetes education programs for adults with type 2 diabetes resulted in improvements in glycated hemoglobin, fasting blood glucose, and diabetes knowl-

edge when monitored at 4–6 months and at 12 months.

In addition, Deakin et al. (2005) recommend more research on the theoretical models underpinning the educational programs. Some of the studies suggested that group education is more effective if based on adult learning principles, client empowerment, and participation. The authors also comment on the need for more research to determine whether this type of program is appropriate for all ethnic backgrounds. Cost effectiveness was included under their implications for future research, which is an especially important factor to be considered in the current healthcare environment.

The difficulty with measuring the effectiveness of different methods of instruction is that many studies do not make a distinction between instructional methods and instructional materials (tools), such as the study conducted by Dougal and Gonterman (1999). Instead the authors treat them as one and the same and therefore the studies' findings cannot be compared nor applied as evidence in this chapter, which deals exclusively with methods of instruction.

There are many empirical studies and expert reviews on the effectiveness of the various instructional methods available to teach different client and staff populations, and this chapter discusses selected reports. Further research needs to be conducted on specific populations in relation to effectiveness of instructional methods for teaching them about specific topics they need to learn. For example, what is the most effective and efficient method to teach healthcare consumers about important safety behaviors for optimal self-care management?

Summary

This chapter presents an in-depth review of the various instructional methods and compares the advantages and limitations of each approach. Also, it briefly addresses the instructional settings in which teaching takes place.

Emphasis is given to the importance of taking into account the learner characteristics, behavioral objectives, teacher characteristics, and available resources prior to selecting and using any of the vast array of methods at the teacher's disposal. In many instances, guidelines are put forth to assist health professional educators in planning and developing their own instructional activities. In addition, the major questions to be considered when evaluating the effectiveness of instructional methods are assessed in detail. Finally, techniques to enhance verbal presentations and some general principles to increase effectiveness of all methods of instruction are discussed.

What must be stressed are the inherent qualities of each method and the fact that no one method is better than another. The effectiveness of any method depends on the purpose for and the circumstances under which it is used. Health professionals in the role of educators are urged to take an eclectic approach to teaching by avoiding reliance on any one particular method. Varying teaching approaches or using them in combination with one another can assist educators in accomplishing the objectives for learning while meeting the different needs and styles of each and every learner.

Multisensory stimulation is best for increasing the acquisition of skills and the retention of information. Research regarding client and staff education is increasing. It is imperative that health professional educators demonstrate a willingness to make decisions on choosing and using instructional methods based on the evidence that is emerging about the most effective ways to teach in relation to learner and situational variables.

REVIEW QUESTIONS

1. How is the term *instructional method* defined?
2. What are the advantages and limitations of each instructional method?
3. Which instructional methods are most effective in encouraging active participation by the learner?
4. Which instructional methods are best for learning cognitive skills? Psychomotor skills? Affective skills?
5. What variables influence the selection of any method of instruction?
6. What major questions should teachers ask themselves when evaluating the effectiveness of an instructional method? Which question is the most important criterion for evaluation?
7. What is the difference between factual/descriptive questions, clarifying questions, and high-order questions?
8. What are the techniques that teachers can use to enhance the effectiveness of teaching?
9. Are teachers born or made? Explain.
10. What are the three classifications of instructional settings?

CASE STUDY

A well-known university in the Boston area offers programs in occupational therapy, physical therapy, athletic training, and exercise physiology. These programs attract a diverse group of students from all over the nation and abroad. Professors at the university meet before the school year to discuss the challenges and opportunities awaiting the incoming entry-level graduate students in their healthcare profession disciplines. One professor remarks, "This is a very eclectic group of students in terms of age, professional experience, ethnicity, and cultural background. I am not sure how to stimulate group interaction in a class with such diversity." The faculty members discuss various instructional methods they have used to facilitate empathy and understanding in groups of students. Mary comments, "I tried role-playing once for team building, but it didn't seem to work too well. Was role-playing a bad choice? What other teaching approaches can be used to actively engage these students?"

1. Discuss the advantages and limitations of the instructional method of role-playing to facilitate group cohesiveness.
2. If professors want to encourage learners to take an active role in their courses, what other instructional methods can they select?
3. An important aspect of evaluating any educational program is to assess the effectiveness of the instructional methods used. What five major questions should be asked to determine if an instructional method was effective?

References

Abruzzese, R. S. (1996). *Nursing staff development: Strategies for success* (2nd ed.). St. Louis, MO: Mosby-Year Book.

Allery, L. A. (2004). Educational games and structured experiences. *Medical Teacher, 26*(6), 504–505.

Babcock, D. E., & Miller, M. A. (1994). *Client education: Theory and practice.* St. Louis, MO: Mosby-Year Book.

Bain, K. (2004, April 9). What makes great teachers great? *The Chronicle of Higher Education,* B7–B9.

Bartlett, T. (2003, May 9). Big, but not bad. *The Chronicle of Higher Education,* 35–38.

Bays, C., & Hermann, C. (1997). Gaming versus lecture discussion: Effects on students' test performance. *Journal of Nursing Education, 36*(6), 292–294.

Beaubien, J. M., & Baker, D. P. (2004). The use of simulation for training teamwork skills in health care: How low can you go? *Quality and Safety in Health Care,* 13, i51–i56.

Begg, M. (2008). Leveraging game-informed healthcare education. *Medical Teacher, 30,* 155–158.

Bender, D., & Randall, K. E. (2006). Description and evaluation of an interactive Jeopardy game designed to foster self-assessment. *The Internet Journal of Allied Health Sciences and Practice, 3*(4), 1–7.

Berbiglia, V. A., Goddard, L., & Littlefield, J. H. (1997). Gaming: A strategy for honors programs. *Journal of Nursing Education, 36*(6), 289–291.

Beylefeld, A. A., & Struwig, M. C. (2007). A gaming approach to learning medical microbiology: Students' experiences of flow. *Medical Teacher, 29,* 933–940.

Billings, D. M., & Halstead, J. A. (2009). *Teaching in nursing: A guide for faculty* (3rd ed.). St. Louis, MO: Saunders Elsevier.

Blakely, G., Skirton, H., Cooper, S., Allum, P., & Nelmes, P. (2008, August 13). Educational gaming in the health sciences: Systematic review. *Journal of Advanced Nursing,* 259–269.

Boyd, M. D., Gleit, C. J., Graham, B. A., & Whitman, N. I. (1998). *Health teaching in nursing practice: A professional model* (3rd ed.). Stamford, CT: Appleton and Lange.

Bradshaw, M. J., & Lowenstein, A. J. (2007). *Innovative teaching strategies in nursing and related health professions* (4th ed.). Sudbury, MA: Jones and Bartlett.

Brookfield, S. D. (2006). *The skillful teacher: On technique, trust, and responsiveness in the classroom.* San Francisco: Jossey-Bass.

Brookfield, S. D., & Preskill, S. (1999). *Discussion as a way of teaching: Tools and techniques for democratic classrooms.* San Francisco: Jossey-Bass.

Burkhart, J. A. (2008). Training nurses to be teachers. *The Journal of Continuing Education in Nursing, 39*(11), 503–510.

Cantillon, P. (2003, Feb. 22). ABC of learning and teaching in medicine: Teaching large groups. *British Medical Journal,* 326, 437–440.

Caputi, L. (2010). *Teaching nursing: The art and science* (2nd ed., Vols. 1, 2, and 3). Glen Ellyn, IL: College of DuPage Press.

Carkhuff, M. H. (1996). Reflective learning: Work groups as learning groups. *The Journal of Continuing Education in Nursing, 27*(5), 209–214.

Childs, J. C., & Sepples, S. (2006). Clinical teaching by simulation: Lessons learned from a complex patient care scenario. *Nursing Education Perspectives, 27*(3), 154–158.

Comer, S. K. (2005). Patient care simulations: Role playing to enhance clinical understanding. *Nursing Education Perspectives, 26*(6), 357–361.

Cook, D., Levinson, A., Garside, S., Dupras, D., Erwin, P., & Montori, V. (2008). Internet-based learning in the health professions: A meta-analysis. *JAMA, 300*(10), 1181–1196.

Cooper, H., Booth, K., Fear, S., & Gill, G. (2001). Chronic disease patient education: Lessons from meta-analyses. *Patient Education and Counseling, 44,* 107–117.

Corbridge, S., McLaughlin, R., Tiffen, J., Wade, L., Templin, R., & Corbridge, T. C. (2008). Using simulation to enhance knowledge and confidence. *The Nurse Practitioner, 33*(6), 12–13.

Cunningham, M. A., & Baker, D. (1986). How to teach patients better and faster. *RN, 49*(9), 50–52.

de Tornyay, R., & Thompson, M. A. (1987). *Strategies for teaching nursing* (3rd ed.). New York: Wiley.

Del Bueno, D. J., Griffin, L. R., Burke, S. M., & Foley, M. A. (1990). The clinical teacher as a critical link in competence development. *Journal of Nursing Staff Development, 6,* 135–138.

Deakin, T., McShane, C. E., Cade, J. E., Williams, R. D. R. R. (2005). Group-based training for self-management strategies in people with type 2 diabetes mellitus. *Cochrane Database of Systematic Reviews,* Issue 2, Art. No.: CD003417. DOI: 10.1002/14651858. CD1858. CD003417.pub2.

DeYoung, S. (2003). *Teaching strategies for nurse educators.* Upper Saddle River, NJ: Prentice Hall.

Dillon, P. M., Noble, K. A., & Kaplan, L. (2009). Simulation as a means to foster collaborative interdisciplinary education. *Nursing Education Perspectives, 30*(2), 87–90.

Dougal, J., & Gonterman, R. (1999). A comparison of three teaching methods on learning and retention. *Journal for Nurses in Staff Development, 15*(5), 205–209.

Editorial. (2009). Games people play could be good for their health, sense of empowerment. *Patient Education Management, 16*(12), 133–135.

Emerson, R. J. (2007). *Nursing education in the clinical setting.* St. Louis, MO: Mosby Elsevier.

Epstein, R. M. (2007). Assessment in medical education. *The New England Journal of Medicine, 346*(4), 387–396.

Evans, M. (2000). Polished, professional presentation: Unlocking the design elements. *Journal of Continuing Education in Nursing, 31*(5), 213–218.

Falvo, D. R. (2004). *Effective patient education: A guide to increased compliance* (3rd ed.). Sudbury, MA: Jones and Bartlett.

Fredette, S. L. (1990). A model for improving cancer patient education. *Cancer Nursing, 13*, 207–215.

Freitas, L., Lantz, J., & Reed, R. (1991). The creative teacher. *Nurse Educator, 16*(1), 5–7.

Gaba, D. M. (2004). The future vision of simulation in health care. *Quality and Safety in Health Care, 13*, i2–i10.

Gaba, D. M. (2009). Do as we say, not as you do: Using simulation to investigate clinical behavior in action. *Simulation in Healthcare, 4*(2), 67–69.

Gaberson, K. B., & Oermann, M. H. (2007). *Clinical teaching strategies in nursing* (2nd ed.). New York: Springer.

Germano, W. (2003, November 28). The scholarly lecture: How to stand and deliver. *The Chronicle of Higher Education,* B15.

Glenn, D. (2009, December 15). Matching teaching style to learning style may not help students. *The Chronicle of Higher Education.* Retrieved from daily-html@chronicle.com.

Haggard, A. (1989). *Handbook of patient education.* Rockville, MD: Aspen.

Hayes, K., Huckstadt, A., & Gibson, R. (2000). Developing interactive continuing education on the Web. *Journal of Continuing Education in Nursing, 31*(5), 199–203.

Henry, J. M. (1997). Gaming: A teaching strategy to enhance adult learning. *Journal of Continuing Education in Nursing, 28*, 231–234.

House, B. M., Chassie, M. B., & Spohn, B. B. (1990). Questioning: An essential ingredient in effective teaching. *Journal of Continuing Education in Nursing, 21*, 196–201.

Irvin, S. M. (1996, May/June). Creative teaching strategies. *The Journal of Continuing Education, 27*(3), 108–114.

Jacobs, K. (2009). Professional presentations and publications. In Creapeau, E., Cohn, E., Boyt Schell, B. (eds.), *Willard and Spackman's Occupational Therapy* (11th ed., pp. 411–417). Philadelphia: Wolters Kluwer/Lippincott Williams & Wilkins.

Jeffries, P. R. (2005). A framework for designing, implementing, and evaluating simulations used as teaching strategies in nursing. *Nursing Education Perspectives, 26*(2), 96–103.

Johnson, D. W., Johnson, R. T., & Smith, K. (2007). The state of cooperative learning in post-secondary and professional settings. *Educational Psychology Review, 19*, 15–29.

Joos, I. R. M. (1984). A teacher's guide for using games and simulation. *Nurse Educator, 9*(3), 25–29.

Kaphingst, K. A., Persky, S., McCall, C., Lachance, C., Lowenstein, J., Beall, A. C., et al. (2009). Testing the effects of educational strategies on comprehension of a genomic concept using virtual reality technology. *Patient Education and Counseling, 77*, 224–230.

Kessels, R. P. (2003). Patients' memory for medical information. *Journal of the Royal Society of Medicine, 96*, 219–222.

Knowles, M. S., Holton, E. F., & Swanson, R. A. (1998). *The adult learner: The defensive classic in adult education and human resource development* (5th ed.). Houston: Gulf Publishing.

Kowalski, K. (2004). The use of set. *The Journal of Continuing Education in Nursing, 35*(2), 56–57.

Lewis, D. J., Saydak, S. J., Mierzwa, I. P., & Robinson, J. A. (1989). Gaming: A teaching strategy for adult learners. *Journal of Continuing Education in Nursing, 20*, 80–84.

Ley, P. (1972). Primacy, rated importance, and recall of medical statements. *Journal of Health and Social Behavior, 13*, 311–317.

Lieberman, D. (2001). Management of chronic pediatric diseases with interactive health games: Theory and research findings. *Journal of Ambulatory Care Management, 24*(1), 26–38.

Lorig, K. R. (2003). Taking patient ed to the next level: Patients with chronic illnesses need more than traditional patient education. They need you to help them develop the self-management skills that they'll use for the rest of their lives. *RN, 66*(12), 35–44.

Lorig, K., & Gonzalez, V. M. (1993). Using self-efficacy theory in patient education. In B. Gilroth (ed.), *Managing hospital-based patient education* (pp. 327–337). Chicago: American Hospital Publishing.

Lowenstein, A. J. (2007). Role Play. In M. J. Bradshaw & A. J. Lowenstein, *Innovative teaching strategies in nursing and related health professions* (4th ed., pp. 173–182). Sudbury, MA: Jones and Bartlett.

Markiewicz, T., & Wells, N. (1997). Mundanatories no more. *Journal of Continuing Education in Nursing, 28*(2), 88–90.

Martin, J. T., Hoffman, M. K., & Kaminski, P. F. (2005). NPs vs. IT for effective colposcopy patient education. *The Nurse Practitioner, 30*(4), 52–57.

Miller, M. A., & Stoeckel, P. R. (2011). *Client education: theory and practice.* Sudbury, MA: Jones and Bartlett.

Murray, E., Burns, J., Tai, S. S., Lai, R., & Nazareth, I. (2005). Interactive health communication applications for people with chronic disease (review). *Cochrane Database of Systematic Reviews, 2005*(4), 70.

Musinski, B. (1999). The educator as facilitator: A new kind of leadership. *Nursing Forum, 34*(1), 23–29.

Musolino, G. M., & Mostrom, E. (2005). Reflection and the scholarship of teaching, learning, and assessment. *Journal of Physical Therapy Education, 19*(3), 52–66.

Narrow, B. (1979). *Patient teaching in nursing practice: A patient and family centered approach.* New York: Wiley.

Oakley, B., & Brent, R. (2004). Turning student groups into effective teams. *Journal of Student Centered Learning, 2*(1), 9–34.

O'Connor, A. B. (2006). *Clinical instruction and evaluation: A teaching resource* (2nd ed.). Sudbury, MA: Jones and Bartlett.

Oermann, M. H. (2003). Effects of educational intervention in waiting room on patient satisfaction. *Journal of Ambulatory Care Management, 26*(2), 150–158.

O'Halloran, V. E. (2003). Instructional settings. In S. B. Bastable (ed.), *Nurse as educator: Principles of teaching and learning for nursing practice* (2nd ed., pp. 465–492). Sudbury, MA: Jones and Bartlett.

O'Leary, S., Diepenhorst, L., Churley-Strom, R., & Magrane, D. (2005). Educational games in an obstetrics and gynecology core curriculum. *American Journal of Obstetrics and Gynecology, 193*, 1848–1851.

O'Very, D. (1999). Self-paced: The right pace for staff development. *Journal of Continuing Education in Nursing, 30*(4), 182–187.

Parrott, T. E. (1994). Humor as a teaching strategy. *Nurse Educator, 19*(3), 36–38.

Peters, F. L., & Connell, K. M. (1991). Incorporating the affective component into an AIDS workshop. *Journal of Continuing Education in Nursing, 22*, 95–99.

Phillips, L. D. (1999). Patient education: Understanding the process to maximize time and outcomes. *Journal of Intravenous Nursing, 22*(1), 19–35.

Prochaska, J., DiClemente, C., Velicer, W., & Rossi, J. (1993). Standardized, individualized, interactive, and personalized self-help programs for smoking cessation. *Health Psychology, 12*(5), 399–405.

Prochaska, J., Velicer, W., Rossi, J., Goldstein, M., Marcus, B., Rakowski, W., et al. (1994). Stages of change and decisional balance for 12 problem behaviors. *Health Psychology, 13*(1), 39–46.

Raines, D. A. (2010). An innovation to facilitate student engagement and learning: Crossword puzzles in the classroom. *Teaching and Learning in Nursing, 5*(2), 85–90.

Ramsey, A. M., & Siroky, A. S. (1988). The use of puppets to teach school-aged children with asthma. *Pediatric Nursing, 14*, 187–190.

Redman, B. K. (2007). *The practice of patient education: A case study approach* (10th ed.). St. Louis, MO: Mosby Elsevier.

Ridley, R. T. (2007). Interactive teaching: A concept analysis. *Journal of Nursing Education, 46*(5), 203–209.

Robinson, K. J., Lewis, D. J., & Robinson, J. A. (1990). Games: A way to give laboratory values meaning. *American Nephrology Nurses Association Journal, 17*(4), 306–308.

Rothwell, W. J., & Kazanas, H. C. (2004). *Mastering the instructional design process: A systematic approach* (3rd ed.). San Francisco: Pfeiffer.

Rowell, S., & Spielvogle, S. (1996). Wanted: "A few good bug detectives." A gaming technique to increase staff awareness of current infection control practices. *Journal of Continuing Education in Nursing, 27*(6), 274–278.

Saarmann, L., Daugherty, J., & Riegel, B. (2000). Patient teaching to promote behavior change. *Nursing Outlook, 48*(6), 281–287.

Salyers, V. L. (2007). Teaching psychomotor skills to beginning nursing students using a web-enhanced approach: A quasi-experimental study. *International Journal of Nursing Education Scholarship, 4*(1), 1–12.

Schmitz, B. D., MacLean, S. L., & Shidler, H. M. (1991). An emergency pursuit game: A method for teaching emergency decision-making skills. *Journal of Continuing Education in Nursing, 22*, 152–158.

Shearer, R., & Davidhizar, R. (2003). Using role play to develop cultural competence. *Journal of Nursing Education, 42*(6), 273–276.

Silberman, M. L. (1990). *Active training: A handbook of techniques, designs, case examples, and tips.* New York: Lexington Books.

Snowman, J., & Biehler, R. (2006). *Psychology applied to teaching.* Boston: Houghton Mifflin Company.

Sorensen, H. A. J., & Yankech, L. R. (2008). Precepting in the fast lane: Improving critical thinking in new graduate nurses. *The Journal of Continuing Education in Nursing, 39*(5), 208–214.

Springer, L., Stanne, M. E., & Donovan, S. S. (1999). Effects of small-group learning on undergraduates in science, mathematics, engineering, and technology: A meta-analysis. *Review of Educational Research, 69*(1), 21–51.

Ridley, R. T. (2007). Interactive teaching: A concept analysis. *Journal of Nursing Education, 46*(5), 203–209.

Tang, T. S., Funnell, M. M., & Anderson, R. M. (2006). Group education strategies for diabetes self-management. *Diabetes Spectrum, 19*(2), 99–105.

Turner, B. (2007). Embracing simulation and virtual reality. *Duke Nursing Magazine, 2*(1), 22–23.

Vander Zanden, J. W., Crandell, T. L., & Crandell, C. H. (2007). *Human development* (8th ed.). Boston: McGraw-Hill.

Wainwright, S. F., Shepard, K. F., Harman, L. B., & Stephens, J. (2010). Novice and experienced physical therapist clinicians: A comparison of how reflection is used to inform the clinical decision-making process. *Physical Therapy, 90*(1), 75–88.

Willingham, D. T. (2004, Spring). Practice makes perfect: But only if you practice beyond the point of perfection. *American Educator,* 31–33, 38.

Woodring, B. C., & Woodring, R. C. (2007). Lecture is not a four-letter word! In M. S. Bradshaw & A. J. Lowenstein (eds.), *Innovative teaching strategies in nursing and related health professions* (pp. 109–130). Sudbury, MA: Jones and Bartlett.

Yoo, M. S., & Yoo, I. Y. (2003). The effectiveness of standardized patients as a teaching method for nursing fundamentals. *Journal of Nursing Education, 42*(10), 444–448.

Young, P., & Diekelmann, N. (2002). Learning to lecture: Exploring the skills, strategies, and practices of new teachers in nursing education. *Journal of Nursing Education, 41*(9), 405–412.

Chapter 12

Instructional Materials

Diane S. Hainsworth

CHAPTER HIGHLIGHTS

KEY TERMS

- ❏ instructional materials
- ❏ characteristics of the learner
- ❏ characteristics of the media
- ❏ characteristics of the task
- ❏ delivery system
- ❏ realia
- ❏ illusionary representations
- ❏ symbolic representations
- ❏ replica
- ❏ analogue
- ❏ symbol
- ❏ audiovisual materials
- ❏ multimedia learning
- ❏ blended learning

OBJECTIVES

After completing this chapter, the reader will be able to

1. Differentiate between instructional materials and instructional methods.
2. Identify the three major variables (learner, task, and media characteristics) to be considered when selecting, developing, and evaluating instructional materials.

3. Cite the three components of instructional materials required to communicate educational messages effectively.
4. Discuss general principles applicable to all types of media.
5. Identify the multitude of instructional materials—printed, demonstration, and audiovisual media—available for client and professional education.
6. Describe the general guidelines for development of printed materials.
7. Analyze the advantages and disadvantages specific to each type of instructional medium.
8. Evaluate the type of media suitable for use depending on such variables as the size of the audience, the resources available, and the characteristics of the learner.
9. Identify where educational tools can be found.
10. Critique instructional materials for value and appropriateness.
11. Recognize the supplemental nature of media's role in client, staff, and student education.

Whereas instructional methods are the approaches used for teaching (as described in Chapter 11), **instructional materials** are the vehicles by which information is communicated. Often these terms are used interchangeably and are frequently referred to in combination with one another as teaching strategies and techniques. But instructional methods and instructional materials are not one and the same, and a clear distinction can and should be made between them. Instructional methods are the way information is taught. Instructional materials, which include printed, demonstration, and audiovisual media, are the adjuncts used to enhance teaching and learning. These multimedia approaches must be examined from a scientific, evidence-based perspective, grounded in theory on how people learn (Mayer, 2005).

Instructional materials, also known as tools and aids, are mechanisms or objects to transmit information that are intended to supplement, rather than replace, the act of teaching and the role of the teacher. These modes by which information is shared with the learner often are not considered in depth, and yet instructional materials represent an important, complex component of the educational process. Given the numerous factors affecting both the teacher and the learner, such as the increase

in staff workloads, the decrease in length of inpatient stays or outpatient visits, the increase in client acuity, the alternative settings in which education is now delivered, and the shrinking resources for educational services, it is imperative that the health professional as educator understand the various types of printed, demonstration, and audiovisual media available to complement teaching efforts efficiently and effectively.

Instructional materials provide the health professional educator with tools to deliver education messages creatively, clearly, accurately, and in a timely fashion. They help the educator reinforce information, clarify abstract concepts, and simplify complex messages. Multimedia resources serve to stimulate a learner's senses as well as add variety, realism, and enjoyment to the teaching/learning experience. They have the potential to assist learners not only in acquiring knowledge and skills but also in retaining more effectively what they learn. Research indicates that a variety of printed, demonstration, and audiovisual materials does, indeed, facilitate teaching and learning.

This chapter provides a systematic overview of the process for selecting, developing, implementing, and evaluating instructional materials. Various types of audiovisual media are examined with an eye to matching them to the particular characteristics of learners, the specific topics to be taught, and the variable situations and settings for teaching and learning. The advantages and disadvantages of each of the media types are discussed. Although the choice of instructional materials often depends on availability or cost, whichever tools are selected should enhance achievement of expected learning outcomes.

This chapter is intended to inform health professional educators about various media options so that they can make informed choices regarding appropriate instructional materials that fit the learner, that affect the motivation of the learner, and that accomplish the learning task. Whether health professionals educate clients and their families, staff, or health professions' students, the same principles apply in making decisions about the type of materials selected for instruction.

General Principles

Before selecting or developing media from the multitude of available options, health professional educators should be aware of the following general principles regarding the effectiveness of instructional materials:

- The teacher must be familiar with the media content before using a tool.
- Printed, demonstration, and audiovisual materials can change learner behavior by influencing cognitive, affective, and/or psychomotor development.
- No one tool is considered better than another in enhancing learning because the suitability of any particular medium depends on many variables.
- The tools should complement the instructional methods.
- The choice of media should be consistent with subject content and match the tasks to be

learned to assist the learner in accomplishing predetermined behavioral objectives.
- The instructional materials should reinforce and supplement—not substitute for—the educator's teaching efforts.
- Media should match the available financial resources.
- Instructional aids should be appropriate for the physical conditions of the learning environment, such as the size and seating of the audience, acoustics, space, lighting, and display hardware (delivery mechanisms) available.
- Media should complement the sensory abilities, developmental stages, and educational level of the intended audience.
- The message imparted by instructional materials must be accurate, valid, authoritative, up-to-date, appropriate, unbiased, and free of any unintended messages.
- The media should contribute meaningfully to the learning situation by adding and diversifying information.

Choosing Instructional Materials

Health professional educators must consider many important variables when selecting instructional materials. The role of the health professional educator goes beyond the dispensing of information only; it also involves skill in designing and planning for instruction. Learning can be made more enjoyable for both the learner and the teacher if the educator knows what instructional materials are available, as well as how to choose and use them so as to enhance the teaching–learning experience.

Knowledge of the diversity of instructional tools and their appropriate use enables the teacher to make education more interesting, challenging, and effective for all types of learners. With current trends in healthcare reform, educational strategies to teach clients, in particular, need to include instructional materials for health promotion and illness prevention, as well as instructional materials for health maintenance and restoration.

Making appropriate choices of instructional materials depends on a broad understanding of three major variables: (1) **characteristics of the learner**, (2) **characteristics of the media**, and (3) **characteristics of the task** to be achieved (Frantz, 1980). A useful mnemonic for remembering these variables is LMAT: learner, media, and task, which is derived from the last letter of the word instructional and the first three letters of the word materials.

1. *Characteristics of the learner:* Many variables are known to influence learning. Therefore, it is important for educators to know their audience so as to choose media that best suit the needs and abilities of various learners. They must consider sensorimotor abilities, physical attributes, reading skills, motivational levels (locus of control), developmental stages, learning styles, gender, socioeconomic characteristics, and cultural backgrounds.
2. *Characteristics of the media:* A wide variety of media—printed, demonstration, and audiovisual—is available to enhance methods of instruction for the achievement of objectives. Print materials are the most common form through which the information is communicated, and nonprint media include a full range of audio and visual possibilities. Because no single medium is most effective, the educator should be flexible in considering a multimedia approach to complement methods of instruction.
3. *Characteristics of the task:* Identifying the learning domain (cognitive, affective, and/or psychomotor) as well as the complexity of those behaviors that are required, which are based on the predetermined behavioral objectives, define the task(s) to be accomplished.

The Three Major Components of Instructional Materials

Depending on the instructional methods chosen to communicate information, educators must decide which media are potentially best suited to assist with the process of teaching and learning. The delivery system (Weston & Cranston, 1986), content, and presentation (Frantz, 1980) are the three major components of media that educators should keep in mind when selecting print and nonprint materials for instruction.

Delivery System

The **delivery system** includes both the software (physical form of the materials) and the hardware used in presentation of information. For instance, the educator giving a lecture might choose to embellish the information being presented using a delivery system, such as PowerPoint slides (software) and a computer (hardware). The content on DVDs (software), in conjunction with DVD players (hardware), and CD-ROM programs (software), in conjunction with the computer (hardware), are other examples of delivery systems.

The choice of the delivery system is influenced by the size of the intended audience, the pacing and flexibility needed for delivery, and the sensory aspects most suitable to the audience. More recently, the geographical distribution of the audience is a significant influence on choice of delivery systems, given the popularity of distance education modalities.

Content

The content (intended message) is independent of the delivery system and is the actual information being communicated to the learner, which might focus on any topic relevant to the teaching–learning experience. When selecting media, the health professional as educator must consider several factors:

- The accuracy of the information being conveyed. Is it up-to-date, reliable, and authentic?
- The appropriateness of the medium to convey particular information. Brochures or pamphlets and podcasts, for example, can be very appropriate tools for sharing information to change behavior in the cognitive or affective domain but not ideal for skill development in the psychomotor domain. Videos, as well as real equipment for demonstrations and return demonstrations, are much more effective tools for conveying information relative to learning psychomotor behaviors.
- The appropriateness of the readability level of materials for the intended audience. Is the content written at a literacy level suitable for the learner's reading and comprehension abilities? The more complex the task, the more important it is to write clear, simple, succinct instructions enhanced with illustrations so that the learner can understand the content (see Chapter 7).

Presentation

Weston and Cranston (1986) state that the form of the message, in other words, how information is presented, is the most important component for selecting or developing instructional materials. However, a consideration of this aspect of the media is frequently ignored. They describe the form of the message as occurring along a continuum from concrete (real objects) to abstract (symbols).

Realia

Realia refers to the most concrete form of stimuli that can be used to deliver information. For instance, an actual woman demonstrating breast self-examination is the most concrete example of realia.

Because this form of presentation might be less acceptable for a wide range of teaching situations, the next best choice would be a manikin. This model, analogous to a human figure, has many characteristics that simulate reality, including size and three-dimensionality (width, breadth, and depth), but without being the true figure that may very well cause embarrassment for the learner. The message is less concrete, yet using an imitation of a person as an instructional medium allows for an accurate presentation of information with near-maximal stimulation of the learners' perceptual abilities. Further along the continuum of realia is a video presentation of a woman performing breast self-examination. The learner could still learn accurate breast self-examination this way, but the aspect of true dimensionality is absent. The message becomes less concrete and more abstract.

Illusionary Representations

The term **illusionary representations** applies to a less concrete, more abstract form of stimuli to deliver a message, such as moving or still photographs, audiotapes projecting true sounds, and real-life drawings. Although many realistic cues, including dimensionality, are missing from this category of instructional materials, the advantages of illusionary media are that they can offer learners a variety of real-life visual and auditory experiences to which they might otherwise not have access or exposure because of such factors as location or expense. For example, pictures of how to stage decubitus ulcers or audiotapes on how to discriminate between normal and abnormal lung sounds, although more abstract in form, do to some degree resemble or simulate realia.

Symbolic Representations

The term **symbolic representations** applies to the most abstract types of messages, yet they are the most common form of stimuli used for instruction.

They include numbers and letters of the alphabet, symbols that are written and spoken as words that are employed to convey ideas or represent objects. Audiotapes of someone speaking, live oral presentations, graphs, written texts, handouts, posters, flipcharts, and whiteboards on which to display words and images are vehicles to deliver messages in symbolic form. The chief disadvantage of symbolic representations stems from their lack of concreteness. The more abstract and sophisticated the message, the more difficult it is to decipher and comprehend. Therefore, these symbolic presentations may be inappropriate as instructional materials for very young children, learners from different cultures, learners with significant literacy problems, and individuals with cognitive and sensory impairments.

When making decisions about which tools to select to best accomplish teaching objectives, the health professional educator should carefully consider these three media components. When choosing from a wide range of print and audiovisual options, the educator must consider the various delivery systems available, the content or message to be conveyed, and the form in which information will be presented. Educators must remember that no one type of media is suitable for all audiences in promoting acquisition and retention of information. Most important, the function of instructional materials is to supplement, complement, and support the educator's teaching efforts for the successful achievement of learner outcomes.

Types of Instructional Materials

Written Materials

Handouts, leaflets, books, pamphlets, brochures, and instruction sheets (all symbolic representations) are the most widely employed and most accessible type of media used for teaching. Printed materials

have been described as "frozen language" (Redman, 2007, p. 34) and are the most common form of teaching tool because of the distinct advantages they provide to enhance teaching and learning.

The greatest virtues of written materials are as follows:

- They are available to the learner as a reference for reinforcement of information when the health professional is not immediately present to answer questions or clarify information.
- They are widely used at all levels of society, so this type of media is acceptable and familiar to the public.
- They are easily obtainable through commercial sources, usually at relatively low cost and on a wide variety of subjects, for distribution by educators.
- They are provided in convenient forms, such as pamphlets, which are portable, reusable, and do not require software or hardware resources.
- They are becoming more widely available in languages other than English as a result of the recognition of significant cultural and ethnic shifts in the general population.
- They are suitable to a large number of learners who prefer reading as opposed to receiving messages in other formats.
- They are flexible in that the information is absorbed at a speed controlled by the reader.

The disadvantages of printed materials include the following facts:

- Written words are the most abstract form in which to convey information.
- Immediate feedback on the information presented may be limited.
- A large percentage of materials are written at too high a level for reading and comprehension by the majority of clients (Doak, Doak, Friedell, & Meade, 1998).
- They are inappropriate for persons with visual or cognitive impairment.

COMMERCIALLY PREPARED MATERIALS

A wealth of brochures, posters, pamphlets, and client-focused texts is currently available from commercial vendors. Whether they enhance the quality of learning is an important question for health professional educators to consider when trying to evaluate these products for content, readability, and presentation. Commercial products may or may not be produced in collaboration with health professionals, which raises the question of how factual the information may be. For example, materials prepared by pharmaceutical companies or medical supply companies might not be free of bias. Educators must ask several questions when reviewing printed materials that have been prepared commercially, including the following:

- Who produced the item? Evidence should make it clear whether input was provided by health professionals with expertise in the subject matter.
- Can the item be previewed? The educator should have an opportunity to examine the accuracy and appropriateness of content to ensure that the information needed by the target audience is provided.
- Is the price of the teaching tool consistent with its educational value? Getting across an important message effectively may justify a significant cost outlay, especially if the tool can be used with large numbers of learners. However, simple printed instruction sheets may do the job just as well at less expense and can provide the educator with the ability to update the information on a frequent basis.

The main advantages of using commercial materials is that they are readily available and can be obtained in bulk for free or at a relatively low cost (Fraze, Griffith, Green, & McElroy, 2010). An educator would need to spend hours researching, writing, and copying materials to create informational materials of equal quality and value. Also, commercial online materials are available, which can be customized to individual clients.

The disadvantages of using commercial materials include issues of cost, accuracy and adequacy of content, and readability of the materials. Some educational booklets are expensive to purchase and impractical to give away in large quantities to learners unless the educator uses materials that can be individualized. Fraze and associates (2010) have developed a checklist to help healthcare providers determine the appropriateness of printed education materials for use by their clients for improvement of health outcomes in various clinical settings.

INSTRUCTOR-COMPOSED MATERIALS

Educators may choose to write their own instructional materials for the purpose of cost savings or the need to tailor content to specific audiences. Advantages to composing materials are many (Brownson, 1998; Doak et al., 1998). By writing their own materials, educators can tailor the information to accomplish the following points:

- Fit the institution's policies, procedures, and equipment
- Build in answers to those questions asked most frequently by clients
- Highlight points considered especially important by the team of physicians and other health professionals
- Reinforce specific oral instructions that clarify difficult concepts

Doak and colleagues (1998) outline specific suggestions for tailoring information to help clients want to read and remember the message and to act on it. These authors define tailoring as personalizing the message so that the content, structure, and image fit an individual client's learning needs. For example, they suggest techniques to tailor information, such as writing the client's name on the cover of a pamphlet, and opening a pamphlet with a client and highlighting the most important information as it is verbally reviewed. In another example, Feldman (2004) describes successful use of child care checklists that had simple line drawings (no more than two to a page) coupled with brief written descriptions that led parents step-by-step through specific care tasks, such as bathing a baby. Audiotapes also accompanied these pictures and simple instructions. Additional studies support the efficacy of tailored instruction over nontailored messages in achieving reading, recall, and follow-through in health teaching (Campbell et al., 1994; Skinner, Strecher, & Hospers, 1994).

There are, of course, disadvantages to composing materials. Educators need to exercise extra care to ensure that materials are well written and laid out effectively, which can be a time-consuming endeavor. Although health professionals as educators are expected to enhance their methods of teaching with instructional materials, few have ever had formal training in the development and application of written materials. Many tools written by health professionals are too long, too detailed, and composed at too high a level for the target audience. Doak, Doak, and Root (1996) and Brownson (1998) suggest the following guidelines to ensure the clarity of self-composed printed education materials:

- Make sure the content is accurate and up-to-date.
- Organize the content in a logical, step-by-step, simple fashion so that learners are being informed adequately but are not overwhelmed with large amounts of information. Avoid giving detailed rationales because they may unnecessarily lengthen the written information. Prioritize the content to address only what learners need to know. Content that is nice to know can be addressed orally on an individual basis.

- Make sure the information succinctly discusses the what, how, and when. Follow the KISS rule: keep it simple and smart. This can best be accomplished by putting the information into a question-and-answer format or by dividing the information into subheadings according to the nature of the content.
- Regardless of format, avoid medical jargon whenever possible, and define any technical terms in laypeople's language. Sometimes it is important to expose clients to technical terms because of complicated procedures and ongoing interaction with the medical team, so careful definitions can minimize misunderstandings. Be consistent with the words used.
- Find out the average grade in school completed by the targeted client population, and write the client education materials two to four grade levels below that level. For individuals who are nonliterate, pictographs can increase recall of spoken medical instruction (Houts et al., 1998; Kessels, 2003). Follow the guidelines in Chapter 7 for decreasing reading level.

Always state things in positive, not negative, terms. Never illustrate incorrect messages. For example, depicting a hand holding a metered-dose inhaler in the mouth not only incorrectly illustrates a drug delivery technique (Weixler, 1994) but reinforces that message by its visual impact alone. **Figure 12–1** illustrates the correct way to use an inhaler and reinforces a positive message.

In addition to the guidelines for clarity and completeness in constructing written materials, format and appearance are equally important in motivating learners to read the printed word. If the format and appearance are too detailed, learners will feel overwhelmed, and instead of attracting the learners, you will discourage and repel them (see **Figure 12–2**). To avoid common pitfalls in writing instructional tools, see Chapter 7 on how to write effective printed materials.

Figure 12-1 Diagram Illustrating Proper Technique for Inhaler Use

Shake inhaler
well.

Hold upright
with cap off.

Hold inhaler 1 to 2
inches from mouth.
Breathe out.

Press down on inhaler. Breathe
in slowly (3 to 5 seconds).

Hold breath 10 seconds,
then repeat puffs.

Figure 12-2 Inadequate Versus Adequate Appearance and Formatting

Cluttered Appearance

Better Visual Appearance

EVALUATING PRINTED MATERIALS

When evaluating printed materials, educators should keep in mind the following considerations.

NATURE OF THE AUDIENCE   What is the average age of the audience? For instance, older adults tend to prefer printed materials that they can read at their leisure. Lengthy materials may be less problematic for older learners, who frequently have enough time and patience for reading educational materials. Children or clients who have low literacy skills, on the other hand, like short printed materials with many illustrations.

Also, what is the preferred learning style of the particular audience? Printed materials with few illustrations are poorly suited to clients who not only have difficulty reading but also do not like to read. Representations of information in the form of simple graphs and charts can be included with the content of printed materials for those who are visual and conceptual learners.

In addition, does the audience have any sensory deficits? Vision deficits are common with older adult clients, and short-term memory may be a problem for comprehension. Having materials that can be reread at their own convenience and pace can reinforce earlier learning and minimize confusion over treatment instructions. To accommodate those individuals with vision impairments, use a large typeface and lots of white space, separate one section from another with ample spacing, highlight important points, and use black print on white paper.

LITERACY LEVEL REQUIRED   The effectiveness of client education materials for helping the learner accomplish behavioral objectives can be totally undermined if the materials are written at a level beyond the comprehension of the learner. The Joint Commission (formerly known as the Joint Commission on Accreditation of Healthcare Organizations) mandates that health information must be presented in a manner that can be understood by clients and family members. This requirement underscores the importance of screening potential educational tools to be used as adjuncts to various teaching methods. A number of formulas (e.g., Fog, SMOG, Flesch, Fry) are available for determining readability (see Chapter 7 and Appendix A).

Linguistic Variety Available Linguistic variety refers to choices of printed materials in different foreign languages. These may be limited because duplicate materials in more than one language are costly to publish and not likely to be undertaken unless the publisher anticipates a large demand. The growth of minority populations in the United States has promoted increasing attention to the need for non-English language teaching materials. Regional differences exist, so there may be more availability of Asian-language materials on the West Coast and more Spanish-language materials in the Southwest and Northeast than in other parts of the country.

Brevity and Clarity In education, as in art, simpler is better. Remind yourself of the KISS rule: keep it simple and smart. Address the critical facts only. What does the client need to know? Choose words that explain how; the why can be filled in by a lecture, one-to-one instruction, or group discussion. Include simple pictures that illustrate step by step the written instructions being given. **Figure 12–3** provides a good example of a clear, easy-to-follow instructional tool used to teach a patient with asthma how to determine when a metered-dose inhaler is empty. Using simple graphics and minimal words, it guides the learner through the procedure with very little room for misinterpretation and is suitable for a wide range of audiences.

Layout and Appearance The appearance of written materials is crucial in attracting learners' attention and getting them to read the information. If a tool has too much wording, with inadequate

Figure 12-3 Example of a Clear, Easy-to-Follow Instructional Tool for an Asthma Client

Full   1/2 Full   Empty

spacing between sentences and paragraphs, small margins, and numerous pages, the learner may find it much too difficult and too time consuming to read (see Figure 12–2).

Doak and colleagues (1996) point out that allowing plenty of white space is the most important step that educators can do to improve the appearance of written materials. This means double spacing, leaving generous margins, indenting important points, using bold characters, and separating key statements with extra space. Inserting a graphic in the middle of the text can break up the print and may be visually appealing, as well as providing a mechanism for reinforcing the narrative information. Redman (2007) states that pictorial learning is better than verbal learning for recognition and recall. For topics that lend themselves to concrete explanations, this is especially true. An example used earlier in this chapter is teaching the psychomotor task of using a metered-dose inhaler (see Figure 12–1). Also, included in **Figure 12–4** are simple step-by-step instructions written in the active voice on the correct inhaler technique to use.

OPPORTUNITY FOR REPETITION Written materials can be read later, again and again by the learner to reinforce the teaching when the educator is not there to answer questions. Thus, it is an advantage if materials are laid out in a simple question-and-answer format. Questions demand answers and this format allows clients to find information easily for repeated reinforcement of important messages. If educators write their own materials, they also must be mindful of the need to keep information current and to update it for changing client populations.

CONCRETENESS AND FAMILIARITY Using the active voice is more immediate, directive, and concrete. For example, "Shake the inhaler very well three times" is more effective than "The inhaler should be shaken thoroughly" (see Figure 12–4). Also, the importance of using plain language instead of medical jargon cannot be overemphasized. Inadequate client understanding of common medical terms used by healthcare providers is a significant factor in noncompliance with medical regimens. A number of studies indicate that clients understand

Figure 12-4 Example of Instructions Written in the Active Voice

STEPS FOR CORRECT INHALER TECHNIQUE

1. Shake the inhaler very well three times.
2. Remove cap and hold inhaler upright.
3. Hold the inhaler 1 to 2 inches from your mouth.
4. Tilt your head back slightly and breathe out fully.
5. Press down on the inhaler and start to breathe in slowly.
6. Breathe in slowly and deeply (3 to 5 seconds) to pull the medicine down into your lungs.
7. Hold your breath for 10 seconds to keep the medicine in your lungs.
8. Take a few normal breaths.
9. Repeat puffs by following steps 1–8 again.

medical terms at a much lower rate than health professionals expect (Estey, Musseau, & Keehn, 1994; Lerner, Jehle, Janicke, & Moscati, 2000).

In summary, instructor-designed or commercially produced printed instructional materials are widely used for a broad range of audiences. They vary in literacy demand levels and may be found written in several languages. **Table 12–1** summarizes their basic advantages and disadvantages.

Demonstration Materials

Demonstration materials include many types of visual, hands-on nonprint media, such as models and real equipment, as well as a hybrid of printed words and visual illustrations (diagrams, graphs, charts, photographs, and drawings) depicted on what are known as displays, such as posters, bulletin boards, flannel boards, flip charts, chalkboards, and whiteboards. These types of media represent unique ways of communicating messages to the learner. Demonstration materials primarily stimulate the visual senses but can combine the sense of sight with touch and sometimes even smell and taste. From these various forms of demonstration materials, the educator can choose one or more to complement teaching efforts in reaching predetermined objectives. Just as with written tools, these aids must be accurate and appropriate for the intended audience. Ideally, these media forms bring the learner closer to reality and actively engage him or her in a visual and participatory manner. As such, demonstration tools are useful for cognitive, affective, and psychomotor skill development. The major forms of demonstration materials—models and displays—are discussed in detail here.

MODELS

Models are three-dimensional instructional tools that allow the learner to immediately apply knowledge and psychomotor skills by observing, examining, manipulating, handling, assembling, and disassembling objects while the teacher provides feedback (Rankin & Stallings, 2005). In addition, these demonstration aids encourage learners to think abstractly and give them the opportunity to use many of their senses (Boyd, Gleit, Graham, & Whitman, 1998). Whenever possible, the use of real objects and actual equipment is preferred, but a model is the next best thing when the real object is not available, accessible, feasible, or is too complex to use. Because approximately 30–42% of people are visual learners and 20–25% are kinesthetic (hands-on) learners, using models not only capitalizes on their learning styles (preference for learning) but enhances their retention and understanding of new information (Aldridge, 2009).

Table 12-1 BASIC ADVANTAGES AND DISADVANTAGES OF PRINTED MATERIALS

Advantages	Disadvantages
Always available	Impersonal
Rate of reading is controllable by the reader	Limited feedback; absence of instructor lessens opportunity to clear up misinterpretation
Complex concepts can be explained both fully and adequately	Passive tool
Procedural steps can be outlined	Highly complex materials may be overwhelming to the learner
Verbal instruction can be reinforced	Literacy skill of learner may limit effectiveness
Learner is always able to refer back to instructions given in print	

The three specific types of models used for teaching and learning, as differentiated by Babcock and Miller (1994), are the following:

- Replicas, associated with the word *resemble*
- Analogues, associated with the words *act like*
- Symbols, associated with the words *stands for*

A **replica** is a facsimile constructed to scale that resembles the features or substance of the original object. The dimensions of the reproduction may be decreased or enlarged in size to make demonstration easier and more understandable. A replica of the DNA helix is an excellent example of a model used to teach the complex concept of genetics. Replicas can be examined and manipulated by the learner to get an idea of how something looks and works. They are excellent for teaching psychomotor skills because they give the learner an opportunity for active participation through hands-on experience. Not only can the learner assemble and disassemble parts to see how they fit and operate, but the pace of learning can also be controlled by the learner.

Replicas are used frequently by the health professional as educator when teaching anatomy and physiology. Models of the brain, limbs, heart, kidney, ear, eye, joints, and pelvic organs, for example, allow the learner to get a perspective on parts of the body not readily viewed without these teaching aids. Resuscitation dolls are a common type of replica used to teach the skills of cardiopulmonary resuscitation (CPR). Learners who regularly refresh their skills using demonstration models as instructional tools are more likely to maintain regular and effective use of the technique than are learners who do not (Pinto, 1993).

Using inanimate objects first is a technique educators can use to desensitize learners before doing invasive procedures on themselves or other human beings. Instructional models have been found to be effective in reducing fear and enhancing acceptance of certain procedures (Cobussen-Boekhorst, Van Der Weide, Feitz, & DeGier, 2000). For example, teaching a client with diabetes how to draw up and inject insulin can best be accomplished by using a combination of real equipment and replicas. Clients first draw up sterile saline in real syringes, practice injecting oranges, and then progress to a model of a person before actually injecting themselves. Sometimes, preliminary use of a video before starting to handle equipment directly may be helpful if learners are very anxious about performing various procedures. For lessons aimed at psychomotor learning, educators can use skills checklists as a mechanism for evaluating the accuracy of return demonstrations. Simulation laboratories use this evaluation method frequently.

The second type of model is known as an **analogue** because it has the same properties and performs like a real object. Unlike replicas, analogue models are effective in explaining and representing dynamic systems. A computer model depicting how the human brain functions is one popular analogue. Although costly, a sophisticated human patient simulator is another analogue. The patient simulator is a manikin that physiologically responds to treatment similar to what would occur in live clients. Web-based patient simulation programs for teaching clinical reasoning to health professionals, such as physical therapists, is growing in popularity and the feasibility of these computer analogues is being investigated (Huhn, Anderson, & Deutsch, 2008).

The third type of model is a **symbol**, which is used frequently in teaching situations. Written words, mathematical signs and formulas, diagrams, cartoons, printed handouts, and traffic signs are all examples of symbolic models that convey a message to the receiver through imaging, convention, or association. International signs, for example, convey a familiar and understandable message to individuals of multilingual or multicultural backgrounds. However, abbreviations and acronyms common to healthcare personnel, such as NPO, PRN, and PO, should be avoided when interacting with consumers because they are likely to be unfamiliar with these abbreviations.

The advantage of models is that they can adequately replace the real object, which may be too small, too large, too expensive, too complex, unavailable, or inappropriate for use in a teaching–learning situation. A vast array of models can be purchased from commercial vendors at varying prices (some for free) or improvised by the teacher. Models do not need to be expensive or elaborate to get concepts and ideas across (Aldridge, 2009; Rankin & Stallings, 2005). In particular, models enhance learning in the following ways:

- Allow learners to practice acquiring new skills without being afraid of compromising themselves or others
- Stimulate active learner involvement
- Provide the opportunity for immediate testing of psychomotor and cognitive behaviors
- Allow learners to receive instant feedback from the instructor
- Appeal to the kinesthetic learner who prefers the hands-on approach to learning

In terms of their disadvantages, some models may not be suitable for the learner with poor abstraction abilities or for audiences with visual impairments, unless each individual is given the chance to tangibly appraise the object using other senses. Also, some models can be fragile, very expensive, bulky to store, and difficult to transport. Unless models are very large, they cannot be observed and manipulated by more than a few learners at any one time. However, this drawback can be overcome by using team teaching and by creating different stations at which to arrange replicas for demonstration purposes (Babcock & Miller, 1994).

DISPLAYS

Whiteboards, posters, story boards, flip charts, and bulletin boards are examples of displays found in most educational settings. In addition, the SMART Board is a large whiteboard that uses touch technology for detecting user input that is similar to personal computing input devices, such as a mouse or keyboard (SMART, 2009). SMART Boards are growing in popularity but are still costly to purchase.

Displays are two-dimensional objects that are useful tools for a variety of teaching purposes. They can be used to convey simple or quick messages and to clarify, reinforce, or summarize information on important topics and themes. Although they have been referred to as static instructional tools because of the fact that they are often stationary (Haggard, 1989), some can be portable and most are alterable. As demonstration materials, these tools can effectively achieve behavioral objectives by vividly representing the essence of relationships between subjects or objects. Whiteboards, flip charts, and SMART Boards are particularly versatile in delivering information. Storyboards, a visual tool that uses pictures and written text to explain a sequence of events, are effective in providing consistent messages to clients in a simple, easy to understand format (Lowenstein, Foord, & Romano, 2009).

These board devices are most useful in formal classes, group discussions, or during brainstorming sessions to spontaneously make drawings or diagrams (with contrasting colored chalk or markers) or to jot down ideas generated from participants while the educator is in the process of teaching. Information can be added, corrected, or deleted quickly and easily while the learners are actively following what the teacher is doing or saying. Such tools are excellent in promoting participation, keeping the learners' attention on the topic at hand, and noting and reinforcing the contributions of others. Flexible and handy, they provide opportunities for the teacher, in an immediate and direct fashion, to organize data, integrate ideas, perform on-the-spot problem solving, and compare and contrast various points of view. Unlike some other types of visuals, these display tools can allow learners to see parts of a whole picture while assisting the teacher in filling in the gaps.

The following are important guidelines suggested by Babcock and Miller (1994) for instructors using chalkboards and whiteboards:

- Be sure writing is legible and discernible.
- Step aside and face the audience after putting notations on the board to maintain contact with the audience.
- Allow learners time to copy the message.
- Enlist a good note taker to capture a creative design or record an idea before the contents on the board are erased or changed.

In particular, the following are some advantages of displays as teaching tools:

- They are a quick way to attract attention and get an idea across.
- Most are flexible, easily modified, and reusable.
- Many are portable and easily assembled or disassembled.
- They stimulate interest or ideas in the observer.
- They are effective for influencing cognitive and affective behaviors.

Some of the disadvantages of displays include the following:

- They may take up a lot of space.
- The more static types, such as posters, can be time consuming to have prepared and for that reason tend to be used as displays for a long time, which increases the risk of their becoming outdated.
- Some (e.g., posters and bulletin boards) can be unsuitable for large audiences if information is to be viewed simultaneously.
- Limited amounts of information can be included at one time.
- They are ineffective for teaching psychomotor skills.
- They may become too cluttered when too much information is placed on them.
- If permanently mounted, they cannot be transported.

- The symbolic nature of the message may be misunderstood, which is a problem that underscores their importance as supplements to learning.

POSTERS

Although they are a type of display material, posters are being addressed separately because they have become an increasingly popular and important educational tool. Essentially hybrids of print and visual media, they heavily employ the written word along with graphic illustrations. Posters are a legitimate and reasonable option for conveying information (Duchin & Sherwood, 1990; Flournoy, Turner, & Combs, 2000; Moneyham, Ura, Ellwood, & Bruno, 1996; Thurber & Asselin, 1999). As a visual supplement to oral instruction of clients and families in various clinical settings, posters are being increasingly accepted as an effective tool to educate staff and students at continuing education meetings and research conferences.

Posters can serve as an independent source of information or can be used in conjunction with other instructional methods and materials. Some critics view the poster as a passive instructional medium, but this conjecture can easily be disputed. Inherent in the design, the message conveyed by a well-constructed poster is brief, constant, and interactive with the audience (Duchin & Sherwood, 1990). Because the primary purpose of a poster is visual stimulation, it is meant to attract attention (Flournoy et al., 2000). Effective posters leave a mental image long after they are seen. This mental image is a cue to the viewer to remember the message being delivered. Much like a bumper sticker on a car, effective poster displays can potentially leave lasting impressions that are easily recalled at some future date. **Figure 12–5** is an excellent example.

The advantages of posters are that they can be used as a cognitive stimulator, as a way to reinforce and synthesize information, and as an ongoing instructional resource. Their value derives from the repetition, individual pacing, and availability of the

Figure 12-5 Example of an Effective Poster for AIDS Awareness

Last night Jennifer had a fatal accident.
She just doesn't know it yet.

Courtesy of artist: Katherine Batruch Meadows. Reprinted with permission.

message across various settings (Bach, McDaniel, & Poole, 1994; Duchin & Sherwood, 1990; Hayes & Childress, 1999; Thurber & Asselin, 1999). Posters serve as an important teaching tool to help bring about a change of behavior by adding knowledge, reinforcing skills, or appealing to attitudes. By forcing content brevity and using eye-catching imagery, a message can be disseminated quickly and simultaneously to a large audience in a variety of settings. Posters also can be used with individuals and small groups to transmit or reinforce information with or without the teacher present. In addition, they are relatively inexpensive and easy to produce.

With practice, and with the availability of today's computer technology, an educator can become skilled at creating attractive, impressive posters in an efficient and timely manner. Software programs such as Print Shop Deluxe, Paint Shop Pro, Adobe Photoshop, and Microsoft Publisher are excellent resources to produce professional-looking visuals. The major disadvantage of posters is that the content is static and, therefore, may become quickly dated. Also, if the same poster is kept on display for too long, the potential audience begins to disregard its message.

The key to a poster's effectiveness lies in its planning and design. Bushy (1991) states that "good ideas do not speak for themselves ... a good poster display cannot rescue a bad idea, but a poor one can easily sink the best idea" (p. 11). She puts forth important aesthetic considerations when preparing and evaluating poster presentations specifically for research purposes. Duchin and Sherwood (1990) and Bach et al. (1994) also provide guidelines that are still relevant today for developing attractive, simple, yet effective posters and include considerations of content, audience needs, and settings. Both Bushy (1991) and Duchin and Sherwood (1990) refer to the application of design elements such as color, spacing, graphics, lettering, and borders required to create presentations that not only catch the eye but also persist in memory. Also, effective imagery can take the form of graphic designs or photographs, and great artistic skill is not required. Simple pictures, such as schematics, outlines, and stick figure drawings, work well and can be created using colored pencils, markers, construction paper, or computer printouts.

The ability of a poster to influence behavior or increase awareness can be greatly enhanced by careful consideration of all of these factors. Because aesthetic appeal is critical in capturing learners' attention, educators should adhere to the following tips when making and critiquing a poster for use as a teaching tool (Bach et al., 1994; Bushy, 1991; Duchin & Sherwood, 1990; Haggard, 1989):

- Use complementary (opposite-spectrum) color combinations, taking into account the three color aspects of hue (wavelength of the light spectrum), saturation (purity of color), and value (brilliance of color). Two colors clash when they are close to each other in these three elements.
- One color should make up as much as 70% of the display. No two colors should be used in equal proportions, and a third color should be used only to accent or highlight printed components such as titles, subheadings, or credits. Too many colors make the design appear cluttered and complicated.

- Because a picture is worth a thousand words, graphics should be used to break up blocks of script or lettering.
- Use simple, high-quality (but not necessarily sophisticated or ornate) drawings or graphics that can be easily interpreted.
- Balance script with white space (or another background color) and graphics to add variety and contrast.
- Use high-quality photographs with colored borders and of different contours, widths, and shapes.
- Convey the message in common, straightforward language, avoiding jargon and unfamiliar abbreviations or symbols.
- Adhere to the KISS principle (keep it simple and smart) when using words to decrease length, detail, and crowding. Simplicity and neatness attract attention.
- Be concise; do not repeat. Include only essential information, but be sure the message is complete.
- Keep objectives in mind for the focus of this display tool.
- Be sure content is current and free of spelling, grammar, and mathematical errors.
- Add textures, if desired, by using a variety of paper and fabrics.
- Make titles catchy and crisp, using 10 words or less (no longer than two lines) and lettering large enough to read from a distance of at least 20 feet.
- Letters should be straight and at least 1 inch in height to be read easily at a distance of four to six feet. Avoid using all-capital letters except for very short titles and labels. Use capitals for only the first letter of each word in titles with more than two to three words or with words longer than four to six letters.
- Use a title or introductory statement that orients readers to the subject.
- Logically sequence the written and graphic components.

- Use letter-quality script or laser print instead of dot matrix if using computer-generated type.
- Use arrows, circles, or directional lines to merge the parts to achieve correct focus, flow, sequence, and unity.
- Achieve balance in visual weight on each side by positioning information around an imaginary central axis running vertically and horizontally.
- Handouts can be used to supplement, highlight, and reinforce the messages conveyed by the poster.
- If a poster is to be transported, use durable backboards and overlays (Styrofoam, heavy cardboard, lamination, or acrylic sprays).

Bushy (1991) has devised a 30-item research poster appraisal tool (R-PAT), still relevant today, that further assists health professionals in critiquing posters specifically designed for research. This tool can be modified for use in preparing and evaluating posters as tools for educational purposes.

The ability of a poster to influence behavior or expand awareness can be greatly enhanced by careful consideration of its content, intended audience, and design elements. The poster for AIDS awareness (Figure 12–5) is a stunning example. The interaction of the viewer with the message is the key to a poster's success. This AIDS awareness poster and the classic World War I poster "Uncle Sam Wants YOU!" are examples of the element of visceral connection between viewer and message that linger in memory.

Table 12–2 summarizes the basic advantages and disadvantages of demonstration materials.

Audiovisual Materials

Technology has changed the traditional approach to teaching. Nowhere is this shift more evident than in the audiovisual arena. **Audiovisual materials** support and enrich the educational process by stimulating the senses of seeing and hearing, adding variety to the teaching–learning experience, and instilling visual memories, which have been found to be more permanent than auditory memories (Kessels, 2003). Audiovisuals have been known to increase retention of information by combining what people hear with what they see. Technology software and hardware are exceptional aids because many can influence all three domains of learning by promoting cognitive development, stimulating attitude change, and helping to build psychomotor skills.

The term **multimedia learning** refers to the use of two or more types of learning modes (e.g., audio, visual, or animation) that can be accessed via a computer to engage the learner in the content. **Blended learning**, a more recent term in

Table 12-2 BASIC ADVANTAGES AND DISADVANTAGES OF DEMONSTRATION MATERIALS

Advantages	Disadvantages
Brings the learner closer to reality through active engagement	Content may be static, easily dated
Useful for cognitive reinforcement and psychomotor skill development	Can be time consuming to make
Effective use of imagery may impact affective domain	Potential for overuse
Many forms are relatively inexpensive	Some forms not suitable for simultaneous use with large audiences
Opportunity for repetition	Not suitable for visually impaired learners or for learners with poor abstraction abilities

education, combines e-learning technology with more traditional instructor-led methodology, such as a lecture or demonstration. Audiovisual technologies often offer learners more control over content as well as the sequencing, pacing, and timing of learning that allows them to tailor their experiences to meet learning objectives. Innovations in instructional media, particularly e-learning technologies, are revolutionizing education, permitting learning to be more individualized and transforming the role of the educator to become "facilitators of learning and assessors of competency" (Ruiz, Mintzer, & Leipzig, 2006).

Because this is an increasingly technological age, educators have to be aware of which audiovisual tools are available, how tools actually and potentially affect the ability to learn, and how to implement the various tools at their disposal effectively and efficiently. When and to what extent educators should use them to augment teaching depends on many variables, not the least of which is the educator's comfort level and expertise in operating these technological devices. Also, it should not be forgotten that some adult learners may have difficulty orienting to the newer modes of learning and that some learners may have physical or cognitive limitations that preclude the use of one or more types of audiovisual tools.

In a riveting article, Prensky (2001) declares that today's young people are no longer the audiences the educational system was originally designed to teach. A growing number of younger learners have been raised in this present digital technology era, surrounded by and oriented to computers, for example, desktop, notebook, and netbooks, smart phones, and many other electronic devices that are integral to their everyday lives. They are known as *digital natives*. Many educators, on the other hand, who were not born during this age of technology, have had to acquire new ways of communicating, somewhat akin to learning a second language. Prensky (2001) refers to them as *digital immigrants*. The challenge, then, for many educators who have for years spoken

a different language is to adapt to as well as adopt the newest forms of instructional tools to teach natives of the digital age. Digital natives are comfortable with multitasking and receiving information rapidly. Use of hypertext and random access comes naturally. Use of streaming video such as YouTube and interactive computer learning modules, as well as video gaming, is commonplace. For educators not well versed in the use of digital technologies to assist and supplement instruction, the challenge is ongoing.

As with any teaching aids, major concerns affecting which media educators choose are accuracy and appropriateness of content, budgetary resources available for the purchase or rental of software programs and hardware equipment, and the time, money, and expertise needed to introduce new technologies or self-produce audiovisual materials.

Audiovisual materials can be categorized into five major types: projected, audio, video, telecommunications, and computer formats. Computer technology is rapidly altering the ways in which educators share information and interact with students. For example, students are using text messaging as a primary means of communication with each other, while educators may be more familiar with using e-mail.

PROJECTED LEARNING RESOURCES

This category of media includes overhead transparencies, PowerPoint slides, SMART Board systems, and other computer outputs that are projected onto a screen. These media types are appropriate for audiences of various sizes.

MICROSOFT POWERPOINT Microsoft's computer-generated slideshow software program, PowerPoint, has replaced conventional slides and overheads for instruction. PowerPoint slides are easy to design, economical to produce, and an impressive medium by which to share information with a large or small audience. The program allows for flexibility to make changes in the slides whenever necessary as well as flexibility during the presentation to repeat slides, add new slides, or skip slides to move ahead to other content. PowerPoint slides have many advantages. They are an excellent medium for conveying a message because they are an attractive mode for learning at all ages in a manner that facilitates retention and recall. They can enhance an oral presentation by adding visual dimensions to the narration. Presentations can be burned onto a CD or DVD, transferred to a flash drive, or downloaded from a server for presentation through a portable notebook computer. Digital photographs and graphics can easily be scanned and added to PowerPoint slides. Animation also can be an additional feature. And finally, slides can be personalized or tailored to meet specific audience needs.

Careful composition of slides is needed to avoid clutter. Too much detail makes it difficult for the viewer to assimilate. DuFrene and Lehman (2004) provide an elegant four-step process for assisting educators to develop and deliver lively PowerPoint presentations designed to avoid the "death by PowerPoint" experience for intended audiences. Educators should adhere to the following suggestions when preparing a PowerPoint slide presentation:

- Illustrate one idea per slide.
- Keep images simple by using clear pictures, symbols, or diagrams. Put long lists of words or complex figures on handouts that supplement the slides.
- Avoid distorted images by keeping the proportion of height to width at 2:3.
- Use large, easily readable, and professional-looking lettering.

Brown (2001) suggests additional important tips on how to employ this innovative tool productively:

- Use this medium to generate interaction between the teacher and the learner rather than as a tool that provides an outline of content to be followed for presenting information only in a traditional lecture format.
- On various slides, leave out some points to be made or ideas that should be included so that the learner must figure out what may be missing. This omission encourages critical thinking by the audience.
- Open a blank slide and type in the main points as they emerge from interactive discussion.
- Use text sparingly on each slide to keep details to a minimum by including no more than six points about any one idea per slide and limiting the word count to approximately six words per point.
- Use contrasting but bold complementary colors so that the text of each slide is clearly visible. Be sure the background color is dark enough that the words in print are not washed out.
- Be sure the print size on each slide is large enough for the audience to read with ease at a distance. The *floor test* is one simple method to determine appropriate print size. That is, can you clearly read a printout of the slide placed on the floor in front of you when in a standing position?
- Minimize or avoid animated text, sounds, and fancy transitions, which can serve to distract the reader from the message being conveyed.
- Keep unity of design from slide to slide by using a master slide as a template.
- Provide audience members with handouts of the slides (three slides per page) for purposes of note taking.
- Limit the number of slides to be projected for teaching to no more than one to two slides per minute (not to exceed 60 slides for a 1-hour presentation) to avoid including too much content in a given period of time. It is important to provide time for cognitive processing that allows learners to internalize the concepts being presented and to give learners a chance to discuss content and ask questions.

Remember, visuals should enrich the message, not become the message. Overuse of slides may flatten out audience participation, potentially sacrificing rich interactive discussions (DuFrene & Lehman, 2004). Dickerson (2005) reminds educators that audiovisual resources are only the tools they use to help achieve teaching objectives. She notes a common complaint that PowerPoint presentations can encourage learners to think only in bullet points and suggests laying out presentations with enough space between bullets for learners to fill in critical information developed during a presentation. For further assistance to the health professional as educator, Schrock (2003) provides a very useful set of resource links to assist in getting started using PowerPoint in the classroom, and deWest (2006) addresses both the advantages and disadvantages, as well as best applications for effective use of PowerPoint.

PowerPoint slides must be used judiciously to avoid overuse and abuse of this medium as a tool for effective teaching and learning. PowerPoint slides can readily be converted to overheads, as needed, especially for use in handling unexpected computer mishaps. A prepared presenter should keep this type of backup (DuFrene & Lehman, 2004).

Overhead Transparencies This medium is still frequently used for teaching in a variety of settings, both in the classroom and for small-group presentations. Since the advent of PowerPoint, however, overheads are used less frequently. Nevertheless, advantages remain for using transparencies and the overhead or doccam (document camera) projector (hardware). As with PowerPoint, large numbers of people can see the projected images at one time, and images can be enlarged for easier viewing. Most important, transparencies can be shown in fully lighted rooms, are inexpensive to produce or purchase, diagrams and figures can readily be photocopied and made into transparencies, and multiple transparencies can be laid over one

another to illustrate changes in the content or build in progression of an idea. With doccam projectors, an actual document can be projected, which eliminates the need to create transparencies.

Among the disadvantages of overhead transparencies are the need for both specialized equipment for projection and the support of verbal feedback. For this reason, they are more conducive for use in a classroom than for purposes of individual self-instruction. Another disadvantage is that it is not easy for the educator to refer back or ahead to a particular transparency, and they are difficult for the presenter to keep in order while he or she is trying to stay focused on a presentation. Also, the projector itself is awkward to transport and for traditional overhead hardware the noise given off by the fan of the machine can be distracting in a small room. The newer doccam projectors, which generate no noise, are preferable.

It is essential that transparencies be viewed ahead of time for an assessment of their readability, specifically related to the size of the lettering. Usually letters 0.25 inch high or letters that can be read at a distance of 10 feet before projection are sufficient for easy reading. Note also that too much content on an overhead transparency decreases its efficacy as a teaching tool. The following helpful guidelines for the use of traditional overhead projectors and transparencies are recommended (Babcock & Miller, 1994; Heinrich, Molenda, Russell, & Smaldino, 2002):

- Do not block the audience's view of the screen by standing in front of the machine. This common error can best be solved by making a habit of sitting or standing to the side to avoid interference with the projected image.
- Turn the projector off when you have finished referring to the transparency so as to keep the learners' attention on you and away from what is being projected. Constant use of the machine is also distracting because of the fan noise.

- Keep the message on the transparency simple. Use handouts to cover complex information as a supplement to your message.
- Display only one point at a time by masking the rest with a piece of paper if you have listed several ideas on one transparency. This approach allows listeners to focus on what you are saying and gives them time for note taking.
- Use a screen large enough for the audience to read the information projected.
- Use a light-colored blank wall if a screen is unavailable or too small.
- Pull the projector closer or farther away from the screen to change the size of the projection. This requires that the room be large enough to accommodate moving the equipment at a distance far enough away for adequate projection.
- Use tinted film to reduce glare of light.
- Use colored pens to help organize information, to provide contrast to images, or make specific points. Color is known to attract attention and help differentiate information for better retention and recall (Cooper, 1990).
- Use overlays to help illustrate complex or sequential ideas. Note, however, that too many overlays can make the picture fuzzy.

Table 12–3 summarizes the basic advantages and disadvantages of projected learning resources.

AUDIO LEARNING RESOURCES

Audio technology, although it has existed for a long time, has not been used to any great extent for educational purposes until recently. For years, it has been a useful tool for people who are blind or for those with serious visual or motor impairment. However, with significant advances in audio software and hardware, as well as the adoption of audio technology for more than purely commercial use, compact discs (CDs), digital sound players (e.g., Mp3 players, iPods), radio, and podcasts have become more popular tools for teaching and learning. These resources can be used to relay many different types of messages, can help learners who benefit from repetition and reinforcement, and are well suited for those who enjoy or prefer auditory learning (Heinrich et al., 2002). They are also useful adjuncts for teaching individuals who are illiterate or low literate.

COMPACT DISCS AND DIGITAL SOUND PLAYERS

Digital sound files and CDs are very popular formats today. Use of these media by educators has been growing. The biggest advantage of digital sound files and CDs is their practicality. These audio media have replaced traditional vinyl records and audiotapes. The major advantage of digital sound files and CDs is their superior fidelity, which does not deteriorate over time. They are small, portable,

Table 12-3 BASIC ADVANTAGES AND DISADVANTAGES OF PROJECTED LEARNING RESOURCES

Advantages	Disadvantages
Most effectively used with groups	Lack of flexibility due to static content for some forms
May be especially beneficial for hearing-impaired, low-literate clients	Some forms may be expensive
	Requires darkened room for some forms
Good for teaching skills in all domains	Requires special equipment for use

inexpensive, simple to operate, and easy to prepare or duplicate. Digital sound files are a powerful tool to augment or reinforce information previously presented in other formats, to receive verbal feedback from instructors, or to be exposed to information not easily available or accessible. For example, recorded lung sounds, which allow comparison between normal and abnormal breathing, are available in both CD and digital sound file form. Such audio media on a variety of health topics, from stress reduction to programs on how to quit smoking, can be prepared specifically to meet the needs of a learner by reinforcing facts, giving directions, or providing support. As an example, Hagopian (1996) describes effective use of audio media for increasing knowledge and self-care behaviors of persons undergoing radiation therapy. Naperstek (1993) developed a large line of CDs on guided imagery that is used by practitioners and clients dealing with illness, surgery, and broad treatment modalities.

If the audio sound files and CDs are instructor-made, the learner derives much comfort from hearing the instructor's familiar voice and reassuring words. This tool has been used extensively by Excelsior College, a distance learning degree program, to provide direct feedback to students on the results of their examinations. Learners can listen to information on digital audio files and CDs at their leisure and can review them as often as necessary. They can be used almost anywhere, such as in the home, office, clinic, or hospital setting, and can be played while simultaneously driving a car or fixing a meal, thus filling in what normally would be considered wasted time. Developing a sizable library of sounds files or CDs is well within the capability of most instructors thanks to this medium's low cost and easy storage. Pictures, diagrams, and printed handouts can accompany these instructional tools to fit the needs of a variety of learners.

The versatility of CDs and digital sound players for application to education is currently growing at a rapid rate in academia as well as for client and staff education in a clinical setting. As with all technologies over time, the cost of digital sound players is becoming very reasonable, and the hardware availability of both these and CD players for healthcare education is rapidly increasing.

The disadvantages of using digital sound files and CDs are few. The biggest drawback is that they address only one sense—hearing—and, therefore, cannot be used by individuals with hearing impairment. Also, some learners may become easily distracted from the information being presented unless they have visuals to accompany the recorded information. There is also no opportunity for interactive feedback between the listener and the speaker. As with any medium, digital sound files and CDs should be used only as supplements to the various methods of instruction.

Radio and Podcasts The radio has tremendously affected all of our lives for many years and is one of the oldest forms of audio technology. Because of its commercial nature and appeal to mass audiences, it has typically been used more for pleasure than for education. In recent years, the medium of radio has been exploited by both public and private radio stations, which have begun airing community service and medical talk shows for public education on health issues. These programs are helpful in delivering a message, and, because of the convenience and popularity of radio as a communication tool, it is a useful vehicle for teaching and learning. Podcasts are becoming an increasingly popular form of student and client education as well. These audiences of learners are able to download lectures and informational sessions about various health topics. They are able to listen to these broadcasts on their computers or digital audio players.

The disadvantage of radio and podcasts relates to the difficulty of consistently delivering information on major topics to general as well as specific populations. That is, the health professional as educator has little control over the variety and depth of topics discussed or how regularly learners listen to a program. In addition, the general nature of radio programs and podcasts is not tailored to meet individual needs. Unlike CDs and digital sound files, radio does not allow the opportunity for repetition of information. However, because of its widespread use and versatility, it has the potential for becoming a major source for important and useful healthcare information, especially if air time is funded by private foundations or sponsored by special groups or agencies dedicated to health teaching.

Table 12–4 summarizes the basic advantages and disadvantages of audio learning resources.

VIDEO LEARNING RESOURCES

Digital video files and DVDs, along with camcorders, DVD recorders, television sets, and computer monitors as electronic devices with which to view them, have become commonplace in homes. Health professional educators are using these resources extensively for teaching in a variety of settings. For example, multimedia streaming video and webinar have satisfied the increasing demand for new ways to educate professional and paraprofessional staff in all types of healthcare and academic settings. Webinar format, which allows for interaction between speaker and participants even though sessions are virtual, and streaming technology, which plays audio and visual files from the Internet, are cost effective, easy to use, time efficient, and available wherever the Internet is accessible (Manny, 2006).

In a review of research studies, Jeste, Dunn, Folsom, and Zisook (2008) found that multimedia DVD and CD aids for educating consumers about illness management and treatment decision making increased their understanding of medical information and enabled both patients and their caregivers to take a more active role in making healthcare choices. In other studies, videos for inservice education were found to be a potentially powerful medium for learning (Brooks, Renvall, Bulow, & Ramsdell, 2000), and Green et al. (2003) reported significant usefulness of streamed video as a resource to support learning by students. Video files and DVDs are one of the major nonprint media tools for enhancing client/family, staff, and student education because tapes can be simultaneously entertaining and educational (Carlson, 2003; Tobolowsky, 2007).

Videos, although a logical technology to use for client care, has been underexploited. Clark and Lester (2000) conducted a research study on video interventions with the older adult population. They found this instructional tool to be as effective in changing behaviors as the success videos have shown in teaching and learning of adolescents and younger adults.

Digital video files and DVDs, which incorporate the sound quality of CDs and superior images of video by way of digital technology, have incredible archival qualities similar to CDs that allow for long-term storage and use. The market for this

---

Table 12-4 BASIC ADVANTAGES AND DISADVANTAGES OF AUDIO LEARNING RESOURCES

Advantages	Disadvantages
Widely available	Rely only on sense of hearing
May be especially beneficial for clients who are visually impaired or low-literate	Some forms may be expensive
May be listened to repeatedly	Lack of opportunity for interaction between instructor and learner
Most forms very practical, cheap, small, and portable	

innovative technology has increased as the cost of the software and hardware has become more reasonable (Heinrich et al., 2002).

Originally designed for entertainment purposes only, today these discs are popular with a wide range of audiences in both the fields of higher education and client/staff education. Healthcare facilities broadcast client education segments via video files and DVDs over in-house televisions. The convenience and flexibility of these instructional tools allow educators to use video learning resources for individual client teaching situations as well as for large-group instruction.

The usefulness of video derives from the combination of color, motion, different angles, and sound that enhances learning through visual as well as auditory senses. The disadvantage of purchased digital video files and DVDs is that they may be beyond the viewers' level of understanding, inappropriate for learner needs, or too long. This digital technology has become very inexpensive and the ready portability of recorders allows the educator to capture situations unavailable elsewhere for reinforcement of learning. Williams, Wolgin, and Hodge (1998) outline detailed steps for creating educational videos. They suggest striving for network-quality production by using the following guidelines:

• Write a script for the program. Rehearse thoroughly.
• For a small budget, a single camera with zoom capacity should be used. A larger budget also may allow employing a professional to edit the final product.
• Consider hiring a video technician on a per hour or per diem basis to yield a quality production in a time-efficient and cost-effective manner. The operator of the recorder needs to be knowledgeable of motion picture technology, such as the use of close-ups, dramatization of situations, and angle effects, which are not in the usual repertoire of many health professional educators.

• Always be mindful of the program's objectives to avoid being seduced by the glamour of the process.
• Keep the program short. The attention spans of learners vary, but the longer the video, the more risk of losing viewer interest. A video that is 5–15 minutes long is ideal.

Digital video cameras, in particular, are also a good means to capture real-life and practice experience situations. Role modeling of specific behaviors, attitudes, and values also may be demonstrated powerfully through this medium. Once scenes are captured on tape, a video can serve as an excellent teaching tool to promote discussion and for analyzing and critiquing behaviors that provide direct feedback to learners in the demonstration or rehearsal of complex interpersonal and psychomotor skills. A study by Hill, Hooper, and Wahl (2000) showed improved performance and learner satisfaction among nursing students using video playback as a learning strategy for enhancing their clinical skills. Similar findings were reported by Winters, Hauck, Riggs, Clawson, and Collins (2003). **Table 12–5** summarizes the basic advantages and disadvantages of video learning resources.

TELECOMMUNICATIONS LEARNING RESOURCES

Telecommunications is a means by which information can be transmitted via television, telephone, related modes of audio and video teleconferencing, and closed-circuit, cable, and satellite broadcasting. Telecommunications devices have allowed messages to be sent to many people at the same time in a variety of places at great distances.

TELEVISION   The television, ubiquitous in American homes, has been used for many years as an entertainment tool. Today, there are more televisions than telephones in private residences. The TV is also well suited for educational purposes and has become

Table 12-5 Basic Advantages and Disadvantages of Video Learning
Resources

Advantages	Disadvantages
Widely used educational tool	Viewing formats limited depending on availability of
Inexpensive, for the most part	DVD and digital videofile equipment
Use visual and auditory senses	Some commercial products may be expensive
Flexible for use with different audiences	Some purchased materials may be too long or
Powerful tool for role modeling, demonstration, teaching psychomotor skills	inappropriate for audience

a popular teaching–learning tool in homes, schools, businesses, and healthcare settings. The power to influence cognitive, affective, and psychomotor behavior is well demonstrated by television commercials, whose messages are simple, direct, and variously repetitive to effectively influence the behavior of intended audiences.

Cable TV is legally obligated to provide public access programming by offering channels for community members and organizations to air their own programs. Health education, if placed on the cable system, can be seen in any home with cable access. The advantage of this international option is that distribution of programs is relatively inexpensive. The disadvantage is that there is no control over who is watching, and this medium cannot serve as an interactive question-and-answer experience unless call-in phone lines are provided.

Closed-circuit TV, on the other hand, allows for education programs to be sent to specific locations, such as patient rooms or staff units. The learner can request a particular program at any given time, much like a guest in a hotel can choose on demand from a variety of movies day and night. This telecommunications technology requires programs to be played intermittently or continuously, with program availability clearly advertised. Because the learner controls program viewing, the health professional as educator must follow up to answer

questions and determine whether learning has, in fact, occurred. Satellite broadcasting, a much more sophisticated form of telecommunications, can reach far more distant locations and carry a number of programs at any one time. Because of its expense, not many institutions send health information via this mode, but many receive it. More types of satellite systems are being developed to make this form of communication for educational purposes available on a worldwide basis.

Video teleconferencing for continuing education and staff development is one strategy used for maintaining quality and viability of continuing education programs in a cost-effective manner (Heidenreiter, 1995). In addition, several health networks, such as Lifetime, transmit to cable companies and hospitals.

TELEPHONES   It is almost impossible to imagine being without the telephone as a daily tool. Americans have come to depend on their land-based phone lines or cell phones as a fundamental means of communication. It is not surprising, therefore, that the telephone can be used effectively for education. In recognition of this fact, many healthcare associations have begun to provide telephone services with messages about disease treatment and prevention. The American Cancer Society, for example, has established a toll-free number for the public to obtain short taped messages about various types of cancer. Hospitals, too, have set up call-in services about a variety of health-related topics and sources for referral.

The advantage is that these services are relatively inexpensive and can be operated by someone with minimal medical knowledge because the taped message contains the substance of the content. Another advantage is that this type of service is available in most cases around the clock. The disadvantage is that there is no opportunity for questions to be answered directly.

Telecommunications as an instructional tool is becoming increasingly popular and sophisticated. Many hospitals and healthcare agencies have already established hotline consumer information centers, which are staffed by knowledgeable healthcare personnel so that information can be personalized and appropriate feedback can be given on the spot. The poison control hotline is a good example of the use of this medium.

Table 12–6 summarizes the basic advantages and disadvantages of telecommunications learning resources.

Computer Learning Resources

In this technological society, the computer has changed lives dramatically and has found widespread application in industry, business, schools, and homes. The computer can store large amounts of information and is designed to display pictures, graphics, and text. The presentation of informa-

tion can be changed depending on user input. Although computer technology is a relatively recent addition to the educational field, it is becoming very common, especially with the rapid increase of computer literacy among students, professionals, and the general public (Rice, Trockel, King, & Remmert, 2004). Computers, as a multimedia approach to teaching and learning, usually stimulate learners and transform learning into "an active, engaging process" that promotes problem solving and the development of critical-thinking skills (Huang, 2005, p. 224).

Computer-assisted instruction (CAI), also called computer-based learning (CBL) and computer-based training (CBT), promotes learning in primarily the cognitive domain (Grunwald & Corsbie-Massay, 2006; Staib, 2003), and research has revealed CAI increases both the efficiency of learning and retention of information (Ruiz et al., 2006). Computers are an efficient instructional tool in that the educator has more time to devote to teaching other tasks not usually taught via computer, such as affective and psychomotor skills (Kaveevivitchai et al., 2009). More research definitely needs to be done to establish its usefulness to change attitudes and behaviors or promote psychomotor skill development.

Retention is improved by an interactive exchange between the learner and the computer, even though the instructor is not actually present. DiGiacinto (2007) applied current learning theories related to instruction via computers and found that illustrations (visual information) along with

Table 12-6 Basic Advantages and Disadvantages of Telecommunications Learning Resources

Advantages	Disadvantages
TV program distribution is relatively inexpensive to wide audiences	Complicated to set up interactive capability
Telephone is relatively inexpensive, widely available	Expensive to broadcast via satellite

narration (verbal information) increase learners' recall and comprehension. For example, telemedicine technology has been found to be as effective an educational tool as in-person teaching for diabetes control (Izquierdo et al., 2003). The increasing use of interactive videodisc (IVD) programs show promise in improving retention and understanding of information (Green et al., 2004).

Also, Flash-based Web resources, available to educators and students for free or at low cost, are high-quality Internet materials for instruction (Lamb & Johnson, 2006). Macromedia Flash is required to access such resources, but if it is not already installed on a computer, it is easily downloaded to run on both Windows and Macintosh platforms with any browser. Three key elements of Flash—animation, interaction, and multimedia—give it great appeal and versatility. QuickTime format also is frequently used for digital video. Smith and Lombardo (2005) describe development of a patient education workshop on CD-ROM that utilized Flash, QuickTime, and Acrobat Reader to provide streaming video clips, audio segments, case studies, and interactive practice activities.

CAI has many unique advantages. Instruction can be individualized to the learner, lessons can be varied readily, and the learner can control the pace (Heinrich et al., 2002). Without time constraints, the learner can move as quickly or as slowly as desired to master content without incurring penalties for mistakes or performance speed. For instance, many educational computer games are designed to teach a subject at a variety of skill levels. Instructions that present to learners more problems with increasing complexity at a pace of the learners' own choosing can be selected. The ability of computers to internally change the rules or the format of games makes them endlessly challenging and novel to the user.

Another advantage of CAI is that an instructor can easily track the level of understanding of the learner because the computer has the ability to ask questions and analyze responses to perform ongoing learner assessment. Computers can be programmed to provide feedback to the educator regarding the learner's grasp of concepts, the speed of learning, and those aspects of learning that need reinforcement. The interactive features of this medium also provide for immediate feedback to the learner. An excellent example of efficacy of CAI is the research conducted on mental health training for long-term staff using computer-based interactive videos (Rosen et al., 2002). These authors partnered with Fox Learning Systems, a company that specializes in eldercare program development using CD-ROM and e-learning formats (http://www.foxlearningsystems.com).

Computers are also a valuable instructional tool for those with aphasia, motor difficulties, visual and hearing impairments, or learning disabilities (see Chapter 9 on learners with disabilities). Assistive technologies, such as screen readers that convert electronic text to spoken language, are available to individuals with learning or visual disabilities. However, learners with various disabilities are likely to have constant challenges in trying to access computer files, software programs, and Web sites. This is because Web pages are created in the HTML file format. Other common file formats include Adobe Acrobat's portable document format (PDF) and PowerPoint. Hoffman, Hartley, and Boone (2005) address specific problems of access for those who are disabled. They provide an excellent resource list for educators and learners who want more information on organizations and Web sites specializing in assistive technologies. In addition, the Center for Applied Special Technology (CAST) is a nonprofit educational, research, and development organization whose mission is to expand opportunities for individuals with disabilities through the development of innovative, technology-based educational resources and strategies (http://www.cast.org). Educators can visit this Web site for further information.

The major disadvantage of CAI is the expense of both the hardware and software, making it infeasible for implementation in some learning situations. In most cases, programs must be purchased because they are too time consuming and too complex for the educator to develop. Even if an educator has programming skills, it can take up to 500 hours to produce 1 hour of instructional material (Boyd et al., 1998). See **Table 12–7** for examples of companies that supply client education materials.

Another barrier to education via a computer is the lack of computer literacy or comfort level with computers by some learners and even some health professionals. Lashley (2005) describes the importance of institutional support for faculty development in the use of technology for the successful design and delivery of computer-based instructional methods and materials. Furthermore, in particular, many older adults are computer shy,

Table 12-7 SOME EXAMPLES OF INTERNET SITES AND COMPANIES THAT PROVIDE TECHNOLOGY-BASED CLIENT EDUCATION MATERIALS ACCESSIBLE ONLINE THROUGH THE INTERNET (AVAILABLE TO THE PUBLIC)

GENERAL RESOURCES

- Health Library from EBSCO Publishing: assists hospitals and other medical facilities to enhance their client education Web sites and services (www.epnet.com).
- Wired.MD (www.wired.md): provides interactive, online videos
- MedlinePlus (www.medlineplus.gov): a service of the U.S. National Library of Medicine and the National Institutes of Health
- NIH.gov (www.nih.gov)
- Mayoclinic.org (www.mayoclinic.org)
- WebMD.com (www.webmd.com)
- National Cancer Institutes (www.nci.org)

VIDEOS AND ANIMATIONS

- Wired.MD (www.wired.md)
- HealthLibrary (from EBSCO Publishing; www.epnet.com)
- Pritchett & Hull: uses extensive graphics with a lower reading level in many formats and subjects. Online ordering available at www.p-h.com. Adobe Reader needed.
- Hazelden: emphasis on addiction, recovery, sobriety, and similar health issues. Adobe Reader needed. To locate videos, go to www.hazelden.org/OA_HTML/ibeCCtpSctDspRte.jsp?section=10021 and use Search Bookstore, selecting Videos under All Products.
- Milner-Fenwick Online (www.milner-fenwick.com): free previews covering most health topics. Many available in Spanish and with closed captioning. Adobe Reader needed.
- MedlinePlus in English (www.medlineplus.gov) and Spanish (www.medlineplus.gov/spanish): interactive tutorials (need a special Flash plug-in, version 6 or later)
    1. Diseases and conditions: specific
    2. Tests and diagnostic procedures

Table 12-7 Some Examples of Internet Sites and Companies That Provide Technology-Based Client Education Materials Accessible Online Through the Internet (Available to the Public) *(Continued)*

    3. Surgery and treatment procedures

    4. Prevention and wellness, e.g., hypertension: slides with audio

- The PatientChannel: GE Healthcare (www.gehealthcare.com)

Accessible Online Through the Internet (Expanded Applications May Be Available Through the Intranet of Individual Organizations)

PRINT RESOURCES

- Krames on Demand (www.krames.com): self-care guides in Spanish and English. Publisher of choice for American Heart Association, American Stroke Association, American Lung Association, and National Cancer Institute.

- Medications

    1. Micromedex (www.micromedex.com): medications, diseases, procedures, home care

    2. Lexi-Comp (www.lexi.com): medications, diseases, procedures

- McKesson (www.mckesson.com)

- Blackboard (for more information, see www.blackboard.com/us/index.Bb and www.delmarlearning.com/healthcare/Index.aspx?cat1ID=HCR)

- ADAM (www.adam.com)

- ExitCare (www.exitcare.com)

- HealthWise (www.healthwise.org)

VIDEO RESOURCES

- Emmi Solutions (www.emmisolutions.com)

DVD COMPANIES FOR PURCHASING INDIVIDUAL TITLES

- Milner-Fenwick.com: videos, digital media, and print resources for health professionals providing direct care; free previews; most have Spanish language and closed captioning. Most healthcare topics covered.

- Aquarius Health Care Media (www.aquariusproductions.com): all videos have an inspirational message of hope and healing. Award-winning videos and DVDs on disabilities, cancer, caregiving, children, diseases and health, death and dying, end of life, bereavement, and mental health.

- NIMCO (www.nimcoinc.com)

- Professional Medical Organizations: e.g., American Academy of Allergy, Asthma, and Immunology (www.aaaai.org/patients/publicedmat/patient_education_videos.stm)

computer illiterate, or lack easy access to computers even if they are technologically savvy. This situation is beginning to change, however, as computers become more of a household item. Unfortunately, people with reading problems experience major difficulty making sense of the information on the screen (see Chapter 7 on literacy) and learners with physical limitations, such as arthritis, neuromuscular disorders, pain, fatigue, paralysis, or vision impairment, also may find computers challenging to use (see Chapter 9 on learners with disabilities). Also, it must be acknowledged that although multimedia resources may be an important tool to enhance learning in the older adult, much more research needs to be conducted on age-related cognitive changes that could have implications on the design and use of multimedia learning environments for this growing population of learners (Pass, VanGerven, & Tabbers, 2005).

Moreover, it should not be forgotten that the computer is a machine, so the learner is necessarily deprived of the personal, compassionate, one-to-one interaction that only a teacher can provide to facilitate learning. Because of the independent nature of the computer learning experience, the CAI format is not recommended for nondirected or poorly motivated learners.

Nevertheless, the tremendous growth of the Internet has opened new doors for many learners to gain access to libraries and to direct learning experiences, such as online discussions with educators at great distances. For more information on technology in education, see Chapter 13.

Table 12–8 summarizes the basic advantages and disadvantages of computer learning resources.

Evaluation Criteria for Selecting Materials

Choosing the right tools for client education calls for judgment on the part of the health professional as educator, who must take into consideration the variables of the learner, the task, and the media. Decisions as to which instructional materials are or are not appropriate depend on the size and characteristics of the audience, the predetermined behavioral objectives to be achieved, and the effectiveness and availability of media resources. Answers to these three variables in combination with one another result in the selection of different teaching tools by the educator, who is faced with multiple situations and varying circumstances on a daily basis. In particular, the evaluation of media involves appraising the content, the instructional design, the technical production, and the packaging of any given instructional materials. **Figure 12–6** depicts an adaptation of Discenza's (1993) checklist, which continues to be a valid instrument for selecting and evaluating instructional materials.

Printed materials, as the most popular tool available for client education, require a determination of

---

Table 12-8 Basic Advantages and Disadvantages of Computer Learning Resources

Advantages	Disadvantages
Interactive potential promotes quick feedback, retention of learning	Primarily promotes learning in cognitive domain; less useful in changing attitudes and behaviors or promoting psychomotor skill development
Potential database enormous	
Instruction can be individualized to suit different types of learners or different paces for learning	Both software and hardware are expensive, therefore less accessible to a wide audience
Time efficient	Must be purchased—too complex and time consuming for most educators to prepare
	Limited use for many elderly, low-literate learners, and those with physical limitations

readability levels. This is an essential factor when selecting print media that will be suitable for a given audience of learners (see Chapter 7 on literacy). **Figure 12–7** is an illustration of the learning pyramid. It depicts an important learning principle that, based on numerous research studies, shows people retain information at a higher rate if they are actively involved in the learning process (National Training Laboratories, n.d.). The effectiveness of teaching and learning is greatly enhanced when instructional materials are used that stimulate multiple senses and modes of learning.

In making final media selections, educators must ask themselves which material(s) best support their teaching to achieve the outcomes for their particular audience. They must remember that active learner involvement is best and realia is best for retention of information. Above all else, educators should remember that instructional materials should be used to support learning only by

Figure 12-6 A Checklist for Selecting and Evaluating Instructional Materials

	Yes	No
A. Content		
Is the content valid?	___	___
Relevant?	___	___
Current?	___	___
Is the purpose of the program stated?	___	___
Are instructional objectives given?	___	___
B. Instructional Design		
Are the ideas and information presented logically?	___	___
Is the format of the program appropriate for the audience?	___	___
Does the instructor actively engage the learner?	___	___
Is there evidence of formative evaluation?	___	___
Is summative evaluation material provided?	___	___
C. Technical Production		
Is the visual material sharply focused and clear?	___	___
Is the image composition clear and uncluttered?	___	___
Is the text legible at the maximum viewing distance?	___	___
Is the audio clear and intelligible?	___	___
Is there any distracting background noise?	___	___
Is the pace of the narration appropriate for the audience?	___	___
D. Packaging		
Is the material available in a format for which equipment is available?	___	___
Is descriptive information provided?	___	___
Is a User's Guide provided?	___	___
Has the instructional material won any awards?	___	___

Source: Modified from Discenza, D. J. (1993). A systematic approach to selecting and evaluating instructional material. *Journal of Nursing Staff Development, 9*(4), 198. Reprinted with permission of J. B. Lippincott Company.

Figure 12-7 Learning Pyramid: Information Retention Based on Level of Active Learner Involvement

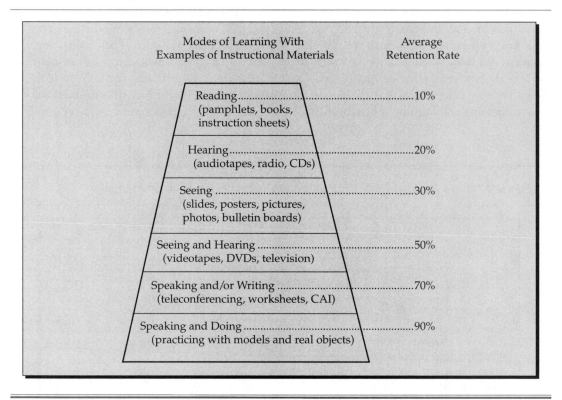

Source: Adapted from National Training Laboratories. (n.d.). Institute for Applied Behavioral Science, 300 N. Lee Street, Suite 300, Alexandria, VA 22314. 1-800-777-5227.

complementing and supplementing the teaching, not by substituting for it.

State of the Evidence

There is broad recognition of the importance that healthcare practice, including client, staff, and student education, be based on supporting evidence of efficacy. Rather than perpetuating practices because they have always been done that way, there is more emphasis on demonstrating that learning has occurred and that care has improved by the way in which information has been taught and received. In education, the focus is on both the processes and the outcomes of teaching and learning.

This chapter focuses on choosing, using, and evaluating instructional materials for client education, as well as for educating health professional staff and students. Some of the newest studies that validate the usefulness of the different media are cited within the chapter. It is only relatively recently that research has been conducted to determine the impact of various types of tools on the acquisition, retention, and recall of information and on the satisfaction with learning. The following are examples of research studies exploring the effectiveness of printed, demonstration, and audiovisual media that stimulate the senses, increase active participation, enhance critical thinking, assist with comprehension and memory of information, and provide opportunities for easier, more rewarding, and more enjoyable learning experiences.

Video recording and playback have become common strategies to help health professional students and staff improve clinical skills performance. Hill et al. (2000) used skill performance checklists to compare initial performance of venipunctures by registered nurses and student nurses with repeat venipuncture performances after they reviewed and evaluated the video recordings of their initial performance. Results showed that with visual reinforcement of the task, performance improved and learner satisfaction increased. Winters et al. (2003) found similar results in a study with baccalaureate nursing students practicing physical assessment techniques.

As another example of the application of video learning resources, Ruston, Canchola, and Lo (2004) used videos of real client scenarios to trigger discussion in medical ethics courses. These recordings brought to life the experiences and views of persons involved in clinical cases, such as patients, families, nurses, and chaplains. Dramatization of the complexity of ethical dilemmas challenged viewers to engage in thought-provoking exchanges. These authors found support for the idea that videos could be used to increase learning, although locating relevant videos for this purpose was cited as a significant barrier.

Learners with low literacy skills or intellectual disabilities are particularly challenging for health professionals as educators. Creativity by an educator can often help overcome barriers to teaching and learning. A study by Leiner, Handal, and Williams (2004) compares the effectiveness of printed information about polio vaccination from the Centers for Disease Control and Prevention (CDC) with the same message converted into a

production of animated cartoons using marketing and advertising techniques. The findings of this study show that the animated cartoon was more effective in delivering the same message as written instructional materials. In another study, Feldman (2004) describes the development, implementation, and evaluation of self-directed learning using pictorial manuals and accompanying audiocassettes to teach basic child-care, health, and safety skills to parents with intellectual disabilities. This study indicates that a significant number of parents with cognitive disabilities are able to improve their parenting skills with these low-cost, low-tech, self-directed materials.

The advent of distance learning via the Internet and various interactive media has begun to blur the lines between instructional methods and instructional materials. It is essential to remember that instructional materials should support learning, not merely be the learning experience altogether. With fewer qualified health professional educators and growing numbers of learners, the challenge of meeting the needs of students is a constant pressure. Lashley (2005) describes development of an online health assessment course for instruction of RN students, both novices and those returning to pursue baccalaureate education. She employed the Web site to display announcements, provide handouts, and explain assignments. A text and CD-ROM were used for readings and testing. She prepared an instructional video of the physical exam that was digitally streamed onto the Web, which allowed students to readily access it from any site and view it repeatedly as needed. CD-ROM and DVD versions of this instructional video also were available. The students reported that completing assignments online did not take any longer than the work required in a traditional class, and 80% reported online learning allowed them to work from home or some other location at their own pace. The interactive features of this modality supported and facilitated this educator's ability to teach an effective course. The reader is referred to other studies that illustrate effective use of interactive video and the Internet to support learning (Green et al., 2003; Jeste et al., 2008; Martin & Klotz, 2001).

Rather than base teaching strategies on assumptions that one vehicle for instruction is superior to another for learning, research has begun to verify the effectiveness of different tools with a variety of audiences under various circumstances. Much more evidence needs to be uncovered, but it is gratifying that educators are taking steps to undertake such investigations. In particular, Mayer (2005) provides a comprehensive examination of multimedia learning based on the latest research and theory in this field.

Summary

This chapter reviews the major categories of instructional materials, identifies how to select media from a range of possible options based on their advantages and disadvantages, and addresses how to evaluate their effectiveness. Health professionals as educators are expected to be able to make media choices every day, whether it be to meet the needs of an individual learner or to design an educational program to satisfy a broader, more diverse group of learners. In this chapter, the importance of considering characteristics of the learner, the media, and the task when choosing instructional materials is emphasized. The supplemental nature of teaching materials is also stressed, as is the need to keep the behavioral objectives in focus when selecting these materials as adjuncts to instruction.

Print media include both commercially prepared and instructor-composed materials. The problem of matching literacy and cognitive levels of learners to printed instructional tools is a relevant concern. The major advantages of printed tools are that they are widely available, clients are able to refer back to these materials for review at any time and at their own pace, and they have potential for reinforcing explanations of complex concepts. Disadvantages include the limited opportunity for learner–educator feedback. For some learners, the readability level and complexity of information may be significant barriers to full utilization of printed tools. The written materials section of the chapter contains several guidelines useful to educators in selecting or developing printed materials appropriate to both the audience and the task.

Demonstration materials include many types of visual, hands-on media, such as models and real equipment as well as displays, such as posters, bulletin boards, and whiteboards. In particular, they stimulate the senses of sight and touch. They are especially useful for cognitive and psychomotor skill development and may even influence attitudes, feelings, and values in the affective domain. Other advantages include bringing the learner closer to reality through active involvement and the opportunity for repetition. The major disadvantage of demonstration materials is the potential for static content or overuse because they are often time consuming to prepare and the educator may be reluctant or unable to revise these materials frequently. In addition, most of these materials are not suitable for simultaneous viewing by large audiences, for learners with visual impairments, or for individuals with poor abstraction abilities.

Audiovisual materials make up the fastest growing category of instructional tools. Their ability to stimulate learners' visual and auditory senses enhances their power to actively engage learners and to potentially increase retention of information. Many audiovisual tools can influence all three domains of learning by promoting cognitive development, stimulating attitude change, and helping to build psychomotor skills. The audiovisual materials section of the chapter examines the five major categories of audiovisual tools—projected, audio, video, telecommunications, and computer formats. The discussion includes audience appropriateness, expense, and convenience of use. Comprehensive guidelines for selecting and developing audiovisual materials are presented. The principal advantages and disadvantages of the five categories are also described. Learners with low literacy skills may benefit from most categories of these media except computer formats. Audio materials are most appropriate for learners with visual impairment, while projected video with captions and computer resources most benefit learners with hearing impairments.

REVIEW QUESTIONS

1. How do instructional materials differ from instructional methods?
2. What are five general principles regarding the effectiveness of printed and nonprinted (audiovisual) tools?
3. What are the three major variables to consider when selecting, developing, and evaluating instructional materials?
4. What are the three primary components of media to be kept in mind when evaluating appropriateness of instructional materials?
5. Which instructional materials are examples of illusionary representations?
6. Why are numbers as well as oral and written words known to be the most abstract forms of messages?
7. What factors must be considered when reviewing commercially prepared print materials for use in instruction?
8. What are three of the guidelines to be followed to ensure the clarity of instructor-composed printed education materials?
9. What are some examples of demonstration materials? Of audiovisual materials?
10. What are the major advantages and disadvantages of computer learning resources?
11. Why is it that instructional materials should not be selected before behavioral objectives are determined?

CASE STUDY

In an effort to educate the public about health and wellness, professional organizations such as the American Occupational Therapy Association (AOTA), the American Physical Therapy Association (APTA), and the American Speech and Hearing Association (ASHA) among others are searching for mechanisms to promote the roles their members play in supporting health, wellness, and quality of life. APTA has decided to go with printed instructional materials to communicate information to clients about health and wellness issues and the physical therapist's role in supporting these quality-of-life goals. The challenge is how to create instructional materials that effectively communicate educational messages to a broad consumer base.

1. What are the three major variables that should be considered by professional organizations when selecting, developing, and evaluating instructional materials for the various consumer audiences they serve?

2. What three components of instructional materials are required to effectively communicate the educational message that healthcare professions support health, wellness, and quality of life?
3. What are the basic advantages and disadvantages of printed instructional materials?

References

Aldridge, M. D. (2009). Using models to teach congenital heart defects. *Dimensions of Critical Care Nursing, 28*(3), 116–122.

Babcock, D. E., & Miller, M. A. (1994). *Client education: Theory and practice.* St. Louis, MO: Mosby–Year Book.

Bach, C. A., McDaniel, R. W., & Poole, M. J. (1994). Posters: Innovative and cost-effective tools for staff development. *Journal of Nursing Staff Development, 10*(2), 71–74.

Boyd, M. D., Gleit, C. J., Graham, B. A., & Whitman, N. J. (1998). *Health teaching in nursing practice: A professional model* (3rd ed.). Stamford, CT: Appleton & Lange.

Brooks, P. A., Renvall, M. J., Bulow, K. B., & Ramsdell, J. W. (2000). A comparison between lecture and videotape inservice for certified nursing assistants in skilled nursing facilities. *Journal of the American Medical Directors Association, 1*(5), 191–196.

Brown, D. G. (2001, March). Judicious PowerPoint. Retrieved August 1, 2007, from http://www.wfu.edu/~brown/Syllabus%20Articles/JudicousPowerPoint.htm

Brownson, K. (1998). Education handouts: Are we wasting our time? *Journal of Nurses in Staff Development, 14*(4), 176–182.

Bushy, A. (1991). A rating scale to evaluate research posters. *Nurse Educator, 16*(1), 11–15.

Campbell, M. K., DeVellis, B., Strecher, V. J., Ammerman, A. S., DeVellis, R. S., & Sandler, R. S. (1994). Improving dietary behavior: The effectiveness of tailored messages in primary care settings. *American Journal of Public Health, 84*, 783–787.

Carlson, S. (2003, August 5). Can *Grand Theft Auto* inspire professors? *Chronicle of Higher Education*, 1931–1933.

Clark, M. C., & Lester, J. (2000). The effect of video-based interventions on self-care. *Western Journal of Nursing Research, 22*(8), 895–911.

Cobussen-Boekhorst, J. G. L., Van Der Weide, M., Feitz, W. F. J., & DeGier, R. P. E. (2000). Using an instructional model to teach clean intermittent catheterization to children. *BJU International, 85*, 551–553.

Cooper, S. S. (1990). Teaching tips, one more time: The overhead projector. *Journal of Continuing Education in Nursing, 21*(3), 141–142.

deWest, C. F. (2006). Beyond presentations: Using Power-Point as an effective instructional tool. *Gifted Child Today, 29*(4), 29–39.

Dickerson, P. S. (2005). Nurturing critical thinkers. *Journal of Continuing Education in Nursing, 36*(3), 68–72.

DiGiacinto, D. (2007). Using multimedia effectively in the teaching–learning process. *Journal of Allied Health, 36*(3), 176–179.

Discenza, D. J. (1993). A systematic approach to selecting and evaluating instructional materials. *Journal of Nursing Staff Development, 9*(4), 196–198.

Doak, C. C., Doak, L. G., Friedell, G. H., & Meade, C. D. (1998). Improving comprehension for cancer patients with low literacy skills: Strategies for clinicians. *CA–Cancer Journal for Clinicians, 48*(3), 151–162.

Doak, C. C., Doak, L. G., & Root, J. H. (1996). *Teaching patients with low literacy.* Philadelphia: J. B. Lippincott.

Duchin, S., & Sherwood, G. (1990). Posters as an educational strategy. *Journal of Continuing Education in Nursing, 21*(5), 205–208.

DuFrene, D. D., & Lehman, C. M. (2004). Concepts, content, construction, and contingencies: Getting the horse before the PowerPoint cart. *Business Communications Quarterly, 67*, 84–88.

Estey, A., Musseau, A., & Keehn, L. (1994). Patient's understanding of health information: A multihospital comparison. *Patient Education and Counseling, 24*, 73–78.

Feldman, M. A. (2004). Self-directed learning of child-care skills by parents with intellectual disabilities. *Infants and Young Children, 17*(1), 17–31.

Flournoy, E., Turner, G., & Combs, D. (2000). Innovative teaching: Read the writing on the wall. *Dimensions of Critical Care Nursing, 19*(4), 36–37.

Frantz, R. A. (1980). *Selecting media for patient education. TCN/Education for self care.* Rockville, MD: Aspen.

Fraze, J., Griffith, J., Green, D., & McElroy, L. (2010). So many materials, so little time: A checklist to select printed education materials for clinical practice. *Journal of Midwifery and Women's Health, 55*(10), 70–73.

Green, M. J., Peterson, S. K., Baker, M. W., Harper, G. R., Friedman, L. C., Rubenstein, W. S., et al. (2004). Effect of a computer-based decision aid on knowledge, perceptions, and intentions about genetic testing for breast cancer susceptibility: A randomized controlled trial. *Journal of the American Medical Association, 492*(4), 442–452.

Green, S. M., Voegeli, D., Harrison, M., Phillips, J., Knowles, J., Weaver, M., et al. (2003). Evaluating the use of streaming video to support student learning in a first-year life sciences course for student nurses. *Nurse Education Today, 23*, 255–261.

Grunwald, T., & Corsbie-Massay, C. (2006). Guidelines for cognitively efficient multimedia learning tools: Educational strategies, cognitive load, and interface redesign. *Academic Medicine, 81*(3), 213–223.

Haggard, A. (1989). *Handbook of patient education*. Rockville, MD: Aspen.

Hagopian, G. A. (1996). The effects of informational audiotapes on knowledge and self-care behaviors of patients undergoing radiation therapy. *Oncology Nursing Forum, 23*(4), 697–700.

Hayes, S. K., & Childress, D. M. (1999). Fairy tales of storyboarding. *Journal for Nurses in Staff Development, 15*(6), 260–262.

Heidenreiter, T. J. (1995). Using videoteleconferencing for continuing education and staff development programs. *Journal of Continuing Education in Nursing, 26*(3), 135–138.

Heinrich, R., Molenda, M., Russell, J. D., & Smaldino, S. E. (2002). *Instructional media and technologies for learning* (7th ed.). Upper Saddle River, NJ: Pearson.

Hill, R., Hooper, C., & Wahl, S. (2000). Look, learn, and be satisfied: Video playback as a learning strategy to improve clinical skills performance. *Journal for Nurses in Staff Development, 16*(5), 232–239.

Hoffman, B., Hartley, K., & Boone, R. (2005, January). Reaching accessibility: Guidelines for creating and refining digital learning materials. *Interventions in School and Clinic, 40*(3), 171.

Houts, P. S., Bachrach, B., Witmer, J. T., Tringali, C. A., Bucher, J. A., & Localio, R. A. (1998). Using pictographs to enhance recall of spoken medical instructions. *Patient Education and Counseling, 35*, 83–88.

Huang, C. (2005). Designing high-quality interactive multimedia learning modules. *Computerized Medical Imaging and Graphics, 29*, 223–233.

Huhn, K., Anderson, E., & Deutsch, J. (2008). Using a Web-based patient simulation program to teach clinical reasoning to physical therapy students: Feasibility and pilot studies. In *Proceedings of World Conference on E-Learning in Corporate, Government, Healthcare, and Higher Education* (pp. 2760–2763). Chesapeake, VA: AACE.

Izquierdo, R. E., Knudson, P. E., Meyer, S., Kearns, J., Ploutz-Snyder, R., & Weinstock, R. S. (2003). A comparison of diabetes education administered through telemedicine versus in-person. *Diabetes Care, 26*(4), 1002–1007.

Jeste, D. V., Dunn, L. B., Folsom, D. P., & Zisook, D. (2008). Multimedia educational aids for improving consumer knowledge about illness management and treatment decisions: A review of randomized controlled trials. *Journal of Psychiatric Research, 42*, 1–21.

Kaveevivitchai, C., Chuengkriankrai, B., Luecha, Y., Thonooruk, R., Panijpan, B., & Ruenwongsa, P. (2009). Enhancing nursing students' skills in vital signs assessment by using multimedia computer-assisted learning with integrated content of anatomy and physiology. *Nurse Education Today, 29*, 65–72.

Kessels, R. P. C. (2003). Patients' memory for medical information. *Journal of the Royal Society of Medicine, 96*, 219–222.

Lamb, A., & Johnson, L. (2006). Flash: Engaging learners through animation, interaction, and multimedia. *Teacher Librarian, 33*(4), 54–56.

Lashley, M. (2005). Teaching health assessment in the virtual classroom. *Journal of Nursing Education, 44*(8), 348–350.

Leiner, M., Handal, G., & Williams, D. (2004). Patient communication: A multidisciplinary approach using animated cartoons. *Health Education Research, 19*(5), 591–595.

Lerner, E. B., Jehle, D. V. K., Janicke, D. M., & Moscati, R. M. (2000). Medical communication: Do our patients understand? *American Journal of Emergency Medicine, 18*(7), 764–766.

Lowenstein, A. J., Foord, L., & Romano, J. C. (2009). *Teaching strategies for health education and health promotion: Working with patients, families, and communities*. Sudbury, MA: Jones and Bartlett.

Manny, R. (2006, Winter). Multimedia streaming: A big part of the future for CHC [Community Health Care Services Foundation]. *Focus, 3*(1), 1, 4.

Martin, P., & Klotz, L. (2001). Implementing a nursing program via live interactive video: Lessons learned. *Nurse Educator, 26*(4), 187–190.

Mayer, R. E. (Ed.). (2005). *The Cambridge handbook of multimedia learning*. New York: Cambridge University Press.

Moneyham, L., Ura, D., Ellwood, S., & Bruno, B. (1996). The poster presentation as an educational tool. *Nurse Educator, 21*(4), 45–47.

Naperstek, B. (1993). Guided imagery: A technique that engages the imagination in the healing process. Health Journeys. (CD). United Kingdom: GlaxoSmithKline.

National Training Laboratories. (n.d.). Learning pyramid. Alexandria, VA: Institute for Applied Behavioral Science. Retrieved January 30, 2007, from http://home pages.gold.ac.uk/polovina/learnpyramid/about.htm

Pass, F., VanGerven, P. W. M., & Tabbers, H. K. (2005). The cognitive aging principle in multimedia learning. In R. E. Mayer (Ed.), *The Cambridge handbook of multimedia learning* (pp. 339–351). New York: Cambridge University Press.

Pinto, B. M. (1993). Training and maintenance of breast self-examination skills. *American Journal of Preventive Medicine, 9*(6), 353–358.

Prensky, M. (2001). Digital natives, digital immigrants. *On the Horizon, 9*(5), 1–6.

Rankin, S. H., & Stallings, K. D. (2005). *Patient education: Principles and practices* (5th ed.). Philadelphia: Lippincott Williams & Wilkins.

Redman, B. K. (2007). *The practice of patient education: A case study approach* (10th ed.). St. Louis, MO: Mosby.

Rice, J., Trockel, M., King, T., & Remmert, D. (2004). Computerized training in breast self-examination: A test in a community health center. *Cancer Nursing, 27*(2), 162–168.

Rosen, J., Mulsant, B. H., Koller, M., Kastango, K. B., Mazumdar, S., & Fox, D. (2002). Mental health training for nursing home staff using computer-based interactive video: A 6-month randomized trial. *Journal of the American Medical Directors Association, 3*(5), 291–296.

Ruiz, J. G., Mintzer, M. J., & Leipzig, R. M. (2006). The impact of e-learning in medical education. *Academic Medicine, 81*(3), 207–212.

Ruston, D., Canchola, J., & Lo, B. (2004). Use of videos by directors of medical ethics courses. *Journal of Clinical Ethics, 15*(2), 201–208.

Schrock, K. (2003). Software to make you look marvelous. *School Library Journal, 49*(9), 38–39.

Skinner, C. S., Strecher, V. J., & Hospers, H. (1994). Physician's recommendations for mammography: Do tailored messages make a difference? *American Journal of Public Health, 84*, 43–49.

SMART. (2009). Home page. Retrieved May 10, 2010, from http://education.smarttech.com/ste/en-us/

Smith, J. A., & Lombardo, N. (2005). Patient education workshop on CD-ROM: An innovative approach for staff education. *Journal of Nursing Staff Development, 21*(2), 43–46.

Staib, S. (2003). Teaching and measuring critical thinking. *Journal of Nursing Education, 42*(11), 498–508.

Thurber, R. F., & Asselin, M. E. (1999). An educational fair and poster approach to organization-wide mandatory education. *Journal of Continuing Education in Nursing, 30*(1), 25–29.

Tobolowsky, B. F. (2007, March–April). Thinking visually: Using visual media in the college classroom. *About Campus*, 21–24.

Weixler, D. (1994). Correcting metered-dose inhaler misuse. *Nursing, 24*(7), 62–65.

Weston, C., & Cranston, P. A. (1986). Selecting instructional strategies. *Journal of Higher Education, 57*(3), 259–288.

Williams, N. H., Wolgin, C. S., & Hodge, C. S. (1998). Creating an educational videotape. *Journal for Nurses in Staff Development, 14*(6), 261–265.

Winters, J., Hauck, B., Riggs, J., Clawson, J., & Collins, J. (2003). Use of videotaping to assess competencies and course outcomes. *Journal of Nursing Education, 42*(10), 472–476.

Chapter 13

Technology in Education

Deborah L. Sopczyk,
Nancy Doyle, and
Karen Jacobs

CHAPTER HIGHLIGHTS

KEY TERMS

- Information Age
- consumer informatics
- information literacy
- Internet
- World Wide Web
- asynchronous

- blogs
- mobile learning (m-learning)
- digital divide
- computer literacy
- e-learning
- distance learning

OBJECTIVES

After completing this chapter, the reader will be able to

1. Describe changes in education that have occurred as a result of Information Age technology.
2. Define the terms *Information Age, consumer informatics, Internet, World Wide Web, information literacy, computer literacy, digital divide, blog, e-learning,* and *distance learning.*
3. Identify ways in which the resources of the Internet and World Wide Web could be incorporated into healthcare education.
4. Recognize the issues related to the use of technology.
5. Describe the role of the health professional as educator in using technology for client, staff, and student education.
6. Discuss the effects that technology has had on education for health professionals.

Life has been greatly influenced by technological advances of the last century. The birth of the Internet and the World Wide Web, the development of information technology, the wide-scale production of computers, and the development of user-friendly software have had an impact on every aspect of people's lives. Some of the most dramatic changes have occurred in the field of education where technology has transformed the way learners learn and the way teachers teach.

Today, students, staff, and clients have a world of information at their fingertips. Computers and the Internet have made it possible to get information from anyone, anywhere, anytime, within the blink of an eye. In today's world, virtually all children begin learning on computers when they are in nursery school and are as young as 3 years of age (National Center for Educational Statistics, 2006). This is a very different beginning from that experienced by most adults who grew up in the 20th century.

Educational technologies, once rare and highly desirable resources, have become commonplace. Both the on-site and distance learner now interact in a multidimensional learning environment. This chapter explores the opportunities and challenges resulting from the use of technology as they pertain to health, health care, and the education

of health consumers and professionals. The use of technology in education has tremendous potential. Through technology health professional educators can increase access to health information, improve educational practices already in place, and create new strategies that transform teaching and learning experiences for healthcare consumers and health professionals.

The use of technology in health education must be implemented with careful planning, monitoring, and evaluation. Although computer-based educational applications have become easier to use and require less technical skill than they did in the past, the decision to use technology as part of an educational program is likely to have significant implications. For example, access, cost, level of support, equipment, process, and outcomes must all be considered. Therefore, the health professional who uses technology to enhance learning must not only have a basic understanding of the technology itself, but he or she must also be able to integrate the technology into a plan that is based on sound educational principles.

This chapter is designed as an introduction to the use of technology in education. Because health professionals provide both healthcare and professional education, it addresses technology-based resources and strategies appropriate for educating clients and health professionals. Although it is not intended to provide detailed instruction on the mechanics of computers and other types of hardware and software, the chapter provides a basic overview of the technology involved and implications for the educator and the learner. This chapter focuses primarily on the Internet, the World Wide Web, and computer-based applications that can be used to enhance learning with clients, students, and staff in face-to-face environments as well as with learners at a distance.

As this chapter begins, it is important for health professional educators to note that the Internet, the World Wide Web, and computer-based technologies are developing at a rapid pace that is accelerating with each new generation of discoveries and applications (Cetron & Davies, 2001). Because of this phenomenon, consumers are often advised that the computers they buy today are not likely to reflect the state-of-the-art technology of tomorrow. The same caution must be given to readers of books on technology. Given the pace of technology and the development cycle of a textbook, it is impossible to capture all that is new and cutting edge in the world of educational technologies in a textbook. Rather, this chapter is meant to serve as a starting point from which readers can begin to investigate the educational technologies and resources available. Ideally, it will generate the interest and skill necessary for readers to continue to search for new and exciting ways to integrate technology into their teaching and learning activities.

Health Education in the Information Age

The use of technology in education is a reflection of what is happening on a much larger scale in American communities. Hence, it is useful to think of educational technology within the broader context of the environment in which people live and work. This era of history is often referred to as the **Information Age**, a period in time characterized by a change in focus from industry to information. Beginning in the 1970s, improvements in information technology and the decreasing cost of computers suddenly made information more accessible, resulting in a dramatically different world (Finnis, 2003). This new access to information has had an enormous impact on the global economy, culture, and people's ways of life. New and powerful industries have emerged, and it is now possible to access people and services from around the world in a blink of an eye and at very low cost.

The demand for technology and for information continues to grow. Twenty-first-century adults and children have come to depend upon pocket-sized telephones, media players, and computer-driven devices. When considering the many ways in which technology has changed the world, it is clear that computers have become more than tools to make life easier—they have become part of human culture.

Computers have also become part of the culture of education. Computers are as common in the educational environment today as chalk and blackboards were in years past. Perhaps the most significant effect computers have on society and on education is related to their capacity to assist in the collection, management, transportation, and transformation of information at high speed. As a result of this newfound ability to handle information, the world has experienced an "information explosion." As a society, Americans have increased both their use and production of information of all kinds.

People living in this information-driven society benefit from the availability of information but also are challenged to keep up with the information that is bombarding them from all directions. Information and knowledge have become valuable commodities, and the ability to gather and evaluate information efficiently and effectively has become a 21st-century life skill.

How has the Information Age changed health education? Consider the following. As a result of technological advances, the infrastructure to link people around the world to one another and to a vast array of Web-based information exists. Internetworldstats.com (2009), an international Web site that provides comprehensive and current information on Internet usage, reports that in North America alone there are more than 246 million Internet users, an increase of 128% between 2000 and 2008. Once a slow and tedious process, connecting to the Internet has become high speed. In April 2008, 55% of adults in the United States had broadband or high-speed Internet access in their homes, up from 47% in March 2007 (Horrigan, 2008). This figure is increasing each year.

For health professionals who provide health and healthcare education, it has never been easier to reach clients. With the use of new technologies, health and healthcare messages can easily extend beyond local communities to a worldwide audience. In addition, educators can provide interactive learning experiences to learners at any time and in any place.

The use of Information Age technology has had such a dramatic influence on health education that a unique and rapidly expanding field of study, **consumer informatics** (also referred to as consumer health informatics), has emerged. The American Medical Informatics Association (AMIA), one of the principal professional organizations for people working in the field of informatics, has established a consumer informatics working group to advance the field through collaboration and dialogue. This group has developed a definition of consumer informatics, which states that it is "a subspecialty of medical informatics which studies from a patient/consumer perspective the use of electronic information and communication to improve medical outcomes and the health care decision-making process" (American Medical Informatics Association, 2009).

Researchers and other professionals in the field of consumer informatics strive to find ways to use technology to strengthen the relationship between client and healthcare provider as well as to use technology to teach and empower clients dealing with issues related to health and wellness. Although much attention has been given to computer-based educational systems, consumer informatics is not restricted to computer-based programs. It includes the study of a wide range of media that can be used to deliver health-related information.

The entire field of consumer informatics is growing rapidly. Many colleges offer courses of study in which health professionals can gain knowledge and skill in using technology to meet the information needs of healthcare consumers. Informaticians and health professionals are conducting research on the use of technology in healthcare education to generate knowledge that will guide future educational endeavors. A review of the literature reveals a growing body of knowledge in the field. Health professionals are using this knowledge to guide practice and improve the quality of the education they are providing to their clients.

Sophisticated technology will continue to make health and healthcare information more accessible and more meaningful to both healthcare consumers and health professionals. Educators in all health disciplines are identifying creative ways to use emerging technology to enhance the teaching–learning process. This trend is reflected in the healthcare literature, where an increasing number of articles on uses of technology in professional and consumer education can be found.

It is important to note, however, that Information Age technology has done more than alter the way in which people teach and learn. Technology has and will continue to prompt dramatic system-wide changes. These changes will be evident in the roles played by health professionals and clients, the relationships they establish, and the environments in which they interact.

The Impact of Technology on the Teacher and the Learner

Information Age technology has had a significant influence on educators and learners for a number of reasons. Most important, access to information bridges the knowledge gap between teacher and learner. When information is widely available, it is no longer necessary for the teacher to "find, filter and deliver" content (Warger, 2006, p. 3). Therefore, the teacher is no longer the person who holds all of the answers or the individual who is solely responsible for imparting knowledge.

Educators in the Information Age are becoming facilitators of learning rather than providers of information and are striving to create collaborative atmospheres in their teaching and learning environments. As information becomes more and more accessible, the need for memorization becomes less important than the ability to think critically. Hence, educators in the Information Age are helping individuals learn how to refine a problem, find the information they need, and critically evaluate the information they find.

Healthcare education can and should follow a similar path. Health professionals must structure their approach to education to be consistent with the needs of Information Age clients. The first step is to reconceptualize the role of the educator as someone who does more than impart knowledge. The health professional must be prepared to be a facilitator of learning by helping clients to access, evaluate, and use the wide range of information that is available. They must be willing to encourage and support clients in their attempts to seek the knowledge they require.

The health professional also must learn how and when to use technology and remain current as new technology-based tools become available to optimize each learning experience. Research studies indicate that this is currently an area that needs improvement. For example, in a study of 454 practicing nurses, Wilbright et al. (2006) found that many nurses only rated themselves as fair to poor in basic information technology skills, such as bookmarking a Web site, conducting a search using Medline or CINAHL, opening more than one computer program at a time, and checking and replying to e-mail messages. The authors of this study identified the age of nurses as one contributing factor. Consistent with national statistics, they found that the majority of their nurse respondents were between the ages of 35 and 50 and entered the workforce prior to the time when computers became prominent.

In another study, Secco et al. (2006) identified additional factors limiting pediatric nurses' use of information technology and their ability to develop **information literacy** skills. These factors included lack of computers with Internet access on clinical units, limited access to bibliographic databases, and lack of time. If health professionals are to be effective facilitators of learning in today's world, these problems must be rectified for all practicing clinicians.

The Information Age has been witness to some dramatic changes in the behavior of healthcare consumers, making the role changes discussed earlier inevitable. Technology and the increased accessibility to information it offers have empowered and enlightened these consumers, encouraging them to form new partnerships with their healthcare providers (Kaplan & Brennan, 2001; Shaw et al., 2006). Even those clients who are reluctant to assume more responsibility for managing their own health care are moving in that direction as changes in the health delivery system have forced them to assume more active roles. As a result, healthcare consumers in the Information Age are eager to learn about and make use of the many information resources available to them.

Today's consumers enter the healthcare arena with information in hand. They are prepared to engage in a dialogue with their providers about their diagnoses and treatments. Surveys of the 113 million clients who have gone online to find health information show that the information they found caused them to make decisions about treatment of a condition and made them confident to ask questions of their care provider (Fox, 2006).

Therefore, health professionals can no longer assume that the clients they see in a hospital or clinic have little information other than what educators have given them or that they haven't explored the treatment options available to them. Furthermore, health professionals cannot assume that clients will unquestioningly accept what they tell them. Research studies show that twice as many online health information seekers go to the Web after a doctor's visit than before (Rainie, 2003).

Whereas healthcare consumers of the past were often isolated from others with similar diagnoses and were dependent upon healthcare providers for information, today's e-consumers and e-caregivers have the means to access networks of other clients and healthcare providers worldwide. Online support groups, blogs, and discussion groups where healthcare consumers can share experiences are readily available. Those who are being treated for health problems can readily find detailed information about their diagnoses, treatments, and prognoses.

Therefore, it is not surprising that the teaching needs of today's healthcare consumers and the expectations they hold for those who will be teaching them are changing. The role of the health professional as educator has not been diminished, but it has changed. Health professionals must now be prepared not only to use technology in education, but also to help clients access information, evaluate the information they find, and engage in discussions about the information that is available.

In addition to altering the educational needs and expectations of healthcare consumers, the Information Age has made a tremendous impact on professional education. Technology has given rise to a dramatic increase in educational opportunities for healthcare providers. Health professionals seeking advanced degrees and credentials or continuing education credits can now study at colleges and universities offering distance education programs in a wide range of subject areas.

Computers have made it possible to provide anytime, anywhere access to job training and continuing education. Virtual reality and computer simulation offer opportunities to learn hands-on skills and develop competencies in areas such as diagnostic reasoning and problem solving. Like consumers, health professionals in the Information Age can use the Internet and the World Wide Web as vehicles for sharing resources and for gaining access to the most current information in their fields of practice.

Strategies for Using Technology in Healthcare Education

The Internet and the World Wide Web

A common misconception is that the Internet and the World Wide Web are two names that describe the same entity. In fact, the Internet and the World Wide Web are related but different. The **Internet** was originally commissioned in 1969 as a program of the Department of Defense to allow the transfer of information from one computer to another (Livinginternet.com, 2009). Today, it is a huge global network of computers that allows for the exchange of information.

In simple terms, the **World Wide Web** is a virtual space to display, rather than exchange, information. It resides on a small section of the Internet and would not exist without the Internet's computer network. In the late 1980s, the first experimental version of the World Wide Web was conceived by Tim Berners-Lee and Robert Cailliau, two scientists working at a laboratory in Switzerland (Livinginternet.com, 2009; Wikipedia, 2009a). From a technical perspective, the World Wide Web is a network of information servers around the world that are connected to the Internet. The servers that make up the World Wide Web support a special type of document called a Web page. Web documents or Web pages are written using Hypertext Markup Language (HTML).

Today, it is almost impossible to track the size of the World Wide Web. Billions of Web pages exist with several million new pages being added every month. These Web pages cover a wide range of topics and display a variety of formats including text, audio, graphic, and video. Links on a Web page allow the user to easily move from one Web page to another with the click of a mouse. A user moves around the World Wide Web by way of a Web browser, a special software program that locates and displays Web pages. Netscape Navigator, Mozilla Firefox, Safari, and Microsoft Internet Explorer are examples of Web browsers.

Search engines and search directories are computer programs that allow the user to search the Web for particular subject areas. Search engines are robots that scour the Web for new Web sites, read them, and put text from them into a database they can access with queries. Google is an example of a search engine. Search directories are hierarchical directories compiled by humans with references to Web sites. These directories are then accessed with a user query. Yahoo! Directory is an example of a search directory. The Web is so large that any one search engine or directory can cover only a small percentage of the Web pages available (Pandia.com, 2009).

The Internet and the World Wide Web both offer a wide range of services, many of which can be used to deliver health information and healthcare education to consumers. The Internet services most likely to be of interest to health professional educators include those that allow computer-facilitated communication between individuals and among groups of people. E-mail, real-time chat, electronic discussions, and listservs are all used to communicate with people about health and health care.

The World Wide Web also provides opportunities to send healthcare messages to large groups of people in the form of educational Web pages. A report produced by the Pew Foundation revealed that 113 million adults, or 80% of all American Internet users, have accessed the World Wide Web to obtain health-related information (Fox, 2006). Web users can find health-related Web sites covering anything from videos of surgical procedures to sites where they can ask questions as well as receive information. There are thousands of health-related Web sites available to consumers offering a wide range of information, products, and services. The number of healthcare sites on the World Wide Web is difficult to capture with any accuracy because new sites are introduced on a daily basis.

Health professionals or healthcare consumers need to go no farther than their computers if they wish to learn how to use the Internet and the World Wide Web. Getting into the Internet or the World Wide Web requires a computer with a telecommunication link and software to connect to an Internet service provider (ISP). Once one is connected, it is simple to find a wide range of Web sites devoted to teaching Internet or World Wide Web navigation skills. With a properly worded command (e.g., World Wide Web and tutorial), a search engine can uncover a number of self-paced tutorials designed to teach novice or intermediate users the desired skills. Most search engines even provide guidance in creating commands that will elicit the information needed.

Knowledge of the World Wide Web is critical for health professionals who work with and educate healthcare consumers. This is true for the following reasons:

• Health professionals can expect to see clients enter the healthcare arena having already searched the Web for information. In fact, a Pew study found that many consumers go to the Web to seek information about a problem they are experiencing to help them determine whether it is necessary for them to see a healthcare provider (Rainie, 2003). Therefore, familiarity with the type of information found on the Web helps direct the assessment of clients prior to teaching to identify the needs of the learner and to determine whether follow-up is necessary.

- The World Wide Web is a tremendous resource for both consumer and professional education. To use the Web effectively, health professionals must possess information literacy skills and be prepared to teach these same skills to clients, including how to access the information on the Web and how to evaluate the information found.

- The World Wide Web provides a powerful mechanism for health professionals to offer healthcare education to a worldwide audience. More and more health organizations are creating Web sites with pages dedicated to presenting healthcare information for consumers. Although health professionals may not be responsible for actually creating the HTML document that will be placed on the Web, they may work with the Web site designers to develop the information it contains, evaluate the accuracy of the information presented, and interact with healthcare consumers who access the site.

The World Wide Web is a vital tool for health professionals. It is a mechanism for keeping up-to-date on professional and practice issues as well as a resource to be shared with clients. If it is to be used effectively, however, a plan to incorporate the World Wide Web into practice must be set in place.

E-Mail

In a discussion of health care in the 21st century, the National Institute of Medicine (2001) proclaimed that both clients and clinicians could benefit from improvements in timeliness through the use of Internet-based communication. Electronic mail, or e-mail, is a commonly used Internet technology that holds great potential for improved health communication and health education. For example, e-mail can provide a simple and efficient way to answer client questions, follow up with clients, and reinforce client education.

Studies suggest that clients are interested in communicating with their healthcare providers via e-mail. One survey found that one third of online health seekers would consider switching healthcare providers if they could communicate with them via e-mail (Kassirer, 2000). Indeed, e-mail is universally used among all age groups and is a very popular form of communication among 90% of Internet users (Fox & Madden, 2005). However, a survey of healthcare consumers revealed that although people in general like to use e-mail, only about 6% actually used e-mail to contact their healthcare provider (Baker, Wagner, Singer, & Bundoff, 2003).

E-mail offers a quick, inexpensive way to communicate with clients. It is very different from the face-to-face interaction typically used by health professionals, but has its own advantages as a form of **asynchronous** communication. This means that the message can be sent at the convenience of the sender and the message will be read when the receiver is online and ready to read it. Messages can be sent and responded to any time, day or night. Such messaging has numerous advantages for both healthcare consumers and professionals.

For clients who identify questions after leaving a healthcare facility, an e-mail message system gives them a chance to get answers from a reliable source familiar with their history. Clients who are not sure how to phrase a question or feel rushed when instructions are being given in a clinical setting have a chance to compose their thoughts at home and prepare an e-mail message. E-mail also provides clients with a venue for asking follow-up questions after a healthcare visit. For example, clients may e-mail their physical therapists with questions after going home and trying to follow instructions for a home strengthening program that they have been given.

Unless there is a mechanism in place for clients to contact the health professional with questions, the client is at risk for making a mistake that may have serious consequences. Simply telling clients to call if they have questions is often inadequate. A call to a busy office or clinic usually results in a call back by the health professional and the client having to wait by the phone for an answer. Even calling hours can be problematic because they imply that the client is free to call at the designated hour.

An e-mail system is also a good alternative to a voice messaging system. For clients who are anxious about asking questions, e-mail allows them all the time they need to gather their thoughts. In addition, clients do not have to remember the answers they are given by the health professional because the e-mail message provides a written recording of the health professional's response.

In contrast, many voice mail systems are time limited. Clients are sometimes cut off in the middle of a voice message if the message is long or if clients are struggling to make themselves understood. Other clients may hesitate to leave a voice mail in the evening or night hours when they know no one is there to respond. However, by virtue of the way e-mail is designed, clients can feel comfortable sending messages at any time.

From the health professional's perspective, an e-mail message system provides a simple way to check on clients to see whether they understood the instructions they were given and to respond to new questions that have arisen. If postteaching follow-up is desired, e-mail offers one way for the health professional to initiate contact after the client has left the healthcare delivery system. The health professional can get in touch with the client via e-mail following a teaching session to convey interest in how he or she is doing with a medication regime, treatment, or other types of instructions given.

For example, the e-mail message could stress important points that were made during a teaching session with a pharmacist, such as, "Remember to take your pill around the same time every day." Also, an e-mail message could be used to assess the client's understanding of what was taught. For example, a social worker might ask, "Do you have insurance coverage or money to pay for your medicine?"

Informational resources also can be shared via e-mail by embedding links to Web sites in the e-mail message. These can be sent out on an as-needed or regular basis. For example, an occupational therapist may elect to send out monthly e-mail reminders to her clients with arthritis about joint protection and energy conservation techniques as well as research updates on pain management and quality-of-life issues.

Any follow-up system such as e-mail takes time and commitment on the part of the organization. Time and resources must be allocated if the system is to work effectively. Client e-mail addresses should be included in the routine information-gathering process for new clients. Because e-mail addresses are likely to change, they need to be updated, just like telephone numbers, whenever a client visits the office, clinic, or other setting within the healthcare delivery system.

Also, the health professional's e-mail address needs to be widely distributed and easy to remember. For example, a mailbox address for a speech-language pathology clinic such as Questions@ SLPClinic.org would be easy to remember because it includes the purpose of the mailbox and the name of the organization. The e-mail address can be easily distributed on appointment cards, written instructions, teaching materials, and other sources of communication with the client.

In addition, a description of the service and instructions for use should be distributed. For example, it may be helpful for clients to know who will be answering their questions, the types of questions that can be submitted, and the typical response time. Also, it is very important that clients understand that an e-mail message system is not intended to replace a visit or phone call when they need to see or talk with a healthcare provider about an immediate problem. These points can be reiterated in an automated reply to each e-mail. For example, the automated message may include: "If this is a medical emergency, please dial 9-1-1 immediately. Thank you for your message. Our goal is to provide you with the best healthcare service possible. We will respond to your message within 48 hours. If you need more immediate assistance, please call our office during business hours. Thank you."

It is a good idea to have more than one person be responsible for responding to e-mail messages so that questions and concerns can be addressed even when a staff member is away because of vacation or other time out of the office. One way to accomplish this goal is to have messages sent to a mailbox rather than to an individual. Another way is to have messages forwarded to a second individual when the primary responder is away from the office. Because more than one person can be given access to an electronic mailbox, continuous coverage can be established. However, if continuous coverage cannot be provided, it is important that clients know how long they can expect to wait to receive answers to their questions.

When sending e-mail messages, it is important for health professionals to remember that electronic communication differs in several ways from face-to-face communication:

- Electronic communication lacks context. Without cues such as facial expressions, tone of voice, and body posture, e-mail messages can appear cold and unfeeling. Although emoticons (symbols like smiley faces used to express emotion) are commonly used by people who send e-mail messages, they may not be appropriate for all professional correspondences. However, a carefully constructed e-mail message can convey the intent of the sender.
- Although electronic communication is convenient, it may take longer in that the sender could wait hours or days before the message is

received and answered. For this reason, it is very important that an e-mail response to a client question be clear and of sufficient detail so that it does not generate more questions that cannot be answered immediately. Furthermore, using e-mail is inappropriate for communicating urgent issues or messages that need to be read or responded to quickly.

- E-mail messages provide a written record. A printed copy can serve as a handy reference for a client and eliminates any question about what information was shared. However, e-mail messages can also serve as documentation of inaccurate or inappropriate information. When responding to a client question, it is vital that the client's record be reviewed and that the response to the question be accurate and carefully thought out. Copies of the e-mail messages sent to clients should be placed in the client's record.
- Finally, it is important to remember that electronic communication can never be assumed to be private. This reminder is especially important in the era of Health Insurance Portability and Accountability Act (HIPAA) regulations. The healthcare provider must take steps to ensure privacy at both the healthcare facility and the client's computer. It is suggested that clients sign a consent form if health-related information is to be shared via e-mail and that they be given instructions for safe use (American Medical Association, 2009).

As physicians and other healthcare providers begin to offer various electronic communication services, such as e-mail and electronic prescription refills, careful planning is necessary to ensure client privacy (Stone, 2007). The American Medical Association has established guidelines for the use of electronic communication with clients that are helpful for health professionals as well. These guidelines are available on the Advocacy Resources section of the AMA Web site at http://www.ama-assn.org/ama/pub/about-ama/our-people/member-

groups-sections/young-physicians-section/
advocacy-resources/guidelines-physician-patient-
electronic-communications.shtml.

Privacy can be ensured at healthcare facilities by requiring a password-protected screen saver at all workstations (American Medical Association, 2009). However, it is important that both health professionals and clients understand that violations of privacy can occur in many ways. For example, clients who send e-mail messages from work may not be aware of the fact that their messages may be stored on servers and hard drives even after they have been deleted. In some cases, the employer may have legal access to this information (Kassirer, 2000). In addition, not all information may be appropriate for an e-mail message. For example, it may not be appropriate to send abnormal test results to a client in electronic form. E-mail messages can also be easily forwarded. Therefore, the health professional should assume that the client may choose to share a response with others.

E-mail communication between health professional and client has tremendous potential to enhance teaching. However, despite the increased use of e-mail among the general population, it is important to remember that not every client has a computer, computer skills, or access to e-mail. A backup system such as voice mail should therefore be made available so that the needs of all clients can be met.

Electronic Discussion Groups

The Internet provides many opportunities for clients and health professionals to participate in electronic discussion groups with other people who share a common interest. In the case of health and healthcare education, common interests can focus on a particular healthcare problem such as cancer, a life circumstance such as death of a spouse, a health interest such as nutrition, or a professional issue such as discipline-specific research.

Although different types of electronic discussion groups are available, all share a common feature—the ability to connect people asynchronously from various locations via computer. People like electronic discussion groups because they are easy to use and are available 24 hours a day. Because electronic discussion involves faceless communication with strangers from all over the world, there is a sense of anonymity even when real names are used. Electronic discussion groups fall into two main categories: those that distribute mail to individual subscribers and those that post messages in a way that makes them accessible to group participants. In the first type of electronic discussion group, messages are sent to the individual. In the second case, the subscriber seeks out the messages that have been posted.

Electronic discussion groups can be structured in many different ways. Some are moderated, whereas others have little or no oversight. Some electronic discussion groups have thousands of subscribers, whereas others are very small closed groups created for specific purposes.

For the health professional, electronic discussion groups can serve a number of purposes. Electronic discussion groups can be used as a vehicle for teaching or as a learning resource to share with clients and other health providers. The health professional who chooses to create an electronic discussion group can use it to reach large or small groups of healthcare consumers or caregivers from within the immediate vicinity or worldwide.

For example, a number of electronic discussion groups have been created and moderated by occupational therapists as a way to promote networking and information sharing among practitioners within a particular specialty area. These groups are open to anyone who is interested and typically have memberships of several hundred people from countries around the world. In comparison, recreational therapists in a hospital or clinic could choose to set up a small private electronic discussion group as a way to facilitate a journal club.

Whether the group is large or small, the asynchronous nature of electronic discussion groups makes it possible for people to communicate with one another despite different time zones and work schedules. And, no matter if the health professional chooses to create an electronic discussion group or uses one already in existence, this form of online communication provides for a creative way to learn and to teach.

Mailing Lists

Automated mailing lists are one of the most common means of setting up an electronic discussion group. With an automated mailing list, people communicate with one another by sharing e-mail messages. The principle by which these groups work is simple. Individuals who have subscribed to the mailing list send their e-mail messages to a designated address, where a software program then copies the message and distributes it to all subscribers. Therefore, when a message is sent to the group, everyone gets to see it.

The most popular of these automated software programs is called "Listserv." In fact, the Listserv program is so commonly used that automated mailing lists are often referred to as "listservs." Other automated programs include Majordomo, Sympa, and Listproc. Although some minor differences exist between these programs, essentially they all work in the same way.

Although mailing lists are owned or managed by an individual, much of the work involved in running the list is automated by the software program used. Subscribers are given two e-mail addresses to use when interacting with the mailing list: one to use when posting messages to the entire group and another to use for administrative issues such as requests to stop mail for a period of time. Both functions—distributing messages and handling routine requests—are automated and handled by the software program rather than by a person. Subscribers must use the correct address and precisely worded commands when attempting to interact with the list because the computer program cannot problem solve.

Upon enrolling, subscribers are sent directions and a list of properly worded commands that should be used when communicating with the software program. New subscribers are encouraged to save the instructions and refer to them as needed. Despite these precautions, new users frequently make mistakes. It is not uncommon to read messages from frustrated subscribers who cannot stop their mail because they are either posting to the wrong address or failing to use the correct command.

Listservs and other automated mailing groups are wonderful tools for the health professional when used as a means for delivering education to large numbers of people or when shared with clients and colleagues as a learning resource. Mailing lists are easy to use once a user understands how the system works. There are also multiple free tutorials available on the Web to help.

With more than 100,000 listservs and mailing lists available, it is possible to find an online group to cover almost any issue. The quality of the messages is usually very high in both health-related and professional mailing lists. Health professionals who choose to create a group rather than to participate in an established one can learn to manage a large or small electronic mailing list without too much difficulty. However, it is helpful for list managers to have either the support of computer professionals in their institution or the knowledge and skill necessary to handle the routine computer issues that arise from time to time.

Listservs or mailing lists can be used effectively as a vehicle for education or information exchange with groups desiring education or information exchange over time. Because mailing lists facilitate group rather than individual communication, they work especially well with groups that are interested in collaborative learning or learning from the experiences of others. Mailing lists designed for professional audiences are good examples. Multiple lists or listservs are available covering everything from, for example, discipline-specific history to evidence-based research to specialty areas of clinical practice. Most lists are quite active, and at any given time, several discussion topics can be addressed by the group. Members post questions, ask advice, and comment on current issues. Relationships between active members are established over time, and group members come to count on others in the group for their counsel.

For these same reasons, listservs and other types of automated mailing lists have become popular as mechanisms for online support for health consumers (Fox & Fallows, 2003; Shaw et al., 2006). With the increased use of computers by the general population, an increasing number of people have turned to their computers to access information and resources that can help them deal with their health issues. As a result, the need for electronic discussion groups devoted to particular health problems was identified and online support groups have been established.

For example, the Association of Cancer On-line Resources (ACOR) has been a major player in the move to bring online support to healthcare consumers. This nonprofit organization devoted to assisting people with cancer has established more than 159 different online support groups since 1996, each devoted to a particular type of cancer or cancer-related problem. Its Web page states that ACOR delivers more than 1.5 million messages per week to its subscribers throughout the world (ACOR, 2009). Memberships in the various groups range from about 25 people in the smaller groups to almost 2,000 individuals in the larger groups.

Other individuals and organizations have established similar online groups covering a wide range of healthcare issues. Sometimes groups are started by individuals who have an interest in a particular topic while others are started by professional or advocacy groups interested in providing service to a particular group of people. In addition to the many public groups that have open enrollments, private groups can be established to meet the needs of a group of people associated with a specific healthcare provider or organization.

Online support groups are particularly relevant to a discussion of technology for education. Han and Belcher (2001) surveyed subscribers of an online support group for parents of children with cancer and found that 76% of participants cited information giving and receiving as the main benefit of the online group. A review of the purposes and goals of several online support groups revealed education and information sharing as the reason for starting and maintaining a group.

The emphasis on information sharing in online support groups is not surprising. Many people join online support groups after they or their loved ones have been diagnosed with a serious illness. They come to the support group not only to receive reassurance and encouragement, but also to gather as much information as possible so that they can begin to make necessary decisions about treatment. By joining an online support group, they are turning to people who know what they are going through and who can give practical advice based on real-life experience. The desire to share the most current information is commonly what brings group members together, and a discussion of new treatments and other discoveries found in the literature is commonplace (Han & Belcher, 2001).

Health professionals may wish to teach their clients about the benefits of online support groups. If an appropriate group is not available, health professionals can start an online support group of their own. Online support groups may be especially helpful to people who find it difficult to leave home because of illness or care responsibilities.

Clients who are unfamiliar with online communication should be reassured that there is no pressure for them to contribute to the discussion and that many people benefit just by reading the comments of others. Clients who are insecure about their ability to express themselves in written format may find it helpful to initially compose their messages using a word processor so that they can take the time to think about what they want to say and use the spelling and grammar check function to edit their remarks. Clients who are unsure whether an online support group will meet their needs should be encouraged to give one a try. There are no costs involved other than the cost of being online, and there are no obligations to continue. Subscribers can withdraw from a group at any time.

Online support groups have some disadvantages that should be shared with clients who are thinking about joining one. Most people who have participated in a listserv or other type of mailing list note that the volume of messages received each day can be problematic (Han & Belcher, 2001). Some lists report an average of 50 or more messages per day.

Experienced users learn to sort messages and delete the unnecessary or irrelevant ones quickly. Others find requesting that messages be sent in digest form (all messages received in a day are combined and sent in one mailing) helps control the volume of e-mails received. In any case, the daily volume of messages initially can be overwhelming and may present a problem for people with low literacy levels or for people for whom English is a second language.

Clients should also be made aware of the fact that most online groups do not have a professional facilitator. Online groups are often run by someone who is interested in the health problem being discussed either because he or she has the condition or has a family member with the healthcare problem. As a consequence, inaccurate information may be shared and problems with group dynamics may not be addressed.

Although this chapter classifies online support groups as part of the category of automated mailing groups, it should be noted that online support groups take many forms. Many groups use the mailing list or listserv format described here. Others use a bulletin board format where messages are posted on a site where they can be reviewed by members of the group. Still others maintain a Web site that provides many avenues for communication, including scheduled and unscheduled chats, bulletin boards, mailing lists, and electronic newsletters. Regardless of the format, online support groups provide a mechanism for meeting the teaching and learning needs of many different client populations.

Other Forms of Online Discussion

Online discussion can take place through many other mechanisms. Although electronic discussion groups and mailing lists are two of the more common approaches to online discussion, others are worthy of mention. When choosing a method for teaching or exchanging information online, it is important to consider all of the options and select the method that is most appropriate for the content to be delivered and the audience to be targeted.

Online forums, message boards, and bulletin boards are systems that provide a way for people to post messages for others to read and respond to. Online forums, message boards, and bulletin boards are found on Web sites that allow users to post directly to the discussion board rather than indirectly via e-mail. Many people may find this system easier to use.

Although most discussion board–type forums require some system of registration, users can often select a user name of their choosing and e-mail addresses are not displayed. This added privacy is a boon to many people who are reluctant to share their names and e-mail addresses with strangers. Online forums, message boards, and bulletin boards for healthcare consumers and health professionals can be found on many health-related sites on the World Wide Web.

Online Chats

Online chats differ from e-mail and the other electronic communication modalities previously discussed in that they provide an opportunity for online conversation to take place in real time. Although chat conversations take the form of text rather than audio, a chat session shares many features with a telephone conference call. In both scenarios, several people from different locations participate in a conversation at the same time. Both allow people to join or leave the session as needed.

Clients and health professionals have many opportunities to engage in online chats related to health issues. A search of the World Wide Web can uncover a vast array of scheduled chats where a particular topic is being discussed at a given time as well as ongoing chats where people are invited to stop in at any time to ask questions or engage in conversation with whomever happens to be in the chat room. In addition to public chat rooms, many organizations sponsor chats for their own clients or staff as a way to offer ongoing educational programs or information exchange among groups.

When leading or facilitating a chat group, it is important to plan ahead. The discussion in a chat room can move quickly, and it is very easy to get so involved in the process of chatting that the content to be covered gets lost or forgotten. Also, without adequate control systems in place, chats can experience a number of communication problems, such as multiple ongoing conversations, lack of focus, and periods of silence. The following suggestions may help to organize a successful chat session:

- E-mail or post the purpose of the chat session in advance. If appropriate, include an agenda, assignments to be completed ahead of time, or other resources that participants will need to prepare for the session.
- Make a list of the discussion points to be covered during the session. The list should be well organized, easy to follow, and placed so that it can be easily seen during the chat. Chat sessions often move so quickly that there is little time for the facilitator to make sense of crumpled or scribbled notes.

- Depending on the topic and the experience of the facilitator, it may be appropriate to limit the number of participants. The larger the group, the more difficult the challenge of running a smooth and productive online chat.
- Sign on to the chat session early and encourage participants to do so as well. You want to be able to handle unexpected problems before the session begins.
- Watch the clock. Time in a busy chat session goes by quickly. If the chat was designed as a question and answer period, it may be helpful to ask people to e-mail important questions ahead of time so that they are not forgotten.
- Help the group to follow the conversation taking place. It is easy for chat discussions to become disjointed or off topic. When responding to a question, refer to the query and the person asking it—for example, "Karen asked about pain management. I think …" If the group is losing focus, bring the participants back to the agenda and the points being discussed.
- Limit the amount of time spent discussing the detailed questions or concerns of any one participant. If someone in the group needs individualized attention, suggest that that person e-mail or call the health professional after the chat has ended.
- If appropriate, ask participants who have not contributed to the discussion whether they have any questions. Some participants choose not to make comments during a chat, which is acceptable. However, there may be others who were not quick enough to get their comments online and who have questions that need to be asked. A statement such as, "Our conversation moved very quickly tonight so I want to give those who haven't had a chance some time to ask their questions" may slow down the conversation long enough for everyone to have an opportunity to contribute.
- Begin to wrap up the session about 10 minutes before the scheduled end time. Announce that

there are 10 minutes left and ask for final questions or comments.

It may also help to prepare participants for the chat experience. Chat sessions can be overwhelming for new users. Health professional educators can share the following guidelines for chat participation with clients or colleagues who will be joining a chat session for the first time:

- Allow enough time before the chat starts to download software if it is needed. First-time users are often required to download software, called a chat client, before beginning. This software is typically offered as freeware or shareware on the Internet and is easy to install.
- Be prepared to choose a user name. Participants in public chats with strangers are often advised not to use their real names so as to protect their privacy.
- Keep comments short and to the point. If a user takes a long time to compose a message, the group may have moved on to an entirely new topic by the time the message gets posted.
- Be prepared for chat lingo in public chat rooms. Abbreviations like BTW (by the way) and emoticons (symbols that represent emotions or facial expressions such as ;) for winking) are commonly used.
- Do not worry about typos and grammar. Chat programs do not have spell checks and not everyone is an experienced typist. People who are frequent chat users learn to overlook spelling errors.

Chat works well as an online communication modality for many people. Clients who are homebound or isolated may benefit from having the opportunity to participate in education programs or to receive answers to their questions without leaving home. Likewise, many health professionals would benefit from being able to access professional education that allows real-time discussion and dialogue.

However, some limitations of chat must be considered. Because chat requires that people be online at the same time, scheduling conflicts and time-zone issues result in less accessibility than asynchronous forms of electronic discussion. Because of the fast pace of most chat discussions, it may be difficult for some clients to keep up with the dialogue. Clients with certain disabilities, clients who are ill, and clients with low literacy levels may find it difficult to participate if the group moves along quickly.

Web Sites

Developing a Web site to share healthcare information is another educational tool for the health professional. Development of a Web site is typically a team effort. In addition to content experts such as health professionals who provide the material to be included on the site, Web designers with technical and layout expertise can provide valuable assistance. There are many resources available to health professionals interested in developing Web sites.

For example the Research Based Web Design and Usability Guidelines Web site (http://www.usability.gov/guidelines) is sponsored by the U.S. Department of Health and Human Services. This resource contains guidelines that can be used in designing health-related Web sites. Not only are the guidelines provided here based on research studies and supporting information from the field, but ratings are also assigned to each guideline according to the strength of the evidence available. For instance, a guideline that is given a rating of 5 is one that is supported by two or more research studies where hypotheses were tested and the guideline was shown to be effective. A score of 0 indicates that although the guideline may be routinely followed on Web pages, there is no evidence to support its effectiveness.

A number of issues must be considered before engaging in health education via a Web site. Web sites have the potential to reach millions of users over an extended period of time. The healthcare consumers who use the Web have varying levels of sophistication. They may or may not know to check the dates on which the Web site was created and modified. Therefore, it is very important that the information on the site be accurate and updated as often as necessary. Depending on the topics covered, it may be necessary to include a disclaimer about the importance of checking with a healthcare provider.

If the site is interactive and the health professional will be responding to questions submitted by users of the site, liability issues must be carefully considered. Health professionals who respond to questions from Web users are providing advice and guidance to people they do not see and cannot assess. Depending on the nature of the site, it may be advisable to include an attorney on the team to provide advice when needed (Hern, Weitkamp, Haag, Trigg, & Gaard, 1997). It is important to determine whether there are relevant legal issues related to practice inherent in the activities of the health professional on the Web site.

Although new technology has opened the door to many new and exciting opportunities, it has also raised many questions about telepractice and licensure. Because technology makes it so much easier than ever before to provide healthcare services to clients across state lines, the provision of nursing, medical, and other types of technology-facilitated healthcare services to clients at a distance has been placed in the spotlight. Multistate licensure and other types of legislation have and will continue to be proposed, and new practice guidelines are likely to be enacted.

Finally, the time commitment required to respond to questions from Web users cannot be underestimated. The health professional educators who respond to questions on NetWellness estimate a time commitment of 20–40 minutes for research and response to each question (Hern et al., 1997). They also suggest that it is important that daily coverage for an interactive Web site be maintained.

Healthcare consumers will use the site 24 hours a day, 7 days a week. Therefore, if the site offers interactive features such as Ask an Expert, it is important that questions be answered on a regular basis so that service is not interrupted for long periods of time.

Blogs

One of the newest forms of online communication is **blogs**. First developed in the late 1990s, blogs, or Web logs, are an increasingly popular mechanism for individuals to share information and/or experiences about a given topic. Although sometimes referred to as Web diaries, blogs are much more than that and include images, media objects, and links that allow for public responses (Maag, 2005). Blog entries are viewed in chronological order and are easy to follow.

The number of blogs available on the Web has increased dramatically in recent years. A report of the Pew Internet and American Life Project (Lenhart & Fox, 2006) states that about 12 million Americans have created a blog and another 57 million read blogs on the World Wide Web. Users can find blogs on any given topic using the search engine technorati.com, where more than 71 million blogs are tracked and rated.

Many of the blogs found on the Web are health related and often tell the story of the creator's experience with a given disease or treatment. For example, a search on technorati.com for blogs on breast cancer revealed more than 500 individual breast cancer–related blogs. These blogs covered everything from the stories of cancer survivors and family experiences to information-based blogs describing various breast cancer treatments. Many blog creators provided a picture with a limited or absent biography.

Given the growing popularity of blogs, it is reasonable to assume that healthcare consumers, particularly young people, will turn to blogs for health-related information and support. The Pew Internet and American Life Project Report on

Blogging (Lenhart & Fox, 2006) notes that bloggers tend to be young men and women under the age of 30 who use a pseudonym rather than their own name. Most are heavy Internet users. Although some blogs are written by health professionals, most are created by healthcare consumers who have a story to tell. Therefore, it is important to warn clients who are getting information from blogs of the importance of evaluating the content.

Wikis

Another new form of online communication is a wiki. In comparison to blogs, wikis are more social in their construction. That is, multiple users come together on a wiki to collaboratively write the content of a collection of Web pages (Wikipedia, 2009c). This collection is easily expanded, and all users have the ability to add to, edit, and remove content. Wikipedia (www.wikipedia.org) is one of the best-known wikis.

Wikis are asynchronous, allowing users to work collaboratively but not necessarily simultaneously. This allows the authors to contribute to the Web pages at their individual convenience. Wikis also have the capacity for multimedia content such as text, videos, audio, and photographs (Erardi & Hartmann, 2008) making them a potentially exciting and engaging source of information.

Health-related wikis such as WikiMD (www .wikimd.org) are promising tools for consumer education (Boulos, Maramba, & Wheeler, 2006; Boulos & Wheeler, 2007). Health practitioners can contribute to or create wikis to disseminate healthcare information and evidence. This communication tool can be open to the general public or accessible to a select group. In the open version of a wiki, anyone can access the information posted to the Web pages. A closed wiki can be used for a specific community to develop a certain resource. For example, an occupational therapy professor may set up a wiki for her online students to develop a resource manual related to

building evidence-based practice in an occupational therapy clinic.

Social Networking Services

Another example of a social communication tool is a social networking service. Usually Web-based, these services work to connect users with similar interests (Boulos & Wheeler, 2007; Wikipedia, 2009b). These networks have the potential to connect individuals with similar health concerns or interests, including health consumers, practitioners, educators, and researchers. This may be another venue, like an electronic discussion group, listserv, or wiki, to build a virtual community to discuss, educate, and/or provide support for health issues.

Webcasts and Webinars

Webcasts, or live broadcasts over the Internet, permit audio and/or video to be transmitted to participants in multiple locations. Webcasts provide a unique mechanism for delivering presentations to users around the globe. Although webcasts do not allow any type of interaction, they are growing in popularity as a training device for sharing lectures and demonstrations. Podcasts are audio-only webcasts, and vodcasts are video-based webcasts (Erardi & Hartmann, 2008).

Webinars, or Web conferencing, are similar to webcasts in that they are Internet-based programs; however, webinars do allow for interaction. Webinars often have two components: a computer-based display, such as a PowerPoint presentation or whiteboard, and a live discussion. Participants typically can join a Web-based conference via telephone or computer.

Mobile Learning

Mobile learning, or **m-learning**, is another new strategy that takes advantage of the many "wireless, mobile, portable and handheld devices" (Traxler, 2007, Introduction, para. 1) that have been developed and widely marketed in recent years (Maag, 2006; Peters, 2007). The word *mobile* refers both to the use of portable technologies such as MP3 players and to the end user, the mobile adult, who can truly learn anytime, anyplace. Mobile devices can be used for a wide range of activities including accessing course materials, searching the Web, listening to lectures or podcasts, recording experiences and assignments, and participating in learning-focused games (Peters, 2007).

Although m-learning has great potential, its use is limited at the present time. Cost is a major factor because portable devices are often expensive. However, the popularity of MP3 players, smart phones, and other portable devices, especially among the young, indicates great promise for future use.

Issues Related to the Use of Technology

Despite the power of computer and Internet technology to enhance learning, the use of these technologies in healthcare education presents some unique challenges. Think for a moment about the many ways in which healthcare education differs from more traditional classroom education. The characteristics of the educational medium, the learners, the setting, and the access to hardware, software, and technological support are all likely to be different. In addition, there are issues related to the information technology itself. These include considerations about the accuracy of online content and the accessibility of electronic resources.

Whereas traditional classroom education is likely to take place in a structured setting, healthcare education takes place in a wide range of settings, many of which are unstructured. Students who are part of an educational system are likely to have some access to the hardware, software, and technological support necessary for facilitating technology-based learning. By comparison, access to resources and support varies considerably among

healthcare consumers and in healthcare organizations. Students in a classroom also often share many common characteristics related to age and ability, whereas clients in healthcare education programs may cover a wide range of ages, abilities, and limitations. As educators, health professionals must be aware of the special issues involved in the use of computer and Internet technology in healthcare education and be prepared to make accommodations as needed.

Despite the rapid growth of technology-based education programs and services, it is important to remember that electronic delivery of health information is still in its infancy. There remain many issues that need to be resolved. One major area of concern is the limited oversight and control over the content that is posted on the Internet and World Wide Web, two of the major vehicles for delivering information to a global audience.

Many people believe that the lack of censorship on the World Wide Web is a freedom of speech issue. However, health professionals are concerned that consumers are making serious healthcare decisions based on information on the Web that has not been reviewed for accuracy, currency, or bias. According to a Pew study (Fox, 2006), 75% of the 85 million Americans who retrieve health-related information from the Web sometimes, hardly ever, or never check the source or date of the information they are retrieving.

Healthcare education and informatics professionals are working together to develop codes to guide practice and safeguard healthcare consumers who use the educational information and services that are delivered via the World Wide Web and the Internet. For example, the Internet Healthcare Coalition (http://www.ihealthcoalition.org), a not-for-profit group, was founded in 1997 for the purpose of identifying and promoting quality educational resources on the Internet. One of the organization's most significant accomplishments was the establishment of the e-Health Code of Ethics, displayed in six languages on its Web site.

The purpose of this code is to ensure confident and informed use of the health-related information found on the Web. The e-Health Code of Ethics is based upon the principles of candor, honesty, quality, informed consent, privacy, professionalism, responsible partnering, and accountability that are described in more detail in **Table 13–1**.

One of the most widely publicized issues related to the use of computers and Internet technology is that of the **digital divide**, or the gap between those individuals who have access to information technology resources and those who do not. According to a Pew Foundation report, one in five Americans is disconnected; that is, they not only have no Internet access in their homes, they report never having been on the Internet (Fox, 2005).

Studies conducted by the Pew Foundation have found that the factors determining the likelihood

---

Table 13-1 Guiding Principles of the E-Health Code of Ethics

CANDOR

- Disclose information about the creators/purpose of the site that will help users make a judgment about the credibility and trustworthiness of the information or services provided.

HONESTY

- Be truthful in describing products/services and present information in a way that is not likely to mislead the user.

QUALITY

- Take the necessary steps to ensure that the information provided is accurate and well supported and that the services provided are of the highest quality.
- Present information in a manner that is easy for users to understand and use.
- Provide background information about the sources of the information provided and the review process used to assist the user in making a decision about the quality of the information provided.

INFORMED CONSENT

- Inform users if personal information is collected and allow them to choose whether the information can be used or shared.

PRIVACY

- Take steps to ensure that the user's right to privacy is protected.

PROFESSIONALISM IN ONLINE HEALTH CARE

- Abide by the ethical code of your profession (e.g., nursing, medicine, physical therapy, social work).
- Provide users with information about who you are, what your credentials are, what you can do online, and what limitations may be present in the online interaction.

RESPONSIBLE PARTNERING

- Take steps to ensure that sponsors, partners, and others who work with you are trustworthy.

ACCOUNTABILITY

- Implement a procedure for collecting, reviewing, and responding to user feedback.
- Develop and share procedures for self-monitoring compliance with the e-Health Code of Ethics.

Source: Adapted from Rippen, H., & Risk, A. e-Health Code of Ethics (May 24), *J Med Internet Res* 2000;2(2):e9, http://www.jmir.org/2000/2/e9/. Accessed April 19, 2010.

that someone will have access to information technology resources are age, income, race or ethnic origin, level of education, and ability (Fox, 2005). These studies revealed that those at risk for limited access included people older than 65, those with household incomes of less than $35,000, African Americans and people of Hispanic descent, adults who did not complete high school, and people with disabilities. In addition, households without children are also not likely to have Internet access.

As a result of the digital divide, many healthcare consumers do not have the resources necessary to gain entry to computer and Internet-based health education programs. Thus, although technology can increase access to healthcare education for some people, educators must be aware that some segments of the population will be denied access if attempts are not made to promote digital inclusion. The first step in promoting digital inclusion is recognizing those groups who are at risk for limited access.

A Pew Foundation study found that although more than half of Americans between the ages of 60 and 69 have Internet access, access to the Internet and online activity diminish with age. As little as 22% of adults older than the age of 70 go online (Fox, 2006). There are many explanations for these statistics. Older adults are more likely to be retired without employer access to a computer, are less likely to have children in the home who typically bring an enthusiasm and knowledge of computers with them, may have less disposable income to purchase computer hardware and software, and never grew up using this technology.

Despite the statistics, it would be a mistake to discount computer-delivered education as a possibility for the older adult population. Research studies have shown that with education and support, older adults enjoy using and learning from computer-based programs (Evangelista et al., 2006; Nahm, Preece, Resnick, & Mills, 2004). Although many older adults have only limited incomes, numerous government and private initiatives are available to provide free or low-cost computer and

Internet access for this population. Whereas some older adults have physiologic and neurologic problems that make computer use difficult, many other older adults enjoy good health and functionality.

Health and healthcare education are important to older adults, and computer- and Internet-based technology holds much promise for this segment of the population. Therefore, it is important that the health professional be prepared to support computer-based learning among older clients. The following interventions may be helpful in encouraging older adults to engage in computer-based learning activities:

- Reinforce principles of ergonomics by making suggestions about equipment and posture that will minimize physical problems related to computer use. Ergonomics is important for everyone but is especially important for older adults who may have visual problems as well as arthritic changes in the neck, hands, and spine. Proper posture, correct positioning of the keyboard and monitor, adjusted screen colors and font size, a supportive chair, and a reminder to get up and walk around three to four times per hour can help older adults to avoid discouraging physical symptoms that may interfere with computer use.

- Identify resources that will provide computer access and support in the older adult's home community. Supply older adults with a comprehensive resource list containing places where free computer and Internet access is available, places where computer training is provided for them, and contact people who will assist if problems are encountered. In addition to public libraries and community centers, numerous projects nationwide are committed to digital inclusion for all segments of the population, including the older adult population.

- Motivate older adults to use a computer by helping them to identify how the computer can meet their needs. It is important to talk to older adults about their needs and abilities. Find out how they like to learn, what kinds of things they enjoy doing, and what their healthcare needs are. Matching a computer program or Web site to the individual's unique circumstances can encourage computer use. For example, an older adult who is caring for a spouse with cancer might appreciate an online support group if he or she enjoys interacting with and learning from the experiences of others. In this way, health professionals can help to generate interest in learning how to use a computer for health education by starting at a place that piques the older adult's interest.

• Create a supportive and nonthreatening environment to teach older adults about using a computer for health education. Today's older adults did not grow up with computers and may not have confidence in their ability to learn this new skill at this point in their lives. The language of computers may seem foreign to them, so teachers should avoid jargon and define new terms. Teachers should pace their teaching according to the older adult learners' responses. Teachers may need to proceed slowly at first and provide opportunities for practice and for reinforcement of skills. Written computer instructions should be reviewed before the teaching session ends so that the older adult clients do not go home with unanswered questions.

Computers can open up a whole new avenue of support and information to older adults who are struggling with their own health problems and those of their partners. Older adults who enjoy good health can find resources to help them maintain their health and to become educated healthcare consumers. It is important that older adults be given the same opportunities to take advantage of the Information Age resources that are available to younger clients. The health professional can play a key role in promoting digital inclusion among this segment of the population.

People with disabilities make up another special population that may require additional planning before using technologies in health and healthcare education. Not only are people with disabilities less likely to have computer and Internet access than are members of the general population, but they may also have difficulty using hardware and software. The ability to use a computer without adaptive devices requires the fine motor coordination and mobility necessary to use a mouse and keyboard, the strength to sit and hold the head in an upright position, and the ability to comprehend information presented on the computer screen.

For example, individuals with visual impairments may have difficulty seeing text or graphics on a computer screen or performing tasks on the computer that require hand–eye coordination. When identifying obstacles related to visual impairments, it is important to think broadly and address the wide range of conditions that affect the way people see. Color blindness, which affects approximately 8% of all males and 0.5% of females, can cause significant problems for computer users if the Web site or software used does not display the correct color combinations, if the contrast between background and foreground is inadequate, and if color rather than text is used to convey directions.

Although hearing impairments cause fewer problems for computer users than do visual impairments, some accessibility issues nevertheless need to be addressed. An individual with a hearing problem may not be able to hear the sounds that are often used as prompts when a wrong key is struck or when an e-mail message is delivered. Accessibility for individuals with hearing impairments is becoming a bigger issue now that it is easier to send audio signals across the Web and audio messages are becoming more commonplace.

Despite the protections offered by the Americans With Disabilities Act and other federal legislation, accessibility issues on the Web and constraints with hardware and software still exist. Federal legislation outlined in Section 508 of the Workforce Investment Act requires government agencies and institutions receiving government funding to make their Web sites accessible to people with disabilities. However, many Web sites and programs do not fall under this umbrella of protection. Chapter 9 describes potential barriers and specific adaptations that can be employed to assist people who have disabilities to use computers.

Health professionals who use the Internet and the World Wide Web to teach also need to consider Web site design when creating or selecting Web sites that might be used by learners who have disabilities. The World Wide Web contains multiple resources that can be used by Web designers or Web users to learn design principles for accessibility. For example, inserting the search command "color blindness" on a search engine produces Web sites that explain color blindness, illustrate how various types of color blindness affect what might be seen on a Web site, describe good Web design principles for promoting accessibility, and provide tools that can be used to select color combinations that will not create barriers for individuals with color blindness.

Several resources are available to assist Web developers in creating Web sites that meet the needs of people with disabilities. The Web Accessibility Initiative Web site (http://www.w3.org/wai) provides guidelines that are recognized by many as the international standard for accessibility. Another Web site of note is a site created by the Center for Applied Special Technology (CAST). CAST provides a program called "Bobby" to assist Web page authors to identify and correct problems that could make their sites inaccessible to individuals with disabilities. Information on Bobby can be found at the CAST Web site (http://www.cast.org).

Age, disabilities, and other factors that place an individual within the digital divide are also factors that can isolate and diminish access to healthcare resources. Therefore, every effort should be made

to help these individuals connect to the wealth of resources that is and can be made available through technology. The health professional can play a vital role in providing the support, education, and advocacy needed to reduce the barriers that still exist for these special groups of people.

Healthcare Consumer Education and the World Wide Web

In years past, healthcare consumers were not encouraged to research health topics or to research options, but rather to rely on their healthcare providers for information. There were fears that clients would not understand the information they found or that they would find information they would not be able to handle. Today, health professionals have more confidence in consumers' ability to manage their own health care.

More and more health professionals are empowering their clients by teaching and encouraging them to take advantage of the resources at their disposal. Health professionals are using a variety of means to expose their clients to the resources on the Web. For example, computers are being placed in waiting rooms set to appropriate Web sites. Also, teaching materials on how to use the Web are being distributed and Web sites are being created for client use. Given concerns about the quality of information available on the Web, some professionals are working together to create trusted Web sites that provide information and resources for specific client populations (Lewis, Gundwardena, & Saadawi, 2005).

There are many reasons why teaching clients where to go on the Web to find information is good practice. Web-based information can be obtained quickly, and the cost of Internet access in the home is minimal, and it is free in libraries and other community service organizations. Many healthcare consumers would benefit from having their questions answered quickly and inexpensively.

For example, families with young children are likely to have frequent questions related to childhood illnesses, growth and development, and behavior problems, and they may not have the time or money to make multiple visits to the pediatrician. Older adults may have questions about the healthcare problems they encounter with aging but may have difficulty getting to a healthcare provider because of transportation and financial issues. People with chronic illness may gain some sense of control over their lives when they are able to access information on the Web about their conditions. Healthy people may have many questions but few opportunities to talk with a health provider to get answers. For those with interest in and access to the Internet, it is important to educate clients about what online resources they can use to research and manage their own health.

Before consumer education of online health resources begins, however, a preteaching assessment must begin with questions about computer use. Despite the widespread use of computers in our society, not everyone has access to a computer or has interest in using a computer. As stated previously, adults older than the age of 65, African Americans, individuals who have less than a high school education, and individuals living in a home without children are less likely to be online than are others (Fox, 2005). Therefore, it is important to determine whether a client has a computer in his or her home, has access to the Internet, is knowledgeable about using a computer, and has interest in using a computer to obtain information and resources regarding his or her health care.

If a client does not have a computer but has interest in using one to access resources on the Web, places where he or she may access a computer should be discussed. Libraries, senior centers, and community centers commonly have computers with Internet access for public use and typically offer instruction and assistance for new users.

Clients who use computers should be asked about their use of the Web. A Pew Foundation study revealed that Web users in the United States found information on the Web that did one of the following:

1. Influenced their decisions about how to treat an illness
2. Led them to ask questions
3. Led them to seek a second medical opinion
4. Affected their decision about whether to seek the assistance of a healthcare provider (Fox, 2006)

Because the Web can be so influential, it is important to determine that the information a client has found is accurate, complete, and fully understood. Only 15% of Web users report that they always check the source and date of the information found, and many report feeling overwhelmed, confused, or frightened by the information presented (Fox, 2006).

These findings are not surprising. The World Wide Web contains information designed for both professional and consumer audiences. Healthcare consumers may not have the background necessary to comprehend professional literature and other types of information designed for health professionals. When healthcare consumers do a search on a topic, they access Web sites designed for them as well as for health professionals. Consumers should not be discouraged from accessing these sites, but health professional educators must help clients find information written for them at their level of readability and comprehension.

The Web also contains information that may be biased, inaccurate, or misleading (Lewis et al., 2005). Many of the health-related Web sites are sponsored by commercial enterprises trying to sell a product. Others contain information posted by nonprofessionals and may be opinion rather than fact based. Because the Web has the potential to change so quickly, it is difficult to regulate. Even Web pages sponsored by physicians, other health professionals, and university medical centers may contain errors or information that is misleading or difficult to decipher.

Clients may find that the Web has provided too much information, information they are not ready to handle, or information they do not fully understand. For example, a client newly diagnosed with a serious illness may be overwhelmed with the detailed information found on the Web regarding the course of the disease, prognosis, and treatment. Therefore, it is important to ask clients if they are using the Web to find health-related information and to explore the types of information they have found.

Clients may or may not initially feel comfortable talking about information they have gathered. They may fear health professionals will interpret their research as a lack of trust in the care they receive. Some may be embarrassed to talk about information they do not fully understand. Others may be anxious about how to bring up information that conflicts with what they have been told or how they are being treated.

For these reasons, it is important for health professionals to establish early in their relationships with clients that they are interested in talking with them about the information they have gathered from the Web or other resources they have available to them. Clients need to feel that health professionals are open to discussing whatever information they find. They need to understand that health professionals are partners in seeking the best information available.

For clients who are being treated for a condition over an extended period of time, it is also important to continue the conversation about their Web searches throughout their treatment. Simply asking, "Have you found any interesting information on the Web lately?" can keep the dialogue open and provide the health professional as educator

with the opportunity to respond to whatever questions or concerns clients may have.

When engaging in online education with a client, it is advantageous to conduct the teaching session in a place where there is computer access. Having a computer available during a teaching session can accomplish several goals. First, it provides the health professional educator with the opportunity to review Web-based information with the client. Not only can the health professional introduce Web sites that are relevant to the client's needs, but the health professional can also review some of the sites the client has been using.

By reviewing the Web sites clients have been visiting, health professional educators can begin to determine the type and amount of information to which clients have been exposed, assess the client's knowledge, and identify areas in which clients may have need for further teaching. Health professionals in their role as educators may also find information that needs further discussion. For example, a client may have visited a Web site that provides distressing information about side effects of treatment, prognosis, or disease progression. Looking at the site together gives the health professional and client the stimulus to talk about what the client has discovered and do additional teaching–learning, if needed.

Another important advantage of reviewing Web sites with a client is that it provides a chance to teach clients information literacy skills. There are many definitions of information literacy. Most agree that individuals who are information literate have the following four competencies:

1. The ability to identify the information they need
2. The skills to access the information they need
3. Knowledge of how to evaluate the information they find
4. The ability to use the information they deem valid

Therefore, if clients are going to make use of the vast array of information on the Web, they must be able to identify the questions they need answered, find the information they are looking for, judge whether the information they find is trustworthy, and decide how they will use the information to meet their needs.

Information literacy is different from **computer literacy**. A client who is information literate knows how to find the information needed and can evaluate the information found for accuracy, currency, and bias. A client who is computer literate has the technical skills and knowledge of computers necessary to use contemporary hardware and software and can adapt to new technologies that emerge (Williams, 2003).

Although healthcare consumers may not have the background knowledge to evaluate information to the same extent as a professional, they can be taught some simple steps to develop their information literacy skills and to help them begin to identify which Web sites are useful and which are problematic. These steps include the following:

1. *Reducing a problem or topic to a searchable command that can be used with a search engine or search directory.* If clients do not know how to narrow their topics or problems to a few words, they will be unable to find the information they desire or may be unable to broaden a search to find comprehensive coverage. Once the search command is identified, using a search engine or search directory is easy, especially if the help function available at most sites is used to solve problems.

2. *Categorizing Web pages according to their purpose.* A client should be taught to look for the person or organization responsible for the Web site and then place the Web site into a category reflective of its purpose. For example, the purpose of a site created by a drug manufacturer could be categorized as marketing, sales, or promotion. Other categories could include, but are not limited to, advocacy, promotion, informational/news, personal, or instructional/tutorial.

3. *Identifying sources of potential bias that may influence the content or the manner in which the content is presented.* For example, an advocacy Web site is likely to present information that favors one side of a debate. A marketing or sales site tends to include information that is supportive of a particular product or service.

4. *Making a judgment as to the likelihood that the information found on the Web page is accurate and reliable.* Clients can be taught to look for the credentials of authors of reports or articles found on the Web. This helps them to determine whether supportive data are provided and to look at more than one site to see if they can find similar claims or suggestions. Some of the more reliable health-related Web sites have links to other sites, such that the original site is not the sole source of information on a particular topic. Likewise, sites maintained by government agencies or educational institutions (sites that end in .gov or .edu) tend to be reliable and contain valid information.

5. *Making a decision as to the completeness or comprehensiveness of the information presented.* Because clients may not have the background knowledge needed to quickly recognize when information is missing, they should be encouraged to look at more than one site when researching an area of interest. If the health professional educator knows that clients are using the Web to investigate a particular topic, they can help them to identify a list of things they should look for in articles or Web pages addressing the topic.

6. *Determining the currency of the information on a Web page.* Consumers need to know the importance of looking for a creation or modification date or other signs that the information on a Web site is up-to-date.

7. *Identifying resources to answer questions or verify assumptions made about the content of a Web page.* If questions arise, healthcare consumers

should be encouraged to check out information with their health provider. If the provider does not have the answers or cannot verify assumptions made, he or she can refer the client to other health professionals.

In the role of educator, the health professional ultimately can teach clients who already access the Web to use it more effectively and can proactively encourage others to give it a try. It may be helpful to compile lists of Web sites appropriate to the needs of different client populations. **Table 13–2** provides examples of the various types of Web sites that are available for consumer use. As illustrated in Table 13–2, a variety of types of Web sites exist, from general sites covering a broad range of topics to sites with a specific focus or theme.

In selecting Web sites to share with clients, it is important that the health professional review them carefully. In recent years, multiple rating scales have been developed to assist in the evaluation of such sites. Most scales include criteria that address the accuracy of the content, design, and aesthetics of the site; disclosure of the authors; sponsors of the site; currency of information; authority of the source; ease of use; and accessibility and availability of the site.

Table 13–3 summarizes the questions that should be asked in evaluating a health-related Web site. Resource lists made up of quality sites not only serve as references for clients but also provide examples of the types of sites they should be accessing.

Finally, health professionals can create Web sites to bring their healthcare messages to Web users around the world. Table 13–2 provides two examples of Web sites that exemplify the types of roles health professionals can play to bring health information to various consumers via the World Wide Web.

For example, Band-Aides and Blackboards is a creative site designed by nurse faculty to facilitate understanding of the problems faced by children growing up with healthcare problems. This site is thought provoking rather than factual. The health professionals who created it use the words and drawings of children and parents to bring a real-life perspective to the thoughts, feelings, and experiences of growing up with illness. Band-Aides and Blackboards teaches important messages about not being alone, about ways to solve common problems, and about what really matters to this population.

NetWellness, another site in which health professionals play a predominant role, is a very different site from Band-Aides and Blackboards. NetWellness is an "electronic consumer health information service developed by the University of Cincinnati Medical Center and more than 35 community partners" (Hern et al., 1997, p. 316). Developed a number of years ago, NetWellness continues to be a wonderful Web resource for healthcare consumers. Nursing faculty at the University of Cincinnati, Ohio State University, and Case Western University assist in maintaining this site by responding to health consumer questions on the site's Ask the Expert feature and by providing information for the section of the site devoted to hot topics.

Professional Education and the World Wide Web

From work-site training to higher education, technology is making professional education more accessible and more meaningful for health professionals. It is no longer necessary for health professionals to quit working or to relocate to earn a higher degree. Technology has contributed to the growth of distance education programs at all degree levels. Likewise, technology is making it possible for health professionals in the workplace to engage in a variety of continuing education activities designed to keep their practice current, to provide career mobility, and to enhance professional development.

The World Wide Web provides a myriad of resources for health professionals to use in practice and in professional education and development. Web sites provide access to bibliographic

Table 13-2 Sample Web Sites for Healthcare Consumers

Title	URL	Sponsor/Author	Description
Medline Plus	http://www.nlm.nih.gov/medlineplus	National Library of Medicine	Example of a government site that provides access to extensive information about specific diseases/conditions, links to consumer health information from the NIH, dictionaries, lists of hospitals and physicians, health information in Spanish and other languages, and clinical trials. There is no advertising on this site.
Aplastic Anemia and MDS International Foundation, Inc.	http://www.aplastic.org	Aplastic Anemia and MDS International Foundation, Inc.	Example of a disease-specific Web site that provides a range of services, including free educational materials and access to a help line where consumer questions will be researched and answered.
MayoClinic.com	http://www.mayohealth.org	Mayo Clinic	Example of a comprehensive hospital site that provides information as well as a variety of interactive tools to help healthcare consumers manage a healthy lifestyle, research disease conditions, and make healthcare decisions. Advertisement helps support this site.
Cancer Net	http://www.nci.nih.gov	National Cancer Institute	Example of a government site devoted to all aspects of cancer. Provides both professional and consumer-oriented information and resources.
Band-Aides and Blackboards	http://www.lehman.cuny.edu/faculty/jfleitas/bandaides/sitemap.html	Nursing faculty at Lehman College	Site provides personal rather than factual information about growing up with health problems from the perspectives of kids, teens, and adults.
NetWellness	http://www.netwellness.org	University of Cincinnati, Ohio State University, and Case Western Reserve University	Non-profit consumer health Web site that provides high-quality information created and evaluated by medical and health professional faculty at several universities.

Table 13-3 CRITERIA FOR EVALUATING HEALTH-RELATED WEB SITES

ACCURACY

- Are supportive data provided?
- Are the supportive data current and from reputable sources?
- Can you find the same information on other Web sites?
- Is the information provided comprehensive?
- Is more than one point of view presented?

DESIGN

- Is the Web site easy to navigate?
- Is the site Bobby Approved?
- Is there evidence that care was taken in creating the site? Do the links work? Are there typos?
- Is the information presented in a manner that is appropriate for the intended audience?
- Do the graphics serve a purpose other than decoration?

AUTHORS/SPONSORS

- Are the sponsors/authors of the site clearly identified?
- Do the authors provide their credentials?
- Do the authors/sponsors provide a way to contact them or give feedback?
- Do the authors/sponsors clearly identify the purpose of the site?
- Is there reason for the sponsors/authors to be biased about the topic?

CURRENCY

- Is there a recent creation or modification date identified?
- Is there evidence of currency (e.g., updated bibliography reference to current events)?

AUTHORITY

- Are the sponsors/authors credible (e.g., is it a government, educational institution, or healthcare organization site versus a personal page)?
- Are the author's credentials appropriate to the purpose of the site?

---

databases, continuing education, online journals, and resources for client teaching and professional practice. Sites established by health professional organizations and publishing companies serve as resource centers where health professionals can find a wide range of information and services addressing any number of educational needs.

Many of the informational sites on the World Wide Web provide both consumer and professional education. Some Web sites provide links on the home page directing users to either consumer or health professional resources. Other sites do not attempt to discriminate and allow users to decide whether consumer material or professional literature is more appropriate to their needs.

It is impossible to list all of the educational opportunities for professionals on the World Wide Web. The Web is constantly changing, with new sites being added and others being removed on a daily basis. **Table 13–4** provides examples of the various types of Web sites that can be used by a variety of health professionals.

Table 13-4 SAMPLE WEB SITES FOR HEALTHCARE PROFESSIONALS

Title	URL	Sponsor/Author	Description
Medline	http://www.nlm.nih.gov/pubs/factsheets/medline.html	National Library of Medicine	Example of a government site providing access to a bibliographic database containing more than 15 million references to journal articles in the life sciences.
SchoolNurse.com	http://www.schoolnurse.com	School Nurse Alert	Example of a site devoted to a specialty area of nursing practice.
National Institutes of Health	http://www.nih.gov	U.S. Department of Health and Human Services	Example of a government sponsored site with information as well as links to a broad range of health and professional issues.
AllNursing Schools.com	http://www.allnursingschools.com	All Star Directory, Inc.	An example of a resource database listing the nursing programs offered by subscribing colleges and universities.

E-Learning

Technology has had such an impact on workforce training that it has given birth to a new industry and a new set of buzzwords that define an Information Age approach to staff education. Professional development and training organizations have capitalized on the power of computer technology to provide businesses with learning solutions referred to as **e-learning**, an abbreviation for electronic learning. Even though the term *e-learning* can be applied to any learning that is delivered via technology, it is most commonly used to describe professional development and training programs. Higher education typically uses the phrase **distance learning** to describe academic programs delivered via computers.

The emphasis on e-learning in industry is on outcomes, with the goal of providing an individual with the information or practice opportunities required to perform a task or solve a problem at the point of need. E-learning has the potential to deliver training programs that are cost effective, promote positive client outcomes, and lead to staff satisfaction. The nature of the work of health care makes workforce training a critical issue, and e-learning appears to have provided a solution to the problem of keeping staff current in a world where new treatments and new techniques are always on the horizon.

What is the e-learning approach to workforce training in health care? First and foremost, e-learning provides learning opportunities at the point of need. In health care, this statement means that training is available 24 hours a day, 7 days a week. Because the point of need in health care is often related to client care, e-learning must be structured in a way that it can be delivered on a clinical unit. Point-of-need training must also be efficient. In this era of health professional shortages and increasing complexity of care, such training must be provided in a way that fits into the schedules of busy healthcare workers. Finally, e-learning in health care must be distributed so that it can be made available to people across any number of environments and situations. Many healthcare organizations have staff in a wide range of settings and locations. A centralized approach to training will not work well if it means that people have to travel to the staff education office for all training programs.

Multiple approaches to e-learning in health care are possible. Although early e-learning training programs took the form of computer-based modules, new technologies are emerging. Some of these technologies allow training to take place in real time. These include webcasts, Web conferencing, and mobile learning (m-learning). Examples of some of the features of e-learning products that have proved attractive to healthcare organizations are as follows:

- E-learning training modules can be delivered via the World Wide Web. Web-based products are attractive because they are easily accessed in a variety of environments and situations. A computer workstation can easily fit into a clinical unit, and laptops can be carried into the field.
- E-learning can be delivered in small modules that can be completed in as little as 15 minutes. Many healthcare workers are unable to leave their work area for long periods of time. However, most can find 15–30 minutes in a given day, particularly if they do not have to leave the unit. Time permitting, staff can complete several modules in one sitting.
- E-learning programs can be customized at a variety of levels: the organization, the staff position, and the individual. Customization personalizes the program and helps to make it relevant to the individual and to the organization.
- E-learning programs can track completion and create a performance report for individual staff members.
- E-learning modules are interactive and reality based. For example, a client simulation that allows the participant to manage the care of a virtual client can be created.

Staff training programs to improve or maintain quality and safety of care and competence of professionals are important to the individual staff members, to the organization, and to the clients served. Therefore, every staff member has a responsibility to do what he or she can to ensure the success of the program. In addition to completing staff continuing education through e-learning, health professionals have many potential roles in the development and implementation of e-learning programs within an institution. As content experts, they may be hired by e-learning companies to create products designed to meet the needs of practicing health professionals. Health professionals within a healthcare organization may be in a position to work with the e-learning company by customizing the training package purchased and developing a plan for its implementation. Those who use the e-learning system can contribute to the program by completing the modules offered and submitting carefully thought-out evaluations of the products used.

Distance Education

As a result of technological advances, distance education for health professionals is flourishing in the 21st century (Billings, 2007). The term *distance learning* means different things to different people. Online courses, correspondence courses, independent study, and videoconferencing are just a few of the techniques that can be used to deliver education to students studying at a distance. The diversity of distance education programs in the United States reflects the myriad approaches that can be used to meet the needs of students who are separated from the traditional classroom setting. In all cases, distance education means that the teacher and the learner are separated from one another (American Association of Colleges of Nursing Task Force on Distance Technology and Nursing Education, 1999).

A variety of strategies is used to provide courses to students who are not in the same location as the teacher. However, online courses are growing at such a rapid pace that the Internet is becoming the primary vehicle for delivering distance education (Institute for Higher Education Policy, 2000). Based on a survey of more than 2,500 higher education institutions in the United States, approximately one third of institutions with health profession and related higher education programs offer online courses in these disciplines (Allen & Seaman, 2008). Some of these courses are totally Internet based, whereas others are hybrid or blended courses that incorporate a mix of classroom instruction and online discussion. It should be noted that online education is not restricted to higher education. Online continuing education programs are also available to health professionals from a variety of sources, such as their own professional organizations.

Research shows that distance education provides much more than a flexible approach to learning. Comparisons of students from distance education courses and from traditional classrooms repeatedly demonstrate that distance education can be a very effective mode for delivering education (Cook et al., 2008; Russell, 1998). A meta-analysis of outcomes in allied health distance education programs indicates that there is a small but significant positive effect for distance versus traditional students (Williams, 2006). In particular, students with professional experiences have significant learning gains in distance education courses that incorporate elements of social interaction, innovation, and introspection into the learning design (Williams, 2006).

In discussions of best practice for online teaching, it is consistently noted that the online environment is only a tool to facilitate teaching and learning (Abel, 2005; Alexander & Boud, 2001; Williams, 2006). The technology itself is not what promotes positive student outcomes. Rather, it is the instructional design and techniques within the online classroom that provide for an enriching learning experience.

Several education organizations have developed guidelines and standards for distance education to assist faculty and to ensure program quality, including the American Council on Education, the National Education Association, the Commission on Higher Education of the Middle States Association of Colleges and Schools, the American Association of Colleges of Nursing, and the Western Interstate Commission on Higher Education (Billings, 2007; Institute for Higher Education Policy, 2000).

The Western Interstate Commission on Higher Education's *Principles of Good Practice for Electronically Offered Academic Degree and Certificate Programs* (http://distance.tamu.edu/faculty_staff/media/documents/thecb_princ_good_pract.pdf) has been used as a guide for the creation and provision of quality higher education online programs since 1995 (Howell & Baker, 2006).

These principles fall under seven main areas:

1. A quality curriculum and instruction
2. An online program consistent with the institution's role and mission
3. Faculty support
4. Resources for learning
5. Students and student services
6. Commitment to support faculty and students
7. Evaluation and assessment of students and the program as a whole

A report by the Alliance for Higher Education Competitiveness (A-HEC) similarly emphasizes the importance of an institution's motivation for and commitment to a full online program as a means of delivering quality online education. Successful programs work with students and faculty to move beyond technological challenges and focus on a better educational product (Abel, 2005).

Online educators and students share responsibility for successful learning. Faculty work to generate the innovation of ideas, introspection by students, integration of concepts, building of information, and social interaction among students and instructors to promote a quality learning experience (Williams, 2006). Students who are satisfied and successful with their online learning engage in discussion with classmates and instructors, believe their education matches their expectations, are satisfied with student services and supports, feel adequately oriented to their online learning program, and strive for learning outcomes that are useful for their career and professional and academic development (SLOAN-C, 2002).

Given the growth and development of online courses in higher education for health professionals, this teaching methodology has the potential to be incorporated into health and healthcare education as well. Health professionals who are responsible for providing education for clients need to begin thinking about how online courses may fit into their programs. Internet-based courses might work very well in areas such as parenting and diabetes education where there is an extended program of instruction and the need for group support.

State of the Evidence

Teaching with technology is not a new concept. Health professionals have been using technology to teach clients and students for many years. However, in the Information Age, the notion of teaching with technology has taken on new meaning. Technology is advancing so quickly that researchers are struggling to keep up with the new products and technology-based strategies that are emerging every day.

There is a large body of research documenting the effects of distance education technologies on student outcomes in higher education. One of the classic and most frequently quoted studies on the impact of technology in education was conducted by Thomas Russell. He reviewed more than 350 studies, reports, dissertations, and papers documenting what he called the "no significant difference phenomenon"; that is, the lack of evidence to support any difference in student outcome for students educated using technology versus traditional methods (Russell, 1998; Young, 2000).

In light of the many new forms of distance education and the numerous research studies that have been conducted in recent years, a Web site has been set up as a companion piece to Russell's work (http://www.nosignificantdifference.org). This Web site provides access to more than 80 years of educational research. The studies included on this site fall into two categories: those that show no difference between traditional and technology-based education and those that show differences in student outcomes based on educational strategy used.

There also is a growing body of research on the use of technology in client or consumer education. A review of the literature reveals studies in a broad range of topics including the use of online support groups and the use of computer-based programs for client education in clinical and home settings. The focus to date has largely been on ways in which clients use technology and the obstacles they face. Most of these studies are small in scope.

Despite a comprehensive body of research on the use of technology in higher education and a growing body of research on client education, there is much yet to learn, particularly in the area of client education. Technology is exciting and has many advantages for both consumers and health professionals. However, technology devoid of teaching and learning principles cannot stand alone in consumer or professional education. The challenge for health professional educators is to keep abreast of the best technology as well as educational principles that together enable and support a quality, enriching consumer learning experience.

Summary

This chapter focuses on Information Age technology and its use in healthcare education. Specifically, this chapter discusses ways in which health professional educators can use the Internet and the World Wide Web to enhance health and health-care education for consumers as well as professional staff and students. Internet and Web-based instructional strategies are introduced and the impact of technology on teachers and learners is addressed. Special considerations for older adults, individuals with disabilities, and other client groups are identified. Trends in e-learning and distance education for health professionals are also explored.

Information Age technology has the potential to transform health and healthcare education. The powerful tool of the computer must be used thoughtfully and carefully, however. Education is about learning, not technology. Technology is merely a vehicle to deliver educational programs and to promote learning. The benefits of technology-based education are numerous, as are the challenges for educators and learners. Health professionals have a responsibility to learn to use new tools to promote health in clients and professional growth and development in themselves, fellow staff, and students. The future looks very bright, and health professional educators can help to shape it by continuing to think creatively about how to use technology in education and by participating in research about its effectiveness.

REVIEW QUESTIONS

1. What is the Information Age and how has it influenced education in general, healthcare education specifically, and healthcare consumers?
2. What Information Age skills are required by health professionals and healthcare consumers?
3. What are the various standards that have been established to ensure quality on the World Wide Web and access by people with disabilities?
4. What are the ways in which resources on the World Wide Web can be used as a health information resource for healthcare consumers and health professionals?
5. What are the various ways in which the Internet can be used to facilitate electronic communication between and among health professional educators and healthcare consumers? What are the advantages and disadvantages of each?
6. When using computer resources with clients, which segments of the population require special considerations because of limited access or special needs? What are those considerations, and how can they be addressed?
7. What is e-learning, and what advantages does it offer in providing training in healthcare settings?
8. How has technology influenced professional and continuing education options for health professionals?

CASE STUDY

Sarah is a speech-language pathologist working with Steve in a rehabilitation outpatient clinic. Steve experienced a stroke 2 months ago and has recently returned home. He is now physically able to live independently but is still working on his ability to communicate effectively with others. Since his stroke, Steve has had difficulty with finding words when speaking with others. A retired human resources specialist, this communication barrier is frustrating to Steve. During an initial client interview with him, Sarah learns that he is hesitant to return to many of his former activities with friends and is feeling socially isolated. Steve feels that his only successful social interactions since returning home are e-mail exchanges with family and friends in different parts of the country. Sarah realizes that because e-mails are written, asynchronous forms of communication, Steve has more time to word-find when composing his messages than he would in a spoken conversation. She asks Steve if he has Internet access at home. He says he has a high-speed Internet connection and computer in his living room that he uses daily. Based on this preassessment of Steve's ability and interest in this technology, Sarah asks him if he has found any online support groups for individuals who have experienced strokes. She explains that this would be a resource for information about others' experience with stroke, a social venue, and another type of written activity to enhance his interaction with others. She suggests that such a group could be educational, socially engaging, and a chance for Steve to continue building his communication skills during his rehabilitation. Steve expresses interest in this idea, and he and Sarah plan to seek out such groups online during their next therapy session.

1. Given Steve's condition and age, how can technology be used to foster social participation? What is Sarah's role in encouraging his social engagement?
2. What potential problems might Steve face when trying to use the Web?
3. As a healthcare educator, what criteria should Sarah use for evaluating health-related Web sites? Explain how she can apply each criterion to determine which Web sites are appropriate for Steve.

References

Abel, R. (2005). Achieving success in Internet-supported learning in higher education: Case studies illuminate success factors, challenges, and future directions. Retrieved May 2, 2009, from http://www.a-hec.org/media/files/A-HEC_IsL0205_6.pdf

Alexander, S., & Boud, D. (2001). Learners still learn from experience when online. In J. Stephenson (Ed.), *Teaching and learning online: Pedagogies for new technologies* (pp. 3–15). London: RoutledgeFalmer.

Allen, I. E., & Seaman, J. (2008). Staying the course: Online education in the United States, 2008. Retrieved May 2, 2009, from http://www.sloan-c.org/publications/survey/pdf/staying_the_course.pdf

American Association of Colleges of Nursing. (1999). *Task force on distance technology and nursing education*. Washington, DC: Author.

American Medical Association. (2009). Guidelines for physician–patient electronic communication. Retrieved April 30, 2009, from http://www.ama-assn.org/ama/pub/about-ama/our-people/member-groups-sections/young-physicians-section/advocacy-resources/guidelines-physician-patient-electronic-communications.shtml

American Medical Informatics Association. (2009). Home page. Retrieved April 30, 2009, from http://www.amia.org/chi-wg

Association of Cancer On-line Resources. (2009). Home page. Retrieved April 30, 2009, from http://www.acor.org

Baker, L., Wagner, T., Singer, S., & Bundoff, K. (2003). Use of the Internet and e-mail for healthcare information. *Journal of the American Medical Association*, *289*, 2400–2406.

Billings, D. (2007). Distance education in nursing: 25 years and going strong. *CIN: Computers, Informatics, Nursing*, *25*, 120.

Boulos, M. N., Maramba, I., & Wheeler, S. (2006). Wikis, blogs, and podcasts: A new generation of Web-based tools for virtual collaborative clinical practice and education. *BMC Medical Education*, *6*, 41.

Boulos, M. N. K., & Wheeler, S. (2007). The emerging Web 2.0 social software: An enabling suite of sociable technologies in health and health care education. *Health Information and Libraries Journal*, *24*, 2–23.

Cetron, M. J., & Davies, O. (2001). Trends now changing the world. *Futurist*, *35*(2), 27–40.

Cook, D. A., Levinson, A. J., Garside, S., Dupras, D. M., Erwin, P. J., & Montori, V. M. (2008). Internet-based learning in the health profession: A meta-analysis. *Journal of the American Medical Association*, *300*(10), 1181–1196.

Erardi, L. K., & Hartmann, K. (2008). Blogs, wikis, and podcasts: Broadening our connections for communication, collaboration, and continuing education. *OT Practice*, *13*, CE1–CE8.

Evangelista, L. S., Stromberg, A., Westlake, C., Galstanyan, A., Anderson, N., & Dracup, K. (2006). Developing a Web-based education and counseling program for heart failure patients. *Progress in Cardiovascular Nursing*, *21*, 196–201.

Finnis, J. A. (2003). Learning in the information age. Retrieved June 18, 2007, from http://dev.twinisles.com/research/learninfoage.pdf

Fox, S. (2005). Digital divisions. Retrieved June 15, 2007, from http://www.pewinternet.org/~/media//Files/Reports/2005/PIP_Digital_Divisions_Oct_5_2005.pdf.pdf

Fox, S. (2006). Online health search. Pew Internet & American life project. Retrieved June 15, 2007, from http://www.pewinternet.org/~/media//Files/Reports/2006/PIP_Online_Health_2006.pdf.pdf

Fox, S., & Fallows, D. (2003). Internet health resources. Retrieved June 15, 2007, from http://www.pewinternet.org/~/media//Files/Reports/2003/PIP_Health_Report_July_2003.pdf.pdf

Fox, S., & Madden, M. (2005). Data memo: Generations online. Retrieved June 18, 2007, from http://www.pewinternet.org/~/media//Files/Reports/2006/PIP_Generations_Memo.pdf.pdf

Han, H.-R., & Belcher, A. (2001). Computer-mediated support group use among parents of children with cancer—An exploratory study. *Computers in Nursing*, *19*(1), 27–33.

Hern, M., Weitkamp, T., Haag, D., Trigg, J., & Guard, J. R. (1997). Nursing the community in cyberspace. *Computers in Nursing*, *15*(6), 316–321.

Horrigan, J. B. (2008). *Home broadband adoption 2008*. Pew Internet & American life project. Retrieved April 15, 2009, from http://www.pewinternet.org/~/media//Files/Reports/2008/PIP_Broadband_2008.pdf

Howell, S. L., & Baker, K. (2006). Good (best) practices for electronically offered degree and certificate programs: A 10-year retrospect. *Distance Learning*, *3*, 41–47.

Institute for Higher Education Policy. (2000). Distance learning in higher education. Retrieved June 1, 2007, from http://ihep.org/assets/files/publications/a-f/DistanceLearningUpdate.pdf

Internetworldstats.com. (2009). Home page. Retrieved April 15, 2009, from http://www.internetworldstats.com

Kaplan, B., & Brennan, P. F. (2001). Consumer informatics: Supporting patients as co-producers of quality. *Journal of the American Medical Informatics Association*, *8*(4), 309–315.

Kassirer, J. P. (2000). Patients, physicians and the Internet. *Health Affairs*, *19*(6), 115–123.

Lenhart, A., & Fox, S. (2006). Bloggers: A portrait of the Internet's new storytellers. Retrieved June 15, 2007, from http://www.pewinternet.org/PPF/r/186/report_display.asp

Lewis, D., Gundwardena, S., & Saadawi, G. (2005). Caring connection: Developing an Internet resource for family caregivers of children with cancer. *CIN: Computers, Informatics, Nursing*, *23*, 265–274.

Livinginternet.com. (2009). Tim Berners-Lee, Robert Cailliau, and the World Wide Web. Retrieved April 30, 2009, from http://www.livinginternet.com/w/wi_lee.htm

Maag, M. (2005). The potential use of blogs in nursing education. *CIN: Computers, Informatics, Nursing*, *23*, 16–26.

Maag, M. (2006). Podcasting and MP3 players: Emerging technologies. *CIN: Computers, Informatics, Nursing*, *24*, 9–13.

Nahm, E., Preece, J., Resnick, B., & Mills, M. (2004). Usability of Web sites for older adults. *CIN: Computers, Informatics, Nursing*, *22*, 326–334.

National Center for Educational Statistics. (2006). *Computer and Internet use by students in 2003: Statistical analysis report*. Washington, DC: U.S. Department of Education Institute of Educational Sciences, NCES 2006-065.

National Institute of Medicine. (2001). *Crossing the quality chasm: A new health system for the 21st century.* Washington, DC: National Academy Press.

Pandia.com. (2009). A short and easy search engine tutorial. Retrieved April 30, 2009, from http://www.pandia.com/goalgetter

Peters, K. (2007). M-learning: Positioning educators for a mobile connected future. *International Review of Research in Open and Distance Learning, 8*(2). Retrieved June 15, 2007, from http://www.irrodl.org/index.php/irrodl/article/view/350/894

Rainie, L. (2003). The online healthcare revolution and the rise of e-patients and e-caregivers. Pew Internet & American life project. Retrieved June 15, 2007, from http://www.pewinternet.org/Presentations/2003/The-Online-Healthcare-Revolution.aspx

Russell, T. L. (1998). The no-significant difference phenomenon. Retrieved July 2, 2007, from http://www.nosignificantdifference.org

Secco, L., Woodgate, R., Hodgson, A., Kowalski, S., Plouffe, J., Rothney, P., et al. (2006). A survey study of pediatric nurses' use of information sources. *CIN: Computers, Informatics, Nursing, 24*, 105–112.

Shaw, B. R., Hawkins, R., Aroroa, N., McTavish, F., Pingree, S., & Gustafson, D. H. (2006). An exploratory study of predictors of participation in a computer support group for women with breast cancer. *CIN: Computer, Informatics, Nursing, 24*(1), 18–27.

SLOAN-C. (2002). *Quick guide: Pillar reference manual.* Retrieved May 2, 2009, from http://www.sloan-c.org/publications/books/dprm_sm.pdf

Stone, J. H. (2007). Communication between physicians and patients in the era of e-medicine. *New England Journal of Medicine, 356*, 2451–2454.

Traxler, J. (2007). Defining, discussing, and evaluating mobile learning: The moving finger writes and having writ.... [Abstract]. *International Review of Research in Open and Distance Learning, 8*(2). Retrieved June 15, 2007, from http://www.irrodl.org/index.php/irrodl/article/viewArticle/346/875

Warger, T. (2006). The changing role of instructors. *Edutech Report, 12*(1), 3–7. Retrieved July 6, 2010, from http://magnapubs.com/issues/magnapubs_etr/22_1/news/598318-1.html

Wikipedia. (2009a). History of the Internet. Retrieved April 30, 2009, from http://en.wikipedia.org/wiki/History_of_the_Internet

Wikipedia. (2009b). Social network service. Retrieved May 1, 2009, from http://en.wikipedia.org/wiki/Social_networking_service

Wikipedia. (2009c). Wiki. Retrieved May 1, 2009, from http://en.wikipedia.org/wiki/Wikis

Wilbright, W. A., Haun, D., Romano, T. A., Krutzfeldt, T., Fontenot, C., & Nolan, T. (2006). Computer use in an urban hospital. *CIN: Computers, Informatics, Nursing, 24*, 37–43.

Williams, K. (2003). Literacy and computer literacy: Analyzing the NCRs being fluent with information technology. *Journal of Literacy and Technology, 3*(1). Retrieved June 15, 2007, from http://www-personal.umich.edu/~katewill/williamsliteracy2003.pdf

Williams, S. L. (2006). The effectiveness of distance education in allied health science programs: A meta-analysis of outcomes. *American Journal of Distance Education, 20*, 127–141.

Young, J. (2000). Scholar concludes that distance ed is as effective as traditional instruction. *Chronicle of Higher Education.* Retrieved July 2, 2007, from http://chronicle.com/article/DistanceClassroom-Educ/15897

Chapter 14

Evaluation in Healthcare Education

Priscilla Sandford
Worral

CHAPTER HIGHLIGHTS

KEY TERMS

- evaluation
- external evidence
- internal evidence
- practice-based evidence
- assessment
- program evaluation

- process (formative) evaluation
- content evaluation
- outcome (summative) evaluation
- impact evaluation
- evaluation research
- reflective practice

OBJECTIVES

After completing this chapter, the reader will be able to

1. Define the term *evaluation*.
2. Discuss the relationships among evaluation, evidence-based practice, and practice-based evidence.
3. Compare and contrast evaluation and assessment.
4. Identify the purposes of evaluation.
5. Distinguish between five basic types of evaluation: process, content, outcome, impact, and program.
6. Discuss characteristics of various models of evaluation.
7. Describe similarities and differences between evaluation and research.
8. Assess barriers to evaluation.
9. Examine methods for conducting an evaluation.
10. Select appropriate instruments for various types of evaluative data.
11. Identify guidelines for reporting results of evaluation.
12. Describe the strength of the current evidence base for evaluation of client and health professions' education.

Evaluation is the process that can provide evidence that what health professionals and educators do makes a value-added difference in the services they provide. **Evaluation** is defined as a systematic process by which the worth or value of something—in this case, teaching and learning—is judged.

Early consideration of evaluation has never been more critical than in today's healthcare environment, which demands that "best" practice is based upon evidence. Crucial decisions regarding learners rest on the outcomes of learning. Can the client go home? Can the health professional provide competent care? If education is to be justified as a value-added activity, the process of education must be measurably efficient and must be measurably linked to education outcomes. The outcomes of education, for the learner and for the organization, must be measurably effective.

Evaluation is a process within processes—a critical component of the healthcare practice decision-making process and the education process. Evaluation is the final component of each of these processes. Because these processes are cyclical, evaluation serves as the critical bridge at the end of one cycle that provides evidence to guide direction of the next cycle.

The sections of this chapter follow the steps in conducting an evaluation. These steps include (1) determining the focus of the evaluation, including use of evaluation models; (2) designing the evaluation; (3) conducting the evaluation; (4) determining methods of analysis and interpretation of data collected; (5) reporting results of data collected, including the use of evaluation results.

Each of these aspects of the evaluation process is important, but all of them are meaningless if the results of evaluation are not used to guide future action in planning and carrying out educational interventions. In other words, the results of evaluation provide "best" practice-based evidence to support continuing an educational intervention as is or revising that intervention to enhance learning.

Evaluation, Evidence-Based Practice, and Practice-Based Evidence

Evidence-based practice (EBP) is "the conscientious, explicit and judicious use of current best evidence in making decisions about the care of [clients]" (Sackett, Richardson, Rosenberg, & Haynes, 1997, p. 2). A similar definition of EBP is also supported by Melnyk and Fineout-Overholt (2005). Most EBP models describe evidence generated from systematic reviews of clinically relevant randomized controlled trials as the strongest evidence upon which to base practice decisions, especially decisions about treatment. Evidence from research is also called **external evidence** because it is intended to be generalizable beyond the particular study setting or sample.

As is discussed later in this chapter, results of evaluation are not considered external evidence. This is because evaluations are not intended to be generalizable, but are conducted to determine effectiveness of a specific intervention in a specific setting with an identified individual or group. Results of a systematically conducted evaluation, although not considered external evidence, are still important from an EBP perspective. When evidence generated from research is not available, the conscientious use of **internal evidence** is appropriate. Results of a systematically conducted evaluation are one example of internal evidence (Melnyk & Fineout-Overholt, 2005).

The health professionals' understanding and use of EBP has evolved and expanded over the past decade. In contrast, the idea of practice-based evidence is only beginning to be defined. In the absence of an official or commonly understood definition of **practice-based evidence**, what might this term mean? Might practice-based evidence—or evidence derived from practice rather than from research—include results of a systematically conducted evaluation? Might practice-based evidence include clients' responses to care delivered on the basis of clinical expertise and an understanding of individual client's values? Might practice-based evidence include results from systematically conducted quality improvement projects?

The results of evaluations, the outcomes of expert-delivered client-centered care, and the results of quality improvement projects all comprise internal evidence gathered by health providers on an ongoing basis as an integral and important component of professional practice. Intentional recognition of these findings about current practice as a source of evidence to guide future practice requires that health professionals critically think before acting and engage in ongoing critical appraisal during and after each health professional–client interaction.

Evaluation Versus Assessment

Although assessment and evaluation are highly interrelated and the terms are often used interchangeably, they are not synonymous. The process of **assessment** is to gather, summarize, interpret, and use data to decide a direction for action. The process of evaluation is to gather, summarize, interpret, and use data to determine the extent to which an action was successful.

The primary differences between these two terms are those of timing and purpose. For example, an education program begins with an assessment of learners' needs. From the perspective of systems theory, assessment data might be called the "input." While the program is being conducted, periodic evaluation lets the educator know whether the program and learners are proceeding as planned. After program completion, evaluation identifies whether and to what extent identified needs were met. Again, from a systems theory perspective, these evaluative data might be called "intermediate output" and "output," respectively.

An important note of caution: Although an evaluation is conducted at the end of a program, that is a bad time to plan it. Evaluation as an afterthought is, at best, a poor idea and, at worst, a dangerous one. Data may be impossible to collect, be incomplete, or even be misleading. Assessment and evaluation planning should ideally be concurrent activities. When feasible, the same data collection methods and instruments should be used. This approach is especially appropriate for outcome and impact evaluations, as is discussed later in this chapter. "If only …" is an all too frequent lament, which can be minimized by planning ahead.

Determining the Focus of Evaluation

In planning any evaluation, the first and most crucial step is to determine the focus of the evaluation. The focus then guides evaluation design, conduct, data analysis, and reporting of results. The importance of a clear, specific, and realistic evaluation focus cannot be overemphasized. Usefulness and accuracy of the results of an evaluation depend heavily on how well the evaluation is initially focused.

Evaluation focus includes five basic components: (1) audience, (2) purpose, (3) questions, (4) scope, and (5) resources (Ruzicki, 1987). To determine these components, ask the following questions:

1. For what audience is the evaluation being conducted?
2. For what purpose is the evaluation being conducted?
3. What questions will be asked in the evaluation?
4. What is the scope of the evaluation?
5. What resources are available to conduct the evaluation?

The audience is the persons or groups for whom the evaluation is being conducted (Ruzicki, 1987). These individuals or groups include the primary audience, or the individual or group who requested the evaluation, and the general audience, or all those who will use evaluation results or who might benefit from the evaluation. Thus, the audience for an evaluation might include clients, peers, the manager of a unit, a supervisor, the staff development director, the chief executive officer of the institution, or a group of community leaders.

When an evaluator reports results of the evaluation, he or she provides feedback to all members of the audience. In focusing the evaluation, however, the evaluator must first consider the primary audience. Giving priority to the individual or group who requested the evaluation makes focusing the evaluation easier, especially if results of an evaluation will be used by several groups representing diverse interests.

The purpose of the evaluation is the answer to the question, "Why is the evaluation being conducted?" The purpose of an evaluation might be to decide whether to continue a particular education program or to determine the effectiveness of the teaching process. If a particular individual or group has a primary interest in results of the evaluation, input from that group can clarify the purpose.

An important note of caution: Why an evaluator is conducting an evaluation is not synonymous with who or what the evaluator is evaluating. For example, literature on client education commonly distinguishes among three types of evaluations: (1) learner, (2) teacher, and (3) program. This distinction answers the question of who or what will be evaluated and is extremely useful for evaluation design and conduct. Why learner evaluation might be undertaken, for example, is answered by the reason or purpose for evaluating learner performance. Determining teaching or program effectiveness is another example of the purpose for undertaking evaluation.

An excellent rule of thumb in stating the purpose of an evaluation is keep it singular. In other words, the evaluator should state, "The purpose is … ," not "The purposes are …" Keeping the purpose audience focused and singular helps avoid the all-too-frequent tendency to attempt too much in one evaluation.

Questions to be asked in the evaluation are directly related to the purpose for conducting the evaluation, are specific, and are measurable. Examples of questions are "To what extent are clients satisfied with the cardiac discharge teaching program?" and "How frequently do staff health professionals use the diabetes teaching reference materials?" Asking the right questions is crucial if the evaluation is to fulfill the intended purpose. As is discussed later in this chapter, delineation of evaluation questions is both the first step in selection of evaluation design and the basis for eventual data analysis.

The scope of an evaluation can be considered an answer to the question "How much will be evaluated?" "How much" includes "How many aspects of education will be evaluated?" "How many individuals or representative groups will be evaluated?" and "What time period is to be evaluated?" For example, will the evaluation focus on one class or on an entire program; on the learning experience for one client or for all clients being taught a particular skill? Evaluation could be limited to the teaching process during a particular client education class or it could be expanded to encompass both the teaching process and related client outcomes of learning.

The scope of an evaluation is determined in part by the purpose for conducting the evaluation and in part by available resources. For example, an evaluation addressing learner satisfaction with educators for all programs conducted by a staff development department in a given year is necessarily broad and long term in scope and will require expertise in data collection and analysis. An evaluation to determine whether a client understands each step in a learning session on how to use principles of good body posture correctly when sitting at a table or desk is narrow in scope, is focused on a particular point in time, and will require expertise in clinical practice and observation.

Resources needed to conduct an evaluation include time, expertise, personnel, materials, equipment, and facilities. A realistic appraisal of what resources are accessible and available relative to what resources are required is crucial in focusing any evaluation. Someone conducting an evaluation should remember to include the time and expertise required to collate, analyze, and interpret data and to prepare the report of evaluation results.

Evaluation can be classified into different types, or categories, based on one or more of the five components just described. The most common types of evaluation identified include process, content, outcome, impact, and program evaluation. A number of evaluation models that help to clarify differences among these evaluation types as well as how they relate to one another have been developed (Abruzzese, 1992; Haggard, 1989; Koch, 2000; Puetz, 1992; Rankin & Stallings, 2005; Suhayda & Miller, 2006; Walker & Dewar, 2000).

Evaluation Models

Abruzzese (1992) constructed the Roberta Straessle Abruzzese (RSA) evaluation model for conceptualizing, or classifying, educational evaluation in different categories or levels. Although developed in 1978 and derived from the perspective of staff development education, the RSA model remains useful for conceptualizing types of evaluation from both staff development and client education perspectives.

The RSA model pictorially places five basic types of evaluation in relation to one another based on purpose and related questions, scope, and resource components of evaluation focus (**Figure 14–1**). The five types of evaluation include process, content, outcome, impact, and total program. Abruzzese describes the first four types as levels of evaluation leading from the simple (process evaluation) to the complex (impact evaluation). Total **program evaluation** encompasses and summarizes all four levels.

Figure 14–1 RSA Evaluation Model

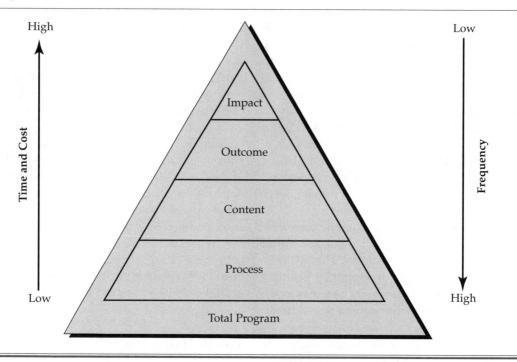

Reprinted by permission of Roberta S. Abruzzese.

Process (Formative) Evaluation

The purpose of **process** or **formative evaluation** is to make adjustments in an educational activity as soon as they are needed, whether those adjustments be in personnel, materials, facilities, learning objectives, or even the health professional educator's attitude. Adjustments may need to be made after one class or session before the next is taught or even in the middle of a single learning experience. Consider, for example, evaluating the process of teaching a person with multiple sclerosis and her family how to modify the home environment to conserve energy while performing cooking and cleaning activities. An occupational therapist (OT) might facilitate learning better by first conducting a home assessment. If the family is reluctant to have

the therapist come to their home, the teaching plan could be revised by having the client and family describe the home environment over the phone rather than hosting a home visit.

Process evaluation is integral to the education process itself. It forms an educational activity because evaluation is an ongoing component of assessment, planning, and implementation. As part of the education process, this ongoing evaluation helps the health professional anticipate and prevent problems before they occur or identify problems as they arise.

Consistent with the purpose of process evaluation, the primary question is, "How can teaching be improved to facilitate learning?" The health professional's teaching effectiveness, the teaching process, and the learner's responses are monitored on an ongoing basis. Abruzzese (1992) describes process evaluation as a "happiness index." While teaching and learning are ongoing, learners are asked their opinions about the educator(s), learning objectives, content, teaching and learning methods, physical facilities, and administration of the learning experience. Specific questions could include the following:

- Am I giving the client time to ask questions?
- Is the information I am giving orally consistent with information included in instructional materials being provided?
- Does the client look bored? Is the room too warm?
- Should I include more opportunities for return demonstration?

The scope of process evaluation generally is limited in breadth and time period to a specific learning experience such as an instruction session, class, or workshop, yet is sufficiently detailed to include as many aspects of the specific learning experience as possible while they occur. Learner behavior, teacher behavior, learner–teacher interaction, learner response to teaching materials and methods, and characteristics of the environment are all aspects of the learning experience within the scope of process evaluation. All learners and all teachers participating in a learning experience should be included in process evaluation. If resources are limited and participants include a number of different groups, a representative sample of individuals from each group rather than everyone from each group may be included in the evaluation. Also, the use of technology, such as a conference call, may be an appropriate tool so as to include more stakeholders.

Resources usually are less costly and more readily available for process evaluation than for other types such as impact or total program evaluation. Although process evaluation occurs more frequently—during and throughout every learning experience—than any other type, it occurs concurrently with teaching. The need for additional time, facilities, and dollars to conduct process evaluation is consequently decreased.

From the perspective of evidence-based practice, process evaluation is important in the use and modification of client-centered clinical practice guidelines or critical pathway guidelines (CPGs). Clinical pathways, also referred to as critical pathways, are tools appropriate for orientation of new healthcare employees, for quality improvement, and for evaluating clinical learning in student-precepted situations. These pathways are used by members of the healthcare team as cost-effective and time efficient measures to note learner progress and the achievement of goal-based outcomes. Implementing this education-focused evaluation method allows educators to choose learning experiences specific to the attainment of clinical outcomes (Bradshaw, 2007). A well-constructed CPG includes not only the specific intervention—but also includes the evidence-based process that should be used to provide that teaching.

Formal development of a CPG requires a high level of rigor and is intended for guiding care to all clients who have similar characteristics and learning needs. As is discussed later in this chapter, CPG development is conducted as evaluation research. Evaluation of the process of using a CPG, however, is focused on its fit for a specific learner or learners. To the extent that a client is the same as those studied in development of the CPG, the client's health professional will follow the guideline as written. To the extent that the client has unique behaviors or responses to teaching, the health professional will use informal process evaluation to vary from the guideline so that the client is able to learn.

Evidence-based practice is not a cookbook approach to providing health care. Similarly, CPGs are not intended to be followed without regard for the individual learner. This does not mean that variance from a CPG is determined in a haphazard manner based on what may be convenient at the moment. As attention to practice-based evidence evolves, the importance of the conscientious use of internal evidence gathered from process evaluation will become an increasingly critical component of every teaching–learning experience.

For instance, Watters and Moran (2006) describe a coordinated approach to care of patients recovering from hip fractures that explains how an interdisciplinary team implemented and modified a hip fracture protocol to be evidence-based and appropriate for a geriatric cohort. Schreurs, Colland, Kuijer, Ridder, and van Elderen (2003) provide an example of process evaluation to examine the benefit of fitting an education intervention to the learner. Using self-regulation theory to support an emphasis on personal goal setting, these clinicians worked with patients to develop an action plan for self-management of their asthma, diabetes, or heart failure, and then continuously reevaluated and adjusted the plan based on clients' success in managing symptoms and maintaining adherence to treatment regimens. Findings demonstrated that both clients and health professionals caring for these individuals were satisfied with the education.

The importance of evidence-based practice to process evaluation encompasses staff education as well as client education. Covell (2005) describes the use of the Iowa model of evidence-based practice to evaluate and modify guidelines for teaching basic cardiac life support (BCLS). Guided by the Iowa model, educators and staff examined their practice environment and searched the literature, and then drafted new guidelines for teaching BCLS that were evidence-based plus reflected key environmental factors. Using process evaluation to revise their guidelines during implementation, educators identified the need for additional equipment and regularly scheduled refresher training for instructors as well as for staff.

Content Evaluation

The purpose of **content evaluation** is to determine whether learners have acquired the knowledge or skills taught during the learning experience. Abruzzese (1992) described content evaluation as taking place immediately after the learning experience to answer the guiding question, "To what degree did the learners learn what was imparted?" or "To what degree did learners achieve specified objectives?" Asking a client to give a return demonstration and asking participants to complete a cognitive test at the completion of a 1-day seminar are common examples of content evaluation.

Content evaluation is depicted in the RSA model as the level in between the process and outcome evaluation levels. In other words, content evaluation can be considered as focusing on how the teaching–learning process affected immediate, short-term outcomes. To answer the question "Were specified objectives met as a result of teaching?" requires that the evaluation be designed differently from an evaluation to answer the question "Did learners achieve specified objectives?" Evaluation designs are discussed in some detail later in this chapter. An important point to be made here, however, is that evaluation questions must be carefully considered and clearly stated because they dictate the basic framework for design and conduct.

The scope of content evaluation is limited to a specific learning experience and to specifically stated objectives for that experience. Content evaluation occurs at a circumscribed point in time, immediately after completion of teaching, but encompasses all teaching–learning activities included in that specific learning experience. Data are obtained from all learners targeted in a specific class or group. For example, if both parents are taught how to help their child with a disability to use assistive devices in the home, both parents are asked to complete a return demonstration. Similarly, all health professionals attending a workshop are asked to complete the cognitive posttest at the end of the workshop.

Resources used to teach content can also be used to carry out evaluation of how well that content was learned. For example, the same equipment included in teaching a client how to change a dressing can be used by the client to perform a return demonstration. In the same manner, a pretest used at the beginning of a continuing education seminar can be readministered as a posttest at seminar completion to measure change.

From the perspective of evidence-based practice, content evaluation, like process evaluation, is focused on collecting internal evidence to determine whether objectives for a specific group of learners were met. Internal evidence must include both baseline data and immediate outcome data so that any change in learning can be identified.

Lott (2006) describes an example of content evaluation in her description of one hospital's creation of a new staff orientation program. Educators in the staff development department constructed an evaluation tool to measure satisfaction of new employees with their orientation experience. Because lack of knowledge about policies in a hospital where staff members had not worked before would have been an unmeaningful baseline, data collected from employees prior to implementation of the new program served as baseline data. These baseline data were compared with data using the same tool given to employees completing the new program. Knowledge of policies and procedures was improved for those employees who participated in the new program. Skill acquisition was evaluated by pre- and postdemonstrations; however, it was evaluated in a manner consistent with traditional content evaluation.

Outcome (Summative) Evaluation

The purpose of **outcome** or **summative evaluation** is to determine the effects or outcomes of teaching efforts. Its intent is to summarize what happened as a result of education. Guiding questions in outcome evaluation include the following:

- Was teaching appropriate?
- Did the individual(s) learn?

- Were behavioral objectives met?
- Did the client who learned a skill before discharge use that skill correctly when at home?

Just as process evaluation occurs concurrently with the teaching–learning experience, outcome evaluation occurs after teaching has been completed or after a program has been carried out. Outcome evaluation measures the changes that result from teaching and learning.

Abruzzese (1992) differentiates outcome evaluation from content evaluation by focusing outcome evaluation on measuring more long-term change that "persists after the learning experience" (p. 243). Changes can include institution of a new process, habitual use of a new technique or behavior, or integration of a new value or attitude. Which changes the health professional educator measures usually are dictated by the objectives established as a result of the initial needs assessment.

The scope of outcome evaluation depends in part on the changes being measured, which, in turn, depend on the objectives established for the educational activity. As mentioned earlier, outcome evaluation focuses on a longer time period than does content evaluation. Whereas evaluating accuracy of a client's return demonstration of a skill prior to discharge may be appropriate for content evaluation, outcome evaluation should include measuring a client's competency with a skill in the home setting after discharge. Similarly, health professionals' responses on a workshop posttest may be sufficient for content evaluation, but if the workshop objective states that health professionals will be able to incorporate their knowledge into practice in the workplace, outcome evaluation should include measuring health professionals' knowledge or behavior some time after they have returned to their work setting. Abruzzese (1992) suggests that outcome data be collected 6 months after baseline data to determine whether a change has really taken place.

Resources required for outcome evaluation are more costly and sophisticated than those for process or content evaluation. Compared to the resources required for the first two types of evaluation in the RSA model, outcome evaluation requires greater expertise to develop measurement and data collection strategies, more time to conduct the evaluation, knowledge of baseline data establishment, and ability to collect reliable and valid comparative data after the learning experience. Postage to mail surveys and time and personnel to carry out observation of health professionals on the clinical unit or to complete client/family telephone interviews are specific examples of resources that may be necessary to conduct an outcome evaluation.

From an evidence-based practice perspective, outcome evaluation might arguably be considered as "where the rubber meets the road." Once a need for change has been identified, the search for evidence upon which to base that change commonly begins with a structured clinical question that will guide an efficient search of the literature. This question is also known as a PICO question. The letters *P*, *I*, *C*, and *O* stand for population (client, staff, or student), intervention, comparison, and outcome, respectively.

For example, occupational or physical therapists caring for an outpatient population of adults with heart failure might discover that many clients are not following their prescribed rehabilitation regimen. Upon questioning these clients, the therapists learn that a majority of the clients do not recognize symptoms resulting from failure to follow recommended protocols on a consistent basis. To search the literature efficiently for ways in which they might better educate their clients, the therapists would pose the following PICO question: Does therapist-directed client education on symptoms and related treatment for heart failure provided to adult outpatients with heart failure result in improved compliance with rehabilitation regimens? In this example, the P is adult outpatients with heart failure, the I is the therapist-directed cli-

ent education on symptoms and related treatment for heart failure, the C is inferred as education currently being provided—or lack of education, if that is the case—and the O is improved compliance with treatment regimens.

A literature search identified an article by Gonzalez and colleagues (2005) that describes an education intervention highly relevant to the PICO question. As presented in the article, health professional–guided education demonstrated significant improvements in understanding of disease, symptoms, purpose of medications, and self-monitoring among 298 outpatients with heart failure. Data were collected at baseline and at 1-year follow-up appointments. Although self-management and knowledge did improve, treatment compliance remained approximately the same. Results from the evaluation published in this article would provide useful suggestions for the health professional to consider. By itself, this article would not be sufficient to dictate change in practice.

Ideally, several well-conducted studies providing external evidence directly relevant to a PICO question should be reviewed prior to making a practice change, especially if that change is resource intensive or, if unsuccessful, might increase client risk. The Gonzalez and colleagues (2005) study is an excellent example of practice-based internal evidence resulting from a 1-year evaluation of specified client outcomes. Such reports should be considered judiciously, but should not be overlooked by health professionals searching for evidence to suggest how they might address clinical issues in their own setting.

Another example of an outcome evaluation was a study conducted by Aldana and colleagues (2006) to examine effectiveness of a worksite diabetes prevention program. Using a sample of at-risk employees who did not have diabetes and who were interested in participating, a team of occupational health nurses and researchers conducted a 1-year program using a protocol and curriculum from the U.S. National Institutes of Health (NIH). Outcomes, including weight, body mass index, oral glucose tolerance testing, fasting blood sugar levels, and aerobic fitness were measured at baseline, after 6 months, after 12 months, and after 2 years. Positive outcomes demonstrated the effectiveness of the NIH protocol and curriculum. Aldana and colleagues (2006) provide not only an example of outcome evaluation, but also an example of evaluation of a critical pathway guideline—in this case, the NIH Diabetes Prevention Program—that was modified for use in a specific setting.

Impact Evaluation

The purpose of **impact evaluation** is to determine the relative effects of education on the institution or the community. Thus, the purpose of impact evaluation is to obtain information that will help decide whether continuing an educational activity is worth its cost. Examples of questions appropriate for impact evaluation include "What is the effect of an orientation program on subsequent health professional staff turnover?" and "What is the effect of a cardiac discharge teaching program on long-term frequency of rehospitalization among clients who have completed the program?"

The scope of impact evaluation is broader, more complex, and usually more long term than that of process, content, or outcome evaluation. For example, whereas outcome evaluation focuses on whether specific teaching results in achievement of specified outcomes, impact evaluation goes beyond that to measure the effect or worth of those outcomes. In other words, outcome evaluation focuses on a learning objective, whereas impact evaluation focuses on a goal for learning. Consider, for instance, a class on the use of body mechanics. The objective is that staff members will demonstrate proper use of body mechanics in providing client care. The goal is to decrease back injuries among the hospital's direct-care providers. This distinction between outcome and impact evaluation may seem subtle, but it is

important to the appropriate design and conduct of an impact evaluation.

Resource requirements for conducting an impact evaluation are extensive and may be beyond the scope of an individual educator. Literature on evaluation (Abruzzese, 1992; Hamilton, 1993; Waddell, 1992) describes impact evaluation as being most like evaluation research. (The distinction between evaluation and evaluation research is addressed later in this chapter.) Eklund, Sonn, and Dahlin-Ivanoff (2004) describe one example of impact evaluation conducted as research. Consistent with the scope and focus of an impact evaluation, the investigators examined long-term outcomes of a health education program for older adults with visual impairment on perceived security in performance of activities of daily living. The study was conducted, not at the site of the education, but where the older adults lived in the community. Using a randomized controlled study design, the researchers collected both observational and survey data over a 28-month period.

Good science is rarely inexpensive and never quick; good impact evaluation shares the same characteristics. The resources needed to design and conduct an impact evaluation generally include reliable and valid instruments, trained data collectors, personnel with research and statistical expertise, equipment and materials necessary for data collection and analysis, and access to populations who may be culturally or geographically diverse. Because impact evaluation is so expensive and time intensive, this type of evaluation should be targeted toward courses and programs where learning is critical to client well-being or to safe, high-quality, cost-effective healthcare delivery (Puetz, 1992).

Conducting an impact evaluation may seem a monumental task, but this reality should not interfere with undertaking the effort. Rather, health professional educators should plan ahead, proceed carefully, and obtain the support and assistance of colleagues. Keeping in mind the purpose for conducting an impact evaluation should be helpful in maintaining the level of commitment needed throughout the process. The current managed care environment requires justification for every health dollar spent. The value of client and staff education may be intuitively evident, but the positive impact of education must be demonstrated if it is to be funded.

A literature search conducted to determine the state of the evidence on impact evaluation in client education found that the term *impact* is used generically to describe both evaluations of client outcomes resulting from education and evaluations of long-term impact from education. What is important to remember when reviewing this literature is not which term the authors use, but what they have as their purpose for evaluation. As noted earlier, the purpose of an outcome evaluation is to determine whether an educational intervention results in intended behavior change, whereas the purpose of an impact evaluation is to determine whether long-term education goals are met. As evidence-based practice continues to grow, impact evaluations will become especially useful in examining the long-term effectiveness of different educational interventions used to disseminate practice guidelines to healthcare providers.

Program Evaluation

The purpose of program evaluation can be generically described as "designed and conducted to assist an audience to judge and improve the worth of some object" (Johnson & Olesinski, 1995, p. 53). The object in this case is an educational program. Using the framework of the RSA model (Abruzzese, 1992), the purpose of total program evaluation is to determine the extent to which all activities for an entire department or program over a specified period of time meet or exceed goals originally established.

Guiding questions appropriate for a total program evaluation from this perspective might be "To what extent did programs undertaken by staff development educators during the year accomplish annual goals established by the department?" or "How well did client education program activities implemented throughout the year meet annual goals established by the institution or agency?"

The scope of program evaluation is broad, generally focusing on overall goals rather than on specific objectives. Although the term *program* could be defined as an individual educational offering (Albanese & Gjerde, 1987), the resource requirements for conducting a program evaluation generally are too extensive to justify the effort on less than a broad scale. Abruzzese (1992) describes the scope of program evaluation as encompassing all aspects of educational activity (e.g., process, content, outcome, impact) with input from all the participants (e.g., learners, teachers, institutional representatives, community representatives). The time period over which data are collected may extend from several months to 1 or more years, depending on the time frame established for meeting the goals to be evaluated.

Resources required for program evaluation may include the sum of resources necessary to conduct process, content, outcome, and impact evaluations. A program evaluation may require significant expenditures for personnel if the evaluation is conducted by an individual or team external to the organization. Additional resources required may include time, materials, equipment, and personnel necessary for data entry, analysis, and report generation.

Suhayda and Miller (2006) provide an excellent example of the scope of program evaluation to establish organized, data-driven, ongoing quality improvement across multiple programs offered by a college of nursing. Using Stufflebeam's content, inputs, process, and product (CIPP) model, the entire infrastructure of the college was included in evaluation of activities ranging from the admissions process to budget decisions to student certification and licensure pass rates. Data tracking was accomplished using a specifically developed data action form completed by members of the evaluation committee with input from program directors, faculty, and students as well as a broad spectrum of stakeholders both internal and external to the college (e.g., accreditation board reviewers).

As stated earlier, the RSA model remains useful as a general framework for categorizing basic types of evaluation: process, content, outcome, impact, and program. As depicted in the model, differences between these types are, in large part, a matter of degree. For example, process evaluation occurs most frequently; program evaluation occurs least frequently. Content evaluation focuses on immediate effects of teaching; impact evaluation concentrates on more long-term effects of teaching. Conduct of process evaluation requires fewer resources compared with impact and program evaluation, which require extensive resources for implementation. The RSA model further illustrates one way that process, content, outcome, and impact evaluations can be considered together as components of total program evaluation.

Health professional educators can find clinical examples of how different types of evaluation relate to one another in Haggard's (1989) description of three dimensions in evaluating teaching effectiveness for the client and in Rankin and Stallings's (2005) four levels of evaluation of client learning. The three dimensions described by Haggard and the four levels identified by Rankin and Stallings are consistent with the basic types of evaluation included in Abruzzese's RSA model, as shown in **Table 14–1**. As depicted in this table, models developed from an education theory base, such as the RSA model, have much in common with models developed from a client care theory base, exemplified by the other two models.

At least one important point about the difference between the RSA and other models needs to be mentioned, however. That difference is depicted in the learner evaluation model shown in **Figure 14–2**. This learner-focused model emphasizes the continuum of learner status determined from needs assessment to learner performance over time once an adequate level of participation has been regained or achieved. This model and the RSA model have value in focusing and planning any type of evaluation but are especially important for impact and program evaluations.

Table 14–1 COMPARISON OF LEVELS/TYPES OF EVALUATION ACROSS STAFF/ CLIENT EDUCATION EVALUATION MODELS

Abruzzese (1992)	Haggard (1989)	Rankin and Stallings (2005)
Process	Client assimilation of information during teaching	Client-education intervention
Content	Client information retention after teaching	Client/family performance following learning
Outcome	Client use of information in day-to-day life	Client/family performance at home
Impact	N/A	Overall self-care and health maintenance
Program	N/A	N/A

Figure 14–2 Five Levels of Learner Evaluation

Based on Rankin, S. H., & Stallings, K. D. (2005). *Patient education in health and illness* (5th ed.). Philadelphia: Lippincott Williams & Wilkins. Reprinted with permission.

Designing the Evaluation

Educators can design an evaluation within the framework, or boundaries, already established by focusing the evaluation. In other words, the design must be consistent with the purpose, questions, and scope and must be realistic given available resources. Evaluation design includes at least three interrelated components: structure, methods, and instruments.

Design Structure

An important question to be answered in designing an evaluation is "How rigorous should the evaluation be?" The obvious answer is that all evaluations should have some level of rigor. In other words, all evaluations should be systematic and carefully and thoroughly planned or structured before they are conducted. How rigor is translated into design structure depends on the questions to be answered by the evaluation, the complexity of the scope of the evaluation, and the expected use of evaluation results. The more the questions address cause and effect, the more complex the scope. Likewise, the more critical and broad-reaching the expected use

of results, the more the evaluation design should be structured from a research perspective.

EVALUATION VERSUS RESEARCH

Evaluation and research are neither synonymous nor mutually exclusive activities. The extent to which they are either very different or indistinguishable from each other depends on the type of evaluation and type of research considered. Ruzicki (1987) makes the following distinction between the two:

> While both research and evaluation involve objective, systematic collection of data, evaluation is conducted to make decisions in a given setting. Research is designed so that it can be generalized to other settings and replicated in other settings. Furthermore, research seeks new knowledge, examines cause and effect relationships, tests hypotheses, whereas evaluation determines mission achievement, examines means-end processes, and assesses attainment of objectives. (p. 234)

For example, this argument holds true when comparing basic research to process evaluation. Basic research is defined as tightly controlled experimental studies of cause and effect conducted for the purpose of generating new knowledge. This new knowledge may or may not eventually influence practice. Process evaluation occurs concurrently with an educational intervention and is conducted in an uncontrolled or real-world setting for the purpose of making change as soon as the need for change is identified. As described earlier in this chapter, this distinction between research and evaluation is analogous to the distinction between external and internal evidence (Melnyk & Fineout-Overholt, 2005).

Differences between research and evaluation have become less distinct over the past several years with the advent of applied research, with the acceptance of qualitative measures and methods as legitimate research, and with the increasing importance given to results of outcome, impact, and program evaluations. This importance is likely to increase as more credibility, and therefore attention, is given to practice-based evidence—or internal evidence—as a legitimate support for evidence-based decision making.

The purpose for conducting applied research is to effect change in practice positively. There is little difference between this purpose and the purpose for conducting evaluation. **Evaluation research**, which is one type of applied research, can be defined as "a process of applying scientific procedures to accumulate reliable and valid data on the manner and extent to which specified activities produce outcomes or effects" (Hamilton, 1993, p. 148).

Using this definition, Hamilton identifies program accreditation, program cost analysis, and outcome of treatment as appropriate for use of evaluation research designs and methods. Hamilton further describes impact evaluation as appropriate for use of quasi-experimental and experimental research design structures. A number of other authors support some use of research designs and data collection methods for outcome, impact, and program evaluations (Albanese &

Gjerde, 1987; Berk & Rossi, 1990; Eklund et al., 2004; Holzemer, 1992; Puetz, 1992; Templeton & Coates, 2004; Waddell, 1992).

Of course, not all outcome, impact, and program evaluations should be conducted as research studies. Some important differences do exist between evaluation and evaluation research. One of the most significant relates to the influence of a primary audience. As discussed earlier in this chapter, the primary audience, or the individual or group requesting the evaluation, is a major component in focusing an evaluation. The evaluator must design and conduct the evaluation consistent with the purpose and related questions identified by the primary audience. Evaluation research, by contrast, does not have an identified primary audience. The researcher has autonomy to develop a protocol to answer a question posed by the researcher.

A second difference between evaluation and evaluation research is one of timing. The necessary timeline for usability of evaluation results may not be sufficient to prospectively develop a research proposal and obtain institutional review board approval prior to beginning data collection.

Given the discussion of evaluation versus evaluation research, how are decisions about level of rigor of an evaluation actually translated into an evaluation structure? The structure of an evaluation design depicts the number of groups to be included in the evaluation, the number of evaluations or periods of evaluation, and the time sequence between an educational intervention and evaluation of that intervention. A group can comprise one individual, as in the case of one-to-one health professional–client teaching, or several individuals, as in the case of an in-service program or workshop.

A process evaluation might be conducted during a single-client education activity where the educator observes client behavior during instruction/demonstration and engages the client in questions and answers upon completion of each new instruction. Because the purpose of process evaluation is to facilitate better learning while that learning is going on, education and evaluation occur concurrently in this case.

Evaluation also may be conducted immediately after an educational intervention. This structure is probably the most commonly employed in conducting educational evaluations, although it is not necessarily the most appropriate. If the purpose of conducting the evaluation is to determine whether after a class learners know specific content that they did not know before attending that class, then a structure that begins with collection of baseline data is more appropriate. Collection of baseline data via a pretest, which can be compared with data collected via a posttest at one or more points in time after learners have completed the educational activity, provides an opportunity to measure whether change has occurred. The ability to measure change in a particular skill or level of knowledge, for example, also requires that the same instruments be used for pre- and posttest data collection at both points in time. Data collection is discussed in more detail later in this chapter.

If the purpose of conducting an evaluation is to determine whether learners know content or can perform a skill as a result of an educational intervention, the most appropriate structure will include at least two groups: one receiving education and one not receiving education. Both groups are evaluated at the same time, even though only one group receives education. The group receiving the new education program is called the treatment or experimental group, and the group receiving standard care or the traditional education program is called the comparison or control group. The two groups may or may not be equivalent. Equivalent groups are those with no known differences between them prior to some intervention, whereas nonequivalent groups may be different from one another in several ways. For example, patients on unit A may receive an educational pamphlet to read prior to attending a class, while patients on unit B attend the class without first reading the pamphlet. Because patients on the two units probably are different in many ways—age and diagnosis, for example—besides which educational intervention they received, they would be considered nonequivalent groups.

Use of the term *nonequivalent* is common to discussions of traditional research designs. Quasi-experimental designs, such as nonequivalent control group designs, should be among those considered in planning an outcome, impact, or program evaluation. Especially if the purpose of an evaluation is to demonstrate that an education program caused fewer client returns to the clinic or fewer health professionals to leave the institution, for example, the evaluation structure must have the rigor of evaluation research.

Another type of quasi-experimental design, called a time-series design, might include only one group of learners from which evaluative data are collected at several points in time both before and after receiving an educational intervention. If data collected before the education consistently demonstrate lack of learner ability to comply with a treatment regimen, whereas data collected after the education consistently demonstrate a significant improvement in client compliance with that regimen, the evaluator could argue that the education was the reason for the improvement in this case.

In recent years, pluralistic designs have appeared in the evidence-based literature as approaches especially suited for evaluation of projects that have a community base, that include participants from diverse settings or perspectives, or that require both program processes and outcomes to be included in the evaluation (Billings, 2000; Gerrish, 2001; Hart, 1999; Suhayda & Miller, 2006). As the term implies, a pluralistic design uses a variety of sources and methods for obtaining evaluative data, often including both qualitative and quantitative evidence. Because these designs are comprehensive, resource intensive, and long term in nature, they are most appropriate for program evaluation.

This chapter does not provide an exhaustive description of evaluation designs. Rather, it is intended to increase awareness of the value and usefulness of these designs, especially when the results of an evaluation will be used to make major financial or programmatic decisions.

A literature search that includes many of the following journals is recommended for planning the evaluation of healthcare education in a cost-conscious and outcome-focused healthcare environment: *Evaluation and the Health Professions, Adult Education Quarterly, Health Education Quarterly, Health Education Research,* and *Patient Education and Counseling*

Evaluation Methods

Evaluation focus provides the basis for determining the evaluation design structure. The design structure, in turn, provides the basis for determining evaluation methods. Evaluation methods include those actions that are undertaken to carry out the evaluation according to the design structure. All evaluation methods deal in some way with data and data collection. Answers to the following questions can assist in selection of the most appropriate, feasible methods for conducting a particular evaluation in a particular setting and for a specified purpose:

- What types of data will be collected?
- From whom or what will data be collected?
- How, when, and where will data be collected?
- By whom will data be collected?

TYPES OF DATA TO COLLECT

Evaluation of healthcare education includes collection of data about people, about the educational program or activity, and about the environment in which the educational activity takes place. Process, outcome, impact, and program evaluations require data about all three: the people, the program, and the environment. Content evaluations may be limited to data about the people and the program, although this limitation is not necessary.

Types of data that are collected about people can be classified as physical, cognitive, affective, or psychomotor. Data that are collected about educational activities or programs generally include such program characteristics as cost, length, number of educators required, amount and type of materials required, teaching–learning methods used, and so on. Data that are collected about the environment in which a program or activity is conducted generally include such environmental characteristics as temperature, lighting, location, layout, space, and noise level.

Given the possibility that an unlimited and overwhelming amount of data could be collected, how do you decide what data should be collected? The most straightforward answer to this question is that data that will answer evaluation questions posed in focusing the evaluation should be collected. The likelihood that the evaluator will collect the right amount of the right type of data to answer evaluation questions can be significantly improved by (1) remembering that any data collected must be used, and (2) using operational definitions.

An operational definition of a word or phrase is a definition that is written in measurement terms. Functional health status, for example, can be theoretically defined as an individual's ability to independently carry out activities of daily living without self-perceived undue difficulty or discomfort. Functional health status can be operationally defined as an individual's composite score on the SF-36 survey instrument (Stewart, Hays, & Ware, 1988; Ware, Davies-Avery, & Donald, 1978). The SF-36, which has undergone years of extensive reliability and validity testing with a wide variety of client populations and in several languages, is generally considered the gold standard for measuring functional health status from the individual's perspective. Continuously updated information about the SF-36 as well as different versions of the actual instrument can be found on the Internet at http://www.sf-36.org.

Similarly, client compliance can be theoretically defined as the client's regular and consistent adherence to a prescribed treatment regimen. For use in an outcome evaluation of a particular educational activity, client compliance might be operationally defined as the client's demonstration of unassisted and error-free completion of all steps in the sterile dressing change as observed in the client's home on three separate occasions at 2-week time intervals.

These examples show that an operational definition states exactly what data will be collected. In the first example, measurement of functional health status requires collection of client survey data using a specific self-administered questionnaire. The second example provides even more information about data collection than does the first, by including where and how many times the client's performance of the dressing change is to be observed, as well as stating that criteria for compliance include both unassisted and error-free performance on each occasion.

In addition to being categorized as describing people, programs, or the environment, data can be categorized as quantitative or qualitative. Quantitative data are numeric and generally are expressed in statistics such as mean, median, ratio, F statistic, t statistic, or chi-square. Numbers can be used to answer questions of how much, how many, how often, and so on in terms that are commonly understood by the audience for the evaluation. Mathematical analysis can demonstrate with some level of precision and reliability whether a learner's knowledge or skill has changed since completing an educational program, for example, or how much improvement in a learner's knowledge or skill is the result of an educational program.

Qualitative data include feelings, behaviors, words, and phrases and generally are expressed in themes or categories. Qualitative data can be described in quantitative terms, such as percentages or counts, but this transformation eliminates the richness and insight that the use of qualitative data can offer. Qualitative data can be used as background to

better interpret quantitative data, especially if the evaluation is intended to measure such value-laden or conceptual terms as satisfaction or quality.

Any evaluation may be strengthened by collecting both quantitative and qualitative data. For example, an evaluation to determine whether a stress reduction class resulted in decreased work stress for participants could include participants' qualitative expressions of how stressed they feel plus quantitative pulse and blood pressure readings. Because collection of both quantitative and qualitative data, although intuitively appealing, is resource-intensive, evaluators must be certain that the focus of the evaluation justifies such an undertaking.

From Whom or What to Collect Data

Data can be collected directly from the individuals whose behavior or knowledge is being evaluated, from surrogates or representatives of these individuals, or from documentation or databases already created. Whenever possible, researchers should plan to collect at least some data directly from individuals being evaluated. In the case of process evaluation, data should be collected from all learners and all educators participating in the educational activity. Content and outcome evaluations should include data from all learners.

Because impact and total program evaluations have a broader scope than do the first three types of evaluation, collecting data from all individuals who participated in an educational program over an extended period of time may be impossible. This is because data collectors may not be able to locate every participant or they may lack sufficient resources to gather data from such a large number of people.

When all participants cannot be counted or located, data may be collected from a subset, or sample, of participants who are considered to represent the entire group. If an evaluation is planned to collect data from a sample of participants, participants who are representative of the entire group should be included. A random selection of participants from whom data are collected can minimize bias in the sample but cannot guarantee representativeness.

For example, an impact evaluation was conducted to determine whether a 5-year program supporting home-based health education actually improved the general health status of individuals in the community served by the program. If all members of the community could be counted, a random sample of community members could be generated by first listing and numbering all members' names, and then drawing numbers using a random numbers table until a 10% sample was obtained. Such a method for selecting the sample of community members would eliminate intentional selection of those individuals who were the most active program participants and who might therefore have a better health status than does the community as a whole. At the same time, the 10% random sample could unintentionally include only those individuals who did not participate in the health education program. Data collected from this sample of nonparticipants would be equally as misleading as data collected from the first sample. A more representative sample for this evaluation should include both participants and nonparticipants, ideally in the same proportions in the sample as in the community.

Preexisting databases should never be used as the only source of evaluative data unless they were created for the purpose of that evaluation. Even though these data were collected for a different purpose, they may be helpful for providing additional information to the primary audience for the evaluation. Data already in existence generally are less expensive to obtain than are original data. The decision whether to use preexisting data depends on whether they were collected from people of interest in the current evaluation and whether they are consistent with operational definitions used in the current evaluation.

HOW, WHEN, AND WHERE TO COLLECT DATA

Methods for how data can be collected include the following:

- Observation
- Interview
- Questionnaire or written examination
- Record review
- Secondary analysis of existing databases

Which method is selected depends, first, on the type of data being collected and, second, on available resources. Whenever possible, data should be collected using more than one method. Using multiple methods provides the evaluator, and consequently the primary audience, with more complete information about the program or performance being evaluated than could be accomplished using a single method.

The evaluator can conduct observations in person or can videotape them for viewing at some later time. In the combined role of educator–evaluator, the health professional educator who is conducting a process evaluation can directly observe a learner's physical, verbal, psychomotor, and affective behaviors so as to respond in a timely manner. Use of videotape or a nonparticipant observer also can be beneficial for picking up the educator's own behaviors of which the educator is unaware, but which might be influencing the learner.

The timing of data collection, or when data collection takes place, has already been addressed both in discussion of different types of evaluation and in descriptions of evaluation design structures. Process evaluation, for example, generally occurs during and immediately after an educational activity. Content evaluation takes place immediately after completion of education. Outcome evaluation occurs some time after completion of education when learners have returned to the setting where they are expected to use new knowledge or perform a new skill. Impact evaluation generally is conducted from weeks to years after the educational program because the purpose of impact evaluation is to determine what change has occurred within the community or institution as a whole as a result of an educational intervention.

Timing of data collection for program evaluation is less obvious than for other types of evaluation, in part because a number of different descriptions of what constitutes a program evaluation can be found both in the literature and in practice. As discussed earlier, Abruzzese (1992) describes data collection for program evaluation as occurring over a prolonged period because program evaluation is itself a culmination of process, content, outcome, and impact evaluations already conducted.

Where an evaluation is conducted can have a major effect on evaluation results. Those conducting an evaluation must be careful not to make the decision about where to collect data on the basis of convenience for the data collector. An appropriate setting for conducting a content evaluation may be in the classroom or skills laboratory where learners have just completed class instruction or training. An outcome evaluation to determine whether training has improved the health professional's ability to perform a skill with a client on the rehabilitation unit, however, requires that data collection—in this case, observation of the health professional's performance—be conducted on the rehabilitation unit.

Similarly, an outcome evaluation to determine whether discharge teaching in the hospital enabled the client to provide self-care at home requires that data collection, or observation of the client's performance, be conducted in the home. What if available resources are insufficient to allow for home visits by the evaluator? To answer this question, keep in mind that the focus of the evaluation is on performance by the client, not performance by the evaluator. Training a family member, a visiting nurse, or even the client to observe and record client performance at home is preferable to bringing the client to a place of convenience for the evaluator.

WHO COLLECTS DATA

Evaluative data are most commonly collected by the educator who is conducting the class or activity being evaluated because that educator is already present and interacting with learners. Combining the role of evaluator with that of educator is one appropriate method for conducting a process evaluation because evaluative data are integral to the teaching–learning process. Inviting another educator or a client representative to observe a class can provide additional data from the perspective of someone who does not have to divide his or her attention between teaching and evaluating. This second, and perhaps less biased, input can strengthen legitimacy and usefulness of evaluation results.

Data can also be collected by the learners themselves, by other colleagues within the department or institution, or by someone from outside the institution. Puetz's (1992) description of data collection using a participant evaluation team is an example of data collection that includes learners. The evaluation team is composed of a small number of randomly selected individuals who are scheduled to attend an educational program. Team members are introduced to other program participants at the beginning of the class, join other participants during the program, and collect data through self-report as well as through observation and interaction with others during breaks.

The individuals chosen to carry out data collection become an extension of the evaluation instrument. If the data that are collected are to be reliable, unbiased, and accurate, the data collectors must be unbiased and sufficiently expert at the task. Use of unbiased expert data collectors is especially important for collecting observation and interview data because these data in part depend on the subjective interpretation by the data collector.

Also, data collectors can influence in other ways the information that is obtained. For example, if health professional staff are asked to complete a job satisfaction survey and their supervisor is asked to collect the surveys for return to the evaluator, what problems might occur? Might some staff be hesitant to provide negative scores on certain items, even though they hold a negative opinion? Likewise, physiological data can be altered, however unintentionally, by the data collector. For example, an outcome evaluation might be conducted to determine whether a series of biofeedback classes given to young executives can reduce stress as measured by pulse and blood pressure. How might some executives' pulse and blood pressure results be affected by a data collector who is extremely physically attractive or overtly acting rushed or frustrated?

Use of trained data collectors from an external agency is, in most cases, not a financially viable option. The potential for a data collector to bias data can be minimized using a number of less expensive alternatives, however. First, the number of data collectors should be limited as much as possible because this step automatically decreases person-based variation. Also, individuals assisting with data collection should wear similar conservative clothing and speak in a moderate tone. Because moderate tone, for example, may not be interpreted the same way by everyone, at least one practice session or dry run should be held with all data collectors prior to actually conducting the evaluation. In addition, data collection should be conducted by someone who has no vested interest in results and who will be perceived as unbiased and nonthreatening by those providing the data. Furthermore, providing interview scripts to be read verbatim by the interviewer can ensure that all clients or staff being interviewed are asked the same questions.

With the advent of continuous quality improvement (CQI) based on evidence as an expectation of daily activity in healthcare organizations, health professionals are obligated to become more knowledgeable about principles of measurement and ways to implement measurement techniques in their work setting (Joint Commission on Accreditation of Healthcare Organizations, 2006).

One benefit that this change in practice has for the health professional as educator is that more people within the organization have some expertise in data collection and are motivated to help with data collection activities. Another potential benefit is that data collection activities already are likely to be a part of practice. Not only might the health professional as educator have readily available individuals to assist with data collection, but the educator also might have readily available and usable instruments and data.

Use of a portfolio as a method for evaluation of an individual's learning over time has been documented in the literature for more than 30 years, primarily from an academic perspective (Appling, Naumann, & Berk, 2001; Ball, Daly, & Carnwell, 2000; Cayne, 1995; Hayes, 2007; Roberts, Priest, & Bromage, 2001). Although formal education of health professional students is not the focus of this text, other uses of portfolios are relevant to the role of the practice-based health professional as educator. For example, currently the National Board for Certification in Occupational Therapy (NBCOT, 2009) recommends occupational therapy practitioners individually complete a professional portfolio for recertification.

Given the growing importance of portfolio documentation for career advancement, the health professional as educator may find several colleagues asking for assistance in creating and maintaining a portfolio that provides a strong base of evaluative evidence demonstrating a health professional's continuing professional development and consequent impact on practice (Byrne et al., 2007; Oermann, 2002). Perhaps the best suggestion the health professional educator might offer—and heed—is to clarify the focus of the portfolio as determined by the requiring organization (in this case, the primary audience) as stated in that organization's criteria for portfolio completion. Is the focus more on process evaluation, outcome evaluation, or both? Specifically, is the health professional expected to demonstrate reflective practice? If so, what does the organization accept as evidence of reflective practice?

One reason why focus clarification is so challenging is because there is no consistent description of how portfolios are to be used or what they are to contain. In its simplest form, a practice portfolio comprises a collection of information and materials about a health professional's practice that have been gathered over time. The issue of whether this collection is intended to demonstrate previous learning or whether the process of collecting is itself a learning experience continues to foster debate (Cayne, 1995; Fitch, Peet, Reed, & Tolman, 2008; Roberts et al., 2001).

Central to this issue is the notion of reflective practice. First coined by Schön (1987), the term **reflective practice** still does not have a commonly agreed-upon definition (Clouder, 2000; Cotton, 2001; Epstein, 2008; Hannigan, 2001; Morgan, 2009; Musolino & Mostrom, 2005; Roche & Coote, 2008; Teekman, 2000; Wainwright, Shepard, Harman, & Stephens, 2010). Noveletsky (2007) offers one definition of reflective practice "as the process of exposing the contradictions in practice … [when] the health professional must first come to understand what he or she defines as ideal practice" (p. 141). Schön describes two key components of reflective practice as reflection-in-action and reflection-on-action. Reflection-in-action occurs when the health professional introspectively considers a practice activity while performing it so that change for improvement can be made at that moment. Reflection-on-action occurs when the health professional introspectively analyzes a practice activity after its completion so as to gain insights for the future (Cotton, 2001). From an evaluation perspective, these components are similar to formative and summative evaluation, indicating that reflective practice has more than one focus (Paschal, Jensen, & Mostrom, 2002).

Given the complexity of attempting to address multiple foci with the use of a single evaluation

method—the practice portfolio—it is not surprising that use of portfolios has inspired such controversy. To the extent that a portfolio is required to include physical documentation as evidence of reflective practice (an introspective activity), the argument by some that portfolios are not adequately reliable or valid for use in evaluation of learning is not at all surprising (Ball et al., 2000; Cayne, 1995).

Evaluation Instruments

In the selection, modification, or construction of evaluation instruments, health professional educators must consider some key points. Whenever possible, an evaluation should be conducted using existing instruments because instrument development requires considerable expertise, time, and expenditure of resources. Construction of an original evaluation instrument, whether it is in the form of a questionnaire or a type of equipment, also requires rigorous testing for reliability and validity (Osborne, Elsworth, & Whitfield, 2007). Timely provision of evaluative information for making decisions rarely allows the luxury of the several months to several years needed to develop a reliable, valid instrument.

The initial step in instrument selection is to conduct a literature search for evaluations similar to the evaluation being planned. A helpful place to begin is with the same journals listed earlier in this chapter. Instruments that have been used in more than one study should be given preference over an instrument developed for a single use because instruments used multiple times generally have been more thoroughly tested for reliability and validity. Once a number of potential instruments have been identified, each instrument must be carefully critiqued to determine whether it is, in fact, appropriate for the evaluation planned.

First, the instrument must measure the performance being evaluated exactly as that performance has been operationally defined for the evaluation. For example, if satisfaction with a continuing education program is operationally defined to include a score of 80% or higher on five specific program components (such as educator responsiveness to questions, relevance of content, and so on), then the instrument selected to measure participant satisfaction with the program must include exactly those five components and must be able to be scored in percentages.

Second, an appropriate instrument should have documented evidence of its reliability and validity with individuals who are as closely matched as possible with the people from whom data will be collected. When evaluating the ability of older adult clients to complete activities of daily living, for example, the evaluator would not want to use an instrument developed for evaluating the ability of young orthopedic clients to complete routine activities. Similarities in reading level and visual acuity also should exist if the instrument being evaluated is a questionnaire or scale that participants will complete themselves.

Existing instruments being considered for selection also must be affordable, must be feasible for use in the location planned for conducting data collection, and should require minimal training on the part of data collectors.

The evaluation instrument most likely to require modification from an existing tool or development of an entirely new instrument is a cognitive test. The primary reason for constructing such a test is that it must be consistent with content actually covered during the educational program or activity. The intent of a cognitive test is to be comprehensive and relevant and to fairly test the learner's knowledge of content covered. Using a test blueprint is one of the most helpful methods for ensuring comprehensiveness and relevance of test questions. A blueprint enables the evaluator to be certain that each area of instructional content is included in the test and that content areas empha-

sized during instruction are similarly emphasized during testing.

Barriers to Evaluation

If evaluation is so crucial to healthcare education, why is evaluation often an afterthought or even overlooked entirely? The reasons given for not conducting evaluations are many and varied but rarely, if ever, insurmountable. To overcome barriers to evaluation, they first must be identified and understood; then, the health professional educator must design and conduct the evaluation in a way that minimizes or eliminates as many identified barriers as possible.

Barriers to conducting an evaluation can be classified into three broad categories:

1. Lack of clarity
2. Lack of ability
3. Fear of punishment or loss of self-esteem

Lack of Clarity

Lack of clarity most often results from an unclear, unstated, or ill-defined evaluation focus. Undertaking any action is difficult if the performer does not know the purpose for taking that action. Undertaking an evaluation certainly is no different. Often evaluations are attempted to determine the quality of an educational program or activity, yet quality is not defined beyond some vague sense of goodness. What is goodness and from whose perspective will it be determined? Who or what has to demonstrate evidence of goodness? What will happen if goodness is or is not evident? Inability to answer these or similar questions creates a significant barrier to conducting an evaluation. Not knowing the purpose of an evaluation or what will be done with evaluation results, for example, can become a barrier for even the most seasoned evaluator.

Barriers in this category have the greatest potential for successful resolution because the best solution for lack of clarity is to provide clarity. Recall that evaluation focus includes five components: (1) audience, (2) purpose, (3) questions, (4) scope, and (5) resources. To overcome a potential lack of clarity, the health professional educator must identify all five components and make them available to those conducting the evaluation.

A clearly stated purpose must explain why the evaluation is being conducted. Part of the answer to this question consists of a statement detailing what decisions will be made on the basis of evaluation results. Clear identification of who constitutes the primary audience is as important as a clear statement of purpose. It is from the perspective of the primary audience that terms such as *quality* should be defined and operationalized. Although the results of the evaluation provide the information on which decisions will be made, the primary audience actually makes those decisions.

LACK OF ABILITY

Lack of ability to conduct an evaluation most often results from insufficient knowledge of how to conduct the evaluation or insufficient or inaccessible resources needed to conduct the evaluation. Clarification of evaluation purpose, questions, and scope is often the responsibility of the primary audience. Clarification of resources, however, is the responsibility of both the primary audience and the individuals conducting the evaluation.

The primary audience members are accountable for providing the necessary resources—personnel, equipment, time, facilities, and so on—to conduct the evaluation they are requesting. Unless these individuals have some expertise in evaluation, they may not know what resources are necessary. The persons conducting the evaluation, therefore, must accept responsibility for knowing what resources are necessary and for providing that information to the primary audience. The person asked or expected to conduct the evaluation may be as uncertain about necessary resources as is the primary audience, however.

Lack of knowledge of what resources are necessary or lack of actual resources may form a barrier to conducting an evaluation that can be difficult, although not impossible, to overcome. Lack of knowledge can be resolved or minimized by enlisting the assistance of individuals with needed expertise through consultation or contract (if funds are available), through collaboration, or indirectly through literature review.

Lack of other resources—time, money, equipment, facilities, and so on—should be documented, justified, and presented to those requesting the evaluation. Alternative methods for conducting the evaluation, including the option of making decisions in the absence of any evaluation, also should be documented and presented.

FEAR OF PUNISHMENT OR LOSS OF SELF-ESTEEM

Evaluation might be perceived as a judgment of personal worth. Individuals being evaluated may fear that anything less than a perfect performance will result in punishment or that their mistakes will be seen as evidence that they are somehow unworthy or incompetent as human beings. These fears form one of the greatest barriers to conducting an evaluation.

Unfortunately, the fear of punishment or of being seen as unworthy may not easily be overcome, especially if the individual has had past negative experiences. Consider, for example, traditional quality assurance monitoring, where results were used to correct deficiencies through punitive measures. As another example, many times an educator has interpreted learner dissatisfaction with a teaching style as learner dislike for the educator as a person. Or many times pediatric clients' parents said, "If you don't do it right, the doctor won't let you go home ... and we will be very disappointed in you." And everyone probably has experienced test anxiety at some point in their education.

The first step in overcoming this barrier is to realize that the potential for its existence may be close to 100%. Individuals whose performance or knowledge is being evaluated are not likely to say overtly that evaluation represents a threat to them. Rather, they are far more likely to demonstrate self-protective behaviors or attitudes that can range from failure to attend a class that has a posttest, to providing socially desirable answers on a questionnaire, to responding with hostility to evaluation questions. An individual may intentionally choose to fail an evaluation as a method for controlling the uncertainty of success.

The second step in overcoming the barrier of fear or threat is to remember that "the person is more important than the performance or the product" (Narrow, 1979, p. 185). If the purpose of an evaluation is to facilitate better learning, as in process evaluation, the focus is on the process. For example, in teaching a patient how to perform urinary self-catheterization using the same clean technique as she will use at home, the educator carefully and thoroughly explains each step in the process of urinary self-catheterization, observing the patient's intent expression and frequent head nods during the explanation. When the patient tries to demonstrate the steps, however, she is unable to begin. Why? One answer may be that the use of an auditory teaching style does not match the patient's visual learning style. Another possibility might be that too many distractions are present in the immediate environment, making concentration on learning all but impossible.

A third step in overcoming the fear of punishment or threatened loss of self-esteem is to point out achievements, if they exist, or to continue to encourage effort if learning has not been achieved. The health professional as educator should give praise honestly, focusing on the task at hand.

Finally, and perhaps most important, communication of information can help prevent or minimize fear. Lack of clarity exists as a barrier for those who are the subjects of an evaluation as much as for those who will conduct the evaluation. If learners or educators know and understand the focus of an evaluation, they may be less fearful than if such information is left to their imaginations.

Also, failure to provide and protect certain information may be unethical or even illegal. For example, any evaluative data about an individual that can be identified with that specific person should be collected only with the individual's informed consent. The ethical and legal importance of informed consent as a protection of human rights must be a central concern and responsibility of anyone involved in collecting data for evaluation purposes.

Conducting the Evaluation

To conduct an evaluation means to implement the evaluation design by using the instruments chosen or developed according to the methods selected. How smoothly an evaluation is implemented depends primarily on how carefully and thoroughly the evaluation was planned. Planning is not a complete guarantee of success, however. Three methods to minimize the effects of unexpected events that occur when carrying out an evaluation are as follows:

1. Conduct a pilot test first.
2. Include extra time.
3. Keep a sense of humor.

Conducting a pilot test of the evaluation entails trying out the data collection methods, instruments, and plan for data analysis with a few individuals who are the same as or very similar to those who will be included in the full evaluation. If the health professional educator plans to use any newly developed instruments for the evaluation, a pilot test must be conducted to assess reliability, validity, interpretability, and feasibility of those new instruments. Also, a pilot test should be carried out prior to implementing a full evaluation that will be expensive or time consuming to conduct or on which major decisions will be based. Process evaluation generally is not amenable to pilot testing unless a new instrument will be used for data collection. Pilot testing should be considered prior to conducting outcome, impact, or program evaluations, however.

Ream, Richardson, and Evison (2005) describe a pilot test conducted to evaluate the feasibility of a multidisciplinary education and support group program for patients with cancer treatment–related fatigue. Results provided important information about how to involve team members from different disciplines to best meet clients' needs from a client-centered perspective. Because only six patients were included in the pilot, findings were not intended to show a significant effect of the education; rather they were intended to indicate whether a more expanded program might be beneficial.

Including extra time while conducting an evaluation means leaving room for unexpected delays. Almost invariably, more time is needed than anticipated for evaluation planning, data collection, and translation of evaluation results into reports that will be meaningful and usable by the primary audience.

Because those delays not only will occur but also are likely to occur at inconvenient times during the evaluation, keeping a sense of humor is vitally important. An evaluator with a sense of humor is more likely to maintain a realistic perspective in reporting results that include negative findings, too. However, it is important to acknowledge that an audience with a vested interest in positive evaluation results may blame the evaluator if results are lower than expected.

Analyzing and Interpreting Data Collected

The purposes for conducting data analysis are twofold: (1) to organize data so that they can provide meaningful information, and (2) to provide answers to evaluation questions. *Data* and *information* are not synonymous terms. That is, a mass of numbers or a mass of comments does not become information until it has been organized into coherent tables, graphs, or categories that are relevant to the purpose for conducting the evaluation.

Basic decisions about how data will be analyzed are dictated by the nature of the data and by the questions used to focus the evaluation. As described earlier, data can be quantitative or qualitative. Data also can be described as continuous or discrete. Age and level of anxiety are examples of continuous data; gender and diagnosis are examples of discrete data. Finally, data can be differentiated by level of measurement. All qualitative data are at the nominal level of measurement, meaning they are described in terms of categories such as health focused versus illness focused. Quantitative data can be at the nominal, ordinal, interval, or ratio level of measurement. The level of measurement of the data determines what statistics can be used to analyze those data. A useful suggestion for deciding how data will be analyzed is to enlist the assistance of someone with experience in data analysis.

Analysis of data should be consistent with the type of data collected. In other words, all data analysis must be rigorous, but not all data analysis needs to include use of inferential statistics. For example, qualitative data, such as verbal comments obtained during interviews and written comments obtained from open-ended questionnaires, are summarized, or themed, into categories of similar comments. Each category or theme is qualitatively described by directly quoting one or more comments that are typical of that category. These categories then may be quantitatively described using descriptive statistics such as total counts and percentages.

Different qualitative methods for analyzing data are emerging as they gain legitimacy in a scientific environment once ruled by traditional experimental quantitative methods. One use of qualitative methods in evaluation is called fourth-generation evaluation (Hamilton, 1993). Perhaps most beneficial in conducting a process evaluation, fourth-generation evaluation focuses on teacher–learner interaction and observation of that interaction by the teachers and learners present. Evaluation is an integral component of the education process; that is, evaluation helps construct the education. Data collection, analysis, and use of results occur concurrently. Teacher and learner questions and responses are observed and recorded during an education program. These observations are summarized at the time of occurrence and throughout the program, and then are used to provide immediate feedback to participants in the educational activity.

The first step in analysis of quantitative data consists of organization and summarization using statistics such as frequencies and percentages that describe the sample or population from which the data were collected. A description of a population of learners, for example, might include such information as response rate and frequency of learner demographic characteristics. **Table 14–2** presents an example of how such information might be displayed.

The next step in analysis of quantitative data is to select the statistical procedures appropriate for the type of data collected that will answer questions posed in planning the evaluation. Again, a good suggestion is to enlist the assistance of an expert statistician.

Reporting Evaluation Results

Results of an evaluation must be reported if the evaluation is to be of any use. Such a statement seems obvious, but many times an evaluation was reportedly being conducted, but its results were never announced. Many times people participate in an evaluation but never see the final report. How many times have health professionals conducted an evaluation but not provided anyone with a report on findings? Almost all health professionals, if they are honest, would have to answer this question with a number greater than zero.

Reasons for not reporting evaluation results are diverse and numerous. The four major reasons for why evaluative data may often never get from the spreadsheet to the customer are these:

1. Ignorance of who should receive the results
2. Belief that the results are not important or will not be used

Table 14–2 Demographic Comparison of Survey Respondents to Total Course Participants Using Group Averages

Learner Demographics	Survey Respondents ($n = 50$)	All Course Participants ($n = 55$)
Age	27.5 years	25.5 years
Length of time employed	3.5 years	7.5 years
Years of post-high school education	2.0 years	2.0 years

3. Inability to translate results into language useful for producing the report
4. Fear that results will be misused

Following a few guidelines when planning an evaluation can significantly increase the likelihood that results of the evaluation will be reported to the appropriate individuals or groups, in a timely manner, and in usable form. These guidelines are as follows:

- Be audience focused.
- Stick to the evaluation purpose.
- Use data as intended.

Be Audience Focused

The purpose for conducting an evaluation is to provide information for decision making by the primary audience. The report of evaluation results must, therefore, be consistent with that purpose. One rule of thumb to use: Always begin an evaluation report with an executive summary or an abstract that is no longer than one page. No matter who the audience members are, their time is important to them.

A second rule of thumb is to present evaluation results in a format and language that the audience can use and understand without additional interpretation. This statement does not mean that technical information should be excluded from a report to a lay audience; rather, it means that such information should be written using nontechnical terms. Graphs and charts generally are easier to understand than are tables of numbers, for example. If a secondary audience of technical experts also will receive a report of evaluation results, the report should include an appendix containing the more detailed or technically specific information in which they might be interested.

A third rule of thumb is that the evaluator should make every effort to present results in person as well as in writing. A direct presentation provides an opportunity for the evaluator to answer questions and to assess whether the report meets the needs of the audience.

A final rule to follow is that the evaluation should include specific recommendations or suggestions for how evaluation results might be used. Often the primary audience will expect these as part of the evaluation. Even if the evaluator is not directly asked to provide specific recommendations, however, doing so may increase the likelihood that the results actually will be used.

Stick to the Evaluation Purpose

Evaluators should keep the main body of an evaluation report focused on information that fulfills the purpose for conducting the evaluation. They should provide answers to the questions asked. They should also include the main aspects of how the evaluation was conducted but avoid a diary-like chronology of the activities of the evaluators.

Use Data as Intended

Evaluators should maintain consistency with actual data when reporting and interpreting findings. A question not asked cannot be answered, and data not collected cannot be interpreted. If evaluators did not measure or observe a teacher's performance, for example, they should not draw conclusions about the adequacy of that performance. Similarly, if the only measures of client performance were those conducted in the hospital, they must not interpret successful inpatient performance as successful performance by the client at home or at work.

These examples may seem obvious, but conceptual leaps from the data collected to the conclusions drawn from those data are an all-too-common occurrence. One suggestion that decreases the opportunity to overinterpret data is to include evaluation results and interpretation of those results in separate sections of the report.

A discussion of any limitations of the evaluation is an important part of the evaluation report. For example, if several clients were unable to complete a questionnaire because they could not understand it or because they were too fatigued, the report should say so. Knowing that evaluation results do not include data from clients below a certain educational level or physical status can help the audience realize that they cannot make decisions about those clients based on the evaluation. Discussion of limitations also provides useful information for what not to do the next time a similar evaluation is conducted.

State of the Evidence

A recent search of the Cumulative Index to Nursing and Allied Health Literature (CINAHL) database using the keywords *evaluation, patient education,* and *health professional* identified 205 articles. Applying *research, English language,* and *2002–2009* as inclusion criteria limited the number of articles to a total of 72. A review of titles and abstracts of these 72 articles to exclude those that did not specifically focus on the evaluation process itself still identified 59 articles directly relevant to the state of evidence in evaluation of client education.

A search conducted in the same manner, but replacing the keywords *health professional* with keywords of individual professions such as *occupational therapy, physical therapy, respiratory therapy,* and *pharmacy,* resulted in identification of a range of 1 to 143 articles. A search conducted in the same manner, but replacing the keyword *patient education* with two keywords, *in-service education* and *continuing education,* resulted in identification of more than 2,000 articles. Using the same search criteria, but changing the time frame to articles published prior to 1992, the year that evidence-based practice first appeared in the literature, no relevant articles were found.

Considering the fact that this search was limited to only those articles published in one database, in English, and during only an 8-year period, the

findings were impressive. Clearly, a body of evidence exists and is growing.

One reason why a body of literature on evaluation has come into being is because journal review boards have accepted evaluation projects and internal evidence generated by such projects as important for publication. Many of the articles providing evidence on evaluation of client and staff development education are not research articles—articles providing external evidence resulting from studies conducted to provide generalizable results. For example, Smith and colleagues (2005) describe their project for evaluating client satisfaction with discharge education, cautioning that their outcomes data cannot be generalized beyond their specific setting. Practice-based evidence from such projects should be considered carefully because clients in one setting may not respond in the same manner as would clients in another setting. However, this information is still valuable for informing practice.

DeSilets (2007) comments that research on evidence-based education activities is still limited. She does summarize one study, however, in which health teams who received an evidence-based educational session demonstrated more appropriate outcome behaviors than did health teams who received traditional education. Other studies and examples of educational evaluation found in the literature have been presented throughout this chapter.

Published evidence can now be found on such topics as content and instructiveness of patient education materials (Johansson, Salentera, Katajisto, & Leino-Kilpi, 2004), computer-based instruction versus instructor-led instruction for staff education (Walker, Harrington, & Cole, 2006), and use of educational videos versus written handouts for clients recovering from surgery (Klein-Fedyshin, Burda, Epstein, & Lawrence, 2005). These studies and others are evaluative in nature and, although rigorous, do not meet traditional criteria for experimental research. Nevertheless, the results of these studies are important for informing health professionals in their role as educators of clients, staff, and students.

Summary

Conducting evaluation in healthcare education involves gathering, summarizing, interpreting, and using data to determine the extent to which an educational activity is efficient, effective, and useful for those who participate in that activity as learners, teachers, or sponsors. The following five types of evaluation are discussed in this chapter: (1) process, (2) content, (3) outcome, (4) impact, and (5) program evaluations. Each of these types focuses on a specific purpose, scope, and questions to be asked of an educational activity or program to meet the needs of those who ask for the evaluation or who can benefit from its results. Each type of evaluation also requires some level of available resources for the evaluation to be conducted.

The number and variety of evaluation models, designs, methods, and instruments are experiencing an exponential growth as the importance of evaluation becomes more evident in today's healthcare environment. A number of guidelines, rules of thumb, and suggestions are included in this chapter's discussion of how a health professional educator might go about selecting the most appropriate model, design, methods, and instruments for a particular type of evaluation.

The importance of evaluation as internal evidence has gained even greater momentum with the movement toward evidence-based practice. Perhaps the most important point to remember is this: Each aspect of the evaluation process is important, but all of them are meaningless if the results of evaluation are not used to guide future action in planning and carrying out educational interventions.

REVIEW QUESTIONS

1. How is the term *evaluation* defined?
2. How does the process of evaluation differ from the process of assessment?
3. How is evidence-based practice related to evaluation?
4. How does internal evidence differ from external evidence?
5. What is the first and most crucial step in planning any evaluation?
6. What are the five basic components included in determining the focus of an evaluation?
7. What are the five basic types (levels) of evaluation in order from simple to complex identified in Abruzzese's RSA evaluation model?
8. How does formative evaluation differ from summative evaluation, and what is another name for each of these two types of evaluation?
9. What is the purpose of each type (level) of evaluation as described by Abruzzese in her RSA evaluation model?
10. What data collection methods can be used in conducting an evaluation of educational interventions?
11. What are the three major barriers to conducting an evaluation?
12. When and why should a pilot test be conducted prior to implementing a full evaluation?
13. What are three guidelines to follow in reporting the results of an evaluation?

CASE STUDY

James, a health professional employed at a middle school, just finished reading an interesting journal article related to his practice discipline. The article was about recently conducted research on middle school students and using notebook computers. More than 40% of the subjects complained of musculoskeletal discomfort while using this technology. He found the results interesting because when working with students in the classroom, he has noticed their posture to be awkward while they are typing on their notebook computers. He overheard students complaining, "My neck, shoulders, and back always hurt when I am on the notebook computer." James also knows from experience that many of his students gravitate toward learning when it incorporates technology. James requests a meeting with the school technology consultant, Andrea. He asks her, "Can you help me design an interactive online course that is fun and engaging for students to educate them about ergonomic principles?" Andrea eagerly agrees to work with James to build such a course, which also links them to Web sites and videos of ergonomic examples. James realizes that he needs to build an evaluation into the design of the interactive online course. He decides to use process (formative) evaluation so that he can make ongoing adjustments in this educational activity as soon as they are needed.

1. What primary question should James be asking that is consistent with the purpose of process evaluation?
2. What type of evaluation should be selected to determine the effects or outcomes of this online teaching effort?
3. If evaluation is so crucial to healthcare education, why is evaluation often an afterthought or even overlooked entirely by the educator?

References

Abruzzese, R. S. (1992). Evaluation in nursing staff development. In R. S. Abruzzese (Ed.), *Nursing staff development: Strategies for success* (pp. 235–248). St. Louis, MO: Mosby–Year Book.

Albanese, M. A., & Gjerde, C. L. (1987). Evaluation. In H. VanHoozer et al. (Eds.), *The teaching process: Theory and practice in nursing* (pp. 269–308). Norwalk, CT: Appleton-Century-Crofts.

Aldana, S., Barlow, M., Smith, R., Yanowitz, F., Adams, T., Loveday, L., et al. (2006). A worksite diabetes prevention program: Two-year impact on employee health. *American Association of Occupational Health Nursing Journal, 54*(9), 389–395.

Appling, S. E., Naumann, P. L., & Berk, R. A. (2001). Using a faculty evaluation triad to achieve evidence-based teaching. *Nursing and Health Care Perspectives, 22*(5), 247–251.

Ball, E., Daly, W. M., & Carnwell, R. (2000). The use of portfolios in the assessment of learning and competence. *Nursing Standard, 14*(43), 35–37.

Berk, R. A., & Rossi, P. H. (1990). *Thinking about program evaluation*. Newbury Park, CA: Sage.

Billings, J. R. (2000). Community development: A critical review of approaches to evaluation. *Journal of Advanced Nursing, 31*(2), 472–480.

Bradshaw, M. J. (2007). The clinical pathway: A tool to evaluate clinical learning. In M. J. Bradshaw & A. J. Lowenstein (Eds.), *Innovative teaching strategies in nursing and related health professions* (pp. 427–436). Sudbury, MA: Jones and Bartlett.

Byrne, M., Delarose, T., King, C. A., Leske, J., Sapnas, K. G., & Schroeter, K. (2007). Continued professional competence and portfolios. *Journal of Trauma Nursing, 14*(1), 24–31.

Cayne, J. (1995). Portfolios: A developmental influence? *Journal of Advanced Nursing, 21*(2), 395–405.

Clouder, L. (2000). Reflective practice in physiotherapy education: A critical conversation. *Studies in Higher Education, 25*(2), 211–223.

Cotton, A. H. (2001). Private thoughts in public spheres: Issues in reflection and reflective practices in nursing. *Journal of Advanced Nursing, 36*(4), 512–559.

Covell, C. L. (2005). BCLS certification of the nursing staff: An evidence-based approach. *Journal of Nursing Care Quality, 21*(1), 63–69.

DeSilets, L. D. (2007). The value of evidence-based continuing education. *Journal of Continuing Education in Nursing, 38*(2), 52–53.

Eklund, K., Sonn, U., & Dahlin-Ivanoff, S. (2004). Long-term evaluation of a health education programme for elderly persons with visual impairment. A randomized study. *Disability & Rehabilitation, 26*(7), 401–409.

Epstein, R. M. (2008). Reflection, perception, and the acquisition of wisdom. *Medical Education, 42*, 1048–1050.

Fitch, D., Peet, M., Reed, B. G., & Tolman, R. (2008). The use of eportfolios in evaluating the curriculum and student learning. *Journal of Social Work Education, 44*(13), 37–53.

Gerrish, K. (2001). A pluralistic evaluation to explore people's experiences of stroke services in the community. *Health & Social Care in the Community, 7*(4), 248–256.

Gonzalez, B., Lupon, J., Herreros, J., Urrutia, A., Altimir, S., Coll, R., et al. (2005). Patient's education by nurse: What we really do achieve? *European Journal of Cardiovascular Nursing, 4*(2), 107–111.

Haggard, A. (1989). Evaluating patient education. In A. Haggard (Ed.), *Handbook of patient education* (pp. 159–186). Rockville, MD: Aspen.

Hamilton, G. A. (1993). An overview of evaluation research methods with implications for nursing staff development. *Journal of Nursing Staff Development, 9*(3), 148–154.

Hannigan, B. (2001). A discussion of the strengths and weaknesses of "reflection" in nursing practice and education. *Journal of Clinical Nursing, 10*(2), 278–283.

Hart, E. (1999). The use of pluralistic evaluation to explore people's experiences of stroke services in the community. *Health & Social Care in the Community, 7*(4), 248–256.

Hayes, J. M. (2007). Evaluation of programmatic learning outcomes. In M. J. Bradshaw & A. J. Lowenstein (Eds.), *Innovative teaching strategies in nursing and related health professions* (pp. 409–426). Sudbury, MA: Jones and Bartlett.

Holzemer, W. (1992). Evaluation methods in continuing education. *Journal of Continuing Education in Nursing, 23*(4), 174–181.

Johansson, K., Salentera, S., Katajisto, J., & Leino-Kilpi, H. (2004). Written orthopedic patient education materials from the point of view of empowerment by education. *Patient Education and Counseling, 52*, 175–181.

Johnson, J. H., & Olesinski, N. (1995). Program evaluation: Key to success. *Journal of Nursing Administration, 25*(1), 53–60.

Joint Commission on Accreditation of Healthcare Organizations. (2006). *Accreditation manual for hospitals.* Oakbrook Terrace, IL: Author.

Klein-Fedyshin, M., Burda, M. L., Epstein, B. A., & Lawrence, B. (2005). Collaborating to enhance patient education and recovery. *Journal of the Medical Librarians Association, 93*(4), 440–445.

Koch, T. (2000). "Having a say": Negotiation in fourth-generation evaluation. *Journal of Advanced Nursing, 31*(1), 117–125.

Lott, T. F. (2006). Moving forward: Creating a new nursing services orientation program. *Journal for Nurses in Staff Development, 22*(5), 214–221.

Melnyk, B. M., & Fineout-Overholt, E. (2005). *Evidence-based practice in nursing & healthcare: A guide to best practice.* Philadelphia: Lippincott Williams & Wilkins.

Morgan, G. (2009). Reflective practice and self-awareness. *Perspectives in Public Health, 129*(4), 161–162.

Musolini, G. M., & Mostrom, E. (2005). Reflection and the scholarship of teaching, learning, and assessment. *Journal of Physical Therapy Education, 19*(3), 52–66.

Narrow, B. (1979). *Patient teaching in nursing practice: A patient and family-centered approach.* New York: Wiley.

National Board for Certification in Occupational Therapy. (2009). Requirements for recertification. Retrieved May 11, 2010, from http://www.nbcot.org/pdf/Renewal-Handbook.pdf

Noveletsky, H. T. (2007). Reflective practice. In M. J. Bradshaw & A. J. Lowenstein (Eds.), *Innovative teaching in nursing and related health professions* (pp. 141–148). Sudbury, MA: Jones and Bartlett.

Oermann, M. H. (2002). Developing a professional portfolio in nursing. *Orthopaedic Nursing, 21*(2), 74–78.

Osborne, R. H., Elsworth, G. R., & Whitfield, K. (2007). The health education impact questionnaire (heiQ): An outcomes and evaluation measure for patient education and self-management interventions for people with chronic conditions. *Patient Education and Counseling, 66*, 192–201.

Paschal, K. A., Jensen, G. M., & Mostrom, E. (2002). Building portfolios: A means for developing habits or reflective practice in physical therapy education, *Journal of Physical Therapy Education, 16*(3), 38–53.

Puetz, B. E. (1992). Evaluation: Essential skill for the staff development specialist. In K. J. Kelly (Ed.), *Nursing staff development: Current competence, future focus.* Philadelphia: Lippincott.

Rankin, S. H., & Stallings, K. D. (2005). *Patient education in health and illness* (5th ed.). Philadelphia: Lippincott Williams & Wilkins.

Ream, E., Richardson, A., & Evison, M. (2005). A feasibility study to evaluate a group intervention for people with cancer experiencing fatigue following treatment. *Clinical Effectiveness in Nursing, 9*, 178–187.

Roberts, P., Priest, H., & Bromage, C. (2001). Selecting and utilizing data sources to evaluate health care education. *Nurse Researcher, 8*(3), 15–29.

Roche, A., & Coote, S. (2008). Focus group study of student physiotherapists' perception of reflection. *Medical Education, 42*, 1064–1070.

Ruzicki, D. A. (1987). Evaluating patient education—A vital part of the process. In C. E. Smith (Ed.), *Patient education: Nurses in partnership with other health professionals*. Orlando, FL: Grune & Stratton.

Sackett, D. L., Richardson, W. S., Rosenberg, W., & Haynes, R. B. (1997). *Evidence-based medicine: How to practice & teach EBM*. New York: Churchill-Livingstone.

Schön, D. A. (1987). *Educating the reflective practitioner. Towards a new design for teaching and learning in the professions*. London: Jossey-Bass.

Schreurs, K. M. G., Colland, V. T., Kuijer, R. G., Ridder, D. T. D., & van Elderen, T. (2003). Development, content, and process evaluation of a short self-management intervention in patients with chronic diseases requiring self-care behaviours. *Patient Education and Counseling, 51*, 133–141.

Smith, C. E., Rebeck, S., Schaag, H., Kleinbeck, S., Moor, J. M., & Bleich, M. R. (2005). A model for evaluating systemic change: Measuring outcomes of hospital discharge education redesign. *Journal of Nursing Administration, 35*(2), 67–73.

Stewart, A. L., Hays, R. D., & Ware, J. E. (1988). The MOS short-form general health survey: Reliability and validity in a patient population. *Medical Care, 26*(7), 724.

Suhayda, R., & Miller, J. M. (2006). Optimizing evaluation of nursing education programs. *Nurse Educator, 31*(5), 200–206.

Teekman, B. (2000). Exploring reflective thinking in nursing practice. *Journal of Advanced Nursing, 31*(5), 1125–1135.

Templeton, H., & Coates, V. (2004). Evaluation of an evidence-based education package for men with prostate cancer on hormonal manipulation therapy. *Patient Education and Counseling, 55*, 55–61.

Waddell, D. (1992). The effects of continuing education on nursing practice: A meta-analysis. *Journal of Continuing Education in Nursing, 23*(4), 164–168.

Wainwright, S. F., Shepard, K. F., Harman, L. B., & Stephens, J. (2010). Novice and experienced physical therapist clinicians: A comparison of how reflection is used to inform the clinical decision-making process. *Physical Therapy, 90*(1), 75–88.

Walker, B. L., Harrington, S. S., & Cole, C. S. (2006). The usefulness of computer-based instruction in providing educational opportunities for nursing staff. *Journal for Nurses in Staff Development, 22*(3), 144–149.

Walker, E., & Dewar, B. J. (2000). Moving on from interpretivism: An argument for constructivist evaluation. *Journal of Advanced Nursing, 32*(3), 713–720.

Ware, J. E., Jr., Davies-Avery, A., & Donald, C. A. (1978). *Conceptualization and measurement of health for adults in the health insurance study: Vol. V. General health perceptions*. Santa Monica, CA: RAND.

Watters, C. L., & Moran, W. P. (2006). Hip fractures—A joint effort. *Orthopaedic Nursing, 25*(3), 157–167.

Tests to Measure Readability and Comprehension and Tools to Assess Instructional Materials

How to Use the Spache Grade-Level Score Formula

1. For short passages, test the entire piece. For longer passages, test a minimum of three randomly selected samples of 100 words each. (If the 100-word mark in the sample falls after the midpoint of the sentence, count the sentence as a part of the sample.)
2. Average sentence length (a) can be determined by counting the number of words in the sample and dividing by the number of sentences. If a sentence is punctuated by a period, question mark, exclamation point, semicolon, or colon, count it as an independent sentence.
3. Count the number of words not on the Dale list (b) according to the following guidelines:
   - Count a word only once, even if it appears again or with variable endings later in the sample.
   - Do not count first names.
   - Do not count plurals or possessive endings of nouns.
   - Do not count regular verb forms (-*ing*, -*ed*, -*es*), but do count irregular verb forms.
   - Count adjective or adverb endings (-*ly*, -*er*, -*est*).
   - Count a group of words that consists of repetition of a single word (e.g., "oh, oh, oh"; "look, look, look") as a single sentence regardless of punctuation.
   - Do not count familiar letters like A, B, C.

4. Apply the formula:

$$GL = 0.141(a) + 0.086(b) + 0.839$$

where GL is grade level, (a) is average sentence length, and (b) is the number of words not listed on the Dale list.

In other words, multiply the average sentence length in a sample of 100 words (a) by 0.141. Then multiply the percent of words outside the Dale easy word list (b) by 0.086. To these figures, add a constant, 0.839. The sum represents the estimated reading difficulty of the book. This will be a figure such as 2.267, which, when rounded off as 2.3, designates a book equal in difficulty to readers of school textbooks commonly used in the third month of second grade. When using this formula, it is suggested that at least three samples from the reading material be scored and the results averaged for a more reliable estimate of reading difficulty (Spache, 1953; Spadero, 1983).

How to Use the Flesch–Kincaid Scale

1. To test a whole piece of writing, take three to five 100-word samples of an article or twenty-five to thirty 100-word samples of a book. For short pieces, test the entire selection. Do not pick good or typical samples, but choose every third paragraph or every other page. In a 100-word sample, find the sentence that ends nearest to the 100-word mark; that may be, for example, at the 94th or the 109th word. Start each sample at the beginning of a paragraph, but do not use an introductory paragraph as part of the sample. Count contractions and hyphenated words as one word; count numbers and letters separated by space as words.
2. Figure the average sentence length (SL) by counting the number of words and dividing by the number of sentences. In counting sentences, follow units of thought marked off by periods, colons, semicolons, question marks, or exclamation points.
3. Determine word length (WL) by counting the number of syllables in each word in the sample as they are normally read aloud (i.e., two syllables for $ ["dollars"] and four syllables for *1918* ["nineteen-eighteen"]). It helps to read silently aloud while counting. Divide the syllables by the number of words in the sample and multiply by 100.
4. Determine the average WL by multiplying it by 0.846 and the average SL by multiplying it by 1.015. Then apply the formula:

$$RE = 206.835 - 0.846 \text{ (WL)} - 1.015 \text{ (SL)}$$

where RE is the reading ease score, after WL and SL have been subtracted from 206.835 (Flesch, 1948; Spadero, 1983; Spadero et al., 1980).

The reading ease score ranges from zero (practically unreadable) to 100 (very easy for any literate person) with interpretations in between (**Table A–1**).

Table A–1 Reading Ease Scores

Reading Ease Score	Syllables per 100 Words	Average Sentence Length	Difficulty Level	Grade Level
0–30	192 or more	29 or more	Very difficult	College graduate
30–50	167	25	Difficult	College
50–60	155	21	Fairly difficult	10–12
60–70	147	17	Standard	8–9
70–80	139	14	Fairly easy	7
80–90	131	11	Easy	6
90–100	123 or less	8 or less	Very easy	5

Source: Adapted from Flesch, R. (1948). A new readability yardstick. *Journal of Applied Psychology, 32*(3), 230; and Spadero, D. C. (1983). Assessing readability of patient information materials. *Pediatric Nursing, 9*(4), 275.

How to Use the Fog Formula

1. Count 100 words in succession (W). If the selection is long, choose several samples of 100 words from the text, and average the results.
2. Count the number of complete sentences (S). If the 100th word falls past the midpoint of a sentence, include this sentence in the count.
3. Divide the words (W) by the number of sentences (S).
4. Count the number of words having three or more syllables (A), but do not count verbs ending in -ed or -es that make a word have a third syllable; do not count capitalized words, and do not count combinations of simple words, such as *butterfly*.
5. Apply the formula:

$$GL = (W/S + A) \times 0.4$$

In other words, to find the GL (grade level), divide the number of words (W) by the number of complete sentences (S) in the sample 100-word passage, add the number of words having three or more syllables (A), and multiply the result by a constant of 0.4 (Gunning, 1968; Spadero, 1983; Spadero et al., 1980).

How to Use the Fry Readability Graph

1. Select three 100-word sample passages from near the beginning, middle, and end of a book, article, pamphlet, or brochure. Skip all proper nouns as part of the 100-word count. Fewer

than three samples and passages of less than 30 sentences can be used, but the user should be aware that there is necessarily a sacrifice in both reliability and validity.

2. Count the total number of sentences in each 100-word sample (estimating to the nearest 10th of a sentence for partial sentences).

3. Average the sentence counts of the three sample passages.

4. Count the total number of syllables in each 100-word sample. Count one syllable per vowel sound; for example, *cat* has one syllable, *blackbird* has two, and *continental* has four. Caution: Do not be fooled by word size (e.g., *polio* [three syllables], *through* [one syllable]). Endings such as *-y, -ed, -el,* or *-le* usually make a syllable (e.g., *ready* [two syllables], *bottle* [two syllables]). Graph users sometimes have trouble determining syllables. The clue is to believe what you hear (speech sounds), not what you see (e.g., *wanted* is a two-syllable word, but *stopped* is a one-syllable word). Count proper nouns, numerals, and initials or acronyms as words. A word is a symbol or group of symbols bounded by a blank space on either side. Thus, *1945, &,* and *IRS* are all words. Each symbol should receive a syllable count (i.e., the date 1945 is one word with five syllables, and the initials *IRS* is one word with three syllables).

5. Average the total number of syllables for the three samples.

6. Plot on the graph the average sentence count and the average word count to determine the appropriate grade level of the material. For example,

	Number of Syllables	Number of Sentences
First 100 words	153	6.3
Second 100 words	161	5.9
Third 100 words	139	5.2
Average count =	453 ÷ 3 = 151	17.4 ÷ 3 = 5.8

In the example, the average number of syllables is 151, and the average number of sentences is 5.8. When plotted on the graph (**Figure A–1**), the point falls within the approximate grade level of 9, which shows the materials to be at the ninth-grade readability level. If the point when plotted falls in the gray area, grade-level scores are invalid (Fry, 1968; Fry, 1977; Spadero et al., 1980).

How to Use the SMOG Formula

Passages Longer Than 30 Sentences

1. Count 10 consecutive sentences near the beginning, 10 consecutive sentences from the middle, and 10 consecutive sentences from the end of the selection to be assessed. A sentence is any independent unit of thought punctuated by a period, question mark, or exclamation point. If a sentence has a colon or semicolon, consider each part as a separate sentence.

Figure A–1 Fry readability graph—extended.

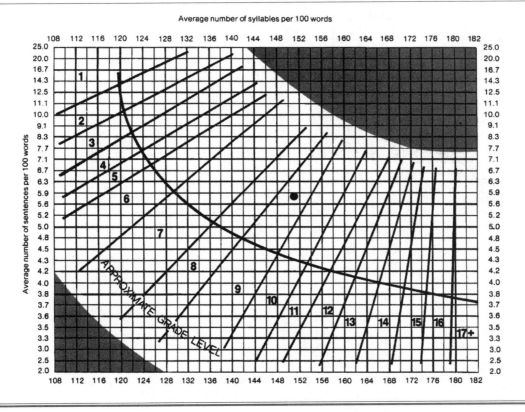

Average number of syllables per 100 words

Source: Edward Fry, Rutgers University Reading Center, New Brunswick, NJ.

2. From the 30 randomly selected sentences, count the words containing three or more syllables (polysyllabic), including repetitions. Abbreviated words should be read aloud to determine their syllable count (e.g., *Sept. = September =* three syllables). Letters or numerals in a string beginning or ending with a space or punctuation mark should be counted if, when read aloud in context, at least three syllables can be distinguished. Do not count words ending in *-ed* or *-es* if the ending makes the word have a third syllable. Hyphenated words are counted as one word. Proper nouns should be counted.

3. Approximate the reading grade level from the SMOG conversion table (**Table A–2**), or calculate the reading grade level by estimating the nearest perfect square root of the number of words with three or more syllables and then adding a constant of 3 to the square root. For example, if the total number of polysyllabic words was 53, the nearest perfect square would

Table A–2 SMOG CONVERSION TABLE

Word Count	Grade Level
0–2	4
3–6	5
7–12	6
13–20	7
21–30	8
31–42	9
43–56	10
57–72	11
73–90	12
91–110	13
111–132	14
133–156	15
157–182	16
183–210	17
211–240	18

Source: Developed by Harold C. McGraw, Office of Educational Research, Baltimore County Public Schools, Towson, MD.

be 49. The square root of 49 would be 7. By adding a constant of 3 (7 + 3 = 10), the reading level would be tenth grade.

Figure A–2 is an example of how to count all the words containing three or more syllables in a set of 10 sentences taken from one of the many pamphlets designed and distributed by the National Cancer Institute.

In Figure A–2, there are 20 words with three or more syllables. Note, the word *United* is not counted as a three-syllable word because only the *-ed* ending makes it polysyllabic (see rule 2). For this passage of 10 sentences, use the conversion table (**Table A–3**) as per the following words for passages shorter than 30 sentences. That is, for 10 sentences the conversion number is 3. Multiply 3 × 20 words = 60. Then using Table A–2, 60 falls at the 11th grade level.

Figure A–2 Example of counting words with three or more syllables.

> [1](Mastectomy:) **A Treatment for Breast Cancer**
>
> [2]You've been(diagnosed)as having breast cancer and your doctor has(recommended)a(mastectomy.)
> [3]If you're like most women, you(probably)have many concerns about this treatment for breast cancer.
> [4](Surgery)of any kind is a(frightening)(experience,)but(surgery)for breast cancer raises special concerns.
> [5]You may be(wondering)if the(surgery)will cure your cancer, how you'll feel after(surgery)—and how you're going to look.
> [6]It's not(unusual)to think about these things. [7]More than(100,000)women in the United States will have(mastectomies)this year. [8]Each of them will have(personal)concerns about the impact of the (surgery)on her life.
> [9]This booklet is designed to ease some of your fears by letting you know what to expect—from the time you enter the(hospital)to your(recovery)at home. [10]It may also help the special people in your life who are concerned about your(well-being.)

Source: National Cancer Institute of the National Institutes of Health, Public Health Service, U.S. Department of Health and Human Services, pamphlet entitled *Mastectomy: A Treatment for Breast Cancer* (1987, p. 1).

Passages Shorter Than 30 Sentences

1. Count the number of sentences in the material and the number of words containing three or more syllables.
2. In the left-hand column of Table A–3, locate the number of sentences. Then in the column opposite, locate the conversion number.
3. Multiply the word count found in step 1 by the conversion number. Locate this number in Table A–2 to obtain the corresponding grade level.
   Example: If the material is 25 sentences long and 15 words of three or more syllables were counted in this material, the conversion number in Table A–3 for 25 sentences is 1.2. Multiply the word count of 15 by 1.2 to get 18. For the word count of 18, the grade level in Table A–2 is 7. Therefore, the material is at a seventh-grade reading level.

Table A–3 SMOG CONVERSION FOR SAMPLES WITH FEWER THAN 30 SENTENCES

Number of Sentences in Sample Material	Conversion Number
29	1.03
28	1.07
27	1.1
26	1.15
25	1.2
24	1.25
23	1.3
22	1.36
21	1.43
20	1.5
19	1.58
18	1.67
17	1.76
16	1.87
15	2.0
14	2.14
13	2.3
12	2.5
11	2.7
10	3

How to Use the Cloze Test

How to Construct a Cloze Test

1. Select a prose passage (one without reference to figures, tables, charts, or pictures) from printed educational materials currently in use such as pamphlets, brochures, manuals, or

instruction sheets. Be sure the material is typical of what is normally given to patients but has not been previously read by them. The chosen passage should include whole paragraphs so that readers benefit from complete units of thought.

2. Leave the first and last sentences intact, and delete every fifth word from the other sentences for a total of about 50 word deletions. Do not delete proper nouns, but delete the word following the proper noun. Replace all deleted words with a line or blank space, all of equal length.

3. Ask the reader to fill in the blanks with the *exact* word replacements.

How to Score a Cloze Test

1. Count as correct only those words that *exactly* replace the deleted words (synonyms are not to be counted as a correct answer).

2. Inappropriate word endings such as *-s, -ed, -er,* and *-ing* should be counted as incorrect.

3. The raw score is the number of exact word replacements.

4. Divide the raw score by the total number of blank spaces to determine the percentage of correct responses. For example, if the passage has 50 blanks and the patient correctly filled in 25 blanks (10 were incorrect responses and 15 spaces were left blank), divide 25 by 50, and the percentage score would be 50%.

5. A score of 60% or above indicates the patient is fully capable of understanding the material. A score of 40–59% indicates the patient needs supplemental instruction. A score below 40% indicates that the material as written is too difficult for the patient to understand.

The following are the words that were deleted from the sample cloze test in **Figure A–3**.

1. it	14. cause	27. oxygen	40. pressure
2. heart	15. a	28. its	41. moment
3. kidney	16. blood	29. to	42. or
4. cases	17. to	30. your	43. are
5. causes	18. the	31. through	44. you
6. chemistry	19. work	32. the	45. arteries
7. a	20. muscle	33. oxygen	46. constrict
8. have	21. pump	34. begins	47. even
9. high	22. your	35. by	48. blood
10. remain	23. from	36. the	49. your
11. been	24. it	37. vessels	50. then
12. risk	25. all	38. pumping	51. return
13. heart	26. supplying	39. creates	52. relax

Note: Words are listed in missing order. Hyphenated words are counted as one word; words in parentheses are counted as a word.

Figure A–3 Sample cloze test.

High Blood Pressure

High blood pressure, also called hypertension, affects 37 million Americans—many of them older than 55. A dangerous, silent killer, __1__ can lead to stroke, __2__ attack and heart or __3__ failure. Yet, in most __4__, no one knows what __5__ high blood pressure. Body __6__, emotions, heredity, overweight, and __7__ high-sodium (salt) diet may __8__ something to do with __9__ blood pressure, but scientists __10__ uncertain. It has long __11__ recognized as a major __12__ factor in stroke and __13__ attack—cardiovascular diseases which __14__ nearly 1 million deaths __15__ year.

To understand high __16__ pressure, it is necessary __17__ know something about how __18__ heart and blood vessels __19__. Your heart is a __20__ that acts like a __21__. The left side of __22__ heart receives oxygen-rich blood __23__ the lungs and pumps __24__ through the arteries to __25__ parts of your body, __26__ it with nutrients and __27__. Blood that has distributed __28__ nutrients and oxygen returns __29__ the right side of __30__ heart which pumps it __31__ the pulmonary artery to __32__ lungs where it absorbs __33__, and then the process __34__ again.

The force exerted __35__ your blood flowing against __36__ walls of the blood __37__ is blood pressure. The __38__ action of your heart __39__ the force. Your blood __40__ varies from moment to __41__ depending upon the situations __42__ activities in which you __43__ involved. For example, when __44__ become excited, the small __45__ that nourish your tissues __46__. The heart must pump __47__ harder to force the __48__ through the arteries, causing __49__ blood pressure to rise. __50__ the blood pressure will __51__ to normal when you __52__. Because of these changes in blood pressure, the doctor will usually take several blood pressure readings over a period of time before making a diagnosis of high blood pressure.

Source: Adapted from American Heart Association. (1983). An older person's guide to cardiovascular health, Dallas, TX: National Center. The information from this booklet is not current and is used for illustrative purposes only.

Figure A–4 Suitability assessment of materials (SAM) scoring sheet.

2 points for superior rating
1 point for adequate rating
0 points for not suitable rating
N/A if the factor does not apply to this material

FACTOR TO BE RATED	SCORE	COMMENTS

1. CONTENT

(a) Purpose is evident
(b) Content about behaviors
(c) Scope is limited
(d) Summary or review included

2. LITERACY DEMAND

(a) Reading grade level
(b) Writing style, active voice
(c) Vocabulary uses common words
(d) Context is given first
(e) Learning aids via "road signs"

3. GRAPHICS

(a) Cover graphic shows purpose
(b) Type of graphics
(c) Relevance of illustrations
(d) Lists, tables, etc. explained
(e) Captions used for graphics

4. LAYOUT AND TYPOGRAPHY

(a) Layout factors
(b) Typography
(c) Subheads (chunking) used

5. LEARNING STIMULATION, MOTIVATION

(a) Interaction used
(b) Behaviors are modeled and specific
(c) Motivation—self-efficacy

6. CULTURAL APPROPRIATENESS

(a) Match in logic, language, experience
(b) Cultural image and examples

    Total SAM score: _____

    Total possible score: _____, Percent score: _____%

Source: Doak, Doak, & Root (1996), *Teaching patients with low literacy skills,* p. 51. Reprinted with permission from Lippincott.

Guidelines for Writing and Evaluating Printed Education Materials (PEMs)

To Reduce Reading Level and Increase Reading Ease,
Do the Following:

1. Write in conversational style with an active voice in the present tense using the second person pronoun *you* or *your*.
2. Use short, simple vocabulary of one- or two-syllable words; avoid multisyllabic words.
3. Spell out words rather than using abbreviations or acronyms, unless they are familiar to the reader or defined.
4. Organize information into chunks or series of numbered and bulleted lists; use statistics sparingly; a question and answer format is an interactive approach to presenting single units of information.
5. Keep sentences short (20 words maximum); avoid complex grammatical sentence structures that contain colons, semicolons, commas, and dashes.
6. Focus on familiar terms; avoid technical jargon and medical terminology; define or spell out difficult words phonetically; include a glossary if "medicalese" is necessary.
7. Use words consistently (repetition) throughout text; avoid synonyms.
8. Use exact terms; avoid value judgment words with many interpretations.
9. Put the most important information first by prioritizing the "need to know."
10. Use advance organizers to cue the reader about the topic being presented.
11. Limit the use of connective words that lengthen and make sentences more complex.
12. Make the first sentence of a paragraph the topic sentence.
13. Reduce concept density by including only one idea per sentence and limiting each paragraph to a single message or action.
14. Keep the density of words low (do not exceed 30–40 characters per line).
15. Provide adequate white space for margins and between lines and paragraphs (use double spacing).
16. Justify left margins and keep right margins unjustified.
17. Use arrows or numbers that give direction and organization to layouts.
18. Select large print (minimum of 12–14-point font) and simple style type (serif); avoid *italics*, all CAPITAL letters, and *fancy lettering*.
19. Rely on bold print or underlining to emphasize key points or words.
20. Attract attention with consistent use of appealing colors to highlight and organize topics.
21. Use a simple, short title that clearly indicates the subject being presented.
22. Keep the length of the document short; avoid including details and extraneous information.
23. Avoid glossy paper to reduce glare; rely on bold primary colors (not pastels) and black print on white paper for the older audience.

24. Use simple, realistic illustrations that convey the intended message; never superimpose typed words on a background design.
25. Include a summary at the end to review key points of information.
26. Put reading grade level (RGL) on the back of the tool for future reference.
27. Determine readability, comprehension, and reading skills by applying at least two formulas or tests.

A. Readability Formulas	B. Comprehension Tests	C. Reading Skills Tests
1. SMOG	1. Cloze procedure	1. WRAT
2. Fog	2. Listening test	2. REALM
3. Fry		3. TOFHLA

References

Doak, C. C., Doak, L. G., & Root, J. H. (1996). *Teaching patients with low literacy skills* (2nd ed.). Philadelphia: Lippincott.

Flesch, R. (1948). A new readability yardstick. *Journal of Applied Psychology, 32*(3), 221–233.

Fry, E. (1968). A readability formula that saves time. *Journal of Reading, 11*, 513–516, 555–579.

Fry, E. (1977). Fry's readability graph: Clarifications, validity, and extension to level 17. *Journal of Reading, 21*, 242–252.

Gunning, R. (1968). The fog index after 20 years. *Journal of Business Communications, 6*, 3–13.

Spache, G. (1953). A new readability formula for primary-grade reading materials. *Elementary School Journal, 53*(7), 410–413.

Spadero, D. C. (1983). Assessing readability of patient information materials. *Pediatric Nursing, 9*(4), 274–278.

Spadero, D. C., Robinson, L. A., & Smith, L. T. (1980). Assessing readability of patient information materials. *American Journal of Hospital Pharmacy, 37*, 215–221.

Resources and Organizations for People With Disabilities

ASSISTIVE TECHNOLOGY

ABLEDATA
8630 Fenton Street
Suite 930
Silver Springs, MD 20910
800-227-0216
E-mail: abledata@verizon.net
www.abledata.com

Alliance for Technology Access
1304 Southpoint Boulevard
Suite 240
Petaluma, CA 94954
707-778-3011
E-mail: ATAinfo@ATAccess.org
www.ataccess.org

AUGMENTATIONS AND ALTERNATIVE COMMUNICATION

American Speech-Language-Hearing
Association (ASHA)
10801 Rockville Pike
Rockville, MD 20852
888-321-ASHA
www.asha.org

International Society for Augmentative and
Alternative Communication (ISAAC)
49 The Donway West, Suite 308
Toronto, ON M3C 3M9
Canada
416-385-0351
www.isaac-online.org

BLINDNESS

American Diabetes Association
1701 N. Beauregard Street
Alexandria, VA 22311
800-342-2383
www.diabetes.org

American Foundation for the Blind
11 Pen Plaza, Suite 300
New York, NY 10001
800-232-5463
www.afb.org

Library of Congress
101 Independence Avenue, S.E.
Washington, DC 20540
202-707-5000
www.loc.gov

Administers a free program of Braille and audio materials

National Braille Press
88 St. Stephen Street
Boston, MA 02115
617-266-6160; 888-965-8965
E-mail: orders@nbp.org
www.nbp.org

National Library Service for the Blind and
    Physically Handicapped
1291 Taylor Street N.W.
Washington, DC 20542
202-707-5100
www.loc.gov/nls/index.html

DEAFNESS

Helen Keller National Center
11 Middleneck Road
Sands Point, NJ 11020-1299
516-944-8900
www.hknc.org

National Academy of Gallaudet College
800 Florida Avenue
Washington, DC 20002-3695
www.gallaudet.edu

National Institutes of Health
National Institute on Deafness and Other
    Communication Disorders
31 Center Drive, MSC 2320
Bethesda, MD 20892-2320
800-241-1044
E-mail: nidcdinfo@nidcd.nih.gov
www.nidcd.nih.gov

Registry of Interpreters for the Deaf, Inc.
333 Commerce Street
Alexandria, VA 22314
703-838-0030
www.rid.org
Provides information on interpreting and interpreters; referral to local agencies and state chapters of the Registry of Interpreters for the Deaf for assistance in locating interpreters.

DEVELOPMENTAL DISABILITIES

National Institute of Child Health and
    Human Development
P.O. Box 3006
Rockville, MD 20847
800-370-2943
TTY: 1-888-320-6942
E-mail:
    NICHDInformationResourceCenter@
    mail.nih.gov
www.nichd.nih.gov

DISABILITY SERVICES

Americans with Disabilities Act (ADA)
P.O. Box 66738
Washington, DC 20035
800-514-0383
www.ada.gov

Autism Speaks
2 Park Avenue
New York, NY 10016
212-252-8584
www.autismspeaks.org

Disability Resources, Inc.
4 Glatter Lane
Centereach, NY 11720-1032
631-585-0290
www.disabilityresources.org

National Council on Disability
1331 F. Street N.W.
Suite 850
Washington, DC 20004
202-272-2004
www.ncd.gov

HEAD INJURY

Brain Injury Association of America
800-444-6443
www.biausa.org

HEALTHCARE-RELATED FEDERAL AGENCIES

Centers for Disease Control and Prevention
1600 Clifton Road
Atlanta, GA 30333
404-639-3311
404-639-3534; 800-311-3455
www.cdc.gov

Health Resources and Services
  Administration
301-443-3376
www.hrsa.gov

National Center for Medical Rehabilitation
  Research, NIHD, NIH
800-370-2943
www.nichd.nih.gov/about/ncmrr

National Institute on Disability and
  Rehabilitation Research (NIDRR)
U.S. Department of Education
400 Maryland Avenue S.W.
Room 3060
Washington, DC 20202
202-245-7640
www.ed.gov/about/offices/list/osers/nidrr

LEARNING DISABILITIES

A.D.D. Warehouse
300 N.W. 70th Avenue, Suite 102
Plantation, FL 33317
305-792-8944
www.addwarehouse.com/shopsite_sc/store/
  html/index.html

Association for Children and Adults With
  Learning Disabilities
4156 Library Road
Pittsburgh, PA 15234
412-341-8077
www.ldanatl.org

Attention Disorders Association of Parents
  and Professionals Together (ADAPPT)
P.O. Box 293
Oak Forest, IL 60452
312-361-4330
www.adappt.org

MENTAL HEALTH

Mental Health America
2000 N. Beauregard Street, 6th Floor
Alexandria, VA 22311
703-684-7722
800-969-6642
TTY: 800-433-5959
www.nmha.org

National Institute of Mental Health (NIMH)
Public Information and Communications
  Branch
6001 Executive Boulevard
Room 8184, MSC 9663
Bethesda, MD 20892-9663
301-443-4513
866-615-6464
TTY: 301-443-8431
TTY toll-free: 866-415-8051
E-mail: nimhinfo@nih.gov
www.nimh.nih.gov

NEUROMUSCULAR DISORDERS

ALS Association National Office
27001 Agoura Road
Suite 150
Calabassa Hills, CA 91301-5104
800-782-4747
www.alsa.org

Epilepsy Foundation of America
4351 Garden City Drive
Suite 500
Landover, MD 20785
301-459-3700
800-332-1000
www.epilepsyfoundation.org

Multiple Sclerosis Foundation
6350 North Andrews Avenue
Fort Lauderdale, FL 33309-2130
800-225-6495
954-776-6805
E-mail: admin@msfocus.org
www.msfacts.org

Muscular Dystrophy Association—USA
National Headquarters
3300 E. Sunrise Drive
Tucson, AZ 85718
1-800-FIGHT-MD (344-4863)
E-mail: mda@mdausa.org
www.mdausa.org

Myasthenia Gravis Foundation of America
1821 University Avenue W., Suite S256
St. Paul, MN 55104
651-917-6256; 800-541-5454
E-mail: mgfa@myasthenia.org
www.myasthenia.org

Parkinson's Disease Foundation, Inc.
1359 Broadway, Suite 1509
New York, NY 10018
800-457-6676
212-457-6676
E-mail: info@pdf.org
www.pdf.org

Program Services Assistance, MS Helpline
888-MSFOCUS
954-776-6805
E-mail: support@msfocus.org
www.msfocus.org

SPINAL CORD

National Spinal Cord Injury Association
6701 Democracy Boulevard, Suite 300-9
Bethesda, MD 20817
800-962-9629
301-214-4006
Email: info@spinalcord.org
www.spinalcord.org

Paralyzed Veterans of America
801 Eighteenth Street N.W.
Washington, DC 20006-3517
800-555-9140
E-mail: info@pva.org
www.pva.org

STROKE

National Aphasia Association
350 Seventh Avenue, Suite 902
New York, NY 10001
800-922-4622
www.aphasia.org

National Institute of Neurological Disorders
and Stroke (NINDS)
P.O. Box 5801
Bethesda, MD 20824
www.ninds.nih.gov

National Stroke Association
9707 E. Easter Lane Building B
Centennial, CO 80112
800-STROKES (787-6537)
E-mail: info@stroke.org
www.stroke.org

Teaching Plans

Postcircumcision Care

Purpose: To provide mothers of male newborns with the information necessary to perform postcircumcision care.

Goal: The mother will independently manage postcircumcision care for her baby boy.

Objectives	Content Outline	Method of Instruction	Time Allotted	Resources	Method of Evaluation
Following a 20-minute teaching session, the mother will be able to:					

1. Demonstrate procedure for postcircumcision care with each diaper change (psychomotor)	A. Definition of circumcision
	B. Circumcision care
	  1. Washing penis
	  2. Applying petroleum jelly and gauze
	  3. Diapering baby
		Demonstration
		
		Return demonstration
			10 minutes	Written/ pictorial flip chart
				Infant doll
				Washcloth
				Warm water
				Petroleum jelly
				Gauze
				Diaper
					Observation of return demonstration

Objectives	Content Outline	Method of Instruction	Time Allotted	Resources	Method of Evaluation
2. Identify three reasons to call the doctor or nurse (cognitive)	Postcircumcision complications 1. bleeding 2. weak or absent stream of urine 3. drainage 4. swollen penis 5. baby acts sick or more fussy than expected	1:1 instruction	5 minutes	Written/ pictorial flip chart	Posttest
3. Express any concerns about circumcision care (affective)	A. Summarize common concerns B. Explore feelings	Discussion	5 minutes	White board	Question and answer

Source: Developed as part of teaching project assignment by Eleanor P. McLees, BSN, RN, CNM and Julie-Lynn Corsoniti, BS, RN in NSG 561 course during Spring 2007 semester at Le Moyne College, Syracuse, NY.

Safe Sleep Positioning of Infants

Purpose: Provide parents with information on safe sleep conditions of infant after discharge from the NICU.

Goal: Parents will maintain safe sleep conditions at home for infant to reduce the risk of SIDS.

Objectives and Subobjectives	Content Outline	Method of Instruction	Time Allotted	Resources	Method of Evaluation
Following a 15-minute teaching session, the parents will be able to:					
1. Explain what SIDS is, its causes, and ways to prevent it with 100% accuracy (cognitive)	Introduce the Back to Sleep Campaign concept Review SIDS definition, including incidence				
– Define sudden infant death syndrome (SIDS)	Discuss risk factors (preterm, low birth weight, smoking, prone/side sleeping, soft bedding, cosleeping, cold months, males)	1:1 instruction	5 minutes	PEM on back to sleep	Pre- and Posttest

Objectives and Subobjectives	Content Outline	Method of Instruction	Time Allotted	Resources	Method of Evaluation
− Identify the most common risk factors − State six ways to reduce SIDS	Review risk reduction— back to sleep, no smoking, no soft bedding, no cosleeping, pacifiers, do not overheat				
2. Demonstrate proper safe sleep techniques with 100% accuracy (psychomotor) − Choose crib items that are safe and unsafe − Position baby in crib with proper clothing	Typical shower gifts to avoid—loose blankets, toys, crib bumpers, rolls, pillows Crib set-up, swaddle blanket for warmth	Demonstration, return demonstration	5 minutes	Portable crib with crib bumpers, quilts, toys, rolls, pacifier, loose blankets, dolls, baby clothes	Skills checklist for return demonstration
3. Express any concerns about placing infant on his or her back to sleep (affective)	Summarize common concerns such as choking, flat heads, inability to sleep as well	Discussion	5 minutes	Worksheets listing concerns filled out by participants prior to discussion session	Completed worksheets on observation of level of learner participation in discussion

Source: Developed as part of a teaching project assignment by Christine A. Aris, CNNP, RN and Carol A. Weeks, BS, RN in NSG 461 course during Spring 2007 semester at Le Moyne College, Syracuse, NY.

Use of Incentive Spirometer

Purpose: To provide patients in a preoperative open-heart surgery class with the information and skills necessary to properly use an incentive spirometer.

Goal: Patients will use the incentive spirometer as directed to prevent postoperative pulmonary complications.

Objectives	Content Outline	Method of Instruction	Time Allotted	Resources	Method of Evaluation
Following three 15-minute consecutive group sessions, the patients will:					
1. Name two postoperative complications that can potentially be prevented by their proper use of the incentive spirometer (cognitive: knowledge level)	a. *Pneumonia*: Inflammation of lungs caused by bacterial growth secondary to an excessive build-up of secretions. b. *Atelectasis*: A collapsed or airless condition of the lung caused by excessive secretions.	Lecture	15 minutes	Simple anatomical poster of lungs within the chest cavity	Posttest
2. Return demonstrate the eight steps in proper use of incentive spirometer (psychomotor: guided response level)	a. Use analogy of drinking a thick liquid through a straw b. The eight steps in using incentive spirometer: 1. Slide arrow to the number ordered by your doctor 2. Blow out all of the air from your lungs 3. Hold mouthpiece and close your lips around it	Demonstration and return demonstration	15 minutes	Milkshake Small cups Straws Incentive spirometers for each patient to practice with PEM on incentive spirometer	Observation of return demonstration

Objectives	Content Outline	Method of Instruction	Time Allotted	Resources	Method of Evaluation
	4. Suck air in through the mouthpiece (like a straw)				
	5. Watch the blue flow rate guide and see the blue riser move up				
	6. When the blue flow rate guide rises between the two arrows, hold it there for 6 seconds				
	7. Look at the number where the blue riser stops				
	8. Blow out and repeat				
3. Explain their feelings regarding mastery of incentive spirometer use preoperatively (affective: responding level)	Discussion of the patients' overall feelings towards use of the incentive spirometer prior to surgery	Group discussions: Patients break into small groups, each group discusses feelings and selects a presenter and then each group presenter summarizes feelings and shares them with the larger group	15 minutes	Paper and pencils to document responses	Question and answer

Source: Developed as part of a teaching project assignment by Diane G. Mather, BS, RN and Diane S. McDermott, BS, RN, CNOR in NSG 561 course during Spring 2007 semester at Le Moyne College, Syracuse, NY.

Glossary

4MAT system A learning style model based on Kolb's model combined with right–left brain research.

abstract conceptualization A term used by Kolb as one of two ways of processing information; known as the thinking mode.

accommodator One of the four learning style types according to Kolb's theory, combining the learning modes of concrete experience and active experimentation.

acculturation Describes an individual's adaptation to the customs, values, beliefs, and behaviors of a new country or culture.

active experimentation A term used by Kolb as one of two ways of processing information; known as the doing mode.

adherence Commitment or attachment to health-promoting regimens.

affective domain One of three domains in the taxonomy of behavioral objectives; deals with attitudes, values, and beliefs.

ageism Prejudice against the older adult that perpetuates the negative stereotyping of aging as a period of decline.

aids See instructional materials/tools.

analogue A type of model that uses analogy to explain something by comparing it to something else. The model performs like the real object, although its actual appearance may differ. A dialysis machine and the use of a description of a pump to explain how the kidneys and heart work respectively are examples of analogues.

andragogy The art and science of helping adults learn; a term coined by Knowles to describe his theory of adult learning.

animistic thinking The tendency of preschoolers to endow inanimate objects with life and consciousness; the belief that objects possess human characteristics.

appearance As an important feature of instructional tools, it is the way printed and display materials look to the reader. Appearance is a vital element in determining the effectiveness of media in capturing and holding the learner's attention through adequate use of white space, minimal use of words to convey the message, use of illustrations to break up blocks of print, and use of contrasts in color or shading.

assess To gather, summarize, and interpret pertinent data about the learner to make a decision or plan.

assessment The process of systematically collecting data to determine the relative magnitude, importance, or value of needs, problems, and strengths of the learner to decide a direction for action.

assessment phase The first phase of the educational cycle, which provides the foundation for the rest of the educational process.

assimilation The willingness of a person emigrating to a new culture to gradually adopt and incorporate the characteristics of the prevailing culture.

assimilator One of the four learning style types, according to Kolb's theory, combining the learning modes of abstract conceptualization and reflective observation.

assistive technologies Technological tools (computers and communication devices) available for people with disabilities that provide access to education, employment, recreation, and communication opportunities that allow them to live as independently as possible.

asynchronous A message that can be sent via the computer at the convenience of the sender and the message will be read when the receiver is online and ready to read it; messages that can be sent and responded to any time, day or night.

attention deficit hyperactivity disorder (ADHD) A disorder of children and adults with prominent attentional difficulties as demonstrated by inattention and impulsivity that are signs of developmentally inappropriate behavior.

audio learning resources Instructional tools that utilize the learner's sense of hearing as a mechanism for teaching; audiotapes and recorders are examples.

audiovisual materials (tools) Nonprint instructional media that can influence all three domains of learning and stimulate the senses of hearing and/or sight to help convey the message to the learner. This category includes five major types: projection, audio, video, telecommunications, and computer formats.

augmentative and alternative communication Devices, such as the computer, that allow people who are unable to speak or whose speech is difficult to understand to be able to communicate with others, which has added a whole new dimension and quality to their lives.

augmented feedback An opinion or conveyance of a message through oral or body language by the teacher to the learner about how well he or she performed a psychomotor skill.

autonomy The right to self-determination.

avoidance conditioning A type of negative reinforcement whereby an unpleasant stimulus is anticipated rather than directly applied, and the person receiving the reinforcement avoids doing something he or she does not want to do when faced with a fearful event.

barriers to teaching Those factors that impede the instructor's ability to deliver educational services.

behavioral (learning) objectives Intended outcomes of the education process that are action-oriented rather than content-oriented and learner-centered rather than teacher-centered.

behaviorist learning One of the five major learning theories. According to behaviorists, the focus for learning is mainly on what is directly observable, and learning is viewed as the product of the stimulus conditions (S) and the responses (R) that follow. It is sometimes termed the S-R model of learning.

beneficence The principle of doing good.

blended learning This type of learning combines e-learning (electronic learning) technology with the more traditional instructor-led methodology; this is a more recent term in education.

blogs One of the newest forms of online communication, also known as Web logs or Web diaries, is an increasingly popular mechanism for individuals to share information and/or experiences about a given topic that include images, media objects, and links allowing for public responses.

bodily kinesthetic intelligence A term used by Gardner to describe children who learn by processing knowledge through bodily sensations.

brain preference indicator (BPI) A learning style instrument used to determine hemispheric dominance.

breach of contract Failure, without legal excuse, to perform a promise. Violation of a binding agreement or obligation in the performance of professional duties.

causal thinking The ability of school-aged children to understand cause and effect through logic, concrete thinking, and inductive and deductive reasoning.

causality The ability to grasp a cause-and-effect relationship between two paired, successive events, which is an elementary concept that begins to develop during toddlerhood.

chronic illness A disease or disability that is permanent and can never be completely cured. It constitutes the number one medical malady of people in this country and affects the physical, psychosocial, economic, and spiritual aspects of an individual's life.

cloze procedure A standardized test to measure comprehension of written materials (particularly recommended for health education literature) based on systematically deleting every fifth word from a portion of a text and having the reader fill in the blanks.

code of ethics An articulation of professional values and moral obligations with regard to the provider–patient relationship and in support of the mission of health professions.

cognitive ability The extent to which information can be processed, indicative of the level at which the learner is capable of learning; of major importance when designing instruction.

cognitive development A series of qualitative cognitive changes in perception, thought, and reason as individuals grow and mature based on how external events are conceptualized, organized, and represented within each person's mental framework or schema. The process of acquiring more complex and adaptive ways of thinking as an individual grows from infancy to adulthood according to Piaget's four stages of cognitive maturation: sensorimotor, preoperational, concrete operations, and formal operations.

cognitive domain One of three domains in the taxonomy of behavioral objectives; deals with

aspects of behavior focusing on the way in which someone thinks in acquiring facts, concepts, principles, etc.

cognitive-emotional perspective A cognitive theory recognizing that emotions must be considered within a cognitive framework to adequately consider affect as an aspect of conceptual change.

cognitive learning One of the five major learning theories. According to a cognitive theorist's perspective, in order to learn, individuals change as a result of the way they perceive, process, interpret, and organize information based on what is already known; the reorganization of information leads to new insights and understanding.

commercially prepared materials Predesigned, cost-effective printed educational materials that are widely available on a range of topics for purchase by educators as supplements to teaching and learning, such as brochures, pamphlets, books, posters, etc.

compliance Submission or yielding to predetermined goals through regimens prescribed or established by others.

comprehension The degree to which individuals understand what they have read or heard; the ability to grasp the meaning of a verbal or nonverbal message.

computer-assisted instruction (CAI) An individualized instructional method of self-study using the high technology of the computer to deliver an educational activity. The interactive capability of CAI holds enormous potential for reinforcing learning, primarily in the cognitive domain, and its efficacy is dependent on programmatic software, hardware, and the learner's familiarity with and motivation to use this technology.

computer literacy The ability to use the necessary computer hardware and software to meet the needs for information.

concept mapping A contemporary educational strategy that can be used to promote motivation by enabling the learner to integrate previous learning with newly acquired knowledge through diagrammatic mapping, which facilitates the gaining of complex knowledge with visual links.

concordance A consultative process that is characterized by mutual respect for the client's and the professional's beliefs and that allows for negotiation to take place about the best course of action for the client.

concrete experience A term used by Kolb to describe a dimension of perceiving; known as the feeling mode.

concrete operations period As defined by Piaget, this is the third stage in the cognitive development of children in middle to late childhood (ages 6 to 11 years) who are capable of logical thought processes and the ability to reason but are still incapable of abstract thinking.

confidentiality A binding social contract or covenant; a professional obligation to respect privileged information between the health professional and the client.

conservation The ability to recognize that the properties of an object stay the same even though its appearance and position may change, which is a concept mastered during middle to late childhood.

constructivism See social constructivism.

consumer informatics A discipline that analyzes consumers' needs for information, studies and implements methods of making information accessible to consumers, and models and integrates consumer preferences into medical information systems. Also referred to as consumer health informatics.

content The actual information that is communicated to the learner through various teaching methods and tools.

content evaluation A systematic assessment taking place immediately after the learning experience to determine the degree to which learners have acquired the knowledge or skills taught during a teaching–learning session.

contextual interference effects Factors during motor learning that make the initial performance of a task more difficult, but often result in more effective learning.

contracting A popular, relatively recent means of facilitating learning through informal or formal agreements that delineate and promote learning objectives.

converger One of the four learning style types according to Kolb's theory, combining the learning modes of abstract conceptualization and active experimentation.

corpus callosum The connector between the two hemispheres of the brain.

cosmopolitan orientation Persons with a worldly perspective on life who are receptive to new ideas and opportunities to learn new ways of doing things; a component of experiential readiness.

cost benefit Money well spent. Cost of services (e.g., education) ensures return of satisfied clients and stability of the economic base of a healthcare facility.

cost-benefit analysis The relationship between cost and outcomes that can be expressed in monetary terms; also called a cost-benefit ratio.

cost-benefit ratio Relationship (expressed as a ratio) of program costs to economic benefits gained by the healthcare institution.

cost-effectiveness analysis The efficiency of an educational offering when an actual monetary value cannot be assigned to a program.

cost recovery Occurs when revenues generated are equal to or greater than expenditures.

cost savings Monies realized through decreased use of expensive services, shortened lengths of stay, or fewer complications resulting from preventive services or patient education.

crystallized intelligence The intellectual ability developed over a lifetime, which includes such elements as vocabulary, general information, understanding of social interactions, arithmetic reasoning, and capacity to evaluate experiences, which tends to increase over time as a person ages.

cuing Using prompts and reminders to get a learner to perform routine tasks by focusing on an appropriate combination of time and situation.

cultural assessment An organized, systematic appraisal of beliefs, values, and practices of an individual or group to determine client needs as a basis for planning healthcare interventions.

cultural awareness The process of becoming sensitive to the interactions with other cultural groups by examining one's biases and prejudices toward others of another culture or ethnic background.

cultural competence The ability to demonstrate knowledge and understanding of another person's culture and accept and respect cultural differences by adapting interventions to be congruent with that specific culture when delivering care.

cultural diversity Interacting with others who represent different cultures from one's own culture.

cultural encounter The process of exposing oneself in healthcare practice to cross-cultural interactions with clients of diverse cultural backgrounds.

cultural knowledge The process of acquiring an educational foundation about various cultural worldviews.

cultural literacy The ability to know how to communicate with someone from another culture without having to explain undertones, voice intonations, and message contexts during a conversation.

cultural relativism The values and behaviors every human group assigns to its conventions, which arise out of its own historical background and can only be accurately interpreted and un-

derstood in the light of that group's cultural worldview.

cultural skill The process of learning how to conduct an accurate cultural assessment.

culturally competent model of care A model for conducting a thorough and sensitive cultural assessment that includes the four components of cultural awareness, cultural knowledge, cultural skill, and cultural encounter.

culture A complex concept that is an integral part of each person's life and includes knowledge, beliefs, values, morals, customs, traditions, and habits acquired by the members of a society.

decision aids Include printed materials, videos, and interactive Web-based tutorials designed to assist clients to make informed choices by providing them with information about specific health issues, particular diagnoses, and treatment risks and benefits. These aids also can be in the form of a questionnaire to determine whether clients need more information.

defense mechanisms Employed to protect the self when an individual's ego is threatened; short-term use is a way of slowly accepting reality, but long-term reliance allows individuals to avoid reality and may act as a barrier to learning and transfer.

delivery system The physical form of instructional materials, including durable equipment used to present these materials, such as videos and projectors, audiotapes and tape players, and computer programs and computers.

demonstration An instructional method by which the learner is shown by the teacher how to perform a particular psychomotor skill.

demonstration materials Tools that stimulate the senses by combining sight with touch, smell, and sometimes even taste with the advantage of helping to teach cognitive and psychomotor skill development. Major forms of media in this category include many types of nonprint media, such as models, real equipment, diagrams, charts, posters, displays, photographs, and drawings.

deontological The ethical notion of the Golden Rule promulgated by the 16th-century philosopher Kant.

desirable needs Learning needs of the client that are not life dependent but related to well-being and can be met by the overall ability of professional staff to provide quality care.

determinants of learning Consist of learning needs, readiness to learn, and learning styles.

developmental disability A disorder that manifests itself during the developmental period when a child demonstrates subaverage general intellectual functioning with concurrent deficits in adaptive behaviors. Sometimes referred to as mental retardation or developmental delay.

developmental stages Milestones marking changes in the physical, cognitive, and psychosocial growth of an individual over time from infancy to old age.

dialectical thinking The ability to search for complex and changing understandings to find a variety of solutions to any given situation (to see the bigger picture) which is characteristic of middle-aged adults.

digital divide The gap between those individuals who have access to information technology resources and those who do not.

direct costs Tangible, predictable costs associated with expenditures for personnel, equipment, etc.

disability Inability to perform some key life functions; often used interchangeably with the term functional limitation.

discrimination learning The ability to differentiate, with more and varied practice, among similar stimuli.

displays Type of demonstration materials, frequently regarded as static, which may be permanently installed or portable. Included in this category are whiteboards, flip charts, and posters.

distance learning A flexible telecommunications method of instruction using video or computer technology to transmit live, online, or taped messages directly between the instructor and the learner, who are separated from one another by time and/or location.

distributed practice Learning information over successive periods of time, which is much more effective for remembering facts and forging memories than massed practice or cramming, which may not allow for long-term recall of information.

diverger One of the four learning style types according to Kolb's theory, combining the learning modes of concrete experience and reflective observation.

domains of learning Cognitive, psychomotor, and affective are the three domains in which learning occurs.

Dunn and Dunn learning style inventory A self-reporting instrument that is used in the identification of how individuals prefer to function, learn, concentrate, and perform in learning activities.

duty Responsibility; professional expectation.

dyscalculia A learning disability that impairs the parts of the brain involved in mathematical processing. This type of disability can be developmental (acquired at birth) or the result of an injury to the brain.

dysarthria Difficulty with voluntary muscle control of speech due to damage to the central or peripheral nervous system that controls muscles essential to speaking and swallowing. Types of dysarthria include flaccid, spastic, ataxic, hypokinetic, or mixed. Persons with degenerative neurologic diseases often suffer with this disorder.

education An overall umbrella term used to describe the process, including the components of teaching and instruction, of producing observable or measurable behavioral changes (in knowledge, attitudes, and/or skills) in the learner through planned educational activities.

education process A systematic, sequential, planned course of action that parallels the nursing process and consists of two interdependent operations, teaching and learning, which form a continuous cycle to include assessment of the learner, establishment of a teaching plan, implementation of teaching methods and tools, and evaluation of the learner, teacher, and education program.

educational contracting See learning contract.

educational objectives See instructional objectives.

educator role The teaching role a health professional assumes in supporting, encouraging, and assisting the learner to put learning of behaviors (knowledge, skills, and attitudes) into meaningful parts and wholes to reach an optimum potential of functioning.

edutainment Computer games as educational software that are disguised in a game format.

e-learning An abbreviation for electronic learning, which professional development and training organizations have capitalized on by using the power of computer technology to provide learning solutions for workforce training; it involves the use of technology-based tools and processes to provide for customized learning anytime or anywhere.

e-mail An Internet-based activity that is a quick, inexpensive, and increasingly popular way to communicate asynchronously via the computer.

embedded figures test (EFT) A test designed to measure how a person's perception of the environment (field independence/dependence) is influenced by the context in which it appears.

emoticons Symbols commonly used to represent emotions, such as a :) (smiley face) or ;) (winking), by people who are sending e-mail messages.

emotional readiness A state of psychological willingness to learn, which is dependent on such factors as anxiety level, support system, motivation, risk-taking behavior, frame of mind, and psychosocial developmental stage.

escape conditioning An individual's response that causes an unpleasant or uncomfortable stimulation to cease.

ethical A term that refers to the norms or standards of behavior of healthcare professionals.

ethics Guiding principles of human behavior.

ethnic group A population of people, also referred to as a subculture, that has different experiences from those of the dominant culture.

ethnicity A dynamic and complex concept referring to how members of a group perceive themselves and how, in turn, they are perceived by others in relation to the population subgroup's common heritage of customs, characteristics, language, and history.

ethnocentrism A concept in which the belief is held that one's own culture is superior and all other cultures are less sophisticated.

ethnomedical A cultural orientation delineating the nature and consequences of illness problems and disease interventions rather than adhering to the biomedical orientation of defining diseases and illness interventions. In this context, the concept of illness incorporates the relationship of humans with their universe, bridging culture with a sensitivity toward the daily practices inherent within specific ethnic groups.

evaluation A systematic and continuous process by which the significance of something is judged; the process of collecting and using information to determine what has been accomplished and how well it has been accomplished to guide decision making.

evaluation research Scientific inquiry applied to a specific program or activity to determine processes, outcomes, and/or their relationship.

evidence-based practice (EBP) The conscientious use of current best evidence in making decisions about client care; most EBP models gather evidence from systematic reviews of clinically relevant, randomized controlled trials upon which to base practice decisions, especially about treatment.

experiential readiness A state of willingness to learn based on such factors as an individual's past experiences with learning, cultural background, previous coping mechanisms, locus of control, orientation, and level of aspiration.

expressive aphasia An absence or impairment of the ability to communicate through speech or writing due to a dysfunction in the Broca's area of the brain, which is the center of the cortex that controls motor abilities.

external evidence Evidence derived from research that is generalizable beyond a particular study setting or sample.

external locus of control An individual's motivation to learn comes from outside oneself, attributing success or failure of an action to luck, the nature of the task, or to the efforts of someone else.

extraversion-introversion (E-I) Terms used to describe behavior that reflects an orientation to either the outside world of people or to the inner world of concepts and ideas; one of four dichotomous preference dimensions in the Myers-Briggs type indicator.

extrinsic feedback A response provided by the teacher through the sharing of opinion or the conveying of a message through body language about how well a learner has performed; often used in relation to psychomotor skill performance.

field dependence One of two styles of learning in the cognitive domain identified by Witkin in which a person's perception of the environment is immersed in and influenced by the surrounding field.

field independence One of two styles of learning in the cognitive domain identified by Witkin in which a person's perception of the environment is separate from the surrounding field.

fixed costs Predictable and controllable expenses that remain stable over time.

Flesch-Kincaid scale An objective, statistical measurement tool for readability of written materials between fifth grade and college level, based on a count of the two basic language elements of average sentence length in words of selected samples and of average word length measured as syllables per 100 words of sample.

fluid intelligence The intellectual capacity to perceive relationships, to reason, and to perform abstract thinking, which declines over time as degenerative changes occur with aging.

focus groups Optimally 4 to 12 potential learners grouped together for the purpose of identifying points of view or knowledge about a certain topic. A facilitator leads the discussion by asking questions.

Fog Index A formula appropriate for use in determining readability of materials from fourth grade to college level based on average sentence length and the percentage of multisyllabic words in a 100-word passage.

formal operations period As defined by Piaget, this is the fourth and final stage of cognitive development in which the adolescent (ages 12 to 19 years) is capable of abstract thought, internalization of ideas, complex logical reasoning, and understanding causality.

formal settings Scheduled sessions in which teaching and learning take place.

format The general physical appearance of a book, pamphlet, or other printed materials, which includes such characteristics as the type face, the margins, the organization of information, the quality of the paper, etc.

formative evaluation Also referred to as process evaluation. It is a systematic and continuous assessment of success of the teaching process made during the implementation of materials, methods, and activities to control, ensure, or improve the quality of performance in delivery of an educational program.

four-step appraisal of needs A systematic approach for assessing learning needs of caregivers and the healthcare organizations in which they practice.

Fry readability graph A measurement tool for testing the readability of materials (especially books, pamphlets, and brochures) at the level of first grade through college by using a graph to plot the number of syllables of words and the number of sentences in three 100-word samples.

functional illiteracy The lack of fundamental education skills needed by adults to read, write, or comprehend information to function effectively in today's society; the inability to read well enough to understand and interpret written information for use as intended.

functional magnetic resonance imaging (fMRI) A type of advanced technology that has revolutionized the field of neuroscience by making colorful images of the brain on computer monitors to determine the possible areas of nerve activity involved in the processes of thinking, emotions, and recall.

gaming An instructional method requiring the learner to participate in a competitive activity (which may or may not reflect reality) with preset rules.

Gardner's eight types of intelligence A theory that describes the styles of learning in children.

gender bias A preconceived notion about the abilities of women and men that prevent individuals from pursuing their own interests and achieving their potentials.

gender gap The behavioral and biological differences between males and females.

gender-related cognitive abilities A comparison between the sexes as to how males and females act, react, and perform in situations affecting every sphere of life as a result of genetic and environmental influences on behavior.

gender-related personality behaviors The observed differences between the sexes in personality and affective behaviors thought to be largely determined by culture, but to some extent are a result of interaction between environment and heredity.

gerogogy The art and science of teaching the older adult.

Gestalt perspective The oldest of psychological theories that emphasizes the importance of perception in learning from a cognitive perspective, with a focus on the configuration or organization of a pattern of stimuli rather than of discrete stimuli. It reflects the maxim that "the whole is greater than the sum of the parts."

goal A desirable outcome to be achieved by the learner at the end of the teaching–learning process; goals are global and more future oriented and long term in nature than the specific, short-term objectives that lead step by step to the final achievement of a goal.

group discussion A commonly employed method of instruction whereby a group of learners (ideally 3 to 20 people) gather together to exchange information, feelings, and opinions with each other and the teacher; the activity is learner centered and subject centered.

habilitation Includes all the activities and interactions that enable individuals with a disability to develop new abilities to achieve their maximum potential.

hardware Part of the delivery system for many types of media (e.g., computers, projectors, tape players).

health belief model A framework or paradigm used to explain or predict health behavior composed of the interaction between individual perceptions, modifying factors, and likelihood of action.

health education A participatory educational approach, often used interchangeably with the term patient education or client education, aimed at preventing disease, promoting positive health, and incorporating the physical, mental, and social aspects of learning needs.

health literacy Refers to how well an individual can read, interpret, and comprehend health information for maintaining an optimal level of wellness.

healthcare-related setting One of three classifications of instructional settings, in which healthcare-related services are offered as a complementary function of a quasi-health agency. Examples: American Heart Association, American Cancer Society, Muscular Dystrophy Association, and Leukemia Society of America.

healthcare setting One of three classifications of instructional settings, in which the delivery of health care is the primary or sole function of an institution, organization, or agency. Examples: hospitals, visiting nurse associations, public health departments, outpatient clinics, physician offices, health maintenance organizations, extended-care facilities, and nurse-managed centers.

healthcare team An interdisciplinary group of healthcare professionals and nonprofessionals who provide services to the patient and family members in an attempt to maximize optimal health and well-being of the client to whom their activities are directed.

hearing impairment A complete loss or a reduction in sensitivity to sounds by persons who are deaf or hard of hearing.

hidden costs Costs that cannot be predicted or accounted for until after the fact.

hierarchy of needs Theory of human motivation based on integrated wholeness of the individual and levels of satisfaction of basic human needs organized by potency.

humanistic learning One of the five major learning theories, which views learning as being facilitated by curiosity, needs, a positive self-concept, and open situations where freedom of choice and individuality are promoted and respected.

ideology Thoughts, attitudes, and beliefs that reflect the social needs and desires of an individual or ethnocultural group.

illiteracy The total inability of adults to read, write, or comprehend information or whose reading and writing skills are at or below the fourth-grade level.

illusionary representations A category of instructional materials that depict realism, such as dimensionality. Examples are photographs, drawings, and audiotapes, which depend on imagination to fill in the gaps and offer the learner experiences that simulate reality.

iloralacy The inability to understand simple oral language.

imaginary audience A type of social thinking that explains the pervasive self-consciousness of adolescents who may feel embarrassed because they believe everyone is looking at them, which has considerable influence over their behavior.

impact evaluation The process of assessing outcomes or effects of an educational activity that extend beyond the activity itself to address organizational and/or societal effects.

indirect costs Costs that may be fixed but are not necessarily directly related to an educational activity (e.g., heating, electricity, housekeeping).

informal settings Unplanned or spontaneous sessions in which teaching and learning take place.

informatics See consumer informatics.

Information Age The present period of time, in which sweeping advances in computer and information technology have transformed the economic, social, and cultural life of society.

information literacy The ability to access, evaluate, organize, and use information from a variety of sources.

information processing A cognitive perspective that emphasizes thinking processes: thought, reasoning, the way information is encountered and stored, memory functioning, and information retrieved.

input disabilities A general category of learning disability that refers to the process of receiving and recording information in the brain, which includes visual, auditory, perceptual, and integrative processing, such as dyslexia and short- and long-term memory disorders.

instruction Often used interchangeably with teaching. Involves the communicating of information about a specific skill in the cognitive, affective, or psychomotor domain with the objective of producing learning.

instructional materials/tools The resources or vehicles used to help communicate information, which include both print and nonprint media, to aid teaching and learning by stimulating the various senses, such as vision and hearing. These are intended to supplement, not replace, actual teaching. Synonymous terms are educational aids and audiovisual materials.

instructional method The way information is taught that brings the learner into contact with what is to be learned; a technique or approach used by the teacher to communicate and share information with the learner. Examples of methods include lecture, group discussion, one-to-one instruction, etc.

instructional objectives Intended outcomes of the education process that are in reference to an aspect of a program or a total program of study that are content oriented and teacher centered; also referred to as educational objectives.

instructional setting A situation or area in which health teaching takes place as classified on the basis of what relationship health education has to the primary function of an organization, agency, or institution in which the teaching occurs.

instructional strategy See teaching strategy.

internal evidence Evidence that is not generated from research but is appropriate for use when, for example, it is derived from a systematically conducted evaluation.

internal locus of control Individuals are motivated from within to learn, attributing success or failure to their own ability or effort.

Internet A huge global computer network, of which the World Wide Web is a component, established to allow transfer (exchange) of information from one computer to another; it provides a diverse range of services used to deliver information to large numbers of people and to enable people to communicate with one another, such as via e-mail, real-time chat, or electronic discussion groups.

interpersonal intelligence A term used by Gardner to describe children who learn best in groups.

intrapersonal intelligence A term used by Gardner to describe children who learn well with independent, self-paced instruction.

intrinsic feedback A response that is generated within the self, giving learners a sense of or a feel for how they have performed; often used in relation to a psychomotor skill performance.

judging-perceiving (J-P) Terms used to describe behavior that reflects the way a person comes to a conclusion about something or becomes aware of something; one of four dichotomous preference dimensions in the Myers-Briggs type indicator.

justice The equal distribution of benefits and burdens.

knowledge deficit A gap in what a learner needs or wants to know; this category of nursing diagnosis can include learning needs in the cognitive, affective, and psychomotor domains.

knowledge readiness A state of willingness to learn dependent on such factors as the learner's present knowledge base, the level of learning capability, and the preferred style of learning.

Kolb's learning style inventory An experiential learning model that includes four modes of learning reflecting the dimensions of perception and processing.

LAD (Literary Assessment for Diabetes) A reading skills test to measure word recognition in adult patients with diabetes. This standardized test, modeled after the REALM test, consists of lists of common words used when teaching self-care management of diabetes.

law A clearly stated pronouncement of a binding custom, enforceable by a controlling body.

layout The arrangement of printed and/or graphic information on a flat surface. Effective use of white space, graphics, and wording will depend heavily on this arrangement.

learner characteristics One of the three major variables that refers to the learner's perceptual abilities, reading ability, self-direction, and learning style, which must be considered when making appropriate choices of instructional materials.

learning A conscious or unconscious permanent change in behavior as a result of a lifelong, dynamic process by which individuals acquire new knowledge, skills, and/or attitudes that can be measured and can occur at any time or in any place due to exposure to environmental stimuli.

learning contract A mutually agreed-on specific plan of action between the learner and educator clearly defining the specific behavioral objectives and predetermined goal to be achieved as a result of instruction. Also referred to as an educational contract.

learning curve Also sometimes referred to as the experience curve, it is a record of an individual's improvement in psychomotor skill development made by measuring his or her ability at different stages during a specified time period, which includes six stages: negligible progress, increasing gains, decreasing gains, plateau, renewed gains, and approach to limit.

learning disability (LD) A generic term that refers to a heterogeneous group of disorders manifested by significant difficulties with learning that affects the ability to listen, think, speak, read, write, spell, or do math.

learning needs Gaps in knowledge that exist between a desired level of performance and the actual level of performance; what the learner needs or wants to know.

learning styles The manner by which individuals perceive and then process information. Certain characteristics of style are biological in origin, whereas others are sociologically developed as a result of environmental influences.

learning theory A coherent framework and set of integrated constructs and principles that describe, explain, or predict how people learn.

lecture The oldest, most commonly used, and most traditional instructional method by which the teacher verbally transmits information in a highly structured format directly to a group of learners.

left-brain thinking The left hemisphere of the brain is vocal and analytic, which is used for verbalization and reality-based, logical thinking according to Sperry.

legal A term that refers to rules governing behavior or conduct of healthcare professionals that are enforceable under threat of punishment or penalty, such as a fine, imprisonment, or both.

legally blind A person's vision is 20/200 or less in the better eye with correction, or if visual field limits in both eyes are within 20 degrees diameter.

linguistic intelligence A term used by Gardner to describe children who have highly developed auditory skills and think in words.

listening test A standardized test to measure comprehension using a selected passage from an instructional material written at approximately the fifth-grade level that is read aloud at a normal rate to determine what a person understands and remembers when listening.

ListServ An automated mailing list software program that copies messages and distributes them to all subscribers.

literacy The ability of adults to read, understand, and interpret information written at the eighth-grade level or above. An umbrella term used to describe socially required and expected reading and writing abilities; the relative ability of persons to use printed and written material commonly encountered in daily life.

literate The ability to write and to read, understand, and interpret information written at the eighth-grade level or above.

locus of control (LOC) The location of control of behaviors as either self-directed or directed by others. Persons with internal or external locus of control differ particularly in the degree of responsibility taken for their own actions (see also internal locus of control and external locus of control).

logical-mathematical intelligence A term used by Gardner to describe children who are strong in exploring patterns, categories, and relationships of objects.

low literacy The ability of adults to read, write, and comprehend information between the fifth- and the eighth-grade level of difficulty (also referred to as marginally literate or marginally illiterate).

m-learning Stands for mobile learning, which is a new strategy that takes advantage of the many wireless, portable, and handheld devices, such as MP3 players, that can access course materials, search the Web, listen to lectures, and record experiences and assignments.

malpractice Failure to exercise an accepted degree of professional skill or knowledge by one rendering professional services that results in injury, loss, or damage to the recipient of those services.

mandatory needs Requisites to be learned for survival or situations where the learner's life or safety is threatened.

marginally literate A term to describe a person with low literacy skills; also known as marginally illiterate.

massed practice Learning information all at once, which is much less effective for remembering facts than learning information over successive periods of time; similar to cramming.

media characteristics One of the three major variables that refers to the form through which information will be communicated that must be considered when making appropriate choices of instructional materials.

media/medium The form in which information or ideas are conveyed to learners.

mental practice The imagining or visualizing of a skill without physical movement that can have positive effects on the performance of a skill.

message See content.

metacognition A person's understanding of his/her way of learning. A concept related to cognitive learning theory.

models Three-dimensional instructional tools that allow the learner to apply knowledge and psychomotor skills by observing, examining, manipulating, handling, assembling, and disassembling objects while the teacher provides feedback. Replicas, analogues, and symbols are all types of models that enhance instruction by means that range from concrete to abstract.

moral A term that refers to an internal value system, a certain moral fabric, that is expressed externally in ethical behaviors of healthcare professionals; often used interchangeably with the terms morality and morals.

motivation A psychological force that moves a person to take action in the direction of meeting a need or goal, evidenced by willingness or readiness to act.

motivational axioms Premises on which an understanding of motivation is based, such as a state of optimum anxiety, learner readiness, realistic goal setting, learner satisfaction/success, and uncertainty-reducing or uncertainty-maintaining dialogue.

motivational incentives Factors that influence motivation in the direction of the desired goal.

motivational interviewing A method of staging readiness to change for the purpose of promoting desired health behaviors, which is an individualized, flexible, client-centered approach that is supportive, empathetic, and goal directed.

motor learning A set of processes associated with practice or experience leading to relatively permanent changes in the capability for movement.

motor performance Involves the acquisition of a skill but not necessarily retention of the skill.

multimedia learning Refers to the use of two or more types of learning modes (e.g., audio, visual, or animation) that can be accessed via a computer to engage the learner in the content being taught.

musical intelligence A term used by Gardner to describe children who are talented in playing musical instruments, singing, dancing, and keeping rhythm and who often learn best with music playing in the background.

Myers-Briggs type indicator (MBTI) A self-report inventory that uses forced-choice questions and word pairs to measure four dichotomous dimensions of behavior.

needs assessment The process of determining through data collection what a person, group, organization, or community must learn or wants to learn to provide appropriate education programs to meet the required or desired needs of the learners.

negligence Doing or nondoing of an act, pursuant to a duty, that a reasonable person in the same circumstances would or would not do; the acting or the nonacting is the proximate cause of injury to another person or property.

noncompliance Nonsubmission or resistance of the individual to follow a prescribed, predetermined regimen.

nonhealthcare setting One of three classifications of instructional settings in which health care is an incidental or supportive function of an organization, such as a business, an industry, or a school system.

nonmalfeasance The notion of doing no harm.

nonprint instructional materials Include the full range of audio and visual instructional materials, including demonstrations and displays.

numeracy The ability to read and interpret numbers.

nursing process A model for nursing practice using the problem-solving approach, which includes the phases of assessment, nursing diagnosis, planning, implementation, and evaluation of patient care that parallels the educational process.

object permanence Toward the end of the second year of life, a child realizes that objects and events exist even when they cannot be seen, heard, or touched.

objective A specific, single, unidimensional behavior that is short term in nature, which should be achievable at the conclusion of one teaching session or within a matter of a few days following a series of teaching sessions.

obstacles to learning Those factors that negatively affect the ability of the learner to attend to and process information.

one-to-one instruction A common instructional method for exchange of information whereby the teacher delivers individual verbal instruction of learning activities in a format designed specifically to meet the needs of a particular learner.

operant conditioning Focuses on the behavior of an organism as a result of a positive or negative reinforcer (stimulus or event) applied after a response that strengthens the probability that the response will be performed again;

nonreinforcement and punishment decrease the likelihood that a response will continue to be performed.

oral literacy The ability to comprehend the spoken word.

outcome The result of actions that may be intended or unintended; synonymous with stated goals.

outcome evaluation See summative evaluation.

output disabilities A general category of learning disability that refers to orally responding and performing physical tasks, which include language and motor disorders.

pacing The speed at which information is presented to a learner.

parochial orientation Persons who demonstrate close-mindedness in thinking, conservativeness, and less willingness to learn new material and who place trust in traditional authority figures; a component of experiential readiness.

patient education A process of assisting consumers of health care to learn how to incorporate health-related behaviors (knowledge, skills, and/or attitudes) into everyday life with the purpose of achieving the goal of optimal health.

pedagogy The art and science of helping children to learn.

PEMs See printed education materials.

people-first language The practice of writing and speaking about a person and not about his or her disability; word choice should refer to what a person has rather than what a person is.

personal fable A type of social thinking that leads adolescents to believe that they are invulnerable or invincible, which can result in them engaging in risk-taking behavior.

physical maturation Change in an individual's physical characteristics as a result of normal body growth and development during the aging process.

physical readiness A state of willingness to learn that is dependent on such factors as measures of physical ability, complexity of task, health status, gender, and environmental effects.

pooled ignorance Lack of knowledge or information about issues or problems during a group discussion session, whereby clients cannot adequately learn from one another if they do not possess a basic, accurate understanding of a subject to draw on for purposes of discourse.

portfolio A method for evaluation of an individual's learning over time.

positron emission tomography (PET) A type of technology that has revolutionized the field of neuroscience by making images of the brain to detect which possible areas of the brain are used for cognating, feeling, and remembering.

possible needs Nice to know information that is not essential at a given point in time or in situations in which learning is not directly related to daily activities.

posters A type of display that combines print and nonprint media to help convey a message.

post-formal operations period The ability to learn during middle adulthood that goes beyond Piaget's last stage of cognitive development (formal operations) to include searching for complex and changing understandings to find a variety of solutions to any given situation or problem; to be able to see the bigger picture.

poverty circle (cycle of poverty) A process whereby parents who are of low income and educational level produce children of low income and educational attainment, who grow up and repeat the process with their own children; a situation in which generation after generation are born into poverty caused by many factors, such as poor health care, limited resources, family stress, and low-paying jobs.

practice acts Documents that define a profession, describe a profession's scope of practice, and provide guidelines for state professional boards regarding entry into a profession via licensure and disciplinary actions that can be taken when necessary; these acts have been developed to protect the public from unqualified practitioners and to protect the professional title.

practice-based evidence Evidence derived from practice rather than from research, such as the results of a systematically conducted evaluation, clients' responses to care delivered on the basis of clinical expertise, or a systematically conducted quality improvement project.

precausal thinking Unawareness by children in early childhood (3 to 5 years of age) of causation by invisible and mechanical forces.

preoperational period As defined by Piaget, this is the second key milestone in the cognitive development of children when in the early childhood stage (3–5 years) they are acquiring language skills and gaining experience but their thinking is precausal, animistic, egocentric, and intuitive, with only a vague understanding of relationships and multiple classifications of objects.

presentation The form in which the message (content) is put forth, occurring along a continuum from real objects to symbols.

primary characteristics of culture Factors that influence an individual's identification with an ethnic group and that cause the individual to share a group's worldview, such as nationality, race, color, gender, age, and religious affiliation.

printed education materials (PEMs) As the most common type of teaching tools, these include handouts, leaflets, books, pamphlets, brochures, and instruction sheets, which may be purchased or instructor developed.

process evaluation See formative evaluation.

Prochaska's change model See stages of change model.

productivity environmental preference survey (PEPS) The assessment tool used in the adult version of the Dunn and Dunn learning style inventory.

program evaluation A systematic assessment to determine the extent to which all activities for an entire department or program over a specified time period have accomplished the goals originally established.

programmed instruction A type of self-study tool, usually printed or computerized, that takes the learner through the learning task step by step.

projected learning resources Audiovisual instructional formats that depend primarily on the learners' sense of sight as the means through which messages are received. These resources require equipment to project images, usually in a darkened room, and include movies, PowerPoint slides, overhead transparencies, and others.

propositional reasoning The ability to think abstractly and use complex logical reasoning, which begins in the adolescent stage of development.

protection motivation theory A linear motivational theory that explains behavioral change in terms of threat and coping appraisal, which leads to intent and ultimately to action.

psychodynamic learning One of the five major learning theories. Largely a theory of motivation stressing emotions rather than cognition and responses; this perspective emphasizes the importance of conscious and unconscious forces derived from earlier childhood experiences and conflicts that guide and change behavior.

psychomotor domain One of three domains in the taxonomy of behavioral objectives, which is concerned with the physical activities of the body, such as coordination, reaction time, and muscular control, related to the acquisition of a skill or task.

psychosocial development The process of psychological and social adjustment as an individual grows from infancy to adulthood according to Erickson's eight stages of the psychological and social maturation of humans: trust versus mistrust, autonomy versus shame and doubt, initiative versus guilt, industry versus inferiority, identity versus role confusion, intimacy versus isolation, generativity versus self-absorption and stagnation, and ego integrity versus despair.

Purnell model for cultural competence A popular organizing framework for understanding the complex phenomenon of culture and ethnicity that provides a comprehensive, systematic, and concise approach to assist healthcare providers in delivering holistic, culturally competent, and therapeutic interventions.

reachable moment A unique opportunity described by Beddoe when health professionals provide emotional support to clients; the time when a provider truly connects with clients by directly meeting them on mutual terms without being inhibited by prejudice or bias, setting the stage for the teachable moment.

readability The level of reading difficulty at which printed teaching tools are written. A measure of those elements in a given text of printed material that influence with what degree of success a group of readers will be able to read and understand the information; the ease, or, conversely, the difficulty, with which a person can understand or comprehend the style of writing of a selected printed passage.

readiness to learn The time when the learner is receptive to learning and is willing and able to participate in the learning process; preparedness or willingness to learn.

reading Also known as word recognition, it is the process of transforming letters into words and being able to pronounce them correctly.

realia The most concrete form of stimuli that can be used to deliver information. Example: a real person or a model being used to demonstrate a procedure such as breast self-examination.

REALM (rapid estimate of adult literacy in medicine) A reading skills test to measure a client's ability to read medical and health-related vocabulary.

receptive aphasia An absence or impairment of the ability to comprehend what is read or heard due to a dysfunction in the Wernicke's area of the brain, which controls sensory abilities. Although hearing is unimpaired, the person is unable to understand the significance of the spoken word and is unable to communicate verbally.

reflective observation A term used by Kolb to describe a dimension of perceiving; known as the watching mode.

reflective practice A notion of evaluation that includes the two components of reflection-in-action, when the health professional introspectively considers a practice activity while performing it so change for improvement can be made at that moment (formative evaluation), and reflection-on-action, when the health professional introspectively analyzes a practice activity after completion so as to gain insights for the future (summative evaluation).

rehabilitation The relearning of previous skills, which often requires an adjustment to altered functional abilities and altered lifestyle.

religiosity An individual's adherence to beliefs and ritualistic practices associated with religious institutions.

repetition A technique that strengthens learning by aiding in retention of information of new or difficult material through reinforcement of important points.

replica A facsimile constructed to scale that resembles the features or substance of the original object. It may be examined or manipulated by the learner to get an idea of how something works. Example: resuscitation dolls.

resistance What people oppose talking about or learning, which is an indicator of underlying emotional difficulties that must be dealt with for them to move ahead emotionally and behaviorally.

respondent conditioning Emphasizes the importance of stimulus conditions and the associations formed in the learning process, whereby, without thought or awareness, learning takes place when a newly conditioned stimulus (CS) becomes associated with a conditioned response (CR); also termed classical or Pavlovian conditioning.

return demonstration An instructional method by which the learner attempts to perform a psychomotor skill, with cues or prompting as needed from the teacher.

revenue generation Income realized over and above costs; also called profit.

right-brain thinking The right hemisphere of the brain is emotional, visual-spatial, and nonverbal, in which thinking is intuitive, subjective, relational, holistic, and time free, according to Sperry.

role modeling The use of self as a role model, often overlooked as an instructional method, whereby the learner acquires new behaviors and social roles by identification with the role model.

role-playing A method of instruction by which learners participate in an unrehearsed dramatization, acting out an assigned part of a character as they think the character would act in reality.

SAM (suitability assessment of materials) An evaluation instrument designed to measure the appropriateness of print materials, illustrations, and video- and audiotaped instructions for a given client population.

secondary characteristics of culture Factors that influence an individual's identification with an ethnic group and that cause the individual to share a group's worldview, such as SES (socioeconomic status), physical characteristics, educational status, occupational status, and place of residence.

selective attention The process of recognizing and selecting appropriate or inappropriate stimuli.

self-composed instructional materials Printed instructional materials composed by individual instructors for the purpose of supplementing teaching.

self-efficacy theory A framework that describes the belief that one is capable of accomplishing a specific behavior.

self-instruction A method of instruction used by a teacher to provide or design teaching materials and activities that guide the learner in independently achieving the objectives of learning.

self-study materials Written materials that are designed to allow the learner to independently master understanding of concepts or tasks.

sensing-intuition (S-N) Describes how individuals perceive the world, either directly through the five senses or indirectly by way of the unconscious; one of four dichotomous preference dimensions in the Myers-Briggs type indicator.

sensorimotor period As defined by Piaget, this is the first key milestone in the cognitive development of children in the age group of infancy to toddlerhood when learning is enhanced through movement and manipulation of objects in the environment via visual, auditory, tactile, olfactory, taste, and motor stimulation.

sensory deficits A category of common physical disabilities that includes, in particular, hearing and visual impairments.

silent epidemic A term used to describe the literacy problem in the United States; also known as the silent barrier or silent disability.

simulation A method of instruction whereby an artificial or hypothetical experience that engages the learner in an activity reflecting real-life conditions but without the risk-taking consequences of an actual situation is created.

simulation laboratories A type of learning laboratory that contains real equipment in a lifelike setting, but that allows the learner to practice manipulating and using this equipment as a prelude to performing a task in a real-life situation. Frequently used to supplement the learning of psychomotor skills.

skill inoculation The opportunity for repeated practice of a behavioral task.

SMOG formula A relatively easy-to-use, popular, valid test of readability based on a set number of sentences and polysyllabic words in printed material from grade four to college level.

social cognition An increasingly popular perspective within cognitive theory that highlights the influence of social factors on perception, thought, motivation, and behaviors.

social constructivism An increasingly popular perspective within cognitive theory proposing that individuals formulate or construct their own versions of reality and that learning and human development are richly colored by the social and cultural context in which people find themselves.

social learning One of five major learning theories, this theory is seen as a mixture of behaviorist, cognitive, and psychodynamic influences; much of learning is a social process that occurs by observation and watching other people's behavior to see what happens to them. Role modeling is a central concept of this theory, with cognitive or psychodynamic aspects of internal processing and motivation sometimes considered in the learning process.

socioeconomic status (SES) Variation in health status, health behavior, or learning abilities among individuals of different social and economic levels.

software Computer programs and other instructional materials such as videotapes, CDs, and overhead transparencies.

Spache grade-level score A readability formula specifically designed to judge materials written for children at grade levels below the fourth grade (elementary grades first through third).

spatial intelligence A term used by Gardner to describe children who learn by images and pictures.

spirituality A belief in a higher power, a sacred force that exists in all things.

spontaneous recovery A response, which appears to be extinguished, reappears at any time (even years later), especially when stimulus conditions are similar to those in the initial learning experience.

staff education A process of assisting healthcare staff personnel to acquire knowledge, skills, or attitudes in practice for the purpose of maintaining or improving their ability to deliver quality care to the consumer.

stages of change model A model developed by Prochaska that forms the phenomenon of health behaviors of the learner, particularly applied to addictive and problem behaviors, and includes the six distinct stages of change: precontemplation, contemplation, preparation, action, maintenance, and termination.

stereotyping An oversimplified conception, opinion, or belief about some aspect of an individual or group.

stimulus generalization The tendency of initial learning experiences to be easily applied to other similar stimuli.

subculture An ethnocultural group of people who have experiences different from those of the dominant culture.

subobjective A specific statement of a short-term behavior that is written to reflect an aspect of the main objective leading to the achievement of the primary objective.

suitability assessment of materials See SAM.

summative evaluation Systematic assessment of the degree to which individuals have learned or objectives have been met as a result of education intervention; also referred to as outcome evaluation.

support system Resources and significant others, such as family and friends, on whom the patient relies or is dependent for information or assistance in managing activities of daily living and who may serve as a positive or negative influence on teaching efforts.

syllogistic reasoning The ability to consider two premises and draw a logical conclusion from them, which is a cognitive skill developed in middle to late childhood.

symbol A type of model that conveys a message to the learner through the use of abstract constructs, like words, that stand for the real thing. Cartoons and printed materials are examples of symbolic forms of a message.

symbolic representations Numbers and words, symbols written and spoken to convey ideas or represent objects, which are the most common form of communication and yet are the most abstract types of messages.

systematic desensitization A technique based on respondent conditioning that is used by psychologists to reduce fear or anxiety by unlearning or extinguishing it through teaching relaxation techniques or introducing a fear-producing stimulus at a nonthreatening level.

tailoring Coordinating a patient's treatment regimens into his or her daily schedule by allowing new tasks to be associated with old behaviors.

task characteristics One of the three major variables defined by the behavioral objectives in the cognitive, affective, and psychomotor domains of learning, which must be considered when making appropriate choices of instructional materials.

taxonomic hierarchy See taxonomy.

taxonomy A form of hierarchical classification of cognitive, affective, and psychomotor domains of behaviors according to their degree or level of complexity.

teachable moment As defined by Havighurst, that point in time when the learner is most receptive to a teaching situation; it can occur at any time that a patient, family member, staff member, or student has a question or needs information.

teaching As one component of the educational process, it is a deliberate, intentional act of communicating information to the learner in response to identified learning needs with the objective of producing learning to achieve desired behavioral outcomes.

teaching plan Overall blueprint or outline for instruction clearly defining the relationship between the essential components of behavioral objectives, instructional content, teaching methods and tools, time frame for teaching, and methods of evaluation that fit together in a logical pattern of flow to achieve a predetermined goal.

teaching strategy An overall plan of action for instruction that anticipates barriers and resources of the learning experience to achieve specific behavioral objectives.

telecommunications Technological devices for the Deaf (TDD).

telecommunications learning resources Instructional tools used to help convey information via electrical energy from one place to another such as telephones, televisions, and computers.

teleological The ethical notion purported by Mill that, given the alternatives, choices should be made that result in the greatest good for the greatest number of people.

telepractice The provision of nursing, medical, and other types of technology-facilitated healthcare services to clients at a distance.

theory of reasoned action A framework that is concerned with prediction and understanding of human behavior within a social context.

therapeutic alliance model An interpersonal provider-client model that addresses the continuum of compliance, adherence, and collaboration in therapeutic relationships.

therapeutic relationship A principle of humanistic theory that emphasizes the healing nature of a relationship between health professionals and their clients.

thinking-feeling (T-F) An approach used by individuals to arrive at judgments through impersonal, logical, subjective, or empathetic processes; one of four dichotomous preference dimensions in the Myers-Briggs type inventory.

TOFHLA (test of functional health literacy in adults) A relatively new instrument for measuring patients' literacy level by using actual hospital materials, such as prescription labels, appointment slips, and informed consent documents, to determine their reading and numeracy skills.

tools See instructional materials/tools.

transcultural care A formal area of study and practice comparing and analyzing different cultures and subcultures with respect to cultural care, health practices, and illness beliefs with the goal of using these insights to provide culture-specific and culture-universal care to diverse groups of people.

transfer of learning The effects of learning one skill on the subsequent performance of another related skill; includes self-transfer, near transfer, and far transfer.

transference Occurs when individuals project their feelings, conflicts, and reactions, especially those developed during childhood, onto authority figures and others in their lives.

triad communication A technique of involving a third person, such as a family member, significant other, or caregiver, in the communication pattern of the health professional and the client to serve as a listener and learner in the teaching situation for the purpose of assisting the client in understanding content, encouraging family or caregiver involvement and support, and enhancing client compliance with treatment regimens.

variable costs Not predictable, volume-related expenses.

VARK learning style A model that describes four categories or preferences—visual, aural, read/write, and kinesthetic—that reflect learning style experiences.

veracity Truth telling; honesty.

vicarious reinforcement A concept from social learning theory that involves determining whether role models are perceived as rewarded or punished for their behavior.

visual impairment A reduction or complete loss of vision due to infection, accident, poisoning, or congenital degeneration of the eye(s). See legally blind.

whole brain thinking When learners are able to use both brain hemispheres in developing their thought processes; a duality of thinking.

worldview The way individuals or groups of people look at the universe to form values and beliefs about their lives and the world around them.

World Wide Web A computer network of information servers around the world that are connected to the Internet; it is a technology-based educational resource that was created as a virtual space for the display of information.

WRAT (wide range achievement test) A word recognition screening test used to assess a person's ability to recognize and pronounce a list of words out of context as a criterion for measuring comprehension of written materials. The level I test is designed for children ages 5–12 years; level II is intended to test persons over 12 years of age.

Index